The Unofficial Guide to Obstetrics & Gynaecology

EDITION

2

The Unofficial Guide to Obstetrics & Gynaecology

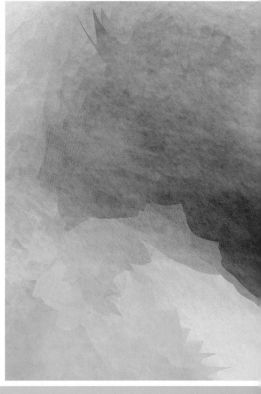

Series Editor:
Zeshan Qureshi, BM, BSc (Hons), MSc, MRCPCH,
FAcadMEd, MRCPS(Glasg)
Paediatric Registrar, London Deanery, United Kingdom

Editors:
Katherine Lattey, BMBS (Dist), MRes (Dist), MRCOG
Obstetrics and Gynaecology Specialist Trainee, Severn Deanery, United Kingdom

Matthew Wood, BM (Dist), MRCOG
Obstetrics and Gynaecology Consultant, Shrewsbury and Telford Hospital NHS Trust,
    West Midlands Deanery, United Kingdom

ELSEVIER

First edition © 2018. Published by Zeshan Qureshi.

Notices

ISBN: 978-0-443-11020-7

Content Strategist: Alexandra Mortimer
Content Project Manager: Shubham Dixit
Cover Designer: Miles Hitchen
Illustrations Coordinator: Akshaya Mohan
Marketing Manager: Deborah Watkins

Printed in India by Manipal Technologies Limited

Last digit is the print number: 9 8 7 6 5 4 3 2 1

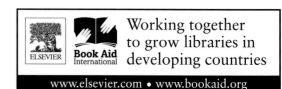

Series Editor Foreword

The Unofficial Guide to Medicine is not just about helping students study; it is also about allowing those that learn to take back control of their own education. Since its inception, it has been driven by the voices of students and, through this, democratised the process of medical education, blurring the line between learners and teachers.

Medical education is an evolving process, and the latest iteration of our titles has been rewritten to bring them up to date with modern curriculums, after extensive deliberation and consultation. We have kept the series up to date, incorporating new guidelines and perspectives from a wide range of students, junior doctors and senior clinicians. There is greater consistency across the titles, more illustrations, and through these and other changes I hope the books will now be even better study aids.

These books, however, are a process of continual improvement. By reading this book, I hope that you not only get through your exams but also consider contributing to a future edition. You may be a student now, but you are also the future of medical education.

I wish you all the best with your future career and any upcoming exams.

Zeshan Qureshi
November 2022

Introduction

This is the second edition of *The Unofficial Guide to Obstetrics and Gynaecology,* and we are proud to have updated this book according to recent changes in national and international guidelines. Obstetrics and gynaecology is a speciality that covers a broad range of medical and surgical presentations in women and girls of all ages that often appear both on the wards and in medical school exams. However, clinical exposure to this speciality at an undergraduate level is often limited. Therefore, it is crucial that educational resources explain and cover this area of medicine in a concise and accessible manner.

Obstetrics and gynaecology is a challenging specialty because of the `grey areas' in clinical practice where management strategies are often led more by clinical experience and preference rather than by clear-cut guidelines. This can be difficult to convey at the undergraduate level, where multiple-choice or short-answer questions do not leave much space for explaining these subtle complexities. The core ethos of this project was therefore to produce a book based on guidelines and evidence, minimising the use of potentially differing clinical opinions or variations in practice.

This book presents a succinct, approachable summary for each section, which covers information that is relevant for both examinations and working on the wards. These summaries lead into over 350 questions, both multiple choice and true/false, or extended matching questions. Answers are then explained in full to help gain an understanding of not only why the correct answer is right but also why incorrect answers are inferior options.

With this textbook we hope that you gain a greater understanding of obstetrics and gynaecology, and, whether you are interested in this specialty as a potential future career choice or you are just learning it to pass exams, we hope you find it a useful resource.

Katherine Lattey and Matthew Wood

Contributors

Halimah Alazzani, BSc (Hons), MBChB, FHEA, MRCOG — (Onco-Gynaecology)
Obstetrics and Gynaecology Specialist Trainee
West Midlands Deanery
Telford, United Kingdom

Suzanne Braggins, BMBS — (Management of labour)
Anaesthetic Registrar
Welsh School of Anaesthesia
Cardiff, United Kingdom

Sarah Channing, MBBS, MA (Cantab), MRCOG, PGCertMedEd — (HPO axis)
University Hospitals Bristol and Weston NHS Foundation Trust
Obstetrics and Gynaecology
St Michael's Hospital
Bristol, United Kingdom

Nish Dalavaye, BSc — (Urogynaecology)
School of Medicine
Cardiff University
Cardiff, United Kingdom

Charlie Dyson, MBBChir, MA (Cantab), MRCOG — (Careers in obstetrics and gynaecology)
Obstetrics and Gynaecology Specialist Trainee
Peterborough City Hospital
Peterborough, United Kingdom

Monisha Edirisooriya, MBChB, BMedSci (Hons), PGCertMedEd — (Multiple pregnancy)
Doctor
London Deanery
London, United Kingdom

Verity Ellis, MBChB — (Medical disorders in pregnancy)
Obstetrics and Gynaecology Specialist Trainee
Severn Deanery
Bristol, United Kingdom

Emily Hotton, BSc, MBChB, PhD, MRCOG — (Obstetric Emergencies)
Obstetrics and Gynaecology Specialist Trainee
Severn Deanery
Bristol, United Kingdom

Sian Jenkins, MBChB, BSc (Hons) — (Benign gynaecology)
Obstetrics and Gynaecology Specialist Trainee
Severn Deanery
Bristol, United Kingdom

Amar Karia, MSc, MBBS, BSc, AKC — (Methods of delivery)
Clinical Fellow – National Maternity and Perinatal Audit Clinical Quality
Royal College of Obstetricians and Gynaecologists
London, United Kingdom

Rosinder Kaur, MBChB, MRCOG — (Pelvic pain)
Doctor, Obstetrics and Gynaecology
University Hospitals Birmingham NHS Foundation Trust
Edgbaston, United Kingdom

Katherine Lattey, BMBS, MRes, MRCOG — (Management of labour)
Obstetrics and Gynaecology Specialist Trainee
North Bristol Trust
Bristol, United Kingdom

Naushabah Malik, MBBS, MCPS, BSCCP, MRCOG — (Onco-Gynaecology)
Obstetrician and Gynaecologist
West Midlands Deanery
Birmingham, United Kingdom

Karolina McDowell, MBChB, PGDip, TLHP — (Obstetric complications)
Obstetrics and Gynaecology Specialist Trainee
Severn Deanery
Bristol, United Kingdom

Hannah Osborne, MBChB, MA — (Ethics)
Obstetrics and Gynaecology Specialist Trainee
Birmingham Women's Hospital
Birmingham, United Kingdom

Kar Yen Phoong, MBChB, BSc (Hons) — (Early pregnancy complications)
Doctor, General Medicine
East Lancashire Hospitals NHS Trust
Blackburn, United Kingdom

Jameela Sheikh, MBChB, BMedSc (Hons) —
    (Antenatal care)
Doctor, Academic Foundation Programme
Guy's and St Thomas' NHS Foundation Trust
London, United Kingdom

Yan Ting Woo, MBChB — (Postnatal complications)
Medical Student
University of Birmingham
Birmingham, United Kingdom

Matthew Wood, BM, MRCOG — (Gynaecological
    anatomy and examination)
Obstetrics and Gynaecology Consultant
Shrewsbury and Telford Hospital NHS trust
Telford, United Kingdom

Abbreviations

17-OHP 17-Hydroxyprogesterone
ABC airway breathing circulation
ABCDE airway breathing circulation disability exposure
AC abdominal circumference
ACE angiotensin-converting enzyme
ACS acute chest syndrome
ACTH adrenocorticotropic hormone
ADH antidiuretic hormone
AED anti-epileptic drugs
AFLP acute fatty liver of pregnancy
AFP alpha fetoprotein
AIDS acquired immunodeficiency syndrome
ALP alkaline phosphatase
ALS advanced life support
ALT alanine transaminase
AMH anti-Mullerian hormone
Anti-HBc antibody to hepatitis B core protein
anti-HBe anti-hepatitis B envelope antibody
AP anteroposterior
APH antepartum haemorrhage
APS antiphospholipid syndrome
APTT activated partial thromboplastin time
ARDS acute respiratory distress syndrome
ARM artificial rupture of membranes
ART assisted reproductive techniques
ART anti-retroviral therapy
AST aspartate aminotransferase
ATP adenosine triphosphate
AVPU alert, voice, pain, unresponsive
B1 thiamine
B6 pyridoxine
BASHH British Association of Sexual Health and HIV
BMI body mass index
BNP B-type natriuretic peptide
BP blood pressure
bpm beats per minute
BSO bilateral salpingo-oophorectomy
BUSOG British Undergraduate Society of Obstetrics and Gynaecology
BV bacterial vaginosis
CA 19-9 cancer antigen 19-9
CA-125 cancer antigen 125
CAH congenital adrenal hyperplasia
CAIS complete androgen insensitivity syndrome
CBT cognitive behavioural therapy
CD4 cluster of differentiation 4
CEA carcinoembryonic antigen
CGIN glandular intra-epithelial neoplasia
CIN cervical intraepithelial neoplasia

cm centimeter
CMV cytomegalovirus
CNS central nervous system
COCP combined oral contraceptive pill
COPD chronic obstructive pulmonary disease
CPR cardiopulmonary resuscitation
CRL crown rump length
CRP c-reactive protein
CRS congenital rubella syndrome
CT computed tomography
CTG cardiotocography
CTPA computer tomography pulmonary angiogram
CTZ chemoreceptor trigger zone
CVS chorionic villous sampling
CYP450 cytochrome P450
DCDA dichorionic diamniotic
DEXA dual-energy X-ray absorptiometry
DHEAS dehydroepiandrosterone
DIC disseminated intravascular coagulopathy
dl decilitres
DM diabetes mellitus
DNA deoxyribonucleic acid
DSD differences of sexual development
DVT deep vein thrombosis
EBRT external beam radiotherapy
EBV Epstein-Barr virus
ECG electrocardiogram
ECT electroconvulsive therapy
ECV external cephalic version
ED emergency department
EEG electroencephalogram
EFW estimated fetal weight
EMQ extended matching question
EPAS early pregnancy assessment service
FAI free androgen index
FBC full blood count
FBS fetal blood sample
FFP fresh frozen plasma
FGM female genital mutilation
FGR fetal growth restriction
FHD fetal haemolytic disease
FHR fetal heart rate
FIGO Fédération Internationale des Gynaecologistes et Obstetristes
FSE fetal scalp electrode
FSH follicle stimulating hormone
g grams
G&S group and save
GABA gamma-aminobutyric acid

Gamma GT gamma-glutamyl transferase
GBS group B streptococcus
GCS Glasgow coma scale
GDM gestational diabetes mellitus
GH growth hormone
GnRH gonadotropin releasing hormone
GP general practitioner
GT glutamyl transferase
GTT glucose tolerance test
GUM genitourinary medicine
H$_2$ molecular hydrogen
HAV hepatitis A virus
HbA haemoglobin A
HbA1c glycated haemoglobin
HBeAg hepatitis B envelope antigen
HBIG hepatitis B immunoglobulin
HbS haemoglobin S
HBsAg hepatitis B surface antigen
HBV hepatitis B virus
hCG human chorionic gonadotropin
HCV hepatitis C virus
HDU high dependency unit
HDV hepatitis D virus
HELLP haemolysis, elevated liver enzyme levels, and low platelet levels
HHV human herpes virus
HIV human immunodeficiency virus
HIV-ab human immunodeficiency virus antibody
HMB heavy menstrual bleeding
HNPCC hereditary non-polyposis colorectal cancer
hPL human placental lactogen
HPO hypothalamic pituitary ovarian
HPT hypothalamus pituitary testes
HPV human papilloma virus
HRT hormone replacement therapy
HSG hysterosalpingogram
HSV herpes simplex virus
IBS irritable bowel syndrome
ICSI intracytoplasmic sperm injection
Ig immunoglobulin
IGF1 insulin-like growth factor 1
IgG immunoglobulin G
IgM immunoglobulin M
IL-6 interleukin-6
IM intramuscular
IMB intermenstrual bleeding
INR international normalised ratio
IOTA international ovarian tumour analysis
IPT interpersonal therapy
IQ intelligence quotient
ITU intensive treatment unit
IU international unit
IUCD intrauterine contraceptive device
IUD intrauterine death
IUD intrauterine device
IUGR intrauterine growth restriction
IUI intrauterine insemination
IUS intrauterine system

IV intravenous
IVF *in vitro* fertilisation
IVIG intravenous immunoglobulin
JVP jugular venous pressure
kg kilograms
L litre
LBW low birth weight
LDH lactate dehydrogenase
LFTs liver function tests
LH luteinising hormone
LHRH luteinising hormone releasing hormone
LLETZ large loop excision of the transformation zone
LMP last menstrual period
LMWH low molecular weight heparin
LSCS lower uterine segment caesarean section
m meter
MAOI monoamine oxidase inhibitor
MC&S microscopy, culture and sensitivity
MCADD medium-chain acyl-CoA dehydrogenase deficiency
MCDA monochorionic diamniotic
mcg microgram
MCMA monochorionic monoamniotic
MCV mean cell volume
MDT multidisciplinary team
mg milligram
min minutes
ml millilitre
mm millimeter
mmHg millimeters of mercury
mmol millimole
MMP matrix metalloproteinase
MMR measels mumps and rubella
mol mole
MRI magnetic resonance image
MRSA methicillin resistant Staphylococcus aureus
MSM men who have sex with men
MSU midstream specimen of urine
MUS mid-urethral sling
NAAT nucleic acid amplification test
ng nanograms
NHS National Health Service
NICE National Institute for Health and Care Excellence
NICU neonatal intensive care unit
nmol nanomoles
NRTI nucleoside reverse transcriptase inhibitors
NSAIDs non-steroidal anti-inflammatory drugs
O&G obstetrics and gynaecology
OA occipitoanterior
OAB overactive bladder
OGTT oral glucose tolerance test
OHSS ovarian hyperstimulation syndrome
OP occipitoposterior
OSCEs objective structured clinical examinations
OT occipitotransverse
PAIS partial androgen insensitivity syndrome
PAPP-A pregnancy associated plasma protein A
PCA patient controlled analgesia
PCB postcoital bleeding

PCOS polycystic ovarian syndrome
PCP pneumocystis carinii pneumonia
PCPwSI primary care physician with special interest
PCR polymerase chain reaction
PE pulmonary embolism
PEG-IFNα-2a pegylated interferon alpha-2a
PET positron electron tomography
PFMT pelvic floor muscle training
pg picograms
PG prostaglandin
PGE2 prostaglandin E2
PID pelvic inflammatory disease
PIGD pre-implantation genetic diagnosis
PKU phenylketonuria
PMB postmenopausal bleeding
PMD premenstrual disorder
PMS premenstrual syndrome
PO per oral
POI premature ovarian insufficiency
POP progestogen-only pill
PHP panhypopituitarism
PPH postpartum haemorrhage
PPROM preterm premature rupture of membranes
PROM prolonged rupture of membranes
PT prothrombin time
PTNS posterior tibial nerve stimulation
PUL pregnancy of unknown location
PVR post-void residual volume
RBC red blood cell
RCOG Royal College of Obstetricians and Gynaecologists
RDS respiratory distress syndrome
RMI risk of malignancy index
ROM rupture of membranes
S1 first heart sound
S2 second heart sound
SCC squamous cell carcinoma
SCCA squamous cell carcinoma antigen
SCD sickle cell disease
SCJ squamous columnar junction
SFH symphysis fundal height
SGA small for gestational age
SHBG sex hormone binding globulin
SIRS systemic inflammatory response syndrome
SMI serious mental illness

SNRIs selective noradrenaline reuptake inhibitors
SNS sacral nerve stimulation
SSRIs selective serotonin reuptake inhibitors
STIs sexually transmitted infections
SUDEP sudden unexpected death in epilepsy
SVR systemic vascular resistance
T2DM type 2 diabetes mellitus
T3 triiodothyronine
T4 thyroxine
TBG thyroid binding globulin
TCA tricyclic antidepressant
TCRE transcervical resection of endometrium
TENS transcutaneous electric nerve stimulation
TFTs thyroid function tests
TORCH toxoplasmosis, other, rubella, cytomegalovirus and herpes
TPO thyroid peroxidase
TSH thyroid stimulating hormone
TTP-HUS thrombotic thrombocytopenic purpura haemolytic uraemic syndrome
TTTS twin to twin transfusion syndrome
TV trichomonas vaginalis
TVS transvaginal (ultrasound) scan
TVT tension free vaginal tape
TVUS transvaginal ulstrasound scan
TZ transformation zone
U&Es urea and electrolytes
UAE uterine artery embolisation
UK United Kingdom
UKMEC United Kingdom Medical Eligibility Criteria
umol micromoles
UTI urinary tract infection
V/Q ventilation/perfusion
VAIN vaginal intraepithelial neoplasia
VBAC vaginal birth after caesarean
VDRL venereal disease research laboratory test
VEGF vascular endothelial growth factor
VIN vulval intraepithelial neoplasia
VTE venous thromboembolism
VZIg varicella zoster immunoglobulin
WCC white cell count
WHO World Health Organisation
β hCG beta human chorionic gonadatropin

Acknowledgement

We would like to thank all of the authors, from the first and second editions, for their dedication and hard work. We would like to thank you, the reader: as a medical student or junior doctor, you have inspired this project, believed in it and continued to promote, contribute to and distribute this book across the UK and further afield. In addition, we are thankful to the support of medical schools, without whom this project would not be possible.

Additional thanks to our friends and family (mostly our long-suffering parents Rachel, Nick, Maurice and Ivy). Finally, a massive thank you to our partners (Greg and Emma) who have put up with us and supported us during this project.

Katherine and Matthew

CONTRIBUTORS FROM THE FIRST EDITION

Stephanie Arrigo—Benign ovarian cysts
Victoria Awobajo—Cardiac disorders in pregnancy
Alexandra Black—Disorders of sexual development; Vulval disorders; Cervical screening; Cervical cancer; Vulval and vaginal cancers; The impact of maternal weight on pregnancy
Darren Chan—Congenital intrauterine infections
Rachel Crane—Preterm labour
Lyndsay Creswell—Monitoring the fetus
Kirsty Dawson—Pelvic organ prolapse; Urinary incontinence
Megan Durant—Ovarian cancer
Patrick Green—Endometriosis
Marcus Hards—Ectopic pregnancy
Sofia Hart—Hepatitis B in pregnancy
Sarah Hobern—Endometrial cancer
Emily Hotton—Secondary amenorrhoea; Polycystic ovarian syndrome; Cord prolapse; Shoulder dystocia; Retained placenta; Postpartum haemorrhage; Amniotic embolism; Maternal collapse

Marie Jasim—Sickle cell disease in pregnancy
Shujing Jane Lim—Preterm labour; Chorioamnionitis
Georgina Martin—Fibroids
Emily Mayo—Monitoring the fetus; Induction and augmentation; Pain relief in labour; Malpresentation and malposition of the fetus; Assisted delivery and instrumental births
Rayna Patel—Epilepsy in pregnancy; Thyroid disease in pregnancy; HIV in pregnancy
Prateush Singh—Fetal haemolytic disease
Yashashwi Sinha—The menstrual cycle and physiology of the HPO axis; Puberty; Diabetes in pregnancy; Chorioamnionitis
Emily Slade—Antepartum haemorrhage
Thivya Sritharan—Infertility
Steve H. Tsang—Pre-eclampsia and pregnancy-induced hypertension
Laura Wharton—Venous thromboembolism; Bacterial sepsis following pregnancy; Perineal trauma; Mastitis; Postnatal mental health

Language Statement

Equality, diversity and inclusivity are aspects of society that are constantly evolving, but also varying amongst different communities. As this happens the language around these topics' changes. The latest edition of the Unofficial Guide to Obstetrics and Gynaecology has been updated with this in mind.

We recognise obstetrics and gynaecology will be accessed by women, gender-diverse individuals and people whose gender identity does not align with the sex they were assigned at birth. Students reading this, as well as doctors, will also come from these same groups. We have used pronouns such as "she" or "woman" but appreciate that some people reading this as a student or accessing healthcare may not identify with this language. As a medical textbook and learning resource we have reviewed our language but want to ensure that our content remains understandable. We believe strongly that care must at all times be appropriate, inclusive and sensitive to the needs of everyone, and that this is applicable to our learning resources as we train doctors of the future.

Language is crucial in breaking down barriers for people accessing care and we have committed to using inclusive language wherever possible. This is a constantly and quickly evolving field so we are aware that the language used in the book may become outdated, potentially soon after publication. We will strive in future editions to update and improve our language use. In obstetrics, we have worked hard to preserve the women-centred language, such as "birth" as a baby is born and not delivered, and to not unnecessarily pathologise the birthing process. We have strived to use language that does not stigmatise but again has clarity of understanding as students use our content to negotiate the often-complex nature of obstetrics and gynaecology.

We hope not to have caused offence in the language we have chosen to use but we welcome comments on how we can improve our inclusivity as a community.

Kind regards,
Katherine Lattey and Matthew Wood

Contents

Introduction

OVERVIEW

Gynaecology is an exciting, wide-ranging speciality. It is predominantly a surgical speciality, but endocrinology plays a crucial role in many of the diseases and treatments offered. Like obstetrics, aspects of the speciality are highly emotive, requiring good communication and interpersonal skills to guide patients through challenging times in their lives. Gynaecologists have the enviable role of making a difference in a panoply of different aspects of patients' lives, for example:

- Creating life – subfertility.
- Prolonging life – oncology, colposcopy.
- Saving life – emergency surgery to treat ectopic pregnancies and heavy bleeding following miscarriage.
- Improving quality of life – treating menstrual disorders, urinary incontinence and chronic pelvic pain from endometriosis.

This introduction will explain the key aspects of the gynaecological examination. As this is a surgical speciality, it will also highlight the important anatomy and provide an overview about obtaining consent for surgery.

EXAMINATION

The pelvic examination is completed in three stages:

- Abdominal examination – similar to a surgical examination.
- Speculum examination – to inspect the vulva, vagina and cervix.
- Bimanual examination – to palpate the internal organs.

Pelvic examination is intimate and invasive. It is essential to communicate well with the patient prior to any examination to adequately prepare them. This can be achieved by completing the following steps:

1 Formally introduce yourself and check the identity of the patient.
2 Ask if the patient has had a pelvic examination before.
3 Explain what the examination involves and the reasons why it is being offered.
4 Gain verbal consent.
5 Ask the patient if they would like to empty their bladder prior to the examination.
6 Introduce the chaperone to the patient. It is imperative for a clinician (regardless of their gender) to be chaperoned for any intimate examination.
7 Ask the patient if they would like a friend or relative with them during the examination for support.
8 Allow the patient to move over to the examination couch. The patient should have privacy so they can remove their clothes from the lower half of their body and be given a sheet so that they can cover themselves while on the examination couch. This limits unnecessary exposure and discomfort.

ABDOMINAL EXAMINATION

Conducting an abdominal examination before a vaginal examination is important, as it enables the patient to get used to being examined prior to the more intimate part of the examination. It also gives information to aid a clinical diagnosis and to inform further examinations, for example, a palpable mass.

1 Wash your hands.
2 Expose the lower abdomen and inspect.
3 Ask the patient if they have any areas of tenderness.
4 Palpate in the four quadrants like in any standard abdominal examination, identifying masses and areas of tenderness. Take particular notice of tenderness or masses palpated over the 'triangle' area (Fig. 1.1) between the anterior superior iliac crests and symphysis pubis, as this is where the ovaries, uterus and bladder will be palpated.
5 Assess other aspects of the standard abdominal examination, as dictated by the history and examination findings, such as balloting the kidneys, palpating the liver and spleen, testing for pain on a straight leg raise and listening for bowel sounds.

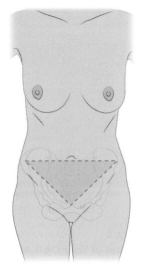

Fig. 1.1 Triangle of palpation between the pubic bone and the anterior superior iliac spines.

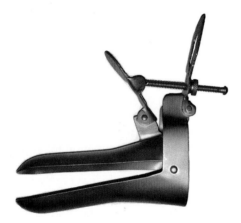

Fig. 1.2 Cusco speculum.

6   Allow the patient to lower their top back down.
7   If a rectal examination is indicated, this can be performed after the bimanual examination.

SPECULUM EXAMINATION

1   Obtain consent for a speculum examination during the introduction.
2   Put on a pair of non-latex gloves.
3   Prepare the trolley – appropriate-sized Cusco speculum (Fig. 1.2), lubricating jelly and any swabs or other investigation tools required, dependent on the case. If the speculum is metal, warm the speculum to avoid patient discomfort. A C-shaped vaginal speculum (formally called a Sims speculum) may be used in some circumstances, such as when examining for vaginal prolapse. The examination technique for a C-shaped speculum is discussed under pelvic organ prolapse.

[See 'Pelvic organ prolapse' page 105.]

4   Put a small amount of lubricant on either side of the speculum.
5   Explain clearly for the patient to *'bring your heels up to your bottom and then move your knees apart'*. It may help to suggest that they concentrate on placing

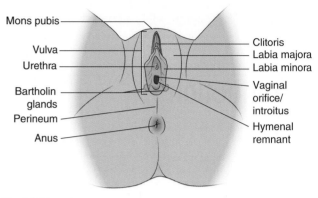

Fig. 1.3 The vulva.

their knees as close to the examination couch as possible, as this maximises space to examine the vagina and it helps keep the patient relaxed.
6   Position the light and switch it on.
7   Inspect the vulva (Fig. 1.3) for any ulceration, masses, erythema, rashes, papules, discharge, bleeding and distortion of the typical anatomy.
8   Carefully part the labia with the non-dominant hand, ensuring all hair and skin is out of the way, and insert the speculum into the vagina with the dominant hand, with the handle of the speculum at around the 2 o'clock position. Once the speculum is a few centimetres into the vagina, turn the speculum so the handles are at 12 o'clock. Swap hands and hold the speculum handles in the non-dominant hand. Apply pressure with the thumb of the dominant hand at the base of the speculum and insert the speculum as far as possible, gently and slowly. This technique reduces patient discomfort.
9   While applying pressure to the speculum base with the dominant thumb, gently open the speculum by squeezing the two handles together using the non-dominant hand.
10   Identify and inspect the cervix and the external os.
11   If required, take vaginal swabs and perform any other investigations or procedures needed; for example, a cervical smear, insertion of an intrauterine device, or taking an endometrial biopsy. To aid this, most Cusco speculums have a screw that locks the speculum in the open position. To minimise discomfort only keep the speculum open for the minimum time required.
12   To remove the speculum, hold the handles tightly in position, undo the screw and then gently release pressure on the handles, letting the speculum close. Apply a little pressure to stop the speculum from fully closing as it can pinch the vaginal tissue and cause pain.
13   Gently pull back the speculum, holding the handles with the non-dominant hand and the base of the speculum with the thumb of the dominant hand. While removing the speculum, view the rest of the vaginal walls for any abnormality.
14   Once the speculum is out, dispose of the speculum, turn off the light and label any swabs taken.
15   Cover the patient with a sheet while preparing for the bimanual examination.

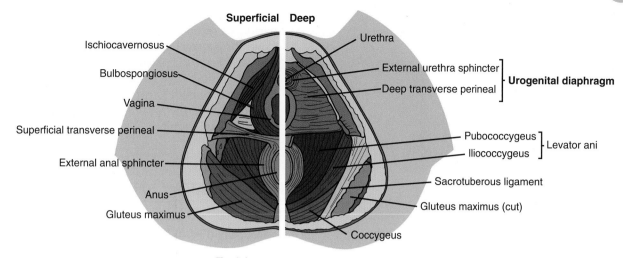

Superficial   Deep

Ischiocavernosus

Bulbospongiosus

Vagina

Superficial transverse perineal

External anal sphincter

Anus

Gluteus maximus

Urethra

External urethra sphincter

Deep transverse perineal

⎤ **Urogenital diaphragm**

Pubococcygeus

Iliococcygeus

⎤ Levator ani

Sacrotuberous ligament

Gluteus maximus (cut)

Coccygeus

Fig. 1.4 The perineum and pelvic diaphragm.

 Speculum Tips

The cervix can sometimes be difficult to visualise on speculum examination. Here are some additional techniques to bring the cervix into view:

- If part of the cervix can be seen but not the full view, getting the patient to cough can push the cervix into the open speculum.
- Ask the patient to make a fist with their hands and then put their hands under their bottom. This alters the angle of the pelvis, bringing the cervix to a more anterior position.
- Use the speculum upside down, particularly if the anterior wall of the vagina is obstructing the view.
- Gently examine with two fingers to feel where the cervix is, and then insert the speculum, aiming for the area felt. It is important to remember that when the patient is lying on the couch, the vagina is not parallel to the couch; instead, it angles upwards.
- Sometimes a longer speculum is required to reach the cervix. Similarly, in adolescents and the elderly, a small speculum will be needed to avoid discomfort.
- In obstetrics and gynaecology (O&G) departments, some examination couches are equipped with leg stirrups so the patient can be placed in the lithotomy position.

BIMANUAL EXAMINATION

1 Clearly explain that an internal examination is going to be done.
2 Wash hands and put on gloves.
3 Lubricate the index and middle finger of the dominant hand. Insert these two fingers gently into the vagina. Place the non-dominant hand on the abdomen in the suprapubic region.
4 Move the fingers inside the vagina behind the cervix and attempt to push the uterus up, while pushing downwards with the non-dominant hand and attempting to palpate the uterus between the examining hands. Comment on the size and mobility of the uterus. The uterus is typically mobile, but if it cannot move, the uterus is fixed; this is usually a result of adhesions. A typically sized uterus (when not pregnant) is roughly the size of a plum.
5 Move the fingers in the vagina, anterior to the cervix, and again try to ballot the uterus between the examining hands. If the bulk of the uterus can be felt, the uterus is anteverted (the most common finding) (Fig. 1.5). If not, then it is likely retroverted.

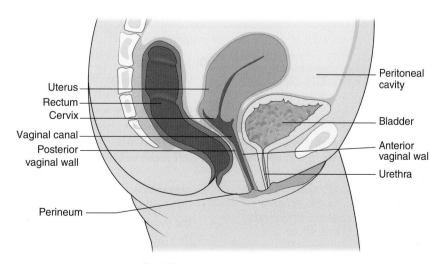

Uterus

Rectum

Cervix

Vaginal canal

Posterior vaginal wall

Perineum

Peritoneal cavity

Bladder

Anterior vaginal wal

Urethra

Fig. 1.5 Sagittal section of the pelvis.

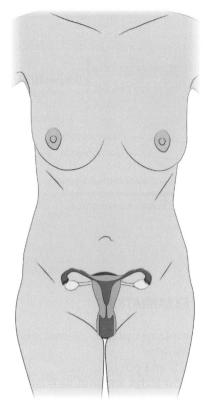

Fig. 1.6 Uterus and ovaries *in situ*.

6 Feel the cervix with a finger. A healthy cervix feels smooth, with a similar texture to the tip of the nose.

7 Gently wobble the cervix from side to side by pushing it with a finger. This stretches the visceral peritoneum of the broad ligaments. If this causes pain, it is referred to as 'cervical excitation'. Ectopic pregnancy, endometriosis and pelvic infection can cause this sign.

8 Move the two fingers to the lateral aspect of the cervix. Move the non-dominant hand to the same side on the abdomen and again push the two hands together, attempting to palpate the ovary and any abnormal masses (Fig. 1.6). Typically ovaries are the size of a large grape, so it is rarely possible to palpate them. Repeat this step on the other side to examine the other adnexa.

> ### 💡 Presenting Reassuring Findings of an Examination
>
> - Inspection of the abdomen was unremarkable. On palpation, the abdomen was soft, with no distension, no areas of tenderness and no palpable masses.
> - Speculum examination revealed no abnormality on inspection of the vulva, vagina and cervix. Typical vaginal discharge was observed.
> - Digital vaginal examination revealed no tenderness of the introitus or vagina. An average-sized, mobile, anteverted uterus was palpated. No adnexal masses or tenderness was identified. The cervix felt smooth and regular and there was no cervical excitation.

9   Remove the examining fingers and, if indicated, perform a rectal exam if consent has been gained.
10 Cover the patient. Explain that the examination is now over, and leave the patient in private to get changed after providing some tissue for self-cleaning.
11 Ensure the patient is comfortable after the examination, explain the findings and discuss the ongoing management plan.

ANATOMY

IMPORTANT ANATOMY FOR PELVIC SURGERY

UTERUS

Blood Supply (Fig. 1.7)

- Uterine arteries – the major blood vessels supplying the uterus. They are branches of the internal iliac arteries.
- Ovarian arteries – supply a collateral blood supply to the uterus with vessels running from the ovary within the ovarian ligament.
- Vaginal arteries – branches of these vessels commonly anastomose with branches of the uterine arteries. The vaginal arteries originate from the internal iliac arteries.

Ligaments (Fig. 1.8)

The uterus is supported by a number of paired ligaments:

- Uterosacral ligaments – the strongest ligaments of the uterus. They attach the posterior aspect of the lower uterus and the cervix to the sacrum.
- Cardinal ligaments – provide support by attaching the cervix to the lateral pelvic wall.
- Round ligaments – provide support running from the top of the uterus to the deep inguinal ring.
- Broad ligaments – these are a double layer of peritoneum which have attachments to the uterus, ovaries, fallopian tubes, round ligaments, ovarian ligaments and pelvic side walls. They do not provide much structural support to the uterus, but they are important surgically as they often need dividing to identify the course of the ureters in the pelvis.

OVARIES

Blood Supply

- Ovarian artery – this is a direct branch off the aorta. Branches from the ovarian artery also supply the fallopian tube and provide a supply to the uterus.
- The right ovarian vein drains into the inferior vena cava, whereas the left ovarian vein drains into the left renal vein.

Ligaments

- Infundibular pelvic ligament – attaches the ovary to the pelvic side wall. The ovarian vessels run within this ligament.
- Ovarian ligament – attaches the ovary to the uterus.

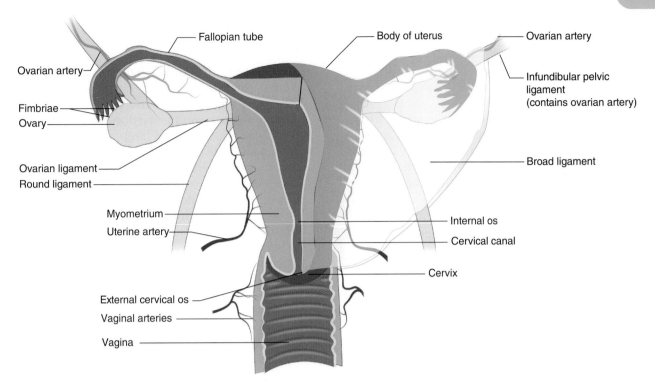

Fig. 1.7 Anterior aspect of the internal gynaecological organs.

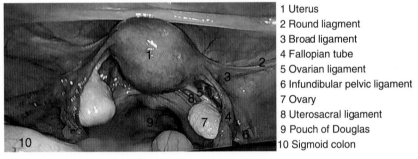

1 Uterus
2 Round liagment
3 Broad ligament
4 Fallopian tube
5 Ovarian ligament
6 Infundibular pelvic ligament
7 Ovary
8 Uterosacral ligament
9 Pouch of Douglas
10 Sigmoid colon

Fig. 1.8 Typical female pelvis at laparoscopy.

URINARY SYSTEM

The most common organ injuries during gynaecology surgery are to the bladder and the ureters, due to their proximity to the reproductive organs. The bladder lies anteriorly to the uterus and is attached to the uterus by a folded piece of visceral peritoneum, the uterovesical fold. At the time of hysterectomy, and at caesarean, this peritoneum is incised and the bladder is reflected away from the uterus to prevent injury.

The ureters are retroperitoneal. They enter the pelvis and can be seen lying anterior to the bifurcation of the common iliac arteries. As they descend into the pelvis, they then run close to the posterior aspect of the ovaries. Then they pass just below the uterine arteries and then laterally to the cervix, before running medially and anteriorly to enter the posterior aspect of the base of the bladder. Therefore, at multiple sites, the ureter lies very close to structures operated on in gynaecology, particularly for hysterectomy. One of the early steps in a hysterectomy is to open the broad ligament to allow a clear view of the course of the ureter.

CONSENT FOR SURGERY

For any surgical procedure, consent can be obtained either by the person doing the procedure or by someone delegated by that person who has sufficient knowledge and experience to provide an adequate explanation of all the relevant aspects of the procedure to the patient. Key items to discuss are:
* The name of the procedure.
* A brief overview of what the procedure involves.
* The recovery period, including the likely length of hospital admission.
* Reasons to undertake the procedure and the perceived benefits.
* The potential risks.
* Alternative options – this should always include no treatment, as well as any other conservative, medical or surgical alternative therapies.

The patient should be given this information in easy-to-understand language, by a combination of methods:
- Verbal discussion with the doctor.
- A copy of the consent form.
- Information leaflets relating to the proposed procedure.

The patient should be given time to weigh up the information, discuss with friends or relatives, and seek any further information they wish, either by researching themselves or by asking further questions of the clinician. Once the patient is satisfied, they can give informed consent.

COMMON GYNAECOLOGY PROCEDURES AND THE RISKS

All common and serious risks of surgical procedures should be explained to the patient, including how likely they are to occur. Generic risks applicable to all gynaecology surgery are:
- Infection – the most common risk for most operations. It may be appropriate to discuss where the infection is likely to occur, for example, the urinary tract, chest, incision sites or uterus.
- Bleeding.
- Venous thromboembolism (blood clot in the leg or lung).
- Pain after the procedure.
- Failure to complete the procedure.
- Injury to adjacent organs – in O&G these occur most commonly to the bladder, bowel, ureters and major blood vessels.
- Blood transfusion.
- Anaesthetic risks – usually discussed in more detail by the anaesthetist.
- Failure of the procedure to achieve intended benefits (such as improving symptoms).
- Death.

The likelihood of a risk occurring will vary depending on the operation (Table 1.1) and the individual patient.

TIPS TO MAKE THE MOST OF YOUR O&G ATTACHMENT

- Gynaecology clinics are where you can see a large variety of non-emergency patients. As well as observing appointments also ask if you can take a history and present it to the doctor.
- The gynaecology ward and acute gynaecology admission suite are where you can experience gynaecology emergencies. It is also where you can learn about the ward management skills you will need as a newly qualified doctor.
- If you wish to learn how to scrub for theatres, ask one of the theatre team to teach or observe you. This is best done when theatres are empty or during an elective theatre case.
- Theatre is the place to learn anatomy, particularly laparoscopic cases where you will have excellent views. It is also an excellent place to undertake supervised speculum and bimanual examinations (but the patient must have consented for this pre-operatively).
- In theatre there is also the anaesthetist who can teach you about their role as well as being experts in many aspects of medicine, including physiology and pharmacology.
- You may scrub for a case, such as a caesarean. Your task will normally be to help the lead surgeon see the operating field. This may involve retracting the abdominal wall and removing blood from the field using suction or a swab. The surgeon will instruct you further.
- Attend the labour ward handover, this will introduce you to the team on the shift and inform you about all the ongoing activity.
- On the labour ward introduce yourself to the midwife co-ordinator. If you would like to observe a spontaneous vaginal birth they will be the most likely team member able to help you with this. Midwives are highly experienced in vaginal birth and are excellent teachers. Ask them questions and help where you can, such as with cleaning the room.

TABLE 1.1 Example Specific Risks of the Common Gynaecological Procedures

PROCEDURE	DESCRIPTION FOR PATIENTS	ADDITIONAL SPECIFIC RISKS
Hysteroscopy	Passing a camera through the cervix to view the inside of the uterus	• Uterine perforation. • Need for additional laparoscopy.
Surgical management of miscarriage	Passing a small tube through the cervix attached to a vacuum, to empty the uterus after a miscarriage	• Uterine perforation. • Laparoscopy. • Retained products of conception.
Laparoscopy	Keyhole surgery – a camera is inserted through the umbilicus (belly button) to view inside the pelvis. Additional small holes are made in the abdomen for insertion of operating instruments	• Incisional hernia. • Undiagnosed bowel injury at the time of procedure. • Laparotomy.
Laparotomy	Open surgery with a large incision on the abdomen	• Large scar. • Incisional hernia.
Vaginal prolapse surgery	Surgery within the vagina to repair damage to the vaginal walls	• Stress incontinence. • Pain on intercourse.

- Most antenatal admissions are young and physically healthy pregnant women. They can be helpful individuals to practice taking histories and performing systems examinations (not just obstetric examinations). They also frequently have positive examination findings such as flow murmurs, palmer erythema, brisk reflexes, and of course, abdominal masses.
- To help you pick a career ask the obstetricians and gynaecologists at various stages in their careers about why they chose O&G. There may also be other doctors rotating through the department (such as foundation doctors and GP trainees), ask them why they have chosen their career route and why they did not choose O&G.

❓ QUESTIONS

Nirja, a 28-year-old, presents to the clinic with acute pelvic pain. After taking a thorough history, it is determined that a bimanual examination is required to determine the cause.

Q1   Answer true or false, regarding the use of chaperones.
  A The chaperone is present only for the benefit of the patient.
  B The chaperone must be a nurse or other qualified doctor.
  C Chaperones should be assumed necessary unless the patient states otherwise.
  D In certain situations, a chaperone may be a family member.
  E Chaperones are not necessary when the doctor performing the examination is female.

Q2   If this patient had a body mass index (BMI) of 35 kg/m^2, which of the following is most correct regarding a discussion of their weight?
  A As a patient's BMI is a clinical matter, this can be discussed at any point in the patient's history or examination.
  B As long as the patient is fully dressed, then comments regarding the patient's weight may be made.
  C Due to the potentially sensitive nature of discussing a patient's weight, the doctor should wait until after the examination, when the patient has dressed and is back in the consultation room.
  D The doctor should discuss the patient's BMI before the examination, as this could be deemed inappropriate if done afterwards.
  E The doctor should not comment on the patient's weight, as it is unrelated to the patient's presentation.

Q3   If pain is experienced on moderate pressure to the cervix, what does this suggest?
  A Appendicitis.
  B Cervical cancer.
  C Fibroids.
  D Pelvic inflammatory disease.
  E This is a typical examination finding.

[Answers on page 163.]

HPO Axis

THE MENSTRUAL CYCLE AND PHYSIOLOGY OF THE HPO AXIS

The hypothalamic-pituitary-ovarian (HPO) axis refers to the interplay of hormones between these areas. The axis is referred to in this way because these glands normally behave in a coordinated manner as one system. The HPO axis controls the menstrual cycle, which is, in turn, responsible for development of the ovarian follicles (folliculogenesis), maturation of the oocyte (egg) within each follicle, ovulation of the oocyte from the dominant follicle and maturation of the uterine environment to facilitate pregnancy (Fig. 2.1).

THE HORMONES INVOLVED IN THE HYPOTHALAMIC-PITUITARY-OVARIAN AXIS

GONADOTROPIN-RELEASING HORMONE

- Peptide hormone.
- Produced by the arcuate nucleus in the hypothalamus, released in a pulsatile manner.
- Stimulates the production of gonadotropins; luteinising hormone (LH) and follicle-stimulating hormone (FSH) from the anterior pituitary (adenohypophysis).

FOLLICLE STIMULATING HORMONE

- Peptide hormone.
- Produced by the anterior pituitary in response to gonadotropin-releasing hormone (GnRH).
- Stimulates growth of the granulosa cells of primordial follicles (primitive follicles which each contain an oocyte) within the ovary, which leads to the development of the ovarian follicles.
- The granulosa cells of the follicles produce oestrogen and inhibin, which act by negative feedback to inhibit GnRH and FSH production. The follicle with the most FSH receptors is able to grow, while other follicles regress as the FSH levels fall in response to

the negative feedback. The one remaining dominant follicle (also called the Graafian follicle or tertiary follicle) is then ready for ovulation.

LUTEINISING HORMONE

- Peptide hormone.
- Produced by the anterior pituitary in response to GnRH.
- Stimulates production of androgens by theca cells of the follicles within the ovaries. Androgens are then converted to oestrogens in the granulosa cells in the follicular phase.
- The granulosa cells of the follicles produce oestrogen and inhibin, which act by negative feedback to inhibit GnRH and LH production in the follicular phase. However, at high concentrations, oestrogen then positively feeds back on the anterior pituitary, causing a sudden release of high concentrations of LH (the LH surge). The LH surge causes prostaglandin synthesis in the dominant follicle, causing the follicle to burst and release the oocyte inside. This event is ovulation.
- After ovulation, LH promotes the luteinisation of the granulosa cells, which then begin to produce progesterone, converting the remnants of the dominant follicle into the corpus luteum.

OESTROGEN

- A steroid hormone.
- Produced by the aromatisation of androstenedione in the granulosa cells of the ovarian follicles in response to FSH.
- Stimulates proliferative changes in the endometrium, building up the lining of the uterus in preparation for a potential pregnancy.
- Increasing levels of oestrogen in the follicular phase has a negative feedback effect on the hypothalamus and pituitary glands, leading to a decreased release of GnRH, FSH and LH. However, when high levels

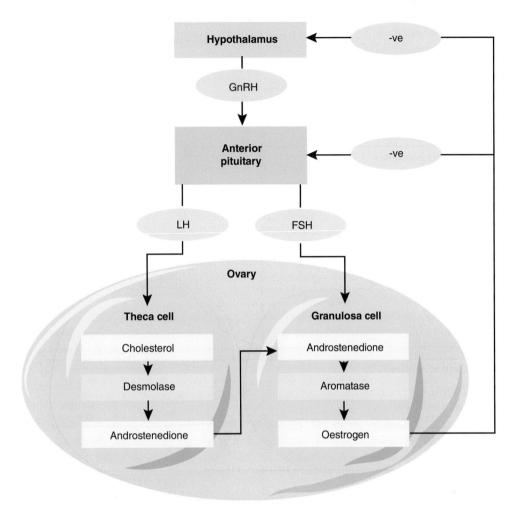

Fig. 2.1 The hypothalamic pituitary ovarian (HPO) axis in the follicular phase. *FSH*, Follicle-stimulating hormone; *GnRH*, gonadotropin-releasing hormone; *LH*, luteinising hormone.

of oestrogen are sustained for approximately 40 to 50 hours, the negative feedback on LH becomes positive feedback and the LH surge occurs.

PROGESTERONE

- A steroid hormone.
- Produced by the granulosa cells of the corpus luteum.
- Stimulates secretory changes of the endometrium, preparing it for blastocyst implantation.

ANDROGENS

- Steroid hormones, such as testosterone and androstenedione.
- Produced by the theca cells of the ovarian follicles in response to LH. Some androgens are also produced by the adrenal cortex.
- Androgens are the precursors of oestrogen. They are converted into oestrogen through aromatase enzyme activity within granulosa cells.

MENSTRUAL CYCLE

The menstrual cycle (Fig. 2.2) is the preparation of the body for pregnancy, whereby the oocyte (egg)

is developed and released and the endometrium is developed to maintain a pregnancy. If pregnancy does not occur, the endometrium is shed (commonly known as 'the period') and the cycle repeats. The classic menstrual cycle is 28 days long.

The phases of a normal 28-day menstrual cycle are summarised in Table 2.1 and Fig. 2.2.

FOLLICULAR PHASE

The first day of menstruation denotes day one of the menstrual cycle and the start of the follicular phase. Rising levels of GnRH released from the hypothalamus increase FSH production by the anterior pituitary. The FSH stimulates the receptors on the ovarian follicles, stimulating up to 20 follicles to mature each cycle.

FSH increases the production of oestrogen from the granulosa cells of the ovarian follicles. Oestrogen has a negative feedback effect on the hypothalamus and pituitary, which decreases FSH and LH levels. As FSH levels fall, follicles with the fewest FSH receptors stop growing and over time degenerate in a process called follicular atresia. The more developed follicles continue to progress, but as the oestrogen levels rise and FSH production is further inhibited, more and more follicles undergo atresia until only a single dominant

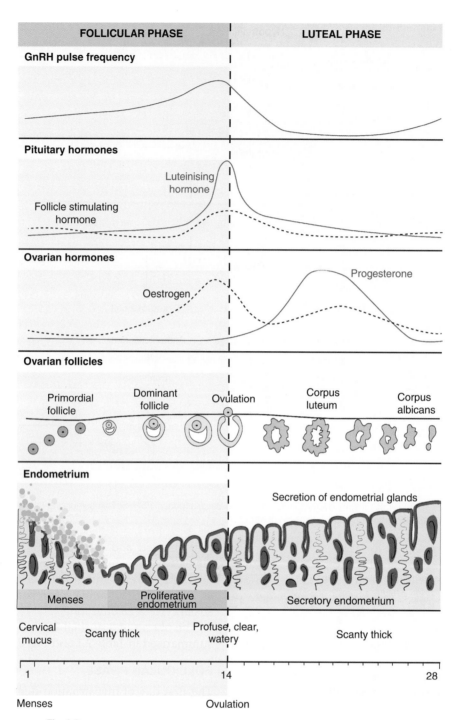

Fig. 2.2 Diagram of the menstrual cycle. *GnRH*, Gonadotropin-releasing hormone.

follicle continues to mature. The dominant follicle will continue to full maturity when it is then referred to as a Graafian follicle, and it will then progress to ovulation.

At the start of the follicular phase, the thickened endometrium from the previous menstrual cycle is expelled (menstruation). Late in the follicular phase, the new endometrium is stimulated to proliferate by the high oestrogen levels.

Ovulation occurs classically at day 14 when oestrogen levels rise to a sustained high level. This causes a shift from negative feedback to a strongly positive feedback on LH production from the pituitary, resulting in

a very high mid-cycle LH concentration, known as the LH surge. LH causes ovulation by activating inflammatory prostaglandin release, which causes the Graafian follicle to burst, releasing the oocyte. The inflammation allows ovulation to be identified clinically as a mild body temperature rise of approximately 0.5°C at the time of ovulation.

LUTEAL PHASE

Following ovulation, the ruptured Graafian follicle luteinises under the influence of LH to become the corpus luteum. Prior to formation of the corpus luteum,

Table **2.1**   **Phases of the Menstrual Cycle**

PHASE	DAYS	KEY PROCESS	MAIN EVENTS
Follicular phase	1–4	Menstruation	**Ovary** • Follicle development begins in response to FSH. **Endometrium** • Endometrium is shed and vaginal bleeding occurs. • First day of menstruation denotes the start of the cycle. • Myometrial contractions occur, which can be painful.
	5–13	Proliferation	**Ovary** • Maturation of the dominant follicle. • Other follicles regress due to the falling levels of FSH, caused by negative feedback from the oestrogen produced by the dominant follicle. **Endometrium** • Proliferation of the endometrium in response to oestrogen.
	14	Ovulation	**Ovary** • Release of the secondary oocyte from the dominant (Graafian) follicle in response to the LH surge from the pituitary.
Luteal phase	15–28	Secretory	**Ovary** • Dominant follicle remnants become the corpus luteum in response to LH. • The corpus luteum produces progesterone, which supports the endometrial lining. **Endometrium** • Secretory changes of the endometrium occur in response to progesterone, preparing for blastocyst implantation. **Outcome** • If the egg is not fertilised, regression of the corpus luteum occurs. The endometrium is no longer supported so it breaks down, leading to menstruation and repeat of the menstrual cycle. The remnant of the corpus luteum, called the corpus albicans, is reabsorbed over time. • If implantation occurs; beta human chorionic gonadotropin (hCG) released by the developing embryo maintains the corpus luteum. In turn, this continues to support the endometrium, and so pregnancy progresses.

very limited synthesis of progesterone occurs. The corpus luteum produces relatively high levels of progesterone and a smaller amount of oestrogen. These hormones act on the endometrium to prepare it for implantation by increasing glandular numbers and secretions. The progesterone and oestrogen produced from the corpus luteum also have a negative feedback on the pituitary, leading to low levels of FSH and LH for the rest of the cycle.

If the egg is fertilised and implantation occurs, hCG produced from the blastocyst maintains the corpus luteum, now called the corpus luteum graviditatis. This ensures synthesis of oestrogen and progesterone to support the endometrium and maintain the pregnancy. Progesterone is secreted by the corpus luteum for up to approximately 10 weeks. After this time, the corpus luteum declines in function, but the placenta fully takes over this role and oestrogen and progesterone levels rise rapidly. LH and hCG are similar in structure and both act on the luteinising hormone choriogonadotrophin receptor (LHCGR) to maintain the corpus luteum at different stages.

If fertilisation does not take place, there is an absence of hCG so the corpus luteum degenerates to its regressed form, called the corpus albicans, and it stops producing progesterone. With a lack of progesterone support from a corpus luteum, the endometrium breaks down and sheds. This is menstruation, and it represents day one of the next menstrual cycle. The cycle is able to restart because the declines in oestrogen and progesterone levels end the negative feedback, allowing the hypothalamus and pituitary to produce GnRH, FSH and LH.

Follicles From Conception to Menopause

Follicular development (Fig. 2.3) begins *in utero*. The first stage of oocyte development is the production of primordial germ cells (oogonia) in large numbers by mitosis. These oogonia become surrounded by granulosa cells, forming primordial follicles containing primary oocytes. The maximal number of follicles occurs at around 7 months' gestation when approximately 7 million oocytes are contained within the primordial follicles. However, through the process of atresia and apoptosis, only 1 million follicles remain at birth. These follicles contain primary oocytes, which are arrested in the prophase stage of meiosis 1.

By menarche, approximately 400,000 primordial follicles remain. High FSH and LH levels at the onset of puberty

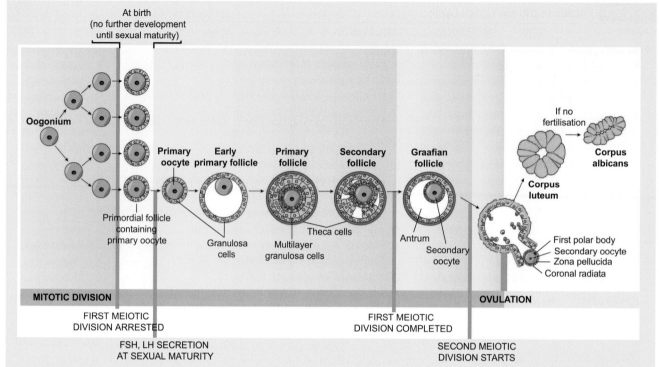

At birth
(no further development
until sexual maturity)

Oogonium

Primordial follicle
containing
primary oocyte

Primary
oocyte

Early
primary follicle

Granulosa
cells

Primary
follicle

Multilayer
granulosa cells

Theca cells

Secondary
follicle

Graafian
follicle

Antrum

Secondary
oocyte

If no
fertilisation

Corpus
albicans

Corpus
luteum

First polar body
Secondary oocyte
Zona pellucida
Coronal radiata

MITOTIC DIVISION

OVULATION

FIRST MEIOTIC
DIVISION ARRESTED

FIRST MEIOTIC
DIVISION COMPLETED

FSH, LH SECRETION
AT SEXUAL MATURITY

SECOND MEIOTIC
DIVISION STARTS

Fig. 2.3 Follicular development.

begins the development into primary and secondary follicles. The primary oocytes remain in the prophase of meiosis 1. Then, during the follicular phase of each menstrual cycle, FSH stimulates approximately 20 primordial follicles to mature further. Of these 20, only one oocyte completes meiosis 1, and that follicle goes on to become the dominant (Graafian) follicle, which contains the secondary oocyte. Half the genetic material is discarded into the first polar body during the process of meiosis.

At ovulation, the secondary oocyte begins meiosis 2, but this is arrested in metaphase. The process only completes when a sperm enters the oocyte, fertilising it. At this time, a further polar body is produced containing discarded deoxyribonucleic acid (DNA).

This process of folliculogenesis continues each cycle until the menopause, at which time there are only approximately 1000 primordial follicles remaining, and these do not respond even to very high FSH levels.

MENSTRUATION

- Menarche is the first episode of menstruation. This occurs, on average, when a girl is 13 years old. Menarche is considered early if it occurs before 10 years of age and late if it has not occurred by age 15.
- Menopause is the natural cessation of menstrual cycles once there are no functional oocytes remaining. The average age of menopause in the UK is 51 years old. Premature menopause occurs at less than 40 years of age and late menopause is at more than 55 years.

There are four specific components to consider regarding menstruation:

- Length of menstrual cycles – the average is 28 days.
  - Frequent if less than 24 days.
  - Infrequent if more than 38 days.
  - The luteal phase of a menstrual cycle is always 14 days. Therefore, any variation in cycle length is due to a change in the length of the follicular phase of the cycle.
- Regularity of menstrual cycles is the variation in the cycle lengths over a 12 month period.
  - Regular: ± 1 to 20 days.
  - Irregular: varying by more than 20 days.
  - Absent: no bleeding in a 90-day period.

Cycle Length Following Menarche and Approaching the Menopause

It is not uncommon for up to 50% of cycles to be anovulatory in the first 2 years following menarche as the HPO axis matures. As a consequence it is not unusual to have irregular cycles at this time, particularly during the first year where cycles of less than 21 days or greater than 45 days can occur without concern. From 1 to 3 years after menarche cycle lengths of 21 to 45 days are normal. By the end of this third year around 80% of adolescents will have menstrual cycles in keeping with adult length.

During the perimenopause, menstrual cycles can again become irregular with an increase in anovulatory cycles.

- Duration of menses – normally 4 to 8 days.
  - Shortened if less than 4 days.
  - Prolonged if more than 8 days.
- Volume of monthly menstrual blood loss – average of 40 mL.
  - Light if less than 5 mL.
  - Heavy if more 80 mL.
  - In clinical practice, blood loss is assessed more practically; for example, the 'number of pads used', experience of any 'flooding' or 'passing of clots'.

PAIN DURING THE MENSTRUAL CYCLE

- Mittleschmerz is pain that occurs in some women when they ovulate. This is a German term meaning 'middle pain' and it occurs in some women due to fluid leaking from the dominant follicle at the same time as the egg is being released. This results in free pelvic fluid which irritates the peritoneum.
- At the time of menstruation, pain ('period cramps') is caused by contraction of the uterine myometrium and by the inflammatory necrosis of the endometrium being shed.

❓ QUESTIONS

Isabella, a 20-year-old girl, comes to the clinic concerned that she is having heavy and painful periods. She has read an article online suggesting that her symptoms may be caused by a hormone imbalance. She would like an explanation as to how these hormones affect her periods, and for her hormone levels to be checked.

Q1 Which of the following statements concerning the HPO axis are true or false?
  A The HPO axis acts to bring about secondary sexual changes.
  B GnRH is released from the anterior pituitary.
  C GnRH is released in a pulsatile manner.
  D GnRH causes the release of FSH alone.
  E Negative feedback from oestrogen occurs in the arcuate nucleus and anterior pituitary.

Q2 Which of the following statements concerning the menstrual cycle are true or false?
  A The average length of a menstrual cycle is 32 days.
  B Ovarian follicles mature during the proliferative phase.
  C Declining FSH levels in the follicular phase can lead to follicular atresia.
  D The mid-cycle LH surge occurs in response to high oestrogen levels.
  E The follicle which released the egg may later become the corpus albicans.

Q3 Which of the following statements regarding the luteal phase are correct?
  A The end of the menstrual cycle occurs secondary to regression of the corpus luteum.
  B Secretory changes of the endometrium are largely due to LH.
  C Increasing levels of progesterone cause a breakdown of the endometrium at the end of the menstrual cycle.
  D The basal body temperature is lower in the luteal phase.
  E If the egg is fertilised, the endometrium is maintained despite falling progesterone and oestrogen levels.

A Asherman syndrome.	G Menopause.
B Dysfunctional uterine bleeding.	H Polycystic ovarian syndrome.
C Endometrial hyperplasia.	I Pregnancy.
D Endometriosis.	J Premature menopause.
E Endometritis.	K Sheehan syndrome.
F Imperforate hymen.	L Turner syndrome.

Select the most appropriate diagnosis from the above list that corresponds to the following statements.

Q4 A 15-year-old presents with cyclical lower abdominal pain for 10 months and denies any history of menstruation. She has normal secondary sexual development.

Q5 A 28-year-old presents to the emergency department following haemorrhagic shock during a spontaneous vaginal birth at home. Following recovery, the patient is unable to lactate for her child.

Q6 A 22-year-old presents with her mother complaining of irregular menstrual cycles. Both the mother and patient are overweight and the girl complains of having to shave very frequently.

Q7 A nulliparous 35-year-old presents with a 2-year history of mild cyclical pelvic pain with a recent onset of pain and bleeding on defecation commencing before menstruation.

Q8 A 51-year-old presents to her primary care physician with a 13-month history of absent periods and palpitations, and she would also like to explore treatment for vaginal dryness.

[Answers on page 165.]

PUBERTY

Puberty is a process that begins in late childhood and leads to the development of secondary sexual characteristics, physical growth and fertility. In females, this is the development of breast tissue (thelarche), body hair (pubarche), a growth spurt and the start of the menstrual cycle (menarche). Puberty is a developmental process led by the maturation of the HPO axis (or the hypothalamic pituitary testes axis in males).

- In females, pubertal changes normally occur in the following order: thelarche, pubarche, growth spurt, and finally menarche.
- Pubertal changes usually take at least 18 months to be complete.
- Thelarche and pubarche occur normally between 8 and 13.5 years of age. Menarche usually commences slightly later, between 10 and 15 years of age, usually 2 to 3 years after thelarche.
- Female precocious puberty is pubertal development at an abnormally early age. It should be investigated if development of secondary sexual characteristics before the age of 8, or if menarche occurs before the age of 10.
- Delayed puberty should be investigated if breast development has not started at age 13. Primary amenorrhoea should be investigated at age 15 if

other secondary sexual characteristics are normal. If there are no signs of puberty by age 13 then investigations should start.

There may be precocious or delayed puberty in all areas of pubertal development, termed complete development, or there may be an isolated presentation; for example, isolated precocious menarche or isolated delayed thelarche. Identification of isolated or global abnormalities in pubertal development is essential to reach the correct diagnosis.

Adrenarche

Adrenarche is the progressive maturation of the adrenal cortex and is associated with rising serum dehydroepiandrosterone (DHEAS).

This process occurs independently to the maturation of the HPO axis.

The rising androgens are marked by the appearance of body odour, acne and pubic or axillary hair (pubarche).

Premature adrenarche can present as isolated premature pubarche with no other secondary sexual characteristics. These are absent as HPO axis maturation has not yet occurred. Gonadotrophin levels will be normal.

Male Puberty

The first sign of puberty in boys is gonadarche (testicular enlargement). The average age of puberty in boys is 11.5 years and follows the sequence of: gonadarche, pubarche, adrenarche (facial hair, acne and voice changes, which are all androgen-driven) and finally the growth spurt. Precocious puberty in boys is any pubertal changes occurring at less than 9 years of age; delayed pubertal development is when changes have not begun by age 14.

PHYSIOLOGY

The HPO axis is active *in utero* but becomes inactive towards the end of the gestation period due to negative feedback from oestrogen and progesterone from the placenta. After birth, the placental hormones are lost and there is a brief reactivation of the HPO axis for a few months. The axis then shuts down and is restarted again in late childhood to commence puberty. What causes the initiation of the HPO axis again is poorly understood. One suggestion is that as the body reaches a certain size and body composition, increasing levels of leptin decreases the level of neuropeptide Y, which inhibits the hypothalamus and pituitary.

The hypothalamus begins secreting GnRH in a pulsatile fashion, initially only at night, but over time this increases to the full 24 hours. GnRH then stimulates the anterior pituitary to release LH and FSH. FSH acts upon the ovarian follicles, stimulating follicular development and oestrogen production from the granulosa cells of the follicles. LH stimulates the theca cells of the ovarian follicles to produce androgens. In addition to the HPO axis, levels of growth hormone releasing hormone (GHRH) from the hypothalamus and growth hormone (GH) from the pituitary dramatically increase at the time of puberty.

Oestrogen appears to be the predominant hormone responsible for thelarche. Androgens, such as testosterone, are important in pubarche. As well as ovarian androgen production, androgens are also made by the adrenal glands outside of the control of the HPO axis. Like the activation of the HPO axis at the time of puberty, it is also unclear what activates the adrenal glands. The growth spurt is predominantly caused by GH, but testosterone is also important in growth and oestrogen influences bone maturation. Menarche occurs last, as high levels of oestrogen are required to allow ovulation. When pregnancy does not occur, the endometrial lining breaks down and sheds, which is the first menstruation.

[See 'The menstrual cycle and physiology of the HPO axis' page 8.]

PRECOCIOUS PUBERTY

Most cases of precocious puberty are idiopathic/constitutional with no sinister cause, particularly in females. It is more common in those with a family history of precocious puberty and obesity. However, pathological causes must be investigated and ruled out. Investigations are usually undertaken by a paediatric endocrinologist, though they may seek support from gynaecology if early menarche has occurred and requires management.

The causes of precocious puberty can be split into central and peripheral (Fig. 2.4).

CENTRAL OR TRUE PRECOCIOUS PUBERTY

Caused by early activation or maturation of the HPO axis.
- Idiopathic or constitutional is the most likely cause.
- Most pathological causes are neurological in origin:
  - Brain tumour.
    - Pituitary adenoma, craniopharyngioma, glioma.
    - Chemotherapy or radiotherapy treatment for a tumour.
  - Following head trauma.
  - Following meningitis or encephalitis.
  - Hydrocephalus – classic symptom triad of normal pressure hydrocephalus is incontinence, unstable gait and confusion.
  - Spina bifida (myelomeningocele).
- Psychosexual abuse is also associated with precocious puberty.

PERIPHERAL OR PSEUDOPRECOCIOUS PUBERTY

Caused by peripheral production of hormones causing puberty, but the HPO axis has not been activated:
- Congenital adrenal hyperplasia (CAH).
- Cushing syndrome.
- Severe hypothyroidism.

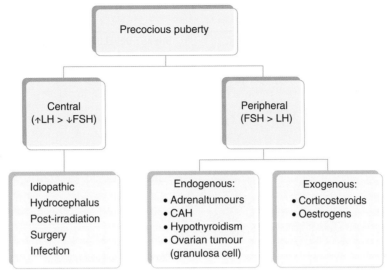

Fig. 2.4 Precocious Puberty. *CAH*, Congenital adrenal hyperplasia; *FSH*, follicle-stimulating hormone; *LH*, luteinising hormone.

- Adrenal cortex or ovarian tumour – may produce oestrogens or androgens.
- McCune-Albright syndrome.
- Exogenous hormones – anabolic steroids, contraceptive pills.

 McCune-Albright Syndrome

This is a congenital genetic abnormality. It causes fibrous dysplasia of the bone, which can cause multiple sites of bone swelling and fracture, café au lait spots and hyperfunction of endocrine tissues. Ovarian hyperfunction is usually the cause of precocious puberty, but any endocrine organ can be affected, so it may also present with a rapid growth spurt caused by excess GH (gigantism or acromegaly).

 Congenital Adrenal Hyperplasia

The term CAH describes a group of autosomal recessive inherited conditions affecting production of enzymes that work in the adrenal glands synthesising steroid hormones. The nature and timing of presentation depends on the severity of the condition.

The more severe "classic" forms are usually detected soon after birth. Female neonates with severe CAH have virilised genitalia as a result of exposure to excess androgens in utero. Those who also have an aldosterone deficiency present with salt-wasting crisis.

Non-classic milder forms of CAH are more common and can present for the first time as precocious puberty. Girls with this condition may develop clitoromegaly, voice deepening and hirsuitism. Delayed puberty and irregular periods can also be features.

[See 'Differences of sexual development' page 20.]

HISTORY

- Age at onset of symptoms.
- Sequence of pubertal symptoms – idiopathic and central causes usually follow the normal sequence of puberty, whereas peripheral causes are more likely to differ.
- Neurological symptoms – tumour, hydrocephalus.

- Endocrine symptoms – hypothyroid, Cushing disease or syndrome.
- Medical history – identify any previous concerns regarding growth, developmental milestones or behaviour throughout childhood. Identify a history of previous infections, head trauma, chemotherapy or radiotherapy. Fractures are common in McCune-Albright syndrome and others where bone age is affected.
- Medication history – exogenous hormone use.
- Family history – idiopathic precocious puberty, CAH, McCune-Albright syndrome.
- Social history – domestic violence and sexual abuse are associated with precocious puberty.

EXAMINATION

Assessment of Pubertal Development
- Growth – height and weight measurements.
  - Plot age and sex-specific growth charts.
  - Repeated measurements will demonstrate growth velocity and help predict further growth.
- Thelarche and pubarche – Tanner stages (Table 2.2) are an objective way of assessing secondary sexual characteristics of thelarche and pubarche.

Systemic Examination
Most examinations will be normal but rarely a cause may be identified.
- Skin inspection.
  - Abnormal injuries and/or the child's behaviour may suggest child abuse.
  - Café au lait spots are brown (milky coffee) coloured macular patches; usually sparing of the midline of the face or trunk may suggest McCune-Albright syndrome.
- Neurology.
  - A neurological examination may reveal a deficit suggestive of an intracranial pathology.

Table 2.2 Tanner Stages

TANNER STAGE		BREAST DEVELOPMENT	PUBIC HAIR GROWTH
1		Preadolescent – elevation of papilla only.	Preadolescent – no pubic hair.
2		Breast budding – small mound.	Sparse growth – long and slightly pigmented.
3		Continued enlargement – no separation of contours.	Darker, coarser and curlier with increased spread.
4		Areola and papilla form second mound.	Inverse triangle distribution, lack of spread to thighs.
5		Mature – projection of papilla only.	Mature – inverse triangle distribution including spread to the thighs.

- Endocrine.
  - Cushing syndrome – central obesity, rounded face, dry skin, hirsutism, male pattern baldness.
  - Hypothyroidism – goitre, cool extremities, dry skin, hair loss, slow heart rate.
- Virilisation.
- CAH – may cause virilised genitalia (clitoromegaly) and hirsutism.

INVESTIGATIONS
Blood Tests
- LH, FSH.
  - If raised into the pubertal range, this suggests the HPO axis is active; therefore, a central cause rather than peripheral cause is more likely.
  - The gold standard test to determine whether the cause of precocious puberty is gonadotropin dependent (central) or gonadotropin independent (peripheral) is a GnRH stimulation test. A GnRH analogue is given and then LH and FSH levels are measured shortly afterwards.

- LH rise greater than FSH suggests a central cause.
- FSH rise greater than LH suggests a peripheral cause.
- If the test is done on a female undergoing typical puberty, FSH is greater than LH when prepubertal and then LH is greater than FSH once pubertal.
- Other blood tests can be considered, depending on clinical suspicion; most of these are looking for peripheral causes of precocious puberty.
  - Hypothyroidism – thyroid stimulating hormone (TSH) and T4.
  - Cushing syndrome – cortisol (further assessed with a dexamethasone suppression test).
  - CAH – 17-Hydroxyprogesterone (17-OHP), sex hormone binding globulin (SHBG), dehydroepiandrosterone (DHEAS), androstenedione, testosterone and a urine steroid profile.
  - Adrenal tumour – oestrogen, testosterone and investigations for CAH.
  - Ovarian tumour – oestrogen and testosterone.

- Acromegaly – insulin-like growth factor 1 (IGF1) (further assessed with a GH level following glucose loading).
- Pituitary adenoma – prolactin may be raised.

Imaging Studies
- Wrist x-ray (non-dominant hand) – compares bone age to chronological age by looking at the development of the carpal bones. Bone age is increased in almost all causes, except hypothyroidism.
  - Oestrogen is involved in the growth spurt. However, high levels in puberty also cause fusion of the epiphyses. In precocious puberty, high oestrogen levels cause early epiphyseal fusion, thereby limiting final adult height.
  - Current height and x-ray findings can be used to predict final adult height.
- Magnetic resonance image (MRI) head – indicated where a central cause of precious puberty is suspected.
- Pelvic ultrasound scan – assess uterine and ovarian size (these organs will enlarge in central precocious puberty). Ovarian tumours can be excluded. An MRI can further assess pelvic abnormalities and can also be performed if adrenal or liver tumours are suspected.

COMPLICATIONS
- Early bone maturation resulting in reduced final adult height. This can sometimes be overlooked as the growth spurt occurs early with precocious puberty, leading to the incorrect assumption that the child will be tall.
- Increased risk of psychological problems.
- If caused by a pathology, the complications of that pathology and treatment for it.

MANAGEMENT
Management will, to a large extent, be determined by the cause. If an endocrine cause, such as hypothyroidism or CAH, is identified, then medications to treat the underlying pathology are required.

If a tumour is identified, resection may be the most appropriate treatment. It is rare that pubertal changes will regress following treatment, but treatment should reduce progression.

In most cases, idiopathic central precocious puberty will be the diagnosis and no underlying pathology will be identified. Treatment will require:
- Emotional and psychological support for the child and parents.
- Serial height measurements and monitoring of the velocity on a growth chart and comparison to mid-parental height.
  - If serial measurements and x-ray findings suggest the likelihood of a significant reduction in final adult height and the child is identified

before 8 years of age, injections of a GnRH agonist can be started.
- GnRH analogues downregulate the HPO axis by over stimulating the axis, as GnRH is usually only released in a pulsatile manner.
- Very occasionally, GH is also used alongside GnRH analogues.

 Calculate Mid-Parental Height

- Female child = (father's height (cm) + mother's height (cm)/2) – 7cm.
- Male child = (father's height (cm) + mother's height (cm)/2) + 7cm.
- 95th percent confidence limits are ± 8cm.

PROGNOSIS

Generally, the aetiology determines morbidity and mortality, and the disease symptoms and progression vary greatly. In idiopathic central precocious puberty, onset after 6 years of age will result in a normal adult height and no long-term sequelae for most girls.

 Partial Precocious Puberty

Here, only one aspect of puberty occurs prematurely. History and examination (including height measurements) will differentiate it from complete precocious puberty. Usually, these changes are without a sinister cause. However, the underlying pathology may need to be investigated. If other pubertal changes occur, then the patient should be tested for complete precocious puberty.
- Premature thelarche – mostly occurs at ages 8 months to 2 years, due to brief reactivation of the HPO axis just after birth. This is a normal variant, is non-progressive and does not require investigation. However, it can sometimes cause emotional distress in some children and parents.
- Premature pubarche – most commonly due to early production of androgens by the adrenal glands, without any HPO activity. It is non-progressive and a normal variant. Investigations to rule out an adrenal tumour should be considered; a mild DHEA rise alone is diagnostic for the benign condition.
- Premature growth spurt – rare and unlikely to be sinister. However, if the growth spurt is excessive, testing for gigantism (acromegaly) should be considered.
- Premature menarche – usually transient due to regression of a benign ovarian cyst, and does not affect the rest of pubertal development. It may cause emotional distress. Examination under anaesthetic and an ultrasound scan may be used to rule out trauma, local infections, tumours and child abuse.

DELAYED PUBERTY

Delayed puberty occurs in approximately 2% of adolescents; 90% of these will be constitutional delay of puberty. This is a temporary delay in pubertal

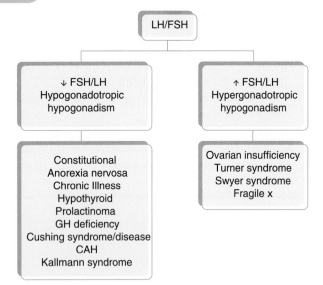

Fig. 2.5 Delayed puberty investigation. *CAH*, Congenital adrenal hyperplasia; *FSH*, follicle-stimulating hormone; *GH*, growth hormone; *LH*, luteinising hormone.

progression, with the majority of children reaching their growth potential. It is essential to exclude pathologies causing delayed puberty, as these are more likely to limit growth potential if left untreated. The most common pathology is anorexia nervosa.

The causes (Fig. 2.5) of delayed puberty could be grouped centrally and peripherally, like precocious puberty. However, it is more useful to subcategorise these into the anatomical levels where there is a problem:

- Constitutional delay.
- Systemic inhibition of HPO or hypothalamus.
  - Puberty is a high energy process (exemplified by the significant food intake of adolescents). If the body does not have surplus energy (either due to low energy intake or increased physical stress), it makes evolutionary sense that the body would not initiate this high energy process until there is surplus energy available. It is not clear how puberty is inhibited, but inhibition is believed to occur at the higher levels, such as inhibition of the hypothalamus. Example causes are:
    - Physical stress – excessive exercise.
    - Mental stress – depression or psychosocial abuse.
    - Chronic disease – inflammatory bowel disease or chronic kidney disease.
    - Chronic infection – tuberculosis, hepatitis or Epstein-Barr virus.
    - Malnutrition – coeliac disease, cystic fibrosis or anorexia nervosa.
- Problem with the hypothalamus or pituitary.
  - Extrinsic failure.
    - Brain tumour causing compression.
    - Head trauma.
    - Cranial surgery, chemotherapy or radiotherapy.
  - Intrinsic failure or genetic cause (rare).
    - Kallmann syndrome.
    - GnRH insensitivity.
    - Prader-Willi syndrome.
- Problem with ovarian function.
  - Genetic causes – Turner syndrome, Fragile X.
  - Swyer syndrome (XY DSD with streak gonads).
  - Acquired ovarian insufficiency – ovarian torsion, damage following infection, autoimmune disease, chemotherapy or radiotherapy.
- Endocrine.
  - Prolactinoma.
  - Hypothyroidism.
  - Cushing syndrome.
  - CAH.
  - GH deficiency – especially if short stature.
- Exogenous hormones – anabolic steroids, contraceptive pills.

GENETIC CAUSES

Hypogonadotropic Hypogonadism (Hypothalamic or Pituitary Failure, Decreased Levels of Follicle-Stimulating Hormone and Luteinising Hormone)

- Kallmann syndrome classically presents with delayed puberty and anosmia. The neurons responsible for transmission of GnRH from the hypothalamus to the pituitary arise in the olfactory placode (as well as the olfactory nerve). This area fails to form in Kallmann syndrome, so GnRH is not released and a sense of smell is absent.
- GnRH insensitivity is caused by a mutation to the GnRH receptors of the pituitary. GnRH is released but FSH and LH are not produced. This is the most likely genetic cause if anosmia is not associated.
- Prader-Willi syndrome is associated with developmental delay, short stature, delayed puberty, over eating and obesity.

Hypergonadotropic Hypogonadism (Impaired Response of Gonads to Gonadotrophins, Increased Level of Follicle-Stimulating Hormone and Luteinising Hormone)

- Turner syndrome – 45 XO (absence of the final sex chromosome). Phenotypical female with classical dysmorphic features, including short stature, broad chest, webbed neck and low-set ears. Children with subtle features may present later with delayed puberty or primary amenorrhoea, which is caused by non-functioning ovaries.
- Fragile X syndrome – X-linked recessive, fragile X messenger ribonucleoprotein 1 (FMR1) gene mutation. Mild to moderate learning difficulties, links to autism spectrum disorders (ASD) and attention deficit hyperactivity disorder (ADHD). Primary ovarian insufficiency is common and can occur in women carrying the pre-mutation.
- Swyer syndrome/gonadal dysgenesis – 46XY (XY DSD). A Y chromosome defect means the

embryological gonads do not differentiate into testes (which are required to produce anti-Mullerian hormone (AMH) and testosterone to cause development of the male *in utero*). The child is phenotypically female, but with non-functioning primitive gonads. They often present with delayed puberty. A gonadectomy is recommended due to increased risk of malignancy.

 Growth Hormone Deficiency

GH deficiency in childhood is usually idiopathic, but in adults is most commonly due to a pituitary tumour. It presents with short stature and delayed puberty. If deficiency is suspected, blood can be tested for levels of IGF-1, which is made in response to GH. If this is low, the diagnosis can be confirmed with an insulin stress test (insulin is given to cause hypoglycaemia which, in a healthy subject, causes the release of glucagon and GH to correct the hypoglycaemia). If there is not a GH rise after hypoglycaemia is induced the diagnosis is made.

HISTORY

- Medical history – identify chronic disease, physical and mental stressors.
- Medication history – exogenous hormone use.
- Neurological symptoms – tumour.
- Endocrine symptoms – hypothyroid, prolactinoma, Cushing syndrome and ask about hirsutism.
- Family history – constitutional delayed puberty or CAH.
- Social history – domestic violence, depression or anorexia.

EXAMINATION

Assessment of Pubertal Development
- Growth – height and weight measurements.
  - Significantly reduced growth suggests Turner syndrome or GH deficiency.
- Thelarche and pubarche.
  - Tanner stages.
  - Constitutional delay should follow the normal developmental pattern.

Systemic Examination
- Inspection.
  - Malnutrition – emaciated, dry skin, dry mucous membranes or lanugo hair.
  - Systemic disease – clubbing, aphthous ulcers or pale conjunctiva.
  - Virilisation – hirsutism or ambiguous genitalia.
  - Dysmorphia – genetic abnormalities, for example, Turner syndrome.
- Systems review.
  - Neurology.
  - Endocrine.
  - Other systems as guided by the history.

INVESTIGATIONS
Blood Tests
Luteinising hormone and follicle-stimulating hormone
- FSH and LH normal or low.
  - Hypothalamus and/or pituitary not functioning.
  - Known as hypogonadotropic hypogonadism.
  - Anorexia, malnutrition or another chronic disease may be the apparent cause from the history.
  - Further blood tests to consider to identify an underlying cause:
    - Evidence of chronic disease – full blood count (FBC), urea and electrolytes (U&Es), liver function tests (LFTs), ferritin, coeliac screen.
    - Hypothyroidism – TSH, T4.
    - Prolactinoma – prolactin.
    - Cushing syndrome – cortisol, dexamethasone suppression test.
    - CAH – 17-OHP, SHBG, DHEA and testosterone.
    - If the child also has short stature, consider growth hormone deficiency – IGF1 (further assessed with an insulin stress test).
  - If no peripheral cause identified, consider a luteinising hormone releasing hormone (LHRH) (similar to GnRH) stimulation test.
    - FSH and LH rise – HPO axis can be stimulated, likely constitutional delay.
    - No FSH or LH rise – HPO axis remains dormant, likely intrinsic deficiency (Kallmann, GnRH insensitivity).
- FSH and LH raised.
  - Hypothalamus and pituitary are working but the ovaries are not.
  - Known as hypergonadotropic hypogonadism.
  - Further testing to identify cause:
    - Karyotyping – essential to rule out Turner syndrome, other rarer causes such as androgen insensitivity can also be investigated.

Imaging Studies
- Wrist x-ray (non-dominant hand) – bone age is delayed in constitutional delay, hypothyroidism and GH deficiency.
- MRI head – indicated where a pituitary or cranial tumour is suspected.
- Pelvic ultrasound scan – indicated to assess for presence of a uterus, vagina and ovaries. Absent uterus in Swyer syndrome and androgen insensitivity.

MANAGEMENT
- Treat any underlying cause for delayed puberty.
- GH injections are given to patients with the hormone deficiency.
- Psychological support is often required for patients with delayed puberty.
- Patients with constitutional delay are monitored for growth spurt and pubertal changes. If a significant

delay occurs, oestrogen can be given in gradually increasing doses to induce puberty (oestrogen is frequently given with cyclical progesterone once a high enough dose has been reached). Oestrogen is increased slowly to reduce the chance of premature closure of the epiphyseal plates.

- For patients with long-term ovarian dysfunction, the combined oral contraceptive pill can be used long-term (once the initial regime as above has been completed). This will reduce the risk of osteoporosis caused by oestrogen deficiency.

PROGNOSIS

The majority of children with constitutional delay will reach their potential adult height, often without treatment. For delayed puberty caused by an underlying condition, the long-term prognosis will be determined by how effectively the condition can be managed. Reduced final adult height and infertility will complicate some of the conditions.

Primary Amenorrhea – Isolated Delayed Menstruation

Patients will present with normal secondary sexual characteristics but never having had a period. All the pathologies of delayed puberty (except GH deficiency) can present as isolated primary amenorrhoea. Therefore, the history, systemic examination and investigations are the same as above, except:

- A wrist x-ray is not needed.
- An MRI head is rarely required unless symptoms are strongly suggestive of a neurological pathology.
- Two additional causes need to be investigated:
  - Polycystic ovarian syndrome (PCOS).

    [See 'Polycystic ovarian syndrome' page 31.]

  - Anatomical anomaly of the genital tract. These either obstruct the flow of menstrual blood due to an anatomical obstruction, or there is a congenital absence of the uterus.

    [See 'Differences of sexual development' page 20.]

 QUESTIONS

Stella, a seven-year-old girl is brought to the primary care physician's practice by her single father because he is worried about his daughter's growth. He says that he thinks the other children in school have been bullying her about her being so tall, and that she's been quiet and feeling sad. On examination, she has a small amount of breast tissue and some hair in her pubic region and axillae. No other significant findings are noted on examination, and she has not begun menstruation.

Q1 What is the most likely cause of her precocious puberty?
  A Central idiopathic precocious puberty.
  B Congenital adrenal hyperplasia.
  C Head trauma.
  D McCune-Albright syndrome.
  E Partial premature thelarche.

Q2 Which of the following regarding puberty are true or false?
  A Precocious puberty is the development of secondary sexual characteristics at less than 8 years old in girls and less than 10 in boys.
  B The first sign of puberty in girls is thelarche.
  C The first sign of puberty in boys is pubarche.
  D Pubic hair extending to the medial surface of the thigh indicates Tanner stage 4 development.
  E One of the first-line investigations in precocious puberty is an x-ray of the wrist.

Q3 Which of the following regarding delayed puberty are true or false?
  A Puberty is delayed if a girl has no breast bud development by 13 years of age.
  B Puberty is delayed if a girl has not had her first period by 14 years of age.
  C The most common cause of delayed puberty is a chronic illness.
  D Turner syndrome is a cause of delayed puberty.
  E Kallmann syndrome is associated with delayed puberty.

[Answers on page 167.]

DIFFERENCES IN SEX DEVELOPMENT

The term disorders in sex development (DSD) was first introduced in 2006. This replaced the previously used 'intersex' and 'hermaphroditism'. It has been recognised that some people may prefer to use an alternative to the word 'disorder' and alternatives 'variations' or 'differences' are now used. In this chapter the term DSD refers to "differences in sex development".

The medical definition of a DSD is 'a condition in which the development of the chromosomal, gonadal or anatomic sex is atypical'. DSD is an umbrella term for a wide range of conditions which can have very different implications for the affected individual. People affected often need input from a wide multidisciplinary team, potentially including both paediatric and adult specialists in gynaecology, psychology, endocrinology and urology.

DSDs can manifest themselves in a number of ways. For example, the person's genitalia may appear atypical, may not match the gender of the person's genotype or may appear typical during childhood but then not develop in the usual manner during puberty. Some cases of DSDs will present as primary amenorrhoea if there are no visible manifestations of the disorder. Some conditions will present a challenge to fertility.

It is best to refer to the particular condition affecting the person and to be aware that two people with the same diagnosis can be affected in different ways and require different types of support. Healthcare professionals must be sensitive and considerate when managing a person with a DSD.

AETIOLOGY

Around 1% of people in the UK are estimated to have a DSD. This figure includes forms of DSDs which do not manifest themselves at birth by atypical genitalia. The incidence of DSDs presenting with atypical genitalia detected at birth is much lower, at 0.02%. This difference is important, as many people with DSDs will not develop symptoms until later in life.

A primary DSD can occur in three ways:

1 The genotype is atypical, for example, Turner syndrome (45 XO).
2 The body does not deal with sex hormones normally, for example CAH.
3 The gonads or genitalia do not develop correctly in the absence of hormonal or genetic abnormalities, for example, gonadal dysgenesis.

CLINICAL FEATURES

The signs and symptoms of DSDs vary depending on the condition that the child has, and the age at which they present. Specific DSDs and their individual signs are discussed later.

PRESENTATIONS AT BIRTH, IN THE NEONATE AND IN INFANCY

Signs may include:

- Atypical genitalia.
- Labial fusion, enlarged clitoris, and labial or inguinal masses.
- Hypospadias (incorrectly placed urethral meatus on the penis), chordee (bending of the penis), undescended testes and a micropenis.
- It may be impossible to ascertain gender without further investigation.
- DSDs may also present with failure to thrive, for example, CAH.

PRESENTATION AT PUBERTY

If a female presents during puberty, they may report the following symptoms:

- Lack of secondary sexual characteristics, such as pubic hair (pubarche) and breast development (thelarche).
- Not starting their period (menarche).
- Short stature compared to peers.

Females may also present even later in life with:

- Difficulty with penetrative intercourse due to structural abnormalities once they become sexually active.
- Infertility – usually associated with normal sexual characteristics and primary amenorrhoea.

Delayed puberty is most commonly caused by constitutional delay, with many endocrine and systemic diseases also causing delay. Similarly, there are many more common causes of infertility than a DSD, but DSDs should be considered when more common causes have been excluded.

INVESTIGATIONS

Investigation of a DSD may include:

- Identifying internal structural abnormalities.
  - Ultrasound scan, MRI and occasionally laparoscopy.
- Karyotyping.
  - A relatively cheap genetic test to ascertain the number of chromosomes.
  - The number and type of sex chromosomes is important in DSDs.
- Specific gene mutations.
  - Genetic testing (can be expensive).
  - Assessing small areas of the genome for each test. A high index of suspicion is required so the correct area of genome can be investigated.
  - Microarrays which can assess multiple gene expressions during a single test are becoming cheaper and more widespread, allowing increased identification of mutations.
- Specific investigations for individual diseases are covered in the differential diagnosis section.

DIFFERENTIAL DIAGNOSIS

For common causes of delayed puberty or amenorrhoea, see chapters on puberty and primary amenorrhoea.

[See 'Puberty' page 13.]

[See 'Primary Amenorrhoea' page 20.]

ISOLATED STRUCTURAL ABNORMALITY OF THE MALE GENITALIA

- Isolated micropenis.
- Undescended testicles.

GENETIC CAUSES

Typically a person has 46 chromosomes. 46XX is usually associated with being female and 46XY is usually associated with being male.

DSDs can be classified by the underlying karyotype:

1 46 XY DSDs – these people have the genes usually seen in males and they have genitals that do not develop in the usual way. The exact differences will depend on the condition and will vary from individual to individual.
2 46 XX DSDs – these people have genes usually seen in females but their genitals may not look like most females due to virilisation *in utero*. The exact differences will depend on the condition and will vary from individual to individual.
3 Sex chromosomal DSDs - these occur due to the loss or gain of a sex chromosome. The genitals will look typical, but sex development is different in other ways.

XY DIFFERENCES IN SEX DEVELOPMENT

Androgen Insensitivity Syndrome

Androgen insensitivity syndrome is the most common cause of 46XY DSD. It occurs in 1:40,000 births. It almost always occurs due to a mutation in the gene for androgen receptors, which is located on the X chromosome. The inability for cells to respond correctly to androgenic hormones leads to the failure of virilisation of the male fetus whilst *in utero*; however, the functioning Y chromosome causes development of the testes, which do not descend but they do produce AMH, preventing development of the uterus, cervix or upper vagina.

In complete androgen insensitivity syndrome (CAIS), the person will be phenotypically female with a normal appearance of the vulva. At the time of puberty, androgens are made and are converted into oestrogen, so usually secondary sexual characteristics occur, with normal breast development, but they may have absent pubic hair. People commonly present during adolescence or adulthood with primary amenorrhoea or with difficulties during intercourse. Examination of a person with CAIS would be expected to show typical female external genitalia and a short vagina. An ultrasound scan would reveal an absent uterus and may see undescended testicles. An MRI scan may be needed to locate the gonads as they can be found anywhere in the line of natural descent from the lower abdomen to the groin.

Management includes:
- Counselling
  - It is potentially very distressing for a person who has been brought up all of their life as a woman, to be told they have male genetics.
  - The absence of a uterus and ovaries means they are infertile.
  - Counselling and psychological support are important in the management of all cases of DSDs, but this will not be repeated in the text for every other cause.
- Surgery
  - The risk of malignancy developing in the gonads is thought to be reported as 3.6–33%, increasing with age, and so removal is recommended. The surgery is delayed until puberty is complete, particularly to allow for normal breast development. Once the gonads have been removed HRT will be required until the age of natural menopause.
  - Vaginal dilation therapy is offered to create a vagina if the person wishes. Psychological support is key to success. If this fails then surgery in the form of a Vecchietti procedure can be performed. This is an operation to create a vagina through traction.

Partial androgen insensitivity syndrome (PAIS) is caused by a similar genetic abnormality, but there is some response to androgens. These people often present with partially masculinised atypical genitalia so are more likely to be identified at birth.

OTHER XY DIFFERENCES IN SEX DEVELOPMENT

Differences in Androgen Synthesis

Examples of these conditions include 5-alpha reductase deficiency (impaired conversion of testosterone to the more potent dihydrotestosterone) and 17-beta hydroxysteroid dehydrogenase deficiency (impaired conversion of androstenedione to testosterone).

These conditions may be detected at birth if the external genitalia appear atypical, but otherwise are not discovered until puberty when high levels of LH increases testicular secretion of androstenedione which can be peripherally converted to testosterone. Vaginal dilator therapy may be possible. LHRH blockers and gonadectomy may be required to prevent further virilisation of genitalia and other changes such as deepening of the voice.

Gonadal Dysgenesis (Swyer Syndrome)

In these conditions, the gonads are non-functioning. AMH will not have been expressed *in utero*, so the Mullerian structures will have developed (uterus, tubes, cervix, upper vagina) as well as the lower vagina. The external genitalia will have a typical female appearance. The person will not go through puberty and will need to have pubertal induction with oestrogen patches. Gonadectomy is advised as the risk of malignancy can be as high as 30%. With oocyte donation they can usually achieve pregnancy.

46 XX DIFFERENCES IN SEX DEVELOPMENT

Congenital Adrenal Hyperplasia

The most common 46XX DSD is CAH (though CAH can also affect males). CAH occurs in around 1:14,000 births. It is an autosomal recessive condition. A gene mutation prevents the functioning of an adrenal gland enzyme which normally produces steroid hormones from cholesterol (Fig. 2.6). The substrates used by the affected enzyme build up and are often converted to androgens by an alternative process. The most common deficiency is in the enzyme 21-hydroxylase. This enzyme is responsible for converting 17-OHP into mineralocorticoids such as aldosterone, and glucocorticoids such as cortisol, but not into androgens. Without 21-hydroxylase, a deficiency in mineralocorticoids and glucocorticoids occurs. However, the common hormone precursors are still produced as normal. As the testosterone production pathway is unaffected by 21-hydroxylase deficiency, an excessive amount of androgens is produced from the high number of precursors.

CAH usually presents either:
- At birth, with atypical genitalia caused by the high androgen levels, giving a masculine appearance of the female genitalia.
- As a neonate, with failure to thrive due to significant electrolyte imbalances, also called salt wasting, due to aldosterone deficiency.
- As a person with mild disease at puberty with amenorrhoea, or even later with hirsutism and subfertility.

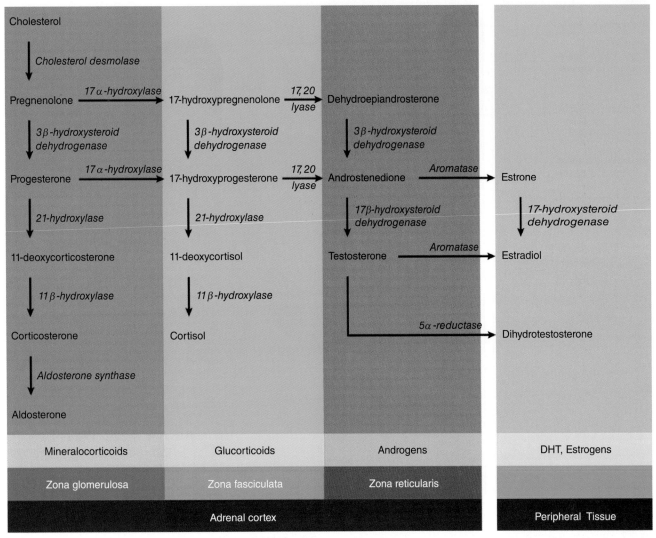

Fig. 2.6 Adrenal synthesis pathway.

Investigations

- 17-OHP – very high levels due to the deficiency in 21-hydroxylase.
- SHBG – low levels as bound to the high concentration of androgens.
- In cases of failure to thrive, electrolytes will be abnormal. Low cortisol and high renin levels are highly suggestive of CAH in this situation and a urine steroid profile can help confirm the diagnosis.

Management

- Glucocorticoids lifelong to replace the cortisol they are lacking.
- Mineralocorticoids lifelong if they have the salt wasting form of CAH.
- Having children is possible, but assisted conception may be required.
- There is debate about the optimal timing of any genital surgery for those with significant virilisation of genitalia presenting in the neonatal period. The surgery is mostly cosmetic in the form of a 'feminising genitoplasty' or 'vaginoplasty' to enable penetrative intercourse, as there tends not to be obstruction to menstrual flow.

 Virilisation in Females

There are other much rarer genetic causes of virilisation in females, such as sulfotransferase deficiency, in which dehydroepiandrosterone (DHEA) is not metabolised correctly, resulting in excess androgen production.

Klinefelter Syndrome

The most common form of sex chromosome DSD is Klinefelter syndrome, 47 XXY. The presence of the Y chromosome means that they are defined as genetically male. Phenotypically, most are male but some have a female (usually virilised) or atypical genitalia phenotype. They may present with abnormal development of secondary sexual characteristics (Fig. 2.7), infertility and poor libido. Men with Klinefelter syndrome are often tall and slim, but may have some central obesity. They can also experience significant gynaecomastia.

Diagnosis is made with karyotyping. Males with Klinefelter may benefit from testosterone replacement,

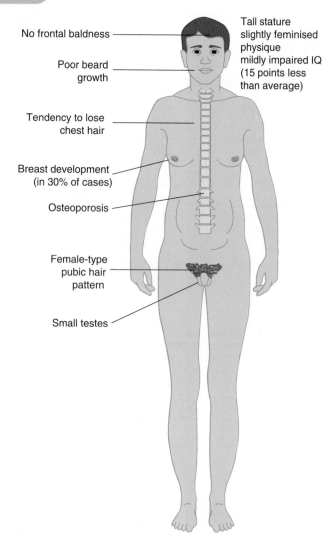

Tall stature
slightly feminised
physique
mildly impaired IQ
(15 points less
than average)

No frontal baldness

Poor beard
growth

Tendency to lose
chest hair

Breast development
(in 30% of cases)

Osteoporosis

Female-type
pubic hair
pattern

Small testes

Fig. 2.7 Klinefelter syndrome.

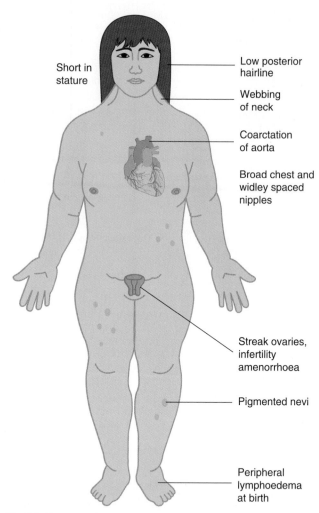

Short in
stature

Low posterior
hairline

Webbing
of neck

Coarctation
of aorta

Broad chest and
widley spaced
nipples

Streak ovaries,
infertility
amenorrhoea

Pigmented nevi

Peripheral
lymphoedema
at birth

Fig. 2.8 Turner syndrome.

to improve muscle bulk and secondary sexual development, and from breast reduction surgery. 3% of male infertility is caused by Klinefelter, but testosterone can improve fertility.

Turner Syndrome

Turner syndrome is a sex chromosome DSD that occurs in 1:2500 births. The person is missing an X chromosome, and their karyotype is most commonly 45 XO. Therefore, like Klinefelter syndrome, karyotyping is the most important investigation for diagnosing someone with Turner syndrome. They are genetically female due to the lack of a Y chromosome and are phenotypically female (Fig. 2.8).

Turner Syndrome Genetics:
• 50% 45 XO (complete absence of an X chromosome).
• 35% to 45% 45 X mosaicism (for example 45X/46XX).
• 5% to 15% structurally abnormal X chromosome.
• 5% have Y-fragments (they are recommended to have a gonadectomy).

People with Turner syndrome often present with primary amenorrhoea and a short stature compared to their peer group. Other common features of Turner

syndrome are a broad chest, short fingers and a webbed neck. They are usually infertile due to primary ovarian insufficiency and are therefore unable to have children without an egg donor. Pre-pregnancy counselling is vital if they have other manifestations of Turner's syndrome, particularly cardiac.

Multidisciplinary management is especially important for people with Turner syndrome as they are at increased risk of several chronic illnesses, particularly those which involve the cardiovascular and genitourinary systems, and also those with an autoimmune cause. As the cardiovascular risk includes serious conditions, including aortic dissection, conduction abnormalities and valvular defects, they should be carefully monitored with a low threshold for referral.

As well as treatment of the complications which arise from Turner syndrome, there may be benefit from recombinant GH during puberty to increase vertical growth. Oestrogen and progesterone therapy may assist in the regulation of menstrual cycles and hormone replacement therapy may be needed if primary ovarian insufficiency occurs. As with all DSDs, psychological support is important, particularly if they are concerned about their fertility.

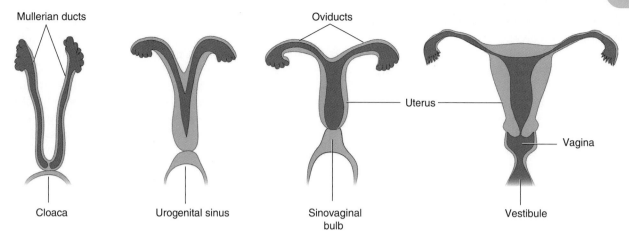

Fig. 2.9 Embryonic formation of the female reproductive system.

STRUCTURAL – MULLERIAN ANOMALIES

In the embryo, the female genital tract is formed from the Mullerian ducts (paramesonephric ducts), which fuse together and differentiate into the fallopian tubes, uterus and upper two-thirds of the vagina (Fig. 2.9). The lower portion of the Mullerian ducts join to the cloaca, which forms the lower third of the vagina and the vulva. The development of these structures can be abnormal. People with structural defects will appear phenotypically female. They often present towards the end of childhood with primary amenorrhoea, or with problems at the time of intercourse.

Transverse Vaginal Septum

Incomplete fusing of the lower third of the vagina (urogenital sinus derived from endoderm) to the upper vagina and uterus (Mullerian ducts derived from mesoderm) causes a thick band of tissue across the vagina. This blocks menstrual flow, therefore presenting as primary amenorrhea. It may also present with difficulties during intercourse. Complex surgery can be required in these cases.

Imperforate Hymen

These are common, occurring in 1:100 births and are not actually a DSD. This may be mistaken for a vaginal septum. The hymen is a thin membrane, present from birth, located just inside the opening of the vagina. There is usually an opening in the hymen which develops before or soon after birth.

If the hymen has no opening at the commencement of menarche, blood can collect behind it, causing pain which is often cyclical, and a bulge in the vagina is visible on examination. Imperforate hymen is the most common cause of obstructive amenorrhoea. A simple day-case surgery is required to correct this.

Mullerian Duct Fusion Defects

Incorrect fusing of the Mullerian ducts in the upper vagina can cause vertical septum formations. These are thick bands which split the vagina into two along its length, often presenting with pain on intercourse. These bands can be treated surgically, but the operation may be complex.

Higher fusion defects of the Mullerian ducts can also occur at the uterus, the most common being a bicornate uterus. The defect can, however, be more severe, causing a large septum within the uterus which increases the risk of preterm birth and miscarriage. Complete failure of fusion of the Mullerian ducts can cause a person to have two distinct uteri, cervixes and upper vaginas (uterine didelphysis).

Mullerian Agenesis

The most severe abnormality of the Mullerian ducts is Mullerian agenesis, often referred to as Mayer-Rokitansky-Kuster-Hauser (MRKH) syndrome. This occurs in 1:4000 births. In this condition, the external genitalia appear normal, but the vagina ends blindly. The vagina is usually shorter than expected, as the upper vagina does not form, and the uterus, cervix and fallopian tubes are absent. Puberty and development of secondary sexual characteristics will occur as normal, but there will be primary amenorrhoea. Affected females will not be able to conceive; however, their ovaries are normal so they could opt for *in vitro* fertilisation (IVF) and surrogacy. In the future, uterine transplantation may offer a fertility option for these people. Whilst Mullerian agenesis is an isolated finding in type 1 MRKH, type 2 MRKH can also be associated with renal or skeletal anomalies.

MANAGEMENT

As DSDs are often extremely distressing for the person and their family, they should be managed in a sensitive manner. Care providers should be open minded and should not pressure the person to abide by social norms. DSDs have numerous psychiatric and physical sequelae; as a result, a multidisciplinary team (MDT) should be involved in the person's care. The team should ideally involve:

- Geneticists to identify any genetic cause of the DSD.
- Neonatologist to care for the child in the early stages of life.
- Paediatric then adult endocrinologists to manage hormonal therapy where required.
- Paediatric and adolescent gynaecologist.
- Psychologists to help support and manage the individual and their family.
- Specialist nurses.
- Paediatric and adult urologists.
- Surgeons with advanced laparoscopic skills.
- Specialist surgeons for any complex genital surgery.

Care of individuals with DSDs rely on all members of the MDT working together to manage the person's psychological wellbeing and explore which treatment options are most appropriate for the individual.

 Gender Assignment

Gender assignment is a very important aspect within the management of DSDs, and if not dealt with appropriately, it can have severe psychosocial consequences, including self-harm, depression and suicide. Most people opt to stay with the gender assigned at birth; however, a number of people do not feel comfortable living their life as this gender and some do not wish to assign themselves to either male or female gender. The issues surrounding gender assignment should be explored openly with the individual to ensure that their needs are met, in order to minimise the chances of long-term psychological problems.

COMPLICATIONS

A DSD can have a significant impact on a persons mental health. Providing adequate psychological support is vital particularly at the time of transition through puberty. These people may have concerns about their appearance, may not feel able to integrate well with society and in some cases feel that they have been assigned to the wrong gender (although this is not a predominant feature). People with some forms of DSDs may not be able to conceive or carry a pregnancy, which may cause significant distress. A person centred approach is important in managing all conditions but should be very closely adhered to for people with DSDs.

People with undescended gonads (including those with Turner syndrome with a Y fragment) have a risk of developing malignancy and are often recommended a gonadectomy at an appropriate time.

PROGNOSIS

People with DSDs can live healthy and fulfilling lives. There may be significant psychological problems if the individual and their family are not treated considerately. Some people may feel that they have been assigned the wrong gender and may require an intervention to treat this. However, most will continue to define themselves as the same gender assigned at birth. Due to the nature of DSDs, infertility due to anatomical or hormonal abnormalities is common. Again, this should be dealt with in a sensitive manner, and people with DSDs should be advised of possible alternative ways to have children if that is their wish.

? QUESTIONS

Ruth is a 29-year-old who is very excited to have just given birth to her first baby, a little girl whom she has named Bethany. When Ruth changes Bethany's nappy for the first time, she notices that Bethany's genitals appear to be swollen. The paediatrician reviews the baby regarding these concerns and notes that the apparent swelling is in fact due to an enlarged clitoris.

Q1 The paediatrician suspects that Bethany has congenital adrenal hyperplasia (CAH). Which of the following tests would be most helpful to confirm the diagnosis?

A 17-OHP.
B Karyotype.
C LH:FSH ratio.
D TSH.
E Ultrasound scan of the pelvic organs.

Q2 Answer true or false: Can surgery form an appropriate part of treatment for these conditions?

A Coeliac disease.
B CAH.
C Constitutional delay of growth and puberty.
D Imperforate hymen.
E Mayer-Rokitansky-Kuster-Hauser syndrome.

Q3 Answer true or false: Do these conditions result from genetic abnormalities?

A Anorexia nervosa.
B CAH.
C Imperforate hymen.
D Polycystic ovarian syndrome.
E Turner syndrome.

[Answers on page 169.]

SECONDARY AMENORRHOEA

Amenorrhoea is the absence of menstruation. Primary amenorrhoea is defined as absence of the onset of menarche by 15 years of age.

Secondary amenorrhoea is the cessation of menstruation in a woman who has previously menstruated. It is defined clinically when a woman who has previously had regular menstrual cycles has not had a period for 3 months, or if a woman who has previously had irregular cycles has not had a period for 6 months.

Around 1% of women are affected by abnormal secondary amenorrhoea. Physiological amenorrhoea is caused by pregnancy and menopause.

PATHOPHYSIOLOGY

The menstrual cycle is tightly controlled by the HPO axis. If any of the endocrine organs involved in this axis are not functioning correctly, the menstrual cycle stops. Therefore, the endometrium of the uterus does not proliferate and menstruation does not occur.

[See 'The menstrual cycle and physiology of the HPO axis' page 8.]

The only other cause that could stop menstruation would be the presence of an anatomical obstruction of the genital tract. In this instance, the HPO axis is working correctly, but no menstrual blood is seen. It is rare for secondary amenorrhoea to be caused by obstruction.

Having a structured way of thinking about the causes helps in remembering them, and then investigating for the underlying reason in a patient.

PREGNANCY

The most common cause of secondary amenorrhoea is the physiological state of pregnancy. Placental hormones, such as hCG and progesterone, inhibit the normal HPO axis, thereby preventing the occurrence of menstruation in early pregnancy and maintaining adequate uterine conditions throughout the pregnancy.

EXOGENOUS CAUSES

- Stress, excessive exercise.
- Chronic disease, infection.
- Anorexia nervosa, sudden weight loss, dieting.
- Medication.

The top three causes stop menstruation for a physiological and evolutionary advantageous reason. Pregnancy requires additional energy and increases the physical demands on the body. When the body is already chronically stressed or low on energy, that is clearly not the best time to conceive, so stopping the menstrual cycle makes sense. This is achieved by complex hormonal interactions; for example, when a woman is stressed or fasting, her levels of cortisol, adrenaline and glucagon rise and act upon her hypothalamus to stop the regular GnRH pulse required to drive the menstrual cycle. When her food supply is returned or the stressor has resolved, normal menstruation can resume and a pregnancy can then take place in an optimum environment.

Another external cause of amenorrhoea is the use of hormonal contraception. Many hormonal contraceptives act by mechanisms involving negative feedback on the HPO axis, resulting in anovulation and cessation of periods. After stopping contraception, normal menstruation can take many months to resume. The depot injection (medroxyprogesterone acetate) is the most likely of the hormonal contraceptives to significantly delay resumption of menstruation after stopping it. Other medications that cause amenorrhoea include anabolic steroids, as these act in the same way as cortisol by promoting the use of the body's energy reserves for building muscle for a fight or flight type response. Similarly, these steroids inhibit the release of GnRH.

ENDOGENOUS HORMONAL CAUSES

The HPO axis is a delicately controlled system with interactions from many hormonal influences within the body, as demonstrated above by the effects of stress and weight loss. Many other hormonal imbalances negatively impact the HPO axis:

- Hypothyroidism – this is the most common single hormone dysfunction which inhibits the HPO axis. The most frequent cause in high income countries is autoimmune thyroiditis, whereas iodine deficiency is the most prevalent cause worldwide.
- Hyperprolactinaemia – a woman's levels of prolactin are high when breastfeeding. Prolactin inhibits GnRH release and so inhibits the HPO axis during breastfeeding. This is a physiological and evolutionarily beneficial process, as the woman with her new baby who requires feeding and full care would benefit from the delay of any future pregnancy until the baby is more independent and the woman has recovered from the stress of her recent pregnancy. The most common pathological cause of a hyperprolactinaemia is a prolactin-secreting pituitary adenoma, typically a microadenoma less than 1 cm in size.

There are other less common hormonal imbalances that can cause secondary amenorrhoea, but these are not routinely investigated unless the patient has symptoms or signs suggestive of them. These include hyperthyroidism, Cushing syndrome, late-onset CAH, androgen-secreting tumours and panhypopituitarism.

 Sheehan Syndrome

Sheehan syndrome is a rare obstetric cause of panhypopituitarism. In pregnancy, the pituitary gland is larger due to hypertrophy, making it more susceptible to ischaemia. After a large postpartum haemorrhage, hypoperfusion can occur, leading to necrosis of the anterior pituitary due to the relatively poor blood supply to the pituitary gland in pregnancy. The first symptom of this may be amenorrhoea following a pregnancy, along with signs of thyroid and adrenal dysfunction. Sheehan syndrome is also called 'empty sella syndrome', as MRI imaging shows that the sella turcica, the region of the skull which would normally house the pituitary, is empty.

OVARIAN CAUSES

Polycystic Ovarian Syndrome (PCOS)

PCOS is a multifactorial condition where the ovaries respond to hormonal stimulation and begin to make follicles as part of the normal menstrual cycle. However, in PCOS, none of these follicles become the dominant follicle, so ovulation does not occur. Without ovulation, the luteal phase of the menstrual cycle cannot occur, so the cycle essentially stops in the follicular phase. PCOS is caused by insulin resistance within the ovary, which reduces the conversion rate of androgens to oestrogen. This affects the way oestrogen negatively feeds back on the HPO axis. Many follicles begin to develop, but none are stimulated appropriately to become the dominant follicle. PCOS accounts for a third of all cases of secondary amenorrhoea.

[See 'Polycystic ovarian syndrome' page 31.]

Primary Ovarian Insufficiency

Ovarian insufficiency has occurred when all the oocytes have been used within an ovary. The rest of the HPO axis is working normally. Therefore, an investigation reveals abnormally high FSH production from the pituitary gland, which is attempting to stimulate the development of non-existent oocytes.

- Ovarian insufficiency can also be described as hypergonadotropic hypogonadism – high gonadotropin levels (FSH and LH), without ovarian activity.
- It can be diagnosed if there is oligo/amenorrhea for at least 4 months and an elevated FSH level greater than 25 IU/l on two occasions more than 4 weeks apart.
- Declining ovarian function is a natural process in menopause, which occurs at an average age of 51 years in the UK. If menopause occurs before the age of 40, it is defined as premature ovarian insufficiency.
- Most commonly, premature ovarian insufficiency is an idiopathic condition. There are associations with genetic conditions, such as Turner syndrome and fragile X; with autoimmune conditions, such as myasthenia gravis; and with infections, such as pelvic tuberculosis. It can also occur following chemotherapy or radiotherapy; therefore, in young women, egg harvesting should be considered prior to starting these treatments to allow the potential for a future pregnancy.
- Premature ovarian insufficiency is often accompanied by the symptoms associated with those experienced at the age of natural menopause.
- Additional investigations to identify the cause of premature ovarian insufficiency include a karyotype, fragile X testing as well as testing for anti-thyroid, anti-ovarian and anti-adrenal antibodies.

OUTFLOW OBSTRUCTION CAUSES

All of the above causes will, in one way or another, have prevented ovulation from occurring, thereby preventing the menstrual cycle from functioning. Outflow obstruction has no effect on the HPO axis, so ovulation and the whole menstrual cycle can occur as normal. However, due to physical obstruction in the genital tract, menstrual blood is not seen even though it is being produced.

Vaginal Obstruction

This is a rare cause of secondary amenorrhoea, as most cases of vaginal obstruction, such as imperforate hymen, vaginal agenesis or a vaginal septum, are congenital. These would not allow menstruation from the start of menarche, so would present as primary amenorrhoea. Occasionally, an obstruction may develop due to fibrosis arising from trauma such as burns or female genital mutilation or as a result of a severe skin condition such as lichen sclerosis.

Cervical Stenosis

Cervical stenosis is most commonly caused by surgery to the cervix, such as a large loop excision of the transformation zone (LLETZ).

[See 'Cervical screening' page 150.]

Uterine Obstruction (Asherman Syndrome)

This syndrome is characterised by adhesions within the uterus, which hold the walls tightly together, obliterating the cavity and preventing the passage of menstrual blood. Uterine surgeries, such as surgical management of miscarriage and dilatation and curettage, are the most common causes in high income countries. In certain low and middle income countries, infections, such as pelvic tuberculosis and schistosomiasis, are common causes of Asherman syndrome.

INVESTIGATIONS

A thorough history and examination will identify possible causes, such as medications, exercise, stress, weight loss, chronic disease, infection, and any florid endocrine disorder.

With only a few tests, together with the history and examination, the correct diagnosis can be identified (Fig. 2.10).

- Urine pregnancy test is the essential first-line investigation.
- TSH and prolactin.
  - Hypothyroidism and prolactinoma.
  - If a rarer endocrine disorder is suspected from the history and examination, this could also be investigated here.
- Progestin challenge.
  - An example regime is medroxyprogesterone acetate 10 mg once daily for 10 days.
  - This test is checking for anovulation. In the normal menstrual cycle, the follicular phase occurs and oestrogen is produced by the ovarian follicles, which causes endometrial proliferation. When ovulation occurs, the cycle enters the luteal phase. Progesterone is made by the corpus luteum and maintains the endometrium. When no pregnancy occurs, the corpus luteum stops making progesterone and menstruation occurs.
  - Giving progestin is equivalent to the corpus luteum making the progesterone. If the ovaries have been actively responding to the higher centres of the HPO axis and producing oestrogen,

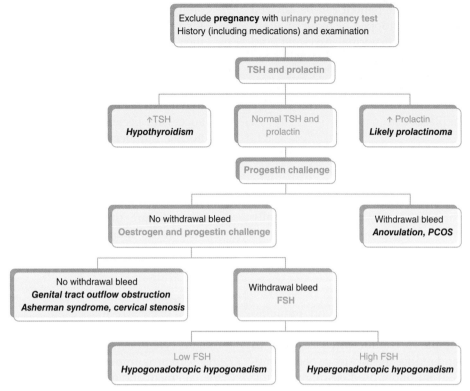

Fig. 2.10 Investigating secondary amenorrhoea. *FSH*, Follicle-stimulating hormone; *PCOS*, Polycystic ovarian syndrome; *TSH*, thyroid-stimulating hormone.

but then not ovulating, the endometrium will be proliferated. Administration of progestin induces secretory changes in the endometrium, like those occurring in the normal luteal phase of the menstrual cycle. When progestin is stopped, the endometrium is no longer supported, so it breaks down and menstruation or a withdrawal bleed occurs.

- If a withdrawal bleed occurs, then the diagnosis is anovulation, which is most likely caused by PCOS.
- If a bleed did not occur, this is either because the endometrium had not been proliferative because the HPO axis is not working at all, or because everything is working fine but there is an obstruction to the blood flow.
- Oestrogen and progestin challenge.
  - Prescribe a combined oral contraceptive for 21 days.
  - The oestrogen component of the pill will act to stimulate the endometrium and the progesterone component will then act on the endometrium as if it is in the luteal phase. The theory is that this challenge will cause menstruation in anyone with a working uterus, regardless of what the HPO axis is doing.
  - When the pill is stopped, if there is no bleed, then there must be an obstruction in the genital tract. In primary amenorrhoea, this test can also be used to demonstrate structural abnormalities such as Mullerian agenesis.

- When the pill is stopped, if there is a withdrawal bleed, this shows that the endometrium and genital tract are working normally, so the diagnosis is failure of the HPO axis.
- FSH.
  - This is released by the anterior pituitary to stimulate the ovaries to commence the follicular phase of the menstrual cycle.
  - If FSH is low, then the failure of the HPO axis is either in the hypothalamus or the pituitary, but the ovaries are likely normal. This is called hypogonadotropic hypogonadism. The exogenous causes, such as stress, anorexia or chronic disease, are examples of hypogonadotropic hypogonadism.
  - If FSH is high, then the hypothalamus and pituitary are working normally, trying to stimulate ovaries which are not responding. This is ovarian insufficiency (hypergonadotropic hypogonadism).

MANAGEMENT

The management of secondary amenorrhoea depends entirely on the diagnosis.

EXOGENOUS CAUSES

- Treat the chronic disease, infection or eating disorder with appropriate medical or psychological treatment.
- Stop any offending medications, such as anabolic steroids or contraceptives.

- If exercise is the cause, the patient can be advised that when the exercise is stopped or reduced, menstrual cycles should return to normal. Advice should be given if they wish to conceive, as they will need to reduce their exercise.

HYPOTHYROIDISM

- Levothyroxine replacement.

HYPERPROLACTINAEMIA

- MRI head to look for prolactinoma.
  - Microprolactinomas are often treated with dopamine agonists, such as cabergoline.
  - Macroprolactinomas are usually surgically resected.
  - Very rarely, a negative MRI may indicate a prolactin-secreting tumour elsewhere in the body.

POLYCYSTIC OVARIAN SYNDROME

- Management is focussed primarily on reducing risks associated with the condition and symptom control. For example, a contraceptive is given to regulate cycles and reduce the incidence of endometrial hyperplasia from unopposed oestrogen acting on the endometrium.

  [See 'Polycystic ovarian syndrome' page 31.]

- If fertility is sought, then medications such as clomiphene may be offered to induce ovulation.

  [See 'Infertility' page 35.]

HYPERGONADOTROPIC HYPOGONADISM OR PREMATURE OVARIAN INSUFFICIENCY

- There is no treatment to reverse complete ovarian insufficiency. Hormone replacement therapy can be offered to treat menopausal symptoms. HRT is advised until the usual natural age of menopause (51 in the UK) to protect women's bones, cardiac and cognitive health and reduce the symptoms of menopause.
- Very occasionally, if there is a small amount of ovarian reserve, medications can be given in an attempt to stimulate follicle development for egg collection for fertility treatments. An AMH (anti-mullerian hormone) level can be taken and used to assess the likelihood of response to ovarian stimulation. Most often at the time of presentation, this is no longer possible.

HYPOGONADOTROPIC HYPOGONADISM

- This represents failure of the HPO axis above the ovary (hypothalamus or pituitary).
- Technically, all the exogenous causes, prolactinoma, hypothyroidism and medications mentioned above fit into this category, as their effects are all on the higher regions of the HPO axis.
- If a low FSH has been identified and no other cause has been elicited from the history, examination or investigation, a referral for an expert endocrinological opinion may be required to assess for rare conditions causing hypothalamic or pituitary failure.
- If fertility is sought, then medications can be given to stimulate the ovaries for the purposes of egg collection, which could then be used for IVF. Compared to ovarian insufficiency, this is far more likely to be successful because the ovaries are likely to have a normal number of oocytes.

GENITAL OUTFLOW OBSTRUCTION

Surgery is usually required to identify and treat an obstruction. Usually, this can be undertaken as a day case procedure under general anaesthetic. Cervical dilatation can open the cervix, and a hysteroscope can be used to view inside the uterus and break down any adhesions due to Asherman syndrome.

PROGNOSIS

Secondary amenorrhoea has many causes. Once the diagnosis has been made, a systematic investigation of the patient is important to determine the cause. The management and outcome of secondary amenorrhoea, as well as the prognosis, are very much dependent on the cause of the amenorrhoea. Some women will not regain normal menstruation and can have trouble with fertility. For others, the treatment is simple and normal menstruation can reoccur.

❓ QUESTIONS

Marlena, a 24-year-old, attends a gynaecology clinic after being referred by her primary care physician for amenorrhoea. Marlena began menstruation at the age of 15 and has had regular periods since. They had cycles lasting 29 days, with menstruation that lasted for 6 days each cycle. Over the last 8 months, they have experienced complete cessation of their periods and are worried about what this may mean. They are usually fit and healthy. They have never used an oral or long-acting contraceptive. They have recently changed jobs and moved house.

Q1 For how many months would Marlena have to experience cessation of their regular menstruation for secondary amenorrhoea to be diagnosed?

  A 2 months.
  B 3 months.
  C 4 months.
  D 6 months.
  E 12 months.

Q2 Answer true or false: Do causes of secondary amenorrhea include?

  A Anorexia nervosa.
  B Asherman syndrome.
  C Edward syndrome.
  D Polycystic ovarian syndrome.
  E Type 2 diabetes mellitus.

Q3   Answer true or false: Which factors are associated with a disturbance of ovulation?
   A Asherman syndrome.
   B Family history of diabetes mellitus.
   C Hypertension.
   D Prolactin secreting pituitary adenoma.
   E Turner syndrome.

A Asherman syndrome.	**G** Prolactin secreting
B History of rubella infection.	pituitary adenoma.
C Hypergonadotropic	**H** Serum β hCG.
hypogonadism.	**I** Serum FSH and LH.
D Hypertension.	**J** Serum thyroxine, TSH
E Oligomenorrhoea.	and prolactin.
F Polycystic ovarian	**K** Sheehan syndrome.
syndrome.	**L** Turner syndrome.

Q4   A 35-year-old presents with secondary amenorrhoea. Which would be your initial investigation?

Q5   A 29-year-old attends the clinic with secondary amenorrhea. They have recently been experiencing headaches and, after visiting their optician, have been diagnosed with bitemporal hemianopia. On questioning, it is revealed that they have also been experiencing some nipple discharge. What is the most likely cause of the symptoms?

Q6   A 32-year-old woman attends the clinic with secondary amenorrhoea. Four years ago, she had her first pregnancy, which was uneventful. She and her partner are trying for a second child but they have experienced some difficulty. She has not menstruated for 8 months and she has a complex past medical history. She had an incomplete termination when she was 16 years old, which required dilation and curettage. She also underwent a difficult hysteroscopy 3 years ago, which diagnosed uterine fibroids, and surgical management of a miscarriage 1 year ago. She is not breastfeeding her child. What is the most likely diagnosis?

Q7   An 18-year-old attends the clinic with secondary amenorrhea. They have always had irregular menstruation but noticed that it has ceased over the last year. They report weight gain despite exercising and reportedly eating a healthy diet. They have been diagnosed with type 2 diabetes and there is a family history of obesity, diabetes and hypertension. What is the most likely diagnosis?

[Answers on page 170.]

POLYCYSTIC OVARIAN SYNDROME

PCOS is a heterogeneous disorder of hyperandrogenic chronic anovulation. It commonly presents with hirsutism, menstrual irregularities and infertility. PCOS affects approximately 7% of premenopausal women in the UK.

AETIOLOGY

The aetiology is unknown. It can present at any age, although it is commonly diagnosed in women in their twenties who present with irregular menstruation and/or abnormal hair growth. No associated genetic or environmental factors have been identified. However, obesity-induced systemic insulin resistance is strongly associated with PCOS. In the long term, patients with PCOS have an increased risk of developing type 2 diabetes mellitus (DM).

PATHOPHYSIOLOGY

A good understanding of the menstrual cycle and HPO axis is required to understand the pathological process in PCOS.

[See 'The menstrual cycle and physiology of the HPO axis' page 8.]

In females, androgens are made by the adrenal glands and by the theca cells of follicles in the ovaries. The granulosa cells of ovarian follicles convert androgens into oestrogens. Insulin is required for this process. Oestrogen is produced by the developing ovarian follicles during the follicular phase of the menstrual cycle. The oestrogens produced have a negative feedback on the hypothalamus and pituitary. The result is a reduction in the concentration of FSH released by the pituitary, which allows only the dominant follicle to continue to develop and go on to ovulate. Ovulation occurs following the LH surge, which is itself caused by positive feedback from high levels of oestrogen.

In PCOS, insulin resistance is seen within all tissues of the body, including the ovaries. The ovaries are less able to convert androgens to oestrogens, resulting in raised serum androgen levels (testosterone is usually measured). It is the high androgen levels which cause the symptoms of hirsutism, acne, and sometimes male pattern hair loss.

Some of the excess androgens are converted in peripheral tissues to oestrogen. This commonly occurs in adipose tissue, which makes oestrone, which may explain why obesity is associated with the condition. This peripheral tissue production is not regulated by the HPO axis, but the oestrogen produced does feed back onto the HPO axis, causing dysregulation. The HPO axis is further dysregulated because the ovarian follicles are not producing the correct oestrogen levels to adequately feed back onto the HPO axis. Consequently, rather than one dominant follicle forming and the others regressing, in PCOS, no dominant follicle forms. Many small immature follicles remain, resulting in the polycystic ovaries seen on ultrasound.

A positive feedback response to the oestrogen levels causes a high LH level; the high LH to FSH ratio is a biochemical marker of PCOS. In a normal menstrual cycle, a high LH level would cause ovulation from the dominant follicle. In PCOS, there is no dominant follicle, so ovulation does not occur. Without ovulation, no corpus luteum can form, so rather than the cycle continuing to the luteal phase and then menstruation, the cycle is essentially stuck in the follicular phase. This clearly explains the symptoms of irregular menstrual cycles and infertility.

Long term, the chronically raised oestrogen levels cause prolonged stimulation of the endometrium, which can increase the risk of endometrial hyperplasia. This is a precancerous change that can progress to endometrial cancer. In a normal menstrual cycle, progesterone in the luteal phase protects the endometrium.

DIAGNOSIS

The diagnosis of PCOS is made after secondary causes have been excluded. PCOS can be diagnosed if a patient has both:
- Irregular menstrual cycles.
- Clinical (hirsutism, acne or male pattern alopecia) and/or biochemical hyperandrogenism (raised free androgen index or testosterone).

If they only meet one of the above criteria, then a pelvic ultrasound can be requested. The diagnosis of PCOS can be made if the scan shows 12 or more follicles in one ovary, measuring 2 to 9 mm, or an ovarian volume of greater than 10 mL.

IRREGULAR CYCLES

- 12 to 36 months post-menarche: less than 21 days or greater than 45 days
- Greater than 36 months post-menarche to perimenopause: less than 21 days, greater than 35 days or less than 8 cycles per year
- If greater than 12 months post-menarche, any cycle greater than 90 days.
- Primary amenorrhoea at age 15, or more than 36 months post-thelarche

Polycystic ovaries are often found incidentally on ultrasound scans performed for other reasons, often to assess for causes of pelvic pain. Unlike other ovarian cysts, polycystic ovaries do not cause pain, so this finding does not explain a patient's symptoms. It is also important to reassure these women that unless one of the other criteria have been met, they do not have PCOS. Normal adolescent ovaries have a high incidence of having a multi-follicular appearance and so ultrasound should not be used to aid diagnosis in the first 8 years post-menarche.

CLINICAL FEATURES

- Hirsutism – this is present in the majority of women with PCOS. It describes male pattern of hair in women, such as facial, chest and back hair (Fig. 2.11). Acne and male pattern baldness are also signs of androgen excess.
- Menstrual irregularities – irregular cycles are present in over three-quarters of women with PCOS.
- Infertility – this can occur in women with PCOS due to chronic anovulation. If a woman is not releasing an egg, pregnancy will not occur.
- Acanthosis nigricans – this is a dermatological manifestation of insulin resistance and hyperinsulinaemia. It is commonly found in women with PCOS. It is an irregular, velvety, hyperpigmentation of the skin, classically located in the axillae and in skin folds.

INVESTIGATIONS

IMAGING

Pelvic ultrasound demonstrating polycystic ovaries. This is diagnosed when there are 12 or more peripheral

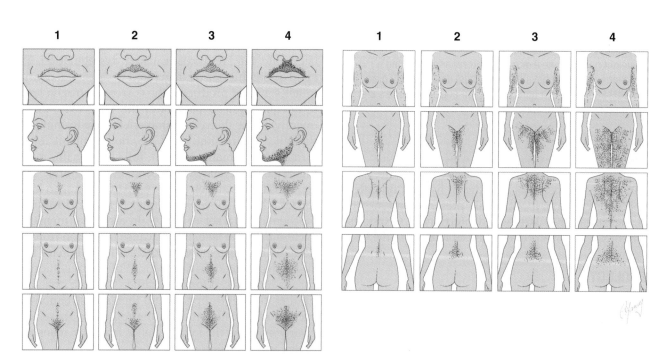

Fig. 2.11 The Ferriman-Gallwey assessment tool for assessing abnormal hair growth. A score more than or equal to seven is diagnostic for hirsutism, with a maximum score of 36.

Table 2.3 Differential Diagnoses for Polycystic Ovarian Syndrome

DIFFERENTIAL	EXCLUSION BLOOD TEST	PRESENTING SYMPTOMS SIMILAR TO PCOS	OTHER CLASSIC CLINICAL FEATURES
Hypothyroidism	TSH	Menstrual irregularities	Tiredness Weight gain Constipation Goitre
Prolactinoma	Prolactin	Menstrual irregularities	Galactorrhoea Visual disturbance
Cushing syndrome	Cortisol	Menstrual irregularities	Irregular fat distribution Bruising Hypertension Striae
Congenital adrenal hyperplasia	17-OHP DHEA	Menstrual irregularities Hirsutism	Family history Virilisation Symptoms start at menarche
Androgen secreting tumour	Testosterone (very high levels) Other tests: • DHEA • Androstenedione	Menstrual irregularities Hirsutism	Male pattern alopecia Clitoromegaly Deepened voice
Hypothalamic dysfunction: for example, anorexia, illness, stress	FSH (low levels)	Menstrual irregularities Anorexic patients may have lanugo hair (fine hair all over the body), grown to retain heat as they have a lack of fat stores due to malnutrition - this hair is not hirsutism	Often underlying stressors: Sudden weight change Excessive exercise Eating disorder Chronic illness
Idiopathic hirsutism	None	Hirsutism	Diagnosis of exclusion Obesity Associated with family history

follicles or increased ovarian volume (more than 10 mL). Another feature of PCOS must be present to make a diagnosis.

BLOOD TESTS

The most reliable biochemical marker for diagnosing PCOS is the free androgen index (FAI). An FAI value of five or greater supports the diagnosis of PCOS. FAI is calculated by:

$$FAI = (total\ testosterone/SHBG) \times 100.$$

The basis for the FAI is that testosterone and other androgens are raised because they are not converted to oestrogens in the ovaries due to insulin resistance. SHBG levels are decreased in PCOS because more of it is bound to the increased level of androgens in the serum.

DIFFERENTIAL DIAGNOSIS

As well as making the diagnosis with blood tests above, these differential diagnoses (Table 2.3) must be excluded to prevent missing important underlying pathology. TSH and prolactin should be requested routinely, and the others based on clinical suspicion.

Good history-taking is essential to identify the need to test for these rare causes. Some medications can also cause similar symptoms to PCOS; anabolic steroid use is a common cause of both menstrual irregularities and hirsutism.

MANAGEMENT

LIFESTYLE MODIFICATION

The initial management strategy should include lifestyle advice. Patients with PCOS should be advised on maintaining a healthy diet and weight and should be encouraged to achieve weight loss if this is required. Losing weight in patients with a raised body mass index (BMI) will improve insulin resistance and assist in losing excess fat, which creates peripheral oestrogen. Patients can be signposted to dietitians and specialist weight loss clinics to aid with this. They may also wish to discuss and consider medications or interventions such as bariatric surgery. Weight loss is the most effective treatment for PCOS in an obese patient, and can resolve all symptoms. All other treatments described below are only treating specific symptoms, not the cause of the disease.

Women should also be screened for other cardiovascular risk factors which can be modified, such as smoking, hypertension, cholesterol, exercise levels and diabetes. All women diagnosed with PCOS with a BMI more than or equal to 25 kg/m², or less than 25 kg/m² with risk factors for diabetes, should have a glucose tolerance test.

PSYCHOLOGICAL SUPPORT

Many patients struggle with the physical effects of PCOS. For young adolescents, hair in the wrong place, even if it seems a small amount, can have a profound effect on their mental health. Psychological support is key to the management of these patients, addressing their concerns and helping them to manage normal living.

MENSTRUATION

In PCOS, patients can have fewer complete menstrual cycles due to anovulation in some cycles, which prevents the luteal phase and then menstruation. Evidence suggests that if patients are having fewer than three menstrual bleeds a year, then they are at increased risk of endometrial hyperplasia and ultimately cancer due to prolonged periods of excess oestrogen exposure. In these patients, it is important to treat with hormonal contraception to reduce the risks. If there are no contraindications, the combined oral contraceptive can be used to generate regular cycles. However, any progesterone-containing contraceptive will confer protection to the endometrium, with the Mirena coil being the most protective. If the patient declines regular contraception, she could use a short course of a progestogen pill (such as medroxyprogesterone acetate 10 mg daily for 10 days) every 3 months, which will induce a bleed each time the medication stops.

FERTILITY

Patients with PCOS may be referred for infertility investigation more readily than others, as they have a known risk factor for fertility problems. The most common cause of infertility in PCOS is anovulation.

The first-line treatments for anovulation are the medications metformin and clomifene. Metformin is a biguanide anti-diabetic drug which is taken every day with the aim to improve insulin sensitivity in the ovaries. Clomifene is taken on days 2 to 6 of the menstrual cycle. It is a selective oestrogen receptor modulator which acts to increase FSH levels, thereby increasing follicular development and the likelihood of ovulation.

Another treatment to improve ovulation in PCOS is ovarian electrocautery (commonly referred to as ovarian drilling). This is a laparoscopic procedure where small holes are made in the ovary. It is not clear how this works, but it increases the likelihood of ovulation for about 6 months after the procedure. It seems particularly effective in PCOS patients with a normal BMI.

If other treatments fail, patients with PCOS can then be referred for IVF.

[See 'Infertility' page 35.]

HIRSUTISM

- Anti-androgens reduce the stimulus for hair growth and also improve acne:
  - Spironolactone – a synthetic anti-mineralocorticoid with weak anti-androgen properties that aims to reduce hair production.
  - Flutamide – a non-steroidal anti-androgen.
  - Finasteride – a 5α-reductase inhibitor that has some anti-androgen properties.
  - Some combined oral contraceptives contain progestogens with anti-androgen effects, such as Dianette (contains cyproterone) and Yasmin (contains drospirenone) and Lucette.
  - Oxytetracycline is an antibiotic sometimes used to treat acne.
- Treatments directly treating the hair:
  - Eflornithine cream – this slows the rate of facial hair growth by interacting with cell division and proliferation in the hair follicle when applied twice a day.
  - Laser hair removal – this method can be beneficial but has short-term side effects including erythema, oedema and pruritus, and long-term use can cause skin pigmentation changes.

METFORMIN

Metformin is a biguanide anti-diabetic drug, which acts to decrease serum glucose levels, primarily by suppressing glucose production by the liver (gluconeogenesis). It also increases insulin sensitivity in other organs, which, in diabetes, results in increased glucose uptake. As PCOS is associated with insulin resistance in the ovary, it was thought that metformin may increase insulin sensitivity and improve PCOS symptoms.

The evidence for metformin use in PCOS outside of fertility treatment is conflicting, so its use is currently not supported by UK guidance. However, some clinicians advocate its use when lifestyle modifications have not improved the symptoms of acne or hirsutism. Research is also ongoing into the long-term use of metformin in PCOS to reduce the chance of developing DM.

LONG TERM COMPLICATIONS

- Obesity.
- Type 2 DM – this is a possible consequence, especially if the patient is obese or has a strong family history of type 2 DM. These women are also at risk of gestational diabetes mellitus (GDM).
- Infertility – this is secondary to anovulation.
- Increased rate of early miscarriage.
- Endometrial hyperplasia or carcinoma – this is a possible consequence of unopposed oestrogen due to reduced menstruation frequency.
- Cardiovascular disease.

PROGNOSIS

PCOS is a lifelong condition. Women diagnosed with PCOS should be counselled regarding treatment and the possible risks associated with their condition. Education regarding healthy living is vital, ensuring they understand the links between obesity, diabetes and hypertension. An improvement in their general health will reduce their risk of long-term complications.

❓ QUESTIONS

Sophie, an 18-year-old, attends the clinic with secondary amenorrhea. Sophie has always had irregular menstruation but noticed that this has ceased over the last year. Additionally, they have experienced weight gain despite exercising and reportedly eating a healthy diet. They have been recently diagnosed with type 2 DM and there is a family history of obesity, DM and hypertension.

Q1   Answer true or false: Can these conditions be a long-term consequence of PCOS?

  A Dyslipidaemia.
  B Endometrial hyperplasia.
  C Hyperthyroidism.
  D Myasthenia gravis.
  E Type 2 DM.

Q2   Answer true or false regarding these statements relating to polycystic ovarian syndrome.

  A PCOS can be diagnosed even in the presence of no ovarian cysts.
  B Complications include infertility and gestational diabetes mellitus (GDM).
  C Anti-androgens are a safe treatment for a woman with PCOS-associated hirsutism who is also trying to conceive.
  D Weight loss has only a small effect on the course of PCOS.
  E In patients with oligomenorrhoea or amenorrhoea, it is recommended that withdrawal bleeds be induced every 3 to 4 months due to the risk of ovarian cancer.

A	Amiodarone.	**F**	Hydrocortisone.
B	Clomifene citrate.	**G**	Insulin.
C	Combined oral contraceptive.	**H**	Metformin.
D	Copper intrauterine device.	**I**	Paracetamol.
		J	Pioglitazone.
E	Eflornithine.	**K**	Ramipril.
		L	Spironolactone.

Q3   Which drug can cause hyperkalaemia, ataxia and renal impairment?

Q4   Which drug offers endometrial protection?

Q5   Which drug can cause hot flushes, mood disturbance and ovarian enlargement?

Q6   Which drugs can be used topically to treat hirsutism?

[Answers on page 172.]

INFERTILITY

Infertility is defined as a failure to conceive after unprotected intercourse two or three times a week for twelve months. Generally, 80% of healthy couples should conceive naturally within 1 year, and this percentage rises to 90% after 2 years. Subfertility is increasingly common, affecting one in seven heterosexual couples in the UK, and it can have a severe psychological impact.

AETIOLOGY

In the simplest terms, a pregnancy can only occur when a female produces an egg (oocyte), a man produces sperm, and the two are able to meet. Infertility investigations are looking for errors in production of either gamete or anatomical blockages to their transport.

The main causes of infertility in the UK are:
- Female aetiologies (40%).
  - Ovulatory disorders.
  - Tubal damage.
  - Uterine or peritoneal disorders.
- Male aetiologies (30%).
  - Sperm production disorders.
  - Obstruction of release.
  - Erectile and ejaculatory dysfunction.
- Combined male and female aetiologies (15%).
- Unexplained infertility (15%).

RISK FACTORS

- Increasing maternal age.
  - This is the most significant risk factor and is becoming more prevalent as women delay conceiving until later in life for a variety of lifestyle reasons.
  - Fertility declines significantly beyond 35 years of age, due to declining numbers and quality of oocytes.
  - In the maternal age groups under age 35, the incidence of subfertility is less than 10%. In the 35- to 39-year age group, subfertility affects 20% and this incidence exponentially increases beyond the age of 40.
  - Increasing male age also affects fertility but to a lesser extent.
- Raised BMI more than or equal to $30 \, kg/m^2$.
  - High BMI increases the likelihood of irregular cycles and anovulation. Anovulation due to PCOS is the underlying cause of infertility in 75% of women.
  - Obese men have reduced fertility due to significantly reduced sperm motility and are also at risk of erectile dysfunction from the associated risk factor DM.
- Low BMI less than $19 \, kg/m^2$ – resulting in irregular menstruation or oligomenorrhoea.
- Active and passive smoking – reduced fertility due to accelerated menopause and poor-quality semen.

- Excessive alcohol intake – risks of fetal harm and detrimental to semen quality.
- Occupation – exposure to chemicals, pesticides or radiation can damage spermatogenesis.
- Medication – for example, chemotherapy, can damage male and female gametes.
- Recreational drugs – cocaine and anabolic steroids can affect sperm production.
- Psychological factors – stress can reduce libido and thus frequency of intercourse. Extreme stress can also inhibit ovulation.

FEMALE INFERTILITY

PATHOPHYSIOLOGY

It can be useful to divide the causes of infertility anatomically.

HYPOTHALAMUS, PITUITARY AND OVARIES

These structures are important for the formation and release of a fertile egg and for preparation of the endometrium for implantation. The WHO refers to infertility problems associated with the HPO axis as ovulatory disorders and splits them into three groups.

[See 'The menstrual cycle and physiology of the HPO axis' page 8.]

Hypothalamic-Pituitary Insufficiency (Group One Ovulatory Disorders)

- Low gonadotropins (FSH, LH) and oestrogen deficiency, also called hypogonadotropic hypogonadism.
- Examples include:
  - Hypothalamic dysfunction caused by anorexia or excessive exercise.
  - Genetic causes such as Kallmann syndrome.
  - Acquired causes such as a pituitary macroadenoma or Sheehan syndrome (panhypopituitarism following PPH).

[See 'Puberty' page 13.]

Hypothalamic Pituitary Ovarian Axis Dysfunction (Group Two Ovulatory Disorders)

- Associated with mild changes in FSH/LH; other investigations confirm the diagnosis.
- PCOS – this is the predominant cause of anovulatory infertility in the UK. Associated with a raised free androgen index and polycystic ovaries on ultrasound scan.

[See 'Polycystic ovarian syndrome' page 31.]

- Other endocrine disorders:
  - Prolactinoma – usually pituitary microprolactinoma. Prolactin suppresses the HPO axis, as it does physiologically during breastfeeding.
  - Hypothyroidism.
  - Cushing disease.
  - Uncontrolled diabetes.

Ovaries (Group Three Ovulatory Disorders)

- High gonadotropins (FSH, LH).
- Ovarian insufficiency – premature ovarian insufficiency, gonadal dysgenesis (Turner syndrome), surgery, chemotherapy and autoimmune causes.

[See 'Secondary amenorrhoea' page 26.]

FALLOPIAN TUBES

Tubal patency is key to successful fertilisation of an ovulated oocyte by approaching sperm, and then for transport of the developing embryo into the uterus for implantation. This transport is achieved by peristaltic movement of the tubes, and by the cilia lining the tubal lumen. The tubes can be damaged by:

- Infection – chlamydia and gonorrhoea are the most common sexually transmitted infections (STIs) to cause pelvic inflammatory disease (PID). The inflammatory process can cause tubal occlusion.
- Inflammation – appendicitis, diverticulitis and Crohn's disease. Due to the proximity to the tubes, inflammation from these conditions can cause tube fibrosis.
- Endometriosis – intra-abdominal inflammation and scarring resulting in anatomical obstruction of the fallopian tubes. Chronic inflammation caused by any of the above causes can also contribute to infertility as cytokines are produced, which are toxic to sperm and embryos.
- Pelvic surgery – previous sterilisation or other pelvic surgery may damage and scar fallopian tubes.

UTERUS

The uterus provides the foundation for implantation, and the sperm must pass through it to reach the oocyte.

- Infection or previous surgery can cause extensive scarring; for example, Asherman syndrome.
- Large fibroids may have a role in infertility.
- Congenital abnormalities – septate uterus, Mullerian agenesis.

[See 'Differences of sexual development' page 20.]

CERVIX

Cervical mucus facilitates sperm entry into the uterus and initiates sperm capacitation (the final step in sperm maturation). During the peri-ovulatory period, the mucus becomes abundant, thin and stretchable.

- Previous cervical surgery – causing scarring, shortening and, rarely, cervical stenosis.
- Cervical infection – can disrupt the cervical glands and/or mucus production.

CLINICAL ASSESSMENT

History

- Menstrual history – regular or irregular.
  - Regular cycles are usually representative of ovulation each cycle.
  - Irregular cycles are usually associated with anovulatory cycles, the most common cause being PCOS.

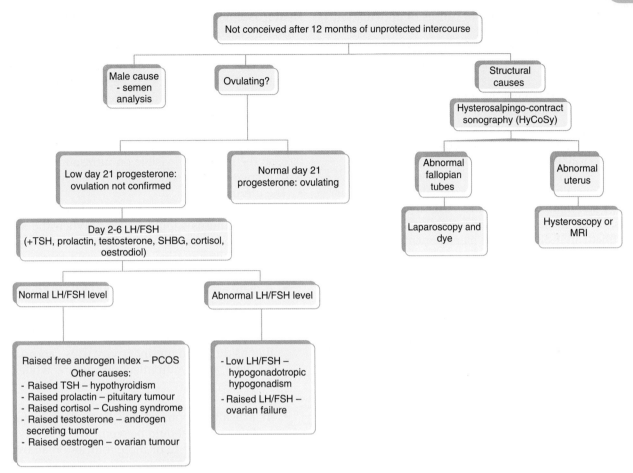

Fig. 2.12 Initial investigations of female subfertility. *FSH,* Follicle-stimulating hormone; *HyCoSy,* hysterosalpingo-contrast sonography; *LH,* luteinising hormone; *PCOS,* polycystic ovarian syndrome; *SHBG,* sex hormone binding globulin; *TSH,* thyroid-stimulating hormone.

- Sexual history – frequency of intercourse and problems with intercourse, including physical problems such as dyspareunia, and psychological issues.
- Current symptoms or history of STIs.
- Previous pregnancies and conception.
- Previous pelvic surgery.
- History of endometriosis.
- Medical co-morbidities, medications, systemic enquiry.
- Social history – smoking, alcohol, drug use.

Examination

Depending on the history, this includes a general examination; for example, BMI, signs of endocrinopathies, acne (PCOS), bitemporal hemianopia (prolactinoma) and a vaginal examination that includes the use of a speculum.

INVESTIGATIONS

Investigations for infertility should be started and referral to a specialist for assessment if a couple has not conceived after 1 year of trying. Earlier referral should be considered if:

- The woman is 36 years old or older.
- Known causes or predisposing factors for infertility exist, for example, PCOS.

- Investigations show a likely poor pregnancy outcome with expectant management, with assisted reproductive techniques such as IVF being the only likely effective treatment.
- If a woman has undergone, or is due to receive, treatment which affects fertility, for example, chemotherapy or radiotherapy.

In simple terms, the whole purpose of investigations is to identify why an egg and sperm are not meeting*:

1 Are the couple having regular intercourse?
   - Assessed in the history – if the answer is no, there is no need to investigate further.
2 Are the gametes being made and released?
   - Male – semen analysis (male factors discussed later).
   - Female (Fig. 2.12) – on day 21 of the menstrual cycle, measure serum progesterone.
     - Normal – ovulating, no further blood test needed (level more than 30 nmol/L).
     - Low – not ovulating: on day 2 of the menstrual cycle, measure FSH, LH, oestradiol, testosterone, SHBG, TSH and prolactin. With these

---

*If a woman is single or in a same-sex relationship and accessing fertility support some investigations will be advised to optimise any assisted reproductive management options that are offered.

results, the majority of causes of anovulation will be identified.

3 Is there an obstruction of the female genital tract?
- Examination of vagina and visualisation of the cervix.
- Ultrasound scan of the uterus, which also visualises the ovaries.
- Hysterosalpingo-contract sonography (HyCoSy), or Hysterosalpingogram (HSG) – demonstrates cervical, uterine and tubal patency.

The investigation process for female subfertility is further summarised in Fig. 2.12. After these investigations, if the cause of a couple's subfertility has been identified, an individualised management plan can be constructed for them.

Day 21 Progesterone

In the normal menstrual cycle, after ovulation, the dominant follicle which has released the oocyte forms the corpus luteum, which produces high levels of progesterone to support the endometrium during implantation. If pregnancy does not occur, the corpus luteum regresses, progesterone levels fall and menstruation occurs. In a normal 28-day menstrual cycle, progesterone is highest on day 21 (mid-luteal phase).

If ovulation occurs in a menstrual cycle, then the luteal phase begins and progesterone levels will be highest mid-luteal phase. If ovulation does not occur, the luteal phase will not begin and progesterone levels will remain low. This is the principle behind the day 21 progesterone test.

Day 21 Progesterone

If someone is having regular menstrual cycles, but the cycle length differs from 28 days, then the progesterone test should be taken 7 days before the end of the cycle is due, for example, day 27 in a 34-day cycle. This is because the luteal phase is fixed at 14 days in length at the end of each cycle, whereas the follicular phase can vary. It is important to make this adjustment to ensure that blood is taken at the mid-luteal point; otherwise, the progesterone level may be falsely low, making an ovulating woman appear anovulatory.

If someone is not ovulating, this does not mean they do not menstruate, as the endometrium can only proliferate in response to oestrogen for so long before it starts to break down. The bleed is more likely to be at random times, creating an irregular menstrual cycle. Irregular cycles can make judging the mid-luteal point difficult for measuring progesterone. The recommended solution is to measure progesterone when ovulation is suspected and then weekly until menstruation occurs. The highest value obtained should be used, which should be 7 days before the start of menstruation.

The downside of the progesterone test is that it tells the clinician if ovulation has occurred in the tested cycle, but not every other cycle. In a woman with a regular cycle and a positive progesterone test, it is highly likely that they ovulate each cycle, but a positive test in a woman with an irregular cycle does not necessarily mean they are ovulating each cycle; they may have sporadic ovulation and may still need ovulatory assistance to treat subfertility.

Hysterosalpingo-Contrast Sonography

This is an examination of the uterus, ovaries, fallopian tubes, and pelvis using transvaginal ultrasound. This is a day case investigation where the woman is awake. Initially, an ultrasound scan is performed to assess the pelvis. A small catheter is then inserted through the cervix. The ultrasound scan is then recommenced while saline is infused into the uterus and fallopian tubes. The saline is mixed with air bubbles or galactose microbubbles, so the infusion is visible on ultrasound. The hysterosalpingo-contrast sonography (HyCoSy) identifies:

- The uterus
  - In a healthy woman, a normal size, shape and mobile uterus should be seen. When the saline is infused clear views of a normally shaped and easily filling uterine cavity should be seen and normal appearance of the endometrium.
  - If there are concerns following HyCoSy, depending on the issue an MRI or a hysteroscopy can be performed. A hysteroscopy involves a small camera being passed through the cervix to view the inside of the uterine cavity. This can usually be done as an outpatient procedure while the woman is awake.
- Ovaries
  - In a healthy woman, two normal sized freely mobile ovaries should be seen.
  - The presence of 12 or more follicles on an ovary, or a volume of more than 10 mL, is diagnostic of polycystic ovaries. Along with other criteria, this finding can diagnose PCOS, which is the most common cause of female infertility.
  - Few or no follicles on small ovaries may suggest ovarian insufficiency.
- Fallopian tubes
  - In a healthy woman, the saline infusion should be seen evenly dilating the fallopian tubes, with the infusion seen spilling out the end of the tubes into the abdominal cavity, which demonstrates the tubes are patent.
  - If one or both tubes appear to be blocked, the woman can then be referred for a day-case laparoscopy and dye test.

In some units, alternative tests to HyCoSy are a standard ultrasound scan and a separate hysterosalpingogram (HSG). A HSG is also performed awake, with a catheter inserted into the cervix, but a radio-opaque dye is then injected into the uterus. A radiograph is taken a few seconds later. In a healthy woman, the dye will be seen outlining the normal shape of the cavity of the uterus, the dye will have passed along both tubes, and it should be seen beginning to spill out of both tubes into the abdominal cavity. The benefit of the HyCoSY is that it is done as one investigation rather than two, and does not use radiation.

Laparoscopy

If one or both tubes appear to be blocked on HyCoSy or HSG, the woman can then be referred for a day-case laparoscopy and dye test. This is a diagnostic laparoscopy performed under general anaesthesia. The fallopian tubes and the rest of the pelvis can be visualised for any abnormality. A catheter is inserted through the cervix and a blue dye is injected. In a woman with normal anatomy, the surgeon can then see blue dye leaking out of both tubes. If a tube appears obstructed, surgery on the tube may be considered.

The drawback of all these tubal investigations is that they check tubal patency but not function. We know there is more to transporting the gametes along the tubes than just tube patency. For example, the cilia within the tubes are an important part of the process, and they can be damaged by many factors, including inflammation and smoking but these are not tested by a HyCoSy, hysterosalpingogram or at laparoscopy.

A laparoscopy may also be considered as part of a fertility investigation if a woman is suspected to have significant adhesions of pelvic organs following HyCoSy or ultrasound scanning, or if significant endometriosis is suspected.

MANAGEMENT
Conservative Management
- Sexual intercourse.
  - Frequency of sexual intercourse should be two to three times a week for 1 year.
  - Counselling for physical or psychological difficulties during sexual intercourse.
- Weight management
  - Aim for a BMI less than 30 kg/m^2 (ideally less than 25 kg/m^2). Healthy diet and exercise (but not excessive) improve ovulation by reducing hyperinsulinaemia and thus hyperandrogenism.
  - Weight gain for those with BMI less than 19 kg/m^2 to increase ovulation.
- Social
  - Stop smoking.
  - Minimise alcohol intake – avoid more than two units a week or intoxication.
  - Advise about the risks in certain occupations, for example, radiation or toxin exposure.
- Drugs
  - Avoid teratogenic medications, switching to alternatives where medication cannot be discontinued, for example, changing warfarin to a low molecular weight heparin.
  - Avoid recreational drug use.
  - Take folic acid – 400 mcg/day pre-conception and up to 12 weeks gestation to avoid neural tube defects; 5 mg/day should be advised for diabetics or those taking antiepileptics.
  - Take vitamin D – 10 mcg/day pre-conception and then throughout pregnancy.

- Screening
  - All woman investigated for subfertility should be offered:
    - Urinary or endocervical swab for chlamydia.
    - Rubella antibodies; if the woman has not been vaccinated they should be offered vaccination.
    - For woman undergoing IVF, serum screening for human immunodeficiency virus (HIV), hepatitis B and hepatitis C infections.

Treatments for the Specific Causes of Subfertility
If a specific cause for subfertility has been identified during investigations, treatment should be commenced. If the cause cannot be treated successfully or no cause is found (unexplained infertility), then assisted reproductive techniques (ART) are offered. If ARTs are not effective or cannot be offered, then alternative choices, such as surrogacy or adoption, are other options.

Inducing Ovulation in Anovulatory Conditions
Polycystic ovarian syndrome (and other group two ovulatory disorders). Weight loss to reduce BMI to less than 30 kg/m^2 is especially helpful in PCOS. The first-line medical treatment for type two disorders is either clomifene or metformin, or both simultaneously.

Clomifene is a selective oestrogen receptor modulator. It antagonistically binds to the oestrogen receptors of the hypothalamus, reducing the negative feedback on GnRH production. GnRH production increases, which increases FSH levels, which increases the chance of a dominant follicle forming and then ovulating.
- Success – 35% probability of pregnancy over 6 months of use.
- If a pregnancy develops, there is a 10% chance of twins (background population risk 1%) because clomifene increases the chance of two dominant follicles forming and two oocytes being released in a single cycle.
- Side effects – results in hot flushes, headaches and visual changes due to the decreased perception of oestrogen by the brain. It can also result in poor endometrial development.
- It is taken in tablet form on days 2 to 6 of the menstrual cycle.
- It is only licensed for 6 months use.
- In the first cycle of use, regular ultrasound scanning is advised to monitor follicular development and ovulation. If there is little evidence of follicular development, then a higher dose can be used for the next cycle. If there is too much development, there is a risk of ovarian hyperstimulation syndrome (OHSS).

Metformin increases insulin sensitivity in tissues including the ovaries, which reduces excess ovarian androgen and oestrogen production. This improves the function of the HPO axis, increasing the chance of ovulation. This raises the likelihood of restoring ovulation in overweight women who have tried weight loss. The most common side effects of metformin are nausea, vomiting, stomach pains and diarrhoea. A rare but severe side effect is persistent lactic acidosis.

- Second-line treatments for type two disorders are:
  - Gonadotropins or pulsatile GnRH.
    - Success – 20% per cycle, but decreases with age greater than 35 years.
    - 30% multiple gestations (twin pregnancies), higher order pregnancies if suboptimal monitoring.
    - Ultrasound monitoring for follicular development is essential to prevent hyperstimulation and multiple pregnancy.
- Laparoscopic ovarian drilling.
  - Using either a laser or electrocautery, multiple holes are made into the stroma of the ovaries. This appears to decrease androgen production by the ovary, which then increases FSH production, increasing the chance of follicle stimulation and ovulation.
  - Up to 80% of women will ovulate and up to 60% of these become pregnant. The effects of the drilling appear to only last for around 6 months.
  - The risks are the same as for a diagnostic laparoscopy.

[See 'Introduction to gynaecology' page 1.]

Hypothalamic pituitary insufficiency (group one ovulatory disorders). Gonadotropins or pulsatile GnRH – risks are as per use in type two ovulatory disorders.

Ovarian insufficiency (group three ovulatory disorders)

- No medical or surgical options are available in true ovarian insufficiency.
- To determine the amount of ovarian reserve (functional oocytes remaining in the ovaries) FSH and AMH blood tests are taken, and ovarian follicle counting on an ultrasound scan is performed.
- Where there is the possibility of some ovarian reserve, either ovulation induction can be attempted, or oocyte retrieval can be undertaken as part of an ART.

Treatment of structural problems

- Tubal surgery.
  - Laparoscopy or hysteroscopy can be used to cannulate the tubes and improve patency. This can improve pregnancy rates, but it also increases the risk of ectopic pregnancy. However, tubal surgery is much less effective than IVF, so this is no longer a common treatment.
  - When a tube is badly damaged, inflamed or filled with fluid (hydrosalpinx), surgeons offer removal of the tube (salpingectomy), since the ongoing

inflammatory process decreases the pregnancy rate even when IVF is used.
  - Laparoscopic treatment of endometriosis is advised in moderate to severe cases, as this treatment appears to improve fertility rates. It is believed that removing endometriosis also removes the associated inflammation of the pelvic peritoneum which reduces fertility rates.
- Uterine surgery.
  - Resection of uterine adhesions using a hysteroscope improves fertility rates.
- Research is ongoing into the benefits of resection of a uterine septum or large fibroids.

PROGNOSIS

- The likelihood of a successful pregnancy depends on the age of the woman, the cause of their subfertility, and what management options are available for them. If the management options already discussed are unsuccessful, the next treatment offered may be ARTs.

MALE INFERTILITY

Again, it may be useful to divide the causes of infertility anatomically.

AETIOLOGY

Hypothalamus, Pituitary and Testes
These structures are required for spermatogenesis via testosterone secretion.

Hypothalamic pituitary failure
- FSH low, testosterone low.
- Testes potentially normal but not being stimulated for spermatogenesis.
- Causes include:
  - Genetic causes, such as Kallmann syndrome.
  - Acquired causes, such as a pituitary macroadenoma or another brain tumour.

Testicular dysfunction. Altered spermatogenesis is the most common cause of male subfertility. Unless otherwise stated, the causes below all affect spermatogenesis and sperm function by reducing the number of sperm made and their morphology and motility.
- Common causes:
  - Trauma, previous testicular torsion, STIs and orchitis.
  - Medical – thyroid dysfunction, prolactinomas, radiotherapy and chemotherapy.
  - Social – obesity, smoking, alcohol, illicit drug use and environmental toxins.
- Chromosomal abnormalities – Klinefelter syndrome (XXY) and Y chromosome deletions.

- Reduced sperm motility specifically:
  - Kartagener syndrome (immotile cilia syndrome).
  - Anti-sperm antibodies.
- Varicocele – a mass of varicose veins within the scrotum. The theory is that the increased temperature caused by the vessels decreases testicular function. These can be treated easily with surgical ligation. However, the evidence for how much varicocoeles affect fertility is in doubt, with National Institute for Clinical Excellence (NICE) guidelines not supporting treatment for them.

Obstructive Causes

The epididymis, vas deferens (spermatic cord), seminal vesicles and ejaculatory ducts are the structures required for the storage, maturation and transportation of spermatozoa.

- Congenital ejaculatory duct obstruction.
  - Bilateral absence of vas deferens – commonly associated with cystic fibrosis or renal tract abnormality, for example, an absent kidney.
  - Hypospadias – urethral defect.
- Acquired ejaculatory duct obstruction – secondary to epididymal or prostatic infections, for example, chlamydia, or surgical procedures, such as a vasectomy.
- Retrograde ejaculation – semen passes into the bladder rather than being expelled at the time of ejaculation. It is then harmlessly passed in the urine. Common causes of this are prostate surgery, drugs such as tamsulosin, spinal cord injury, multiple sclerosis and DM.

Penis

Erectile and ejaculatory dysfunction may be associated with:

- Hypogonadism resulting in low testosterone and low libido.
- Psychological factors.
- Neurovascular complications, for example, DM, prostate surgery and spinal cord disease.

CLINICAL ASSESSMENT

Similar to female subfertility:

- Medical, surgical, medication, social, and previous conception history.
- A focussed sexual history should also assess desire for intercourse, maintenance of erection, and symptoms of infection.
- General examination for systemic disease.
- Examine the penis, spermatic cord and testicular volume and consistency. Consider a rectal examination if prostatic pathology suspected.

INVESTIGATIONS

Semen Analysis

- This is the essential investigation in male subfertility; if normal no other investigation is required.
- Men should abstain from ejaculation for 3 days prior to providing a sample.
- If a first sample is abnormal, a second sample should be repeated 3 months later, as transient changes are observed in sperm production (Fig. 2.13).
- If repeated semen samples are abnormal, further investigation may be required, depending on the abnormality.

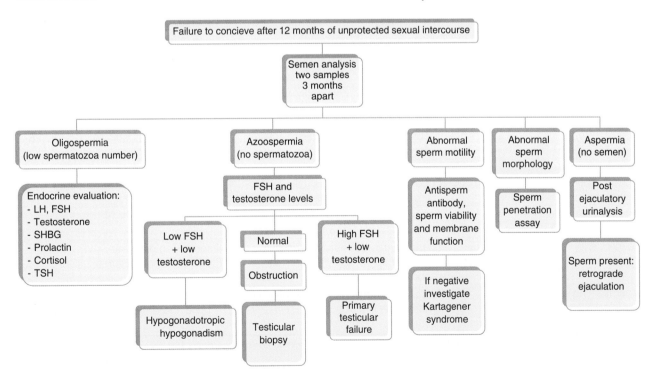

Fig. 2.13 Initial investigations of male subfertility. *FSH*, Follicle-stimulating hormone; *LH*, luteinising hormone; *SHBG*, sex hormone binding globulin; *TSH*, thyroid-stimulating hormone.

Table 2.4 Normal Values for Semen Analysis (World Health Organization Criteria)

CRITERION	NORMAL VALUE
Semen volume	≥15 mL
Semen pH	≥7.2
Sperm concentration	≥15 million per mL
Vitality (live spermatozoa)	≥58%
Progressive motility (sperm that move forwards)	≥32%
Sperm morphology (% of normal forms)	≥4%

For sperm to be effective in conception, there must be a large enough number of them in the ejaculate, as most will not reach the oocyte. They have to be able to swim, and they also have to be able to enter the oocyte when they reach it, which require normal morphology. It is worth noting that, based on the 'normal values' for semen (Table 2.4), the majority of spermatozoa in a healthy man's semen are in fact abnormal

Definitions of semen analysis diagnoses
- Oligospermia – low levels of spermatozoa in semen analysis.
- Azoospermia – no spermatozoa in semen analysis. Either sperm are not produced or the vas deferens or epididymis are obstructed. The analysed semen still contains seminal fluid from the seminal vesicles.
- Aspermia – no spermatozoa or seminal fluid, caused by damage to the ejaculatory tract at, or distal to, the prostate. This is usually confirmed by

urine analysis showing retrograde ejaculation into the bladder.

MANAGEMENT
Conservative
- General healthy lifestyle advice, as discussed in female infertility management.
- Advise wearing loose underwear – the evidence is uncertain, but there is an association between raised scrotal temperature and reduced semen quality.

Other management options are dependent on semen analysis (Table 2.5)

PROGNOSIS
- Dependent on diagnosis.
- ART is the most effective option in male infertility.
- An abnormal semen analysis (see Table 2.5) increases the testicular cancer risk by 20-fold.

Table 2.5 Semen Analysis Results, Further Investigations and Treatment of Subfertility

POTENTIAL RESULT	FURTHER TESTS	TREATMENT
Normal	None	None or conservative
No spermatozoa (azoospermia)	FSH low and testosterone low – hypogonadotropic hypogonadism	GnRH analogue and or gonadotropins (dependent on cause)
	FSH high and testosterone low – primary testicular failure	Likely donor sperm with IVF (may also require testosterone for libido)
	FSH and testosterone normal – likely obstruction, biopsy testes to confirm spermatozoa present	Repair obstruction with microsurgery, or perform sperm retrieval to use in IVF with intracytoplasmic sperm injection (ICSI)
Reduced spermatozoa (oligospermia)	Endocrine tests: FSH, LH, TSH, prolactin, cortisol, testosterone and SHBG	Treat any medical cause identified If not successful – IVF
Predominantly reduced motility	Anti-sperm antibodies, sperm function tests	IVF with or without ICSI
Predominantly reduced morphology	Sperm penetration assay (to assess whether sperm can penetrate an oocyte)	If sperm can penetrate – IVF If sperm cannot penetrate – ICSI
Aspermia – no spermatozoa or seminal fluid	Test urine to confirm presence of semen retrograde ejaculation	Sperm retrieval from post ejaculatory urine, then intrauterine insemination (IUI) or IVF

FSH, Follicle-stimulating hormone; *IVF, in vitro* fertilisation; *LH,* luteinising hormone; *SHBG,* sex hormone binding globulin; *TSH,* thyroid-stimulating hormone.

ASSISTED REPRODUCTION TECHNIQUES

ARTs require the collection of oocytes, spermatozoa or both. These may be from the couple themselves or one or both of the gametes may come from donors. The UK has strict criteria for who can be offered these treatments on the National Health Service (NHS). Couples who do not meet these criteria often choose to have treatment privately, which can be very costly.

SPERMATOZOA RETRIEVAL

- In most cases, semen can be collected following ejaculation. In retrograde ejaculation, spermatozoa can be extracted from the next urination. Where there is an obstruction, a testicular biopsy can be performed to retrieve spermatozoa.
- Tests can be done to check the quality of the spermatozoa and then high-quality specimens can be selected for use in the treatments.

OOCYTE RETRIEVAL (EGG COLLECTION)

This is an intensive and invasive procedure occurring over a number of weeks. There are many different protocols used, the following is a common example:
- Day one of the follicular phase must be established. This is done either with:
    - A combined contraceptive pill to regulate cycles. Day one is the first day of menstruation.
    - Suppression of the natural cycle via daily injection of GnRH analogues or nasal spray for 2 weeks. This places the woman at day one of the follicular phase of the menstrual cycle.
- Daily gonadotropins (FSH analogues) are then given for 12 days to stimulate the ovaries to produce multiple follicles with maturing oocytes; hCG is then used to mimic the LH surge.
    - Medication doses are decided by the likelihood of an ovarian response. Levels of FSH and AMH and the number of ovarian follicles on a baseline ultrasound scan are used to assess this.
- The stimulation process is then monitored with regular transvaginal ultrasound scans to identify the optimal time to collect the oocytes.
    - If stimulation of follicles does not occur, then the cycle may need to be abandoned and higher doses of medication used next cycle.
    - If stimulation is too great, OHSS may occur.
- Eggs are then retrieved using a long needle inserted through the vagina, guided by ultrasound, under sedation. The needle is simply inserted into the ovarian follicles and the contents aspirated.
- Oocytes are then examined and the best quality specimens are used in the ARTs.

IN VITRO FERTILISATION

Indication – first-line treatment for unexplained infertility and second-line in other cases where initial management has failed.

Procedure
- Sperm are collected as above.
- Oocytes are collected as above. At this point, the female is in the ovulation phase of the menstrual cycle.
- Progesterone is then given to simulate the luteal phase of the menstrual cycle, preparing the endometrium for implantation and then supporting the implanted embryo.
- Each individual oocyte is placed in a separate container with sperm. The sperm then naturally penetrate the oocyte. The fertilised eggs (zygote) are then incubated for a few days. At this point, the best embryos are selected for use.
- The embryo is then transferred to the uterus.
    - This is a simple process that is essentially injection of the embryo in through the cervix. The embryo is then left to naturally implant.
    - Where possible, only one embryo is transferred, as this reduces the chance of having multiple births. Where embryos are not thought to be of the best quality and therefore less likely to develop into a successful pregnancy, more than one embryo can be transferred. In the UK, up to two embryos can be transferred in women less than 40 years old and three in women older than 40.
- Any remaining embryos can be frozen for use in future IVF attempts. Any subsequent attempt with frozen embryos is cheaper because the egg harvesting, fertilisation and embryo selecting steps are not repeated.

The success (live birth) rate for each IVF cycle in women younger than age 35 is over 30%. This rate drops to less than 15% by age 40 and less than 2% over the age of 45.

IVF complications
- Multiple pregnancy – up to 20% rate in the UK, reduced by single embryo transfer.
- OHSS.
- Ectopic pregnancy – higher rates of abnormal implantation sites compared to spontaneous conception.
- Psychological and in some cases financial cost of unsuccessful attempts.

In Vitro Fertilisation With Intracytoplasmic Sperm Injection
- Indication – where sperm are present in very low numbers, have poor forms that are unable to penetrate the oocyte themselves or when sperm have been collected by testicular biopsy and there are only limited numbers.
- Procedure – the same process IVF as described above but, at the time of fertilisation, a single spermatozoa is injected into the oocyte, rather than using the classic IVF technique where sperm are simply placed near the oocyte and allowed to naturally fertilise.

- Success rates are similar for IVF, but this procedure is associated with increased genetic and congenital abnormalities in the resultant child, probably representing the fact that a child has been produced that would naturally not have occurred because ineffective sperm would have been prevented from fertilising the egg.

 Implantation Failure

A proposed mechanism for failure in some cases of both spontaneous and IVF pregnancies is due to failure of the blastocyst to implant correctly into the endometrium. Research is ongoing to identify effective treatments to improve implantation, the most common being endometrial scratching, where a plastic stick with a sharp edge is passed through the cervix into the uterus and moved around to make some incisions in the endometrium prior to embryo transfer. This is thought to induce an inflammatory response and increase the vascular supply to the endometrium, which may improve implantation.

In Vitro Fertilisation With Pre-Implantation Genetic Diagnosis

- Indication – previous pregnancies or family history of a serious inheritable genetic condition.
- Procedure – the same process as for IVF, but at the time of embryo selection, a needle is used to take a single cell from each embryo. The embryo may only be eight cells in size at this point. DNA is extracted from the cell for analysis. Embryos unaffected by the genetic condition are then used in the same way as traditional IVF.
- Risks – decreased success rate compared to IVF, likely due to the trauma caused by removing a cell for analysis. Analysis is not always 100% reliable or conclusive. Its simplest use is in sex selection to avoid genetic disease; for example, Duchenne muscular dystrophy, which is an X-linked recessive disorder.

INTRAUTERINE INSEMINATION

- Indications:
  - Same-sex couples or single women using donor sperm, where the female being inseminated is not known to have fertility problems.
  - Where physical or psychological problems prevent vaginal intercourse.
  - HIV infection (after sperm washing).
  - Unexplained infertility, where the woman, for personal reasons, decline IVF treatment.
- Method – sperm is obtained and inserted into the uterus during the time of ovulation. Controlled ovarian stimulation – for example, pulsatile GnRH analogues or clomifene with ultrasound monitoring can be used in some cases to improve fertility rates.

- Success rate – 50% over six cycles in women younger than age 40, with 75% success in 12 cycles.

OTHER OPTIONS FOR CHILDREN WHERE ASSISTED REPRODUCTIVE TECHNIQUES ARE NOT POSSIBLE OR HAVE BEEN UNSUCCESSFUL

- Surrogacy.
  - Indications – absent or damaged uterus, recurrent pregnancy loss or failed IVF procedures.
  - Gametes from the couple, or gametes from a donor/s can be collected, fertilised by IVF, and then implanted in a donor (surrogate) woman's uterus.
  - Under UK law, all parental rights belong to the surrogate regardless of whether any of the fetal DNA belongs to her. Technically, she can choose to terminate the pregnancy, or not to give the child to the couple after delivery. The donor couple gain parental rights only after birth by adopting the child.
- Adoption or fostering.

PROGNOSIS

Most couples who require fertility treatment have a successful pregnancy. However, the whole process can take a long time and IVF can be intensive and invasive, which can be psychologically draining. For couples who are unable to conceive despite treatment, the psychological effects can be even greater. For couples who choose to undergo private fertility treatment, the financial cost can also be considerable.

PRESERVING FERTILITY FOR THE FUTURE

For individuals who have been diagnosed with cancer and are about to undergo chemotherapy or radiotherapy, which could destroy their fertility, there is the possibility of collecting their gametes and freezing them for the future.

- Sperm collection is straightforward, and freezing equally so. There appears to be little difference in pregnancy outcomes using fresh or frozen sperm.
- The egg collection process is the same as is needed for IVF. This is an onerous process, which takes time and could delay treatment for cancer; it can also worsen oestrogen-dependent cancers because of the high oestrogen levels produced during the ovarian stimulation. The other problem is that oocytes freeze very poorly, with poor outcomes from frozen eggs at present, although new freezing techniques are being developed. Freezing embryos is far more effective. However, the downside of this is that social situations may change over time and consent is required from both the egg and sperm donor to use the embryos.

Ovarian Hyperstimulation Syndrome

This occurs in 20% of ovarian stimulation procedures for egg collection using gonadotropins, with less than 5% of cases being severe. It is more likely to occur in women with PCOS and in younger women, as they have a greater ovarian response to stimulation. It is not clear why it happens, but the ovaries release vasoactive substances, which increase the vascular permeability throughout the body, leading to leakage of intravascular fluid into the third space.

- Presentation and clinical diagnosis:
  - Mild to moderate OHSS – mild abdominal bloating, nausea and vomiting due to mild ascites. Ovarian size less than 12 cm. These women usually require symptomatic treatment only and can be managed outside of the hospital.
  - Severe and critical OHSS:
    - Severe intravascular dehydration.
      - Oliguria and renal failure.
      - Haemoconcentration (haematocrit more than 45%, greatly raised white cell count (WCC)).
      - Thromboembolism.
    - Severe third space shifts.
      - Tense ascites causing severe pain.
      - Rarely, pleural effusions or pericardial effusions can cause acute life-threatening complications.
    - Ovary size more than 12 cm.
- Investigations – FBC, U&Es, LFTs, serum osmolality, abdominal ultrasound. In severe cases, additional investigation such as a chest x-ray, arterial blood gas, electrocardiogram (ECG) and an echocardiogram may be required.
- Management – supportive treatment is all that is required, as OHSS will resolve over time.
  - Analgesia and anti-emetics.
  - Thromboprophylaxis.
  - Drain symptomatic severe ascites, and in the severe cases pleural and pericardial effusions.
  - Close fluid balance monitoring, including careful use of intravenous fluids and tight urine output monitoring.
  - In severe cases, intensive care support is required for central venous pressure monitoring and dialysis.
  - Beware of severe acute pain, as enlarged ovaries have a risk of ovarian torsion.

[See 'Benign ovarian cysts' page 133.]

❓ QUESTIONS

Mr and Mrs Fletcher have come to the infertility clinic after failing to conceive for over a year. They have lots of questions, including what will be done to investigate the cause of their infertility, whether IVF is right for them, and what the risks are with IVF.

A	Day 21 progesterone levels.	G	Semen analysis.
B	Endocervical swab.	H	Testicular biopsy.
C	Hysteroscopy.	I	Testosterone levels.
D	Hysterosalpingo-contrast sonography (HyCoSy).	J	Thyroid stimulating hormone (TSH).
E	Karyotyping.	K	Transrectal ultrasound.
F	Post ejaculatory urinalysis.	L	Transvaginal ultrasound.

For each of the following cases, select the next most appropriate investigation for subfertility.

Q1 A 35-year-old woman presents to the infertility clinic. On history taking, she says she has always had irregular periods. She has a BMI of 30 kg/m².

Q2 A 34-year-old woman is referred by her primary care physician, as she has had difficulty conceiving for the last year. On further questioning of her past obstetric history, she reveals that she has had one successful pregnancy 20 years ago. She has also been previously investigated with laparoscopy for chronic pelvic pain and was given a diagnosis of endometriosis. A test has confirmed she is ovulating.

Q3 A 30-year-old women presents with difficulties conceiving. On further consultation, she reports she has regular periods, but has suffered with menorrhagia and dysmenorrhoea for many years and is on ferrous sulphate for anaemia. Tests have confirmed she is ovulating and has patent fallopian tubes, however, there was a possible abnormality identified within the uterine cavity.

Q4 A 28-year-old man and his wife present with difficulty conceiving. His wife has previously conceived; however, he has not. When asking for past genitourinary history, he mentions that he had previously suffered from epididymo-orchitis, which was treated with antibiotics.

Q5 A 29-year-old man attends a follow-up appointment for the results of his initial investigation for subfertility. It showed that he has aspermia.

Q6 Answer true or false to the following statements.
  A Surgical ablation of endometriosis is as effective as IVF in improving fertility rates in women with endometriosis.
  B Metformin is a first-line medical management for subfertility in women with PCOS.
  C Clomifene is an oestrogen receptor modulator that works by increasing oestrogen levels to increase GnRH levels.
  D Ovarian drilling is used in clomifene-resistant PCOS.
  E Letrozole is a competitive reversible agonist of testosterone.

Q7 Answer true or false to the following statements.
  A For IUI, sperm samples can be obtained from post ejaculatory urinalysis.
  B After an IVF cycle, remaining embryos are disposed of.
  C For egg collection in IVF, ovaries are stimulated with daily FSH injections to produce multiple follicles.
  D After egg collection in IVF, oestrogen pessaries are used to prepare the endometrium for embryo transfer.
  E The success of IVF is not age related.

Q8 Answer true or false to the following statements.
  A Multiple pregnancy rates are reduced by single embryo transfer.
  B OHSS is more common in women with PCOS.
  C Tense ascites, reduced haematocrit and bleeding are signs of critical OHSS.
  D Diuretics are key in the management of OHSS.
  E OHSS has a risk of ovarian torsion.

[Answers on page 173.]

KEY REFERENCES

THE MENSTRUAL CYCLE AND PHYSIOLOGY OF THE HYPOTHALAMIC PITUITARY OVARIAN AXIS

Christian, C.A, Moenter, S.M., 2010. The neurobiology of preovulatory and estradiol-induced gonadotropin-releasing hormone surges. Endocr. Rev. 31 (4), 544–577.

Farage, M.A., Neill, S., MacLean, A.B., 2009. Physiological changes associated with the menstrual cycle: a review. Obstet. Gynecol. Surv. 64 (1), 58–72.

Munro, M.G., Critchley, H.O., Fraser, I.S., 2018. The two FIGO systems for normal and abnormal uterine bleeding symptoms and classification of causes of abnormal uterine bleeding in the reproductive years: 2018 revisions. Int. J. Gynecol. Obstet. 143, 393–408.

Royal College of Obstetricians and Gynaecologists, 2014. Long term consequences of polycystic ovarian syndrome. RCOG green top guideline (GTG 33).

Tsutsumi, R., Webster, N., 2008. GnRH pulsatility, the pituitary response and reproductive dysfunction. Endocr. J. 56 (6), 729–737.

PUBERTY

National Institute for Health and Clinical Excellence, 2021. Heavy menstrual bleeding. NICE guideline (CG 44).

Parker, M.A., Sneddon, A.E., Arbon, P., 2010. The menstrual disorder of teenagers (MDOT) study: determining typical menstrual patterns and menstrual disturbance in a large population-based study of Australian teenagers. BJOG 117, 185–192.

Tirumuru, S.S., Arya, P., Latthe, P., Kirk, J., 2012. Understanding precocious puberty in girls. Obstet. Gynecol. 14, 121–129.

DIFFERENCES IN SEX DEVELOPMENT

Michala, L., Creighton, S.M., 2010. The XY female. Best Pract. Res. Clin. Obstet. Gynaecol. 24, 139–148.

National Health Service, 2010. NHS Choices: Differences of Sex Development [Internet]. Available from: https://www.nhs.uk/conditions/differences-in-sex-development/.

Ocal G., Current concepts in disorders of sexual development. J. Clin. Res. Pediatr. Endocrinol 3 (3), 105–114.

SECONDARY AMENORRHOEA

Baird, D.T., 1997. Amenorrhoea. Lancet. 350 (9073), 275–279.

Crouch, N., Creighton, S., 2004. Amenorrhoea in adolescents: diagnosis and management. Prescriber 15 (2), 4–5.

ESHRE, 2015. Management of Women With Premature Ovarian Insufficiency.

National Institute for Health and Care Excellence, 2014. Clinical Knowledge Summaries: Amenorrhoea [Internet]. Available from: http://cks.nice.org.uk/amenorrhoea.

POLYCYSTIC OVARIAN SYNDROME

Azziz, R., Carmina, E., Dewailly, D., Diamanti-Kandarakis, E., Escobar-Morreale, H.F., Futterweit, W., et al., 2009. The Androgen Excess and PCOS Society criteria for the polycystic ovary syndrome: the complete task force report. Fertil. Steril. 91 (2), 456–488.

Monash, 2018. International Evidence-Based Guideline for the Assessment and Management of Polycystic Ovarian Syndrome.

Royal College of Obstetricians and Gynaecologists, 2014. Long-term consequences of polycystic ovarian syndrome. RCOG green top guideline (GTG 33).

INFERTILITY

National Institute for Health and Care Excellence, 2017. Assessment and treatment for people with fertility problems. NICE clinical guideline (CG 156).

Royal College of Obstetricians and Gynaecologists, 2014. Long-term consequences of polycystic ovarian syndrome. RCOG green top guideline (GTG 33).

Royal College of Obstetricians and Gynaecologists, 2016. Management of ovarian hyperstimulation syndrome. RCOG green top guideline (GTG 5).

3

Early Pregnancy Complications

Outline

HYPEREMESIS GRAVIDARUM

Hyperemesis gravidarum is nausea and vomiting in early pregnancy with symptoms severe enough to cause clinical dehydration or a significant reduction in the patient's quality of life. Weight loss of more than 5% of body weight and electrolyte imbalance is also commonly used as part of the definition.

AETIOLOGY

Mild nausea and vomiting in pregnancy affects over 70% of pregnancies, with symptoms classically worse in the morning, leading to the popular colloquialism 'morning sickness'. Hyperemesis affects around 1% of pregnancies.

PATHOPHYSIOLOGY

The cause of nausea and vomiting in early pregnancy is not fully understood. The best-established theory suggests the hormone human chorionic gonadotropin (hCG) causes hyperemesis. Produced by the placenta, β hCG is at its maximum maternal serum level in the first 8 to 12 weeks of pregnancy. It is believed this high level of hCG has a direct stimulatory effect on the chemoreceptor trigger zone (CTZ) and vomiting centres of the midbrain.

The β hCG levels fall sharply in the second trimester. For this reason, hyperemesis usually resolves around or before 16 weeks of gestation. Ongoing or new vomiting beyond 20 weeks of gestation is unlikely to be attributable to hyperemesis gravidarum, and further investigation should be undertaken to identify an alternative cause.

CLINICAL FEATURES

SYMPTOMS

- Nausea.
- Vomiting or retching.
- 'Unable to keep food and drink down'.
- Decreased urinary frequency.
- General exhaustion.

SIGNS

- Prolonged capillary refill time.
- Tachycardia.
- Dry mucous membranes.
- Weight loss.
- In rare severe cases – decreased conscious level, seizures and coma.

Hyperemesis gravidarum is a diagnosis of exclusion. The purpose of the clinical review should be to exclude alternative diagnoses. Identification of other signs and symptoms should prompt further investigation for an alternative diagnosis.

DIAGNOSTIC CRITERIA

The Royal College of Obstetricians and Gynaecologists (RCOG) recommended the following triad is present before diagnosis:
- More than 5% pre-pregnancy weight loss.
- Dehydration.
- Electrolyte imbalance.

INVESTIGATIONS

- Urinalysis:
  - Ketones – demonstrate starvation (metabolism of fatty acids and amino acids rather than glucose).
  - Leucocytes and nitrites – exclude a urinary tract infection.
  - Glucose – consider diabetic ketoacidosis or renal pathology.
  - Colour and concentration are subjective markers of dehydration.
- Urinary pregnancy test – to confirm the patient's report of being pregnant.
- Weight – 5% to 10% loss of body weight may indicate severe dehydration, which increases the risk of metabolic disturbance.

- Blood tests – these tests are useful to exclude alternative causes of vomiting, and haematocrit and urea and electrolytes (U&Es) are also useful to assess the severity of dehydration:
  - Full blood count (FBC).
  - U&Es.
  - Liver function tests (LFTs).
  - C-reactive protein (CRP).
  - Thyroid-stimulating hormone (TSH).
  - Glucose.
- Ultrasound scan – identifies twin or molar pregnancy, both of which can cause significantly elevated hCG levels.

DIFFERENTIAL DIAGNOSIS

- Infective cause – gastroenteritis, urinary tract infection.
- Pain – appendicitis, renal colic.
- Gastrointestinal – reflux, peptic ulceration, liver disease.
- Endocrine – severe hyperthyroidism, diabetic ketoacidosis.
- Psychiatric – bulimia nervosa, anxiety.
- Raised intracranial pressure.
- Molar pregnancy.

COMPLICATIONS

- Severe dehydration.
- Iatrogenic Wernicke-Korsakoff encephalopathy.
  - A neurological emergency resulting from thiamine deficiency.
  - The triad of symptoms include mental status changes, gait and oculomotor dysfunction.
  - Korsakoff encephalopathy is a long-term condition when Wernicke encephalopathy is left untreated, causing symptoms such as psychosis, confabulation and amnesia.
- Refeeding syndrome.
- Fetal complications (in severe cases) – fetal growth restriction and preterm birth.

MANAGEMENT

- Rehydration – obtain intravenous (IV) access and prescribe a crystalloid fluid. The choice is dependent on serum electrolytes; however, carbohydrate containing fluids are usually avoided initially.
- Anti-emesis:
  - Anti-emetics
    - An intramuscular or IV antihistamine anti-emetic, such as cyclizine or promethazine, is usually the first-line anti-emetic therapy. This is then switched to the oral route for ongoing prevention of emesis once oral intake is tolerated. If patients would prefer a non-pharmaceutical alternative for mild symptoms of nausea, ginger is recommended.
    - If symptoms are not adequately controlled with the initial anti-emetic therapy, a second-line anti-emetic can be given in addition to the first-line therapy. Prochlorperazine or metoclopramide are commonly used as second-line therapies.
    - If symptoms are still not controlled, ondansetron can be prescribed. Limited safety data are available, but this compound is not known to be harmful to the fetus.
    - If, despite all other treatments, vomiting persists, senior obstetricians can consider treatment with other anti-emetics such as domperidone or dexamethasone.
- Treating reflux
  - Often gastro-oesophageal reflux and the symptom of water brash can complicate hyperemesis. Treatment with a type 2 histamine receptor (H2) antagonist, such as ranitidine, or a proton pump inhibitor, such as omeprazole, can relieve these symptoms.
  - Antacid liquids and tablets can also offer good symptomatic relief.
- Thiamine supplement – prevent the occurrence of Wernicke encephalopathy.
- Thromboprophylaxis – dehydration and pregnancy are both independent risk factors.
- Encourage oral intake of food and liquid – this returns the body to normal metabolism, stopping gluconeogenesis.

TREATING THE SEVERE COMPLICATIONS

In severe cases of hyperemesis with prolonged starvation and weight loss, patients are at risk of serious complications of routine treatment. In these patients, vitamin B1 (thiamine) should be given prior to the patient receiving IV fluids containing carbohydrates or attempting to eat again. Thiamine is essential in the metabolism of glucose, and in these patients, serum levels are often low. If carbohydrates are given, thiamine is rapidly depleted, which prevents further glucose metabolism. Neurones are reliant on glucose, so severe thiamine deficiency can cause neuronal cell death. This can result in Wernicke encephalopathy which, if not urgently treated with specialist assistance, can progress to permanent Korsakoff psychosis.

Patients with severe hyperemesis are also at risk of refeeding syndrome. Prolonged starvation prevents ingestion of electrolytes. To maintain serum levels of electrolytes, such as magnesium, phosphate, potassium and calcium, these ions are shifted from inside cells to the serum. When feeding restarts, insulin is released in response to increased carbohydrate levels. Insulin drives electrolytes back into cells, resulting in sudden dangerously low serum concentrations of electrolytes, which can result in seizures, arrhythmias, confusion, coma and death. To prevent this, regular electrolyte levels should be taken and low levels treated with intravenous replacements.

PROGNOSIS

Most patients' symptoms resolve quickly after administration of IV fluids and simple antiemetic therapy. Symptoms usually resolve by around 16 weeks gestation. There is also evidence that pregnancies with episodes of hyperemesis have a reduced risk of spontaneous early miscarriage compared to pregnancies without.

❓ QUESTIONS

Sandra, a 24-year-old woman, gravida one, is around 8 weeks pregnant. She has suffered from nausea and occasional vomiting for the last 4 weeks. However, over the last week, she has been unable to eat, is only drinking small amounts and has been unable to work due to the frequency of her symptoms. She is exhausted and very upset. She has no past medical history and is taking no medication.

A Dopamine receptor agonist.	**G** Hydrogen/sodium ATPase inhibitor.
B Dopamine receptor antagonist.	**H** Irreversible proton pump inhibitor.
C Histamine H1 receptor agonist.	**I** Nicotinic receptor agonist.
D Histamine H1 receptor antagonist.	**J** Nicotinic receptor antagonist.
E Histamine H2 receptor agonist.	**K** Serotonin 5-HT3 receptor agonist.
F Histamine H2 receptor antagonist.	**L** Serotonin 5-HT3 receptor antagonist.

The following medications can be used in the management of hyperemesis gravidarum. To what class of drug do they belong?

Q1 Cyclizine.

Q2 Metoclopramide.

Q3 Omeprazole.

Q4 Ondansetron.

Q5 Prochlorperazine.

Q6 Promethazine.

Q7 Which of the following is the major cause of hyperemesis gravidarum?
   A Mass effect of the uterus pressing on the bowel and stomach.
   B β hCG affecting the vomiting centres of the brain.
   C Progesterone relaxing the lower oesophageal sphincter.
   D Oestrogen delaying gastric emptying.
   E Insulin-like growth factor (IGF1) causing insulin resistance and ketoacidosis.

Q8 Answer true or false to these statements regarding hyperemesis gravidarum.
   A Ketonuria supports the diagnosis of hyperemesis.
   B A raised haematocrit is a common investigation result in hyperemesis gravidarum.
   C Ultrasound scanning should form part of first-line investigations in hyperemesis to diagnose molar pregnancies.
   D Pregnancies troubled by hyperemesis are more likely to end in miscarriage.
   E Hyperemesis commonly presents in the second trimester.

[Answers on page 175.]

MOLAR PREGNANCY

Gestational trophoblastic disease is the collective term for types of abnormal proliferation of placental tissue:
- Molar pregnancy (also called hydatidiform pregnancy).
  - Partial molar pregnancy.
  - Complete molar pregnancy.
- Choriocarcinoma.

Molar pregnancies are pregnancies with abnormal cell proliferation of the placental tissue, which occur as a result of two copies of paternal DNA entering the ovum. They can remain within the uterus, but if they invade through the uterus into local structures they are then defined as invasive molar pregnancies (Fig. 3.1). Invasive moles can also metastasise to distant organs.

Cells of a molar pregnancy can subsequently undergo neoplastic change and become the malignant condition choriocarcinoma. Choriocarcinomas, like any cancer, can invade local structures and metastasise.

AETIOLOGY

- Molar pregnancy occurs in 1:700 pregnancies.
- Choriocarcinoma is a very rare condition, only diagnosed after a live birth in 1:50,000 deliveries.

Gestational trophoblastic disease risk factors:
- Extremes of maternal age.
  - Pregnancy at less than 16 years old – 10 times increased risk.
  - Pregnancy at more than 45 years old – 100 times increased risk.
- Previous personal history of molar pregnancy – 10 times increased risk.

PATHOPHYSIOLOGY

Molar pregnancies do not form a normal fetus, so will not progress to delivery of a baby. They are chromosomally abnormal, caused by two copies of paternal DNA being included in the ovum (Fig. 3.2). The simplest way to understand the pathogenesis of molar pregnancy is that it occurs when two sperm enter an ovum. If the ovum was empty (no maternal DNA), then the resulting pregnancy has 46 chromosomes (all of paternal origin), which is a complete mole. However,

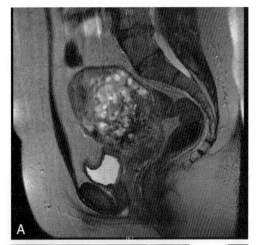

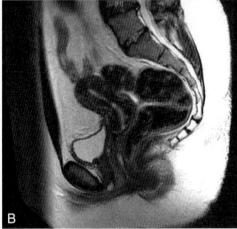

Fig. 3.1 Invasive complete molar pregnancy. (A) Magnetic resonance imaging appearance prior to chemotherapy treatment. (B) Follow-up scan performed three months after chemotherapy completion.

A histological examination of a complete molar pregnancy usually reveals no evidence of any fetal development, with only abnormal placental tissue present. Partial molar pregnancies usually show some evidence of fetal development.

Complete molar pregnancies are more likely than partial moles to become invasive and therefore invade local structures or metastasise to distant organs. They are also more likely to develop into a choriocarcinoma.

Choriocarcinoma is the name given to malignant placental tissue. It most commonly occurs as a result of metaplastic change from a complete molar pregnancy, but it can occasionally develop following changes in a partial molar pregnancy. Rarely, a choriocarcinoma can occur from the placental tissue of an uncomplicated pregnancy, and in this situation may not be diagnosed until after the birth of an otherwise healthy baby. Extremely rarely choriocarcinomas can also form without a pregnancy, as a form of ovarian cancer arising from a malignant growth of a germ cell in the ovary.

The placental tissue of molar pregnancies and choriocarcinoma are endocrinologically active, producing the hormones usually produced by a placenta. As there is substantially more placental tissue made in these conditions than in a healthy pregnancy, the amount of hormone produced is also greater. High levels of β hCG is a diagnostic marker and is also responsible for some of the symptoms associated with the conditions.

CLINICAL FEATURES

Almost all molar pregnancies present in early pregnancy with the same symptoms of a threatened miscarriage:

- Vaginal bleeding.
- Abdominal pain – usually mild and non-specific.
- Abdominal distension – uterine enlargement consistent with pregnancy, sometimes the uterus can be far larger than would be expected for the presumed gestation based on last menstrual period (LMP).
- Miscarriage – following a miscarriage the presence of an ongoing molar pregnancy should be excluded if symptoms are ongoing. If there is clinical suspicion, this can be achieved by either sending products of conception for histology or repeat urinary β hCG test 3 weeks after the miscarriage. If the test is

if the ovum contained maternal derived DNA and two sperm enter, then the resulting pregnancy has 69 chromosomes (one set of maternal haploid DNA and two sets of paternal haploid DNA). This is a partial mole.

In reality, in 90% of cases of complete molar pregnancy, only one sperm enters an empty ovum, but it then duplicates to form the double paternal DNA. In the remaining 10% of cases, it is in fact two sperm which enter. In partial moles, almost all arise as a result of two sperm entering the ovum.

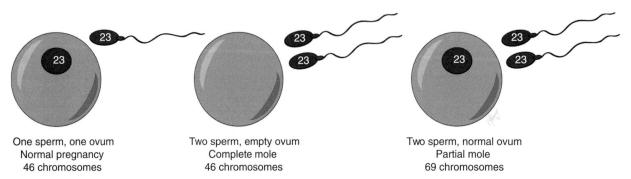

One sperm, one ovum	Two sperm, empty ovum	Two sperm, normal ovum
Normal pregnancy	Complete mole	Partial mole
46 chromosomes	46 chromosomes	69 chromosomes

Fig. 3.2 Molar and Partial Molar Pregnancies.

positive, a further scan is required to look for the cause.

- Hyperemesis – molar pregnancies may also present in early pregnancy (without miscarriage symptoms) as hyperemesis due to the raised β hCG levels. This is the reason patients with hyperemesis receive an early pregnancy ultrasound.
- Rare early pregnancy presentations – these are due to raised β hCG levels and include hyperthyroidism and early onset pre-eclampsia.

Rarely, choriocarcinoma can present after the birth of a baby. Like any tissue with rapidly dividing cells, normal cells of the placenta can potentially undergo neoplastic change at any time during the pregnancy. Checking β hCG levels and an ultrasound should be considered for any patient with persistent irregular vaginal bleeding for many weeks after pregnancy. If missed, a choriocarcinoma could also present with symptoms of local invasion and metastatic spread; for example, haematuria, bowel obstruction, respiratory failure or seizures, depending on the organs involved.

INVESTIGATIONS

- Urine β hCG – confirms the pregnancy, but beware this can be falsely negative with very high β hCG levels.
- Serum β hCG – quantifies the level, also useful for reassurance if concerned despite a negative urine β hCG.
- FBC and group and save (G&S) – taken in preparation for excessive vaginal bleeding.
- Abdominal or transvaginal pelvic ultrasound scan – often the primary diagnostic test. Findings include:
  - Excessive placental tissue.
  - Cystic spaces in placental tissue.
  - Anembryonic pregnancy.
  - Classically described as either 'a bunch of grapes' or a 'snowstorm' appearance (Fig. 3.3).

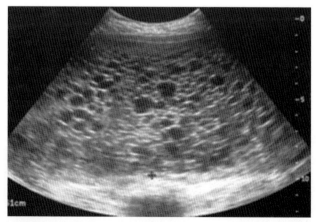

Fig. 3.3 'Bunch of Grapes' or 'Snowstorm' Appearance on Ultrasound.

DIFFERENTIAL DIAGNOSIS

The diagnosis is only confirmed Table 3.1 after the pregnancy tissue is removed and sent for histological analysis.

MANAGEMENT

- Molar pregnancies are non-viable; surgical removal is advised to reduce the chance of metastasis.
  - As with surgical management of a miscarriage, a suction curette is passed through the cervix into the uterus and the contents of the uterus sucked and scraped away.
  - The use of uterotonics (misoprostol and oxytocin) should be avoided where possible, as they may increase the chance of tissue embolisation (tissue entering the vascular or lymphatic systems) and metastatic spread.
  - Anti-D Immunoglobulin injection is given to rhesus negative mothers after the surgery, although this is not needed for a complete mole as no fetal tissue or blood will be present, but treatment is usually given before histology is reported.
- Histology – all products of a suspected molar pregnancy (this includes any miscarriage) should be sent for histology to confirm the diagnosis and the type of trophoblastic disease present, see Table 3.2.

FOLLOW-UP

- Once the molar pregnancy has been surgically evacuated, follow-up is required to monitor for any tissue remaining. In the United Kingdom, this is done by one of three specialist centres (Dundee, Sheffield and London Charing Cross).
- Initially, urine or serum β hCG levels are taken every 2 weeks until levels drop to zero. Tests are then repeated monthly for at least 6 months to confirm there is no recurrence of disease.
- If the β hCG level does not fall or begins to rise during monitoring, then the patient is diagnosed as having persistent gestational trophoblastic disease and is offered chemotherapy.

Table 3.1 Differential Diagnosis of Molar Pregnancy	
PRESENTING COMPLAINT	**OTHER DIFFERENTIAL DIAGNOSES**
Bleeding in early pregnancy	• Threatened miscarriage. • Miscarriage. • Ectopic.
Vomiting in early pregnancy	• Hyperemesis gravidarum. • Twin pregnancy.
Persistent vaginal bleeding, after delivery	• Retained products of conception. • Uterine infection. • Irregular menstrual bleeding.

Table 3.2   Histological Findings in Molar Pregnancy

	COMPLETE MOLE	PARTIAL MOLE
Macroscopic appearance	Bunch of grapes	Fetal tissue visible
Histopathology	Diffuse trophoblast hyperplasia	Focal trophoblastic hyperplasia
	Diffuse villous hydrops	Focal villous hydrops
	No fetal tissue	Fetal tissue
Immunohistochemistry	P57 not expressed	P57 expressed (allele on trophoblast only present in maternal DNA)
Chromosome analysis	Diploid (46 chromosomes)	Triploid (69 chromosomes)

CHEMOTHERAPY

- Required in 5% cases overall: 15% of complete moles, 0.5% of partial molar pregnancies.
- Most cases are treated with methotrexate alternate weeks, with twice weekly β hCG measurements until 6 weeks after the β hCG levels have normalised.
- High-risk patients or patients who do not respond to methotrexate can have a multi-drug regimen of up to five agents at once.

COMPLICATIONS

- Psychological impact of the diagnosis and follow-up.
- Side effects of chemotherapy – low risk of side effects with a short course of methotrexate.
- Symptoms from metastatic disease.
  - Lungs are the most commonly affected site.
  - Liver, spleen, kidney, brain and bowel are also common sites.
  - Chest x-ray is the first investigation to look for metastasis, but a whole-body CT may also be indicated.

PROGNOSIS

- The overall cure rate of molar pregnancy is over 99%.
- The relapse rate is 2% to 3%, but over 95% of these patients are cured.
- Cure rate of gestational choriocarcinoma is 90%.

FUTURE PREGNANCIES

- If chemotherapy is not used, the patients are advised to wait until follow-up has been discontinued before trying to conceive again, as a rising β hCG would be difficult to distinguish between a new pregnancy and a recurrence. If chemotherapy was given, patients are advised to wait for a year after completion of chemotherapy due to potential teratogenic effects.
- Neither molar pregnancy nor methotrexate chemotherapy affect fertility. However, chemotherapy does bring the onset of menopause forward 3 years earlier, on average.
- Risk of a molar pregnancy in a subsequent pregnancy is 1%.

? QUESTIONS

Amy is approximately 8 weeks pregnant. She reports small amounts of vaginal bleeding. Her sister has had a molar pregnancy which presented with vaginal bleeding and Amy is understandably worried.

Q1 Which of these would be the single most useful investigation to diagnose a molar pregnancy?
   A Abdominal ultrasound scan.
   B Analysis of partner's semen.
   C Serum β hCG.
   D Serum human placental lactogen.
   E Urine β hCG.

Q2 Which one of these statements is correct regarding a partial molar pregnancy?
   A Fetal tissue may be seen on ultrasound scan.
   B Most commonly diagnosed after the birth of an otherwise healthy baby.
   C It contains 46 chromosomes.
   D It is caused by two sperm entering an empty ovum.
   E Chemotherapy treatment is likely to be offered after a partial molar pregnancy.

Q3 What is the approximate 5-year survival after treatment of a molar pregnancy?
   A 0%.
   B 25%.
   C 50%.
   D 75%.
   E Over 99%.

[Answers on page 177.]

ECTOPIC PREGNANCY

An ectopic pregnancy is a pregnancy that occurs anywhere outside of the endometrial cavity (Fig. 3.4).

AETIOLOGY

The incidence of ectopic pregnancy is roughly 1:100 pregnancies. The vast majority of ectopic pregnancies will implant in one of the fallopian tubes; rarely, the pregnancy may implant in the ovaries, cervix or

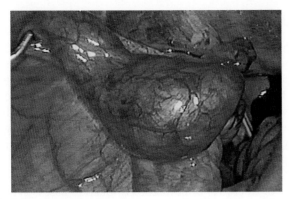

Fig. 3.4 An ectopic pregnancy in the ampulla of the fallopian tube.

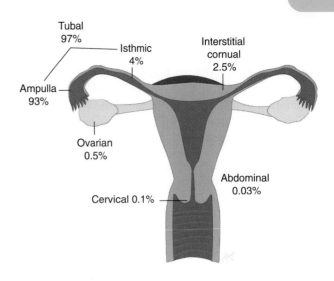

Fig. 3.5 Incidence of Ectopic Pregnancy at Each Site.

even the abdomen (Fig. 3.5). Ectopic pregnancies cannot be moved into the uterus, so cannot lead to a normal pregnancy. However, the ectopic pregnancy can continue to grow, potentially causing life-threatening complications for the pregnant woman.

RISK FACTORS

In a normal pregnancy, the oocyte and sperm join in the fallopian tube. Cilia within the tube transport the pregnancy down the tube so the embryo can implant in the cavity of the uterus. The majority of risk factors lead to an ectopic pregnancy by damaging or blocking the fallopian tubes, which delays the passage of the embryo along the fallopian tube, meaning that if a pregnancy does occur, the implantation is more likely to occur in the fallopian tube (Table 3.3).

CLINICAL FEATURES

LOWER ABDOMINAL PAIN

Stretching of the fallopian tube causes generalised abdominal discomfort which, like most organ pain in the body, does not localise well because there are no somatic nerves in the tubes. However, the pain is more likely to localise to the side of the ectopic.

PELVIC PAIN AND SUPRAPUBIC TENDERNESS

Like appendicitis, the localising pain occurs when there is peritoneal irritation, as the peritoneum does have somatic sensory nerves. Irritation is caused by direct pressure from the ectopic or from irritation from blood leaking intra-abdominally from the ectopic.

Table 3.3 Risk Factors for Ectopic Pregnancies	
RISK FACTOR	**CAUSE OF INCREASED RISK**
Previous ectopic pregnancy	If a woman has had a previous ectopic pregnancy, whatever caused the first one may cause another. Also, the ectopic pregnancy will have resulted in inflammation and damage to the fallopian tube, further increasing the risk.
Pelvic inflammatory disease (PID)	Active or past infection causes inflammation, fibrosis and adhesions to the fallopian tubes, resulting in a higher chance of the embryo implanting there.
Smoking	Smoking reduces the cilia activity within the fallopian tube, meaning the passage of the embryo is slowed.
Previous female sterilisation surgery	Female sterilisation involves intentionally damaging the fallopian tubes by either cutting or blocking them. This means that if conception does occur, it is very likely that transportation of the embryo along the tubes will be obstructed. The failure rate for sterilisation is 1:200.
Any surgery on the fallopian tubes	Any surgery performed on the fallopian tubes will cause damage, increasing the chance of the embryo implanting there.
In vitro fertilisation (IVF)	The fact that patients require IVF suggests that they might have tubal problems. When embryos are inserted into the uterus during the IVF cycle, some will enter a fallopian tube. Movement of tubal cilia should move an embryo back into the uterus, but if this does not occur, then implantation occurs in the tube.
Age over 35	As age increases, cilia activity within the tubes decreases, causing poor transport of the embryo.
Intrauterine contraceptive device (IUCD)	IUCDs cause a decreased chance of pregnancy overall, but if they fail, there is a higher chance of the pregnancy being an ectopic pregnancy (5%), as IUCDs prevent intrauterine pregnancies.

SHOULDER TIP PAIN

Shoulder tip pain can be caused by irritation of the diaphragm from blood leaking intra-abdominally from the ectopic and tracking up in the abdomen to underneath the diaphragm. In the same way that cardiac chest pain classically radiates to the left side of the chest and left arm, diaphragmatic irritation radiates to the shoulder tip.

VAGINAL BLEEDING

Bleeding from an ectopic could possibly track down a fallopian tube and out of the uterus; however, this is very unlikely, so bleeding from an ectopic goes into the abdomen. Vaginal bleeding in an ectopic pregnancy is often small amounts of old blood, which is more likely as a result of the breakdown of the endometrium. In a normal intrauterine pregnancy, the corpus luteum initially maintains the endometrium and the placental tissue gradually takes over this role. However, an ectopic pregnancy rarely grows well and so cannot support the endometrium with progesterone as the corpus luteum fails, so endometrial shedding occurs. It is important to remember that the amount of vaginal bleeding in no way correlates to the amount of intra-abdominal bleeding from a potentially life threatening ruptured ectopic.

PRESYNCOPE, SYNCOPE, HYPOTENSION AND HYPOVOLAEMIC SHOCK

Embryos invade the tissue they implant in. The thick endometrium in the uterus allows for this to occur safely so the placental unit can form, allowing for sufficient nutrient supply to the fetus without compromising the mother. However, in an ectopic pregnancy, the embryo implants in tissue that is not designed for invasion, so the ectopic can invade surrounding blood vessels leading to vessel rupture. In the case of fallopian tubes, their blood supply arises from the ovarian arteries (which are direct branches of the aorta) and the uterine arteries. Therefore, when fallopian tube vessels are ruptured, significant blood loss can occur. Presyncopal episodes should alert the clinician to the significant possibility of ongoing bleeding, and of course syncope and hypovolaemic shock are an emergency situation, requiring immediate resuscitation and stabilisation of the patient to prevent death.

EARLY PREGNANCY ASSESSMENT SERVICE

Most ectopic pregnancies in the United Kingdom are diagnosed at an early stage in their course, before they rupture and compromise the patient. This is achieved by hospitals running daily early pregnancy assessment service (EPAS) clinics, where patients with a positive pregnancy test can be quickly referred when they get any pain or bleeding which could signify the early stages of an ectopic pregnancy.

Clinics are usually run by a specialist nurse, midwife or doctor. A brief history is taken to assess symptoms and likely gestation. A transvaginal ultrasound scan is then performed:

- If the scan confirms a viable intrauterine pregnancy, the patient is usually reassured and discharged, although very rarely there can be an intrauterine pregnancy and a concomitant ectopic pregnancy.
- If the scan confirms an ectopic pregnancy, the patient is referred to the on-call gynaecology team for further investigations and management.
- If the scan does not show a pregnancy, this is termed a pregnancy of unknown location (PUL) and further investigation is needed.

PREGNANCY OF UNKNOWN LOCATION

When a pregnancy cannot be seen on an ultrasound scan, there are three possible causes:

1. A viable intrauterine pregnancy is at an early gestation but is too small to see on ultrasound. Most intrauterine pregnancies can be identified from 5 weeks' gestation.
2. A miscarriage has occurred. The pregnancy test may still be positive because β hCG can remain in the serum for some time after a miscarriage.
3. An ectopic pregnancy which is too small to see on a scan.

To make a diagnosis, a serum β hCG is taken, and then a repeat sample is taken 48 hours later. The levels are then compared between the two samples. The management plan for different levels of β hCG is summarised in Table 3.4 below.

The principle behind serum β hCG monitoring is that a pregnancy in the correct place within the uterus has a good blood supply, so it grows well and produces rapidly increasing levels of β hCG from the growing

Table 3.4 Management of Pregnancy of Unknown Location

β hCG LEVELS	PREGNANCY OUTCOME	MANAGEMENT PLAN
Risen by more than 63%	Likely to be a viable intrauterine pregnancy	An ultrasound scan is repeated after a week to confirm this
Fallen by more than 50%	Likely to be a miscarriage	A urine pregnancy test is checked in 2 weeks, which should be negative
Neither risen nor fallen by the above	Likely to be an ectopic pregnancy	The patient is referred to the early pregnancy assessment services within 24 h for further investigation and management

placental tissue. Conversely, in a failing pregnancy, the placental tissue that is forming is dying, so the β hCG levels fall. An ectopic pregnancy has implanted in a location with a poor blood supply, so although the pregnancy will grow, it will not grow as well as a pregnancy within the uterus, therefore the β hCG levels rise less quickly. However, there are exceptions to the rule, and rarely, an ectopic can grow quickly and produce rapidly increasing β hCG levels like an intrauterine pregnancy. These can be particularly dangerous as the clinician can be falsely reassured by the blood tests, but these rapidly growing ectopics have a high chance of invading into tissues, perforating blood vessels and causing maternal collapse. For this reason, it is imperative to treat any PUL as an ectopic until proven otherwise. All patients being investigated by EPAS should be advised that if they have any increase in pain or bleeding or if they feel dizzy, they should contact the hospital for rapid assessment.

INVESTIGATIONS

DIAGNOSTIC INVESTIGATIONS (USUALLY DONE BY EPAS)

- Urine test for β hCG – to confirm the pregnancy. Any woman of childbearing age presenting in a healthcare setting with vaginal bleeding or abdominal pain should be offered a urinary pregnancy test to exclude the possibility of ectopic pregnancy.
- Transvaginal ultrasound – to assess for evidence of intrauterine or ectopic pregnancy and the evidence of free fluid (Fig. 3.6).
- Serum β hCG levels – when a scan has been unable to identify the location of a pregnancy, repeated β hCG measurements can aid diagnosis and guide management.

INVESTIGATIONS TO MANAGE AN ECTOPIC

- FBC – to assess the haemoglobin level. Anaemia, along with other clinical features, may indicate an

ongoing bleed. Remember, in acute hypovolaemic shock, the haemoglobin concentration may be normal, as acute bleeding causes a reduction in blood volume not concentration. Only after fluid resuscitation will the level fall, as the blood is diluted.
- G&S – taken in preparation should a stable patient become unstable and require a blood transfusion, or taken prior to theatre and cross matched blood ordered in the unstable patient.
- Laparoscopy or laparotomy – in the acutely unwell patient, after initial resuscitation and stabilisation, and if ectopic pregnancy is suspected or has been confirmed, the definitive procedure to identify and treat a ruptured ectopic is via a laparoscopy or laparotomy.

DIFFERENTIAL DIAGNOSIS

- Threatened miscarriage.
- Molar pregnancy.
- Ovarian cyst accident.
- Any other cause of abdominal pain; for example, appendicitis, gastroenteritis, diverticulitis or pelvic inflammatory disease.

COMPLICATIONS

RUPTURED ECTOPIC PREGNANCY

If the diagnosis is not made promptly, an ectopic pregnancy may rupture. This occurs when the pregnancy develops and grows inside the fallopian tube, stretches it and invades the tissues. Eventually, blood vessels are invaded into, causing bleeding that can be heavy and result in massive internal bleeding. Patients with a ruptured ectopic pregnancy usually present much more shocked than can be accounted for by the visible blood loss; this is because the majority of blood loss is internal and has pooled inside the abdomen. This is a very serious complication and may lead to death, so it is important to be vigilant when suspecting an ectopic pregnancy.

IMPAIRED FERTILITY

Impaired fertility may be a complication of ectopic pregnancy. The cause of the ectopic may be damaged tubes, but the ectopic itself, or the management of the ectopic, may further damage the fallopian tube, thereby reducing the prospect of a successful subsequent pregnancy.

MANAGEMENT

There are three main management strategies for ectopic pregnancy. Expectant management which includes careful monitoring with repeat β hCG levels, observations and clinical follow-up. Medical management involves giving medication to terminate the pregnancy, and surgical management removes the ectopic pregnancy Table 3.5.

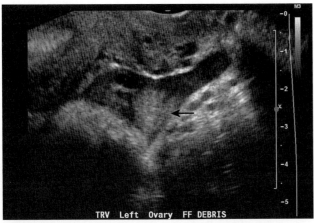

Fig. 3.6 An ultrasound impact of a ruptured ectopic. The free fluid containing echogenic debris representing blood is seen in the cul-de-sac.

Table **3.5** Summary of the Management for Ectopic Pregnancy

EXPECTANT MANAGEMENT	MEDICAL MANAGEMENT	SURGICAL MANAGEMENT
Adnexal mass <35 mm	Adnexal mass <35 mm	Adnexal mass >35 mm
Unruptured ectopic pregnancy	Unruptured ectopic pregnancy	Ruptured ectopic pregnancy
Asymptomatic	No significant pain	Significant pain
No fetal heartbeat	No fetal heartbeat	Visible fetal heartbeat
β hCG level <1000 IU/L	β hCG level <1500 IU/L Consider with β hCG level <5000	β hCG level >5000 IU/L

hCG, Human chorionic gonadotropin.

STABLE ECTOPIC PREGNANCY

Expectant management is the first line for patients who are well, serum β hCG level is less than 1000 IU/L, the ectopic is small in size and appears to be failing. In these cases, close clinical and β hCG monitoring is carried out to confirm complete resolution. If the β hCG level does not fall by over 15% over 48 hours medical or surgical management is then considered.

Medical Management

Medical management is offered as an option in clinically stable women. Classically, these women are clinically well, presenting with a small amount of pain or vaginal bleeding, and ultrasound has then confirmed the presence of an ectopic pregnancy. Methotrexate is the drug of choice. It is a folate analogue that disrupts folate metabolism, which is essential for cell replication. Rapidly replicating cells (such as a developing embryo) are most affected by this compound, which results in cell death. The common side effects of methotrexate are gastrointestinal upset and stomatitis, as the gastrointestinal system is a site of rapidly replicating epithelial cells.

Methotrexate is given intramuscularly as a one-off dose and serum β hCG levels are checked on days 4 and 7 after treatment. If β hCG levels have fallen by at least 15% between days 4 and 7 β hCG is then monitored weekly until it has fallen below 15 IU/L. If β hCG levels have failed to drop by at least 15% between days 4 and 7, then a further dose of methotrexate will be required, although the majority of women will only need one dose. If a second dose still fails to cause a drop in the β hCG levels, then surgical management may be required. The higher the β hCG level and the larger the ectopic, the more likely it is that methotrexate will fail.

Surgical management should be offered first line to stable women in the following circumstances, where methotrexate is less likely to be effective:
- Significant pain.
- A fetal heartbeat visible on ultrasound scan.
- An adnexal mass more than 35 mm.
- Serum β hCG level of more than 5000 IU/L.

Methotrexate should also not be used:
- In women who are either unwilling or unable to attend regular follow-up to ensure methotrexate has been effective.
- Where there is an intrauterine pregnancy as well as the ectopic pregnancy (this is called a heterotopic pregnancy), as the methotrexate would also kill the viable pregnancy.
- In women with liver failure.

Surgical Management

A laparoscopic approach is preferred to an open approach, as patient recovery is much quicker. The aim of surgery is to identify the ectopic, remove it and stop any bleeding. If the ectopic pregnancy is in the fallopian tube, the surgeon will look at the unaffected tube to decide on the operation. If the unaffected tube appears normal, the surgeon will most likely remove the entire affected tube (salpingectomy), in the hope that the appearance of a normal tube on the other side will preserve fertility. Where the unaffected tube appears damaged, the surgeon may consider opening the affected tube and removing the ectopic while leaving the tube in place (salpingotomy). This may preserve fertility, but it increases the chance that some of the ectopic may be left, which could continue to grow and bleed. For this reason, patients who have had a salpingotomy should have a urine pregnancy test 2 weeks after the procedure to confirm it is negative. Any woman who has a surgically treated ectopic pregnancy and is rhesus negative should be offered anti-D prophylaxis.

After an ectopic pregnancy has been removed, it cannot then be implanted into the womb. Ectopic pregnancies can never result in viable pregnancies.

UNSTABLE ECTOPIC PREGNANCY

A patient with a ruptured ectopic may present for the first time with collapse or severe abdominal pain. They may not even know that they are pregnant; hence, every female of childbearing age is offered a pregnancy test on hospital admission. If a patient presents with a history consistent with an ectopic and a positive pregnancy test, and is clinically haemodynamically unstable, then they need to be treated as a presumed ruptured ectopic.

An unstable ectopic pregnancy is a medical emergency and should be treated as such:

- Like any emergency, use an airway, breathing, circulation, disability and exposure (ABCDE) approach.
- Call the appropriate healthcare professionals quickly: senior O&G team members and the anaesthetic team should be involved quickly to enable plans for theatre. If haemodynamically unstable call the cardiac arrest team.
- IV access should be obtained by inserting two large bore cannulas.
- Take a FBC, G&S, crossmatch and a venous blood gas.
- Give rapid intravenous fluids: up to 2.5 L of crystalloid may be used to maintain blood pressure. If not stable with crystalloid, then packed red cells will be needed to replace the massive blood loss. The foot of the bed can be raised to maintain cerebrovascular pressure.
- If the patient does not readily pass urine, pass a catheter to obtain urine for a pregnancy test.
- Transvaginal ultrasound, if there is a machine immediately available, can rapidly confirm the presence of blood in the abdomen. However, this is not essential and if not available, this should not delay transfer of the patient to theatre.

Surgical management is required to treat an unstable patient with a suspected ectopic pregnancy. In most cases, the patient can be stabilised with the ABC approach, and then a laparoscopy can be undertaken to remove the ectopic and control the bleeding. In rare cases, laparotomies may be performed for ectopic pregnancy, usually where there are complications and the surgeon cannot achieve haemostasis during laparoscopy.

PROGNOSIS

The development of sensitive β hCG measurements and reliable transvaginal ultrasound have meant that the majority of ectopic pregnancies are diagnosed and managed before rupture, so prognosis is now usually good. However, ectopic pregnancy has a mortality rate of 1:5000 in the United Kingdom.

Most women who have had an ectopic pregnancy are able to conceive again, and most likely it will be an intrauterine pregnancy. However, they are at increased risk of another ectopic, so they are advised to have an early ultrasound scan at around 6 weeks gestation in subsequent pregnancies to check the location of the pregnancy. Subsequent fertility rates are similar for expectant, medical or surgical management of an ectopic pregnancy, unless the contralateral tube is damaged in which case salpingectomy decreases fertility. Women treated with methotrexate should wait 3 months before trying to conceive again due to potential teratogenic effects.

? QUESTIONS

Emma, a 22-year-old woman, presents to the emergency department with a 3-hour history of cramping lower abdominal pain, predominantly in the left iliac fossa. A few days ago, she had some mild vaginal bleeding, and her last menstrual period was 7 weeks ago. She has no significant past medical history and has previously been well. On examination, there is some tenderness in the suprapubic region. Her urine test is β hCG positive.

Q1   Given this presentation, what would be the most suitable investigation?
   A Abdominal CT scan.
   B Abdominal ultrasound.
   C Abdominal x-ray.
   D Progesterone level.
   E Transvaginal ultrasound.

Q2   Which of these is not a risk factor for ectopic pregnancy?
   A Combined oral contraceptive pill.
   B Intrauterine contraceptive device.
   C Pelvic inflammatory disease.
   D Previous ectopic pregnancy.
   E Smoking.

Q3   Which of these drugs is used first line in the medical management of ectopic pregnancy?
   A Actinomycin D.
   B Methotrexate.
   C Mifepristone.
   D Oestrogen.
   E Progesterone.

A Laparoscopy.	H A serum β hCG concentration static.
B Laparotomy.	
C Medical management of ectopic.	I A serum progesterone rise of more than 50%.
D No further investigations or treatment.	J Urine β hCG rise of more than 63%.
E Repeat ultrasound scan.	K Urine β hCG fall of more than 50%.
F A serum β hCG rise of more than 63%.	L Urine β hCG concentration static.
G A serum β hCG drop of more than 50%.	

Q4   For the patient above, an ultrasound scan is inconclusive. Which investigation above would best indicate a diagnosis of miscarriage?

Q5   For the patient above, an ultrasound scan is inconclusive. Further tests are performed and the patient is then given methotrexate. Which test is most likely to have resulted in this management?

Q6   For the patient above, an ultrasound scan is inconclusive. Blood tests are then performed and following the tests the doctor suggests that this is likely to be an intrauterine pregnancy. Which test is required to confirm this?

Q7   For the patient above, an ultrasound scan is inconclusive. While talking to the patient, she complains of increased pain and briefly loses consciousness. Which option would represent the next step in her management?

Q8   For the patient above, an ultrasound scan shows a hetero-topic pregnancy. Which option would represent the next step in her management?

[Answers on page 178.]

MISCARRIAGE

Miscarriage is defined as a spontaneous pregnancy loss before 24 weeks' gestation. After 24 weeks' gestation, a pregnancy loss is termed a stillbirth. An intended pregnancy loss is a termination. The term spontaneous abortion was previously used for miscarriage but is no longer acceptable due to its interchangeable use colloquially with termination.

Miscarriage is the process from a viable pregnancy, to a fetus which has died, to a fetus which is expelled from the body. A combination of clinical findings and ultrasound scanning help define what stage of the process the miscarriage is at (Table 3.6).

AETIOLOGY

Miscarriage early in pregnancy is common, with approximately 20% of pregnancies ending in miscarriage in the first trimester (up to 12 weeks' gestation).

Miscarriages do occur in the second trimester (up to 24 weeks' gestation), but they are much less common than the first trimester, with around 1% to 2% of pregnancies miscarrying in the second trimester.

PATHOPHYSIOLOGY

The majority of first trimester miscarriages are caused by a non-recurring problem in early development. The most likely cause is one of the following embryonic factors:

- A one-off genetic abnormality.

- A problem with placental implantation and development.

Other causes are responsible in very few cases:
- External causes:
  - Trauma – such as contact sports and high-speed road traffic accidents.
  - Toxin ingestion – such as large quantities of alcohol or cocaine.
- Undiagnosed medical problems in the patient can also cause miscarriage. However, because these are rarely the cause, and the birth of a live baby in a subsequent pregnancy is likely, it is not a common practice to investigate for these causes after an early pregnancy loss. Patients are offered investigation to look for these causes if they have three first trimester recurrent miscarriages or one second trimester miscarriage. However, patients with known medical conditions, such as diabetes or systemic lupus erythematosus, should have their condition optimised before trying to conceive.

[See 'Recurrent Miscarriage' page 63.]

CLINICAL FEATURES

- Vaginal bleeding.
- Abdominal pain – usually lower, cramping, intermittent, period like pain.
- No symptoms – missed miscarriage.

Bleeding occurs in a miscarriage due to shedding of the thickened endometrium. The endometrium is maintained in pregnancy by progesterone initially from the corpus luteum, followed by the developing placenta, which produces β hCG, and then by

Table 3.6   Types of Miscarriage and Their Clinical Features

TYPE OF MISCARRIAGE	CERVICAL OS	FETAL HEARTBEAT ON ULTRASOUND	HISTORY OF PAIN OR BLEEDING	DESCRIPTION
Threatened miscarriage	Closed	Yes	Yes	The fetus remains viable, and may go on to a normal birth or may progress to another type of miscarriage.
Inevitable miscarriage	Open	Yes	Yes	The fetus is currently alive, but it is definitely going to go on to miscarry, as the cervix is open.
Incomplete miscarriage	Open	No	Yes	No viable pregnancy is present, but the products of conception remain in the uterus.
Complete miscarriage	Closed	No	Yes	Ultrasound may have previously shown a pregnancy in the uterus, but now the uterus is empty. The products of conception are completely delivered out of the uterus and the cervix is closed again.
Missed miscarriage	Closed	No	No	Ultrasound scan confirms the products of conception in the uterus, but no heartbeat is detected, indicating the fetus has died. No pain or bleeding has occurred, and the cervix has not yet opened.

progesterone produced by the placenta. When the pregnancy fails, the placenta stops functioning so progesterone no longer maintains the endometrium.

Heavy bleeding can also occur during a miscarriage. As the placenta and the endometrial layer detaches from the rest of the uterus, maternal blood vessels can bleed. Uterine blood vessels run perpendicular to the muscle fibres of the uterus, so that when the uterus contracts, the blood vessels are constricted. However, with the fetus remaining within the cavity, the uterus is unable to fully contract so bleeding can continue until the uterus is empty.

Abdominal pain is caused by the uterine muscle (myometrium) contracting to expel the fetus and shed the endometrial layer. Also, the dead cells of the endometrial layer and the fetus release inflammatory cytokines, which activate pain fibres. The pains are very similar to, but often more painful than, a patient's normal menstrual cycle pains, which is expected given they are the same physiological process.

DIFFERENTIAL DIAGNOSIS

- Ectopic pregnancy.
- Molar pregnancy.
- Any other cause of abdominal pain can present while a patient is also pregnant.
- Other causes of bleeding:
  - Menstruation.
  - Vaginal laceration following trauma or assault.
  - Cervical cause; for example, ectropion.
  - Sexually transmitted infections (STIs).

A urine pregnancy test is essential to confirm the patient is pregnant.

INVESTIGATIONS

In the United Kingdom, most patients will have access to an EPAS in one of their local hospitals. These services are set up to investigate, diagnose and manage the common early pregnancy problems: miscarriage, ectopic pregnancy and the diagnosis of molar pregnancies.

Unfortunately, to make a diagnosis of either a viable pregnancy, miscarriage or ectopic pregnancy, due to the limits of our existing investigation modalities, this commonly takes between a few days to a few weeks, and repeated testing, to reach a final diagnosis.

The main diagnostic tool to assess for fetal viability is ultrasound scanning. Ultrasound probes can either be used abdominally or vaginally to assess the uterus. A transvaginal ultrasound scan can give better views of the inside of the uterus at early gestations, but due to its invasive nature, it is not acceptable to all patients.

The only way to confirm fetal viability is to see the fetal heart beating on ultrasound. However, depending on the gestation, the fetal heart may not be visible, even in a viable fetus. The last menstrual period is unfortunately not an accurate way to assess gestation.

Table 3.7 Ultrasound Scan Findings and Clinical Action in Threatened Miscarriage	
ULTRASOUND SCAN FINDING	**LIKELY DIAGNOSIS AND ACTION**
No evidence of intrauterine pregnancy	Manage as a PUL; further investigation is required, such as serum β hCG.
Gestation sac diameter less than 25 mm	Could be a miscarriage, could be an early intrauterine pregnancy, rescan in 7–14 days.
Gestation sac diameter more than 25 mm but no fetal pole seen	Miscarriage – ask for a second opinion to confirm the diagnosis, if in doubt rescan in 7 days.
Fetal pole seen but CRL less than 7 mm, and no heartbeat	Could be a miscarriage, could be an early intrauterine pregnancy, but too small to see heartbeat. Rescan in 7–14 days.
Fetal pole seen and CRL more than 7 mm and no heartbeat	Miscarriage – a heartbeat should be visible at this size – ask for a second opinion to confirm the diagnosis, if in doubt rescan in 7 days.
Fetal heartbeat seen	Viable intrauterine pregnancy confirmed.

CRL, Crown rump length; hCG, human chorionic gonadotropin; PUL, pregnancy of unknown location.

The first signs of a pregnancy on scan can usually be seen at around 4 weeks' gestation, but viability can often not be confirmed until 6 weeks' gestation.

On ultrasound, the first sign of an intrauterine pregnancy is the gestation sac seen within the uterus. If the fetus is further along in its gestation, the yolk sac may be visible within the gestation sac. If the fetus is further along still, then the fetus itself may be seen within the gestation sac, although the fetus simply looks like a thin white line on the scan in early pregnancy. Once the fetus has grown to a length of 7 mm, the fetal heart is normally visible. If the fetal heart is not seen on the first scan with a crown rump length (CRL) less than 7 mm, then a repeat scan is undertaken, usually 2 weeks later. If on that scan there is still no fetal heart, or there has not been any progression in the pregnancy, then a miscarriage has been diagnosed. Other findings on ultrasound scanning in early pregnancy are described in (Table 3.7).

PREGNANCY OF UNKNOWN LOCATION

When a scan shows no evidence of an intrauterine pregnancy and no evidence of a mass suggestive of an ectopic pregnancy in the adnexa, the patient must be treated as a PUL. Essentially, the patient is treated as a potential ectopic:

- Symptoms and signs of ectopic pregnancy are assessed.

- A serum β hCG is taken, and then a repeat sample taken 48 hours later:
  - If the β hCG has fallen by 50% or more, this is likely to represent a miscarriage.
  - If the β hCG has risen by 63% or more in 48 hours and the patient is well, then the pregnancy is likely to be intrauterine. A repeat ultrasound will likely confirm this.
  - If the β hCG has remained static, or risen or fallen only a small amount, the patient is likely to have an ectopic pregnancy.

[See 'Ectopic Pregnancy' page 52.]

MANAGEMENT

THREATENED MISCARRIAGE

If the patient has had pain or bleeding but has a viable intrauterine pregnancy, then she should be advised that she should carry on with routine antenatal care, but return if the bleeding or pain continues beyond 2 weeks from the scan or if the symptoms get worse.

There is evidence that one of the causes of miscarriage can be low levels of progesterone. Current UK guidance advises commencing vaginal progesterone pessaries in women who have had a previous miscarriage if they develop bleeding in the first trimester of the current pregnancy. The progesterone is continued until 16 weeks of pregnancy.

CONFIRMED MISCARRIAGE

There are three management options available:
1 Expectant management.
2 Medical management.
3 Surgical management.

Expectant Management

Expectant management is waiting for the uterus to contract and naturally pass the products of conception. The advantage of expectant management for some patients is that it is a natural process, thereby not 'medicalising' the patient. The disadvantage is that the timing of pain (uterine contractions), bleeding and miscarriage are unpredictable, and in around 25% of patients, the miscarriage does not occur. As a result, another management option is then required. There is also a risk of heavy bleeding occurring, requiring emergency admission for treatment.

If a patient opts for expectant management, she is advised that bleeding is likely to be similar to that of a very heavy period. Pain is typically worse than a period. Bleeding lightens after the products have passed, and often settles completely over 1 to 2 weeks.

If the miscarriage occurs and symptoms settle, patients are advised to check a pregnancy test in 3 weeks. If negative, the miscarriage is complete; if positive, they should contact the early pregnancy assessment unit as this suggests retained products of conception.

If the miscarriage has not occurred after 2 weeks or symptoms persist, the patient is advised to be reviewed again in the early pregnancy assessment unit. She can then decide whether to continue expectant management or choose one of the other options. If she chooses expectant management, she can be reviewed again in a further 2 weeks.

Expectant management is recommended as the first-line management for most miscarriages, but particularly those of less than 6 weeks' gestation. However, one of the other options with a quicker resolution of the miscarriage should be considered in patients who are bleeding heavily or who have a risk of heavy bleeding, and for patients that have signs of an intrauterine infection. If a patient is having expectant management, she should be advised to attend the assessment unit urgently if she develops signs of an infection. The risk of infection increases if the miscarriage has not been resolved after around 6 weeks of expectant management, and one of the other treatments should be strongly recommended after this time.

Medical Management

If expectant management has failed or is not acceptable to the patient, medical management can be offered. This involves giving medication either orally or vaginally to start uterine contractions and cervical dilatation, with the intention of expediting the miscarriage. There are many different regimes practiced, some requiring an inpatient stay while other patients are managed as outpatients. The regime recommended by NICE is giving 800 µg misoprostol per vagina and then allowing the patient to go home. Misoprostol is a prostaglandin analogue, which acts upon the uterus causing inflammation, uterine contractions and cervical dilation.

The benefits of medical management are that it is more likely to be successful than expectant management (around 85% success), is more predictable as to when the miscarriage will occur, and patients who have failed expectant management see medical management as less invasive than surgery. The downside to medical management is that the medication can cause contractions that are too painful for a patient to cope with at home, thereby requiring admission for analgesia. Heavy bleeding requiring emergency admission is also a risk.

In most cases, bleeding begins within 24 hours and the miscarriage should complete in a similar time period. If the miscarriage is successful, the patient should check that they have a negative pregnancy test 3 weeks later. The patient should reattend for assessment if bleeding does not start within 24 hours, bleeding or pain are too much to manage at home, symptoms do not settle after 2 weeks, or the pregnancy test after 3 weeks is positive.

Surgical Management

Surgical management of miscarriage, previously called evacuation of retained products of conception, involves passing a hollow plastic tube (suction curette) through the cervix into the uterus. The curette is then gently moved around the uterus, while the other end of the tube is attached to a vacuum so the products can be pulled out. The procedure can be performed as an outpatient using local anaesthetic on the cervix, or under general anaesthetic.

The benefit of the surgical procedure is that the date and time of the miscarriage is planned, and it has the lowest failure rate of all the options – less than 5% of cases have retained products after the procedure. The disadvantages are that it is a surgical procedure, and as well as the risk of bleeding and infection (like the other options), there is also a risk of perforating the uterus with the suction curette, which then requires an emergency laparoscopy to check for damage to internal organs such as the bladder and bowel which lie adjacent to the uterus. There is evidence that repeated surgery on the uterus can reduce fertility. There is also a rare complication of the procedure called Asherman syndrome, which is characterised by extensive scarring of the endometrium due to surgical adhesion formation so that all the walls of the cavity are fused together, obliterating the cavity, which prevents fertility.

Patients having the procedure will have a FBC and G&S taken prior to the procedure. If the patient is Rhesus negative, an IM injection of 250 IU anti-D Rhesus prophylaxis will be given, as there is a theoretical risk of fetal blood entering the maternal circulation during the procedure.

[See 'Fetal Haemolytic Disease' page 321.]

After the procedure, the patient's bleeding should settle over the following week. The patient is advised to return if bleeding does not settle or if she develops signs of an infection.

COMPLICATIONS

ECTOPIC PREGNANCY

Although rare, around 1:10,000 patients with an intrauterine pregnancy also have an ectopic pregnancy (heterotopic pregnancy). Clinicians need to consider this diagnosis if a patient has a persistently positive pregnancy test after miscarriage, or ongoing pain and bleeding.

MOLAR PREGNANCY

A miscarriage can also be a presentation of a molar pregnancy. Even after an apparently complete miscarriage (by whichever management), some of the molar pregnancy can remain and grow, which, if not identified, could be fatal. A positive pregnancy test after expectant or medical management necessitates further investigation to assess for molar pregnancy. After surgical management, the products are usually sent to histology to check for molar pregnancy.

[See 'Molar Pregnancy' page 49.]

RETAINED PRODUCTS

A number of symptoms can suggest retained products following an apparent complete miscarriage:

- Persistent bleeding beyond 2 weeks post miscarriage.
- Bleeding which had settled but then restarts heavily. This can sometimes be difficult to distinguish from the first menstruation following the miscarriage.
- Symptoms of infection.
  - Chills, fevers or rigors.
  - Abdominal pain.
  - Offensive vaginal discharge.

An ultrasound scan to look for retained products can be helpful. Depending on the amount of retained products seen and the clinical condition of the patient, oral or IV antibiotics may be prescribed, and medical or surgical management may be offered to complete the miscarriage. Clinical assessment of the patient is needed to decide on ongoing management.

PATIENT COLLAPSE AND EMERGENCY ADMISSION

- Hypovolaemic shock.
  - Tachycardia, hypotension, cold peripheries (vasoconstriction) and visible heavy blood loss.
- Cervical shock.
  - Bradycardia, hypotension and clots or products seen in the cervical os on speculum examination. These cause a vasovagal response, activating the parasympathetic nervous system, causing vasodilation, and the vagus nerve slows the heart rate.
- Septic shock.
  - Tachycardia, hypotension and warm peripheries.

Emergency admissions will need to be assessed and stabilised using an ABCDE approach for assessment. IV access, FBC and G&S are essential in all acute admissions. An assessment of blood loss can be made looking at the patient's clothes, sanitary pads and bed sheets. A speculum examination should then be performed to assess for blood in the vagina and any blood clots or products of conception passing through the cervix which may be causing cervical shock. Once stabilised, a senior gynaecologist can decide on management of the patient. An emergency surgical management of miscarriage is a likely treatment strategy if retained products cause haemorrhage or sepsis.

It is not uncommon for an emergency admission with a miscarriage to be in shock as a result of all three types of shock described above, so IV fluid resuscitation, antibiotics and removal of products from the os may all be needed to optimise the patient's condition.

PROGNOSIS

COMPLETE MISCARRIAGE

Early pregnancy loss is very difficult for the patient and their relatives. By using good communication skills to break the news and guide the patient through the process, the psychological impact on the patient can be limited.

It is important to explain to the patient that the first period after a miscarriage is likely to be 'different' from their normal period. This may be heavier, lighter, shortened, prolonged, intermittent or a combination. This is because the endometrium is returning to a non-pregnant state, and the HPO axis may take time to normalise after being altered by the hormones produced by the placental tissue.

Most clinicians advise if the patient is planning to conceive again to wait until at least one menstrual cycle. This allows time for the endometrium and HPO axis to normalise, it gives the patient time to recover physically and emotionally from the miscarriage and makes dating the pregnancy from the last menstrual period easier. Some limited evidence also suggests that pregnancies conceived very quickly after miscarriage are at a higher risk of miscarriage themselves.

Patients can be reassured that, in general, the live birth rate in a subsequent pregnancy following a miscarriage is around 80%.

Following miscarriage, there is an opportunity to optimise a patient for a future pregnancy with preconception counselling. This may simply be advice on pre-conception folic acid and vitamin D supplementation, but could include dietary advice for patients with a raised body mass index (BMI), alterations of teratogenic medications for patients on long-term medication and reviewing long-term medical conditions, such as diabetes or hypothyroidism, to optimise disease control.

THREATENED MISCARRIAGE

A small vaginal bleed in the first and second trimesters in a viable pregnancy is called a threatened miscarriage. A threatened miscarriage slightly increases the risk of this pregnancy progressing to a complete miscarriage, although the majority progress to a live baby.

A threatened miscarriage associated with heavy bleeding (like a period) in an early pregnancy which remains viable is at risk of intrauterine growth restriction later in pregnancy. This is thought to be due to poor placental function. Serial fetal growth scans should be organised to monitor for growth restriction from 28 weeks' gestation.

❓ QUESTIONS

Shana, a 22-year-old woman, presents to her primary care physician. She missed a period 4 weeks ago and has only had a small amount of bleeding over the last few days when her current period was due. The doctor takes a urine sample and performs a pregnancy test, which is positive. On further questioning, the patient states that her last menstruation was 8 weeks ago, and she has been experiencing cramping suprapubic abdominal pain for the last week. The GP refers the patient to the early pregnancy assessment.

A Asherman syndrome.	H Molar pregnancy.
B Complete miscarriage.	I Munchausen
C Ectopic pregnancy.	pregnancy.
D Incomplete miscarriage.	J Pregnancy of unknown
E Indelible miscarriage.	location.
F Inevitable miscarriage.	K Threatened miscarriage.
G Missed miscarriage.	L Viable pregnancy.

Select the most likely diagnosis from the choices above.

Q1 A patient with a confirmed 8 week intrauterine pregnancy presents with vaginal bleeding; the cervical os is closed.

Q2 A patient with a confirmed 8 week intrauterine pregnancy presents with vaginal bleeding; the cervical os is open.

Q3 A patient who believes she is 8 weeks pregnant presents with light vaginal bleeding. An ultrasound scan reveals no pregnancy. A pregnancy test was positive 2 days ago.

Q4 A patient who believes she is 8 weeks pregnant presents with light vaginal bleeding, but had a heavy bleed the day before when she thinks she passed some products of conception; the cervical os is closed. An ultrasound scan reveals disorganised products of conception.

Q5 A patient attends for a dating scan at 12 weeks' gestation. A 12 week size fetus is seen within the uterus, but there is no fetal heartbeat.

Q6 Which of the following statements regarding miscarriage are true or false?

A Prostaglandin E_1 can be used to manage a miscarriage.

B Surgical management of miscarriage is the best treatment option for miscarriage.

C Miscarriage is complete when there is no longer a fetal heartbeat seen on ultrasound.

D An incomplete miscarriage on ultrasound excludes the diagnosis of ectopic pregnancy.

E A threatened miscarriage may occur in a pregnancy which goes on to full term.

Q7 In an emergency admission to the emergency department (ED), a patient who is miscarrying has profound hypotension and a heart rate of 50 bpm. Which is the most likely cause of these signs?

A Beta blockade.

B Cervical shock.

C Electrolyte disturbance.

D Hypovolaemic shock.

E Septic shock.

[Answers on page 181.]

RECURRENT MISCARRIAGE

Recurrent miscarriage is defined as the loss of three or more pregnancies before 24 weeks' gestation.

AETIOLOGY

Recurrent miscarriage affects 1% of couples trying to conceive. Miscarriage early in pregnancy is common, with approximately 20% of pregnancies ending in miscarriage in the first trimester (up to 12 weeks' gestation). After a couple has had three consecutive first trimester miscarriages, their risk of a subsequent miscarriage is 40%. Investigation and treatment is offered to improve the chance of a successful subsequent pregnancy.

Miscarriages do occur in the second trimester (12 to 24 weeks gestation), but it is much less common than the first trimester, with around 1% to 2% of pregnancies miscarrying in the second trimester. Investigations to identify the cause of miscarriage are offered after one second trimester miscarriage.

PATHOPHYSIOLOGY

Below is an explanation of potential causes of recurrent miscarriage. All these potential causes are investigated, and if any of the investigations reveal a possible cause, treatment can be started to improve subsequent pregnancy outcome.

AGE AND GENETICS

Increasing parental age increases the risk of genetic abnormalities, which can be fatal and end in miscarriage (Table 3.8). As previously stated, the population average risk of a single pregnancy ending in a first trimester miscarriage is 20%. When this figure is split by maternal age, it is clear the risk dramatically increases with a maternal age over 40.

There is also a trend for miscarriage rates to increase if the paternal age is greater than 40, but the evidence is not as clear as for maternal age.

The reason for this increase is due to the increased risk of meiotic non-disjunction. During meiosis I or meiosis II of gamete production, a set of chromosomes does not separate, resulting in one gamete having one extra chromosome and one gamete having one less. The resulting pregnancy using one of these gametes will then either be aneuploid (e.g Turner syndrome, XO) or triploid (e.g. Down trisomy 21, Edward trisomy 18 and Patau trisomy 13). The most common chromosomal abnormality identified in miscarriage is Turner syndrome. Up to 50% of recurrent miscarriages are caused by these sporadic chromosomal abnormalities.

Up to 5% of recurrent miscarriages are caused by a genetic abnormality in one of the parents. This is most commonly a result of a balanced translocation. This is where the patient has a full set of chromosomes but two or more chromosomes have swapped pieces off each other. The patient has the correct number of chromosomes but they are in the wrong place. The parent is usually phenotypically normal. Unfortunately, when they make gametes, the translocation often does not remain balanced, so in the resulting pregnancy, the embryo has an unbalanced translocation, an incorrect amount for at least one chromosome. This is almost always fatal and results in miscarriage (Fig. 3.7).

After three consecutive first trimester miscarriages or one second trimester miscarriage, the products of miscarriage should be sent for karyotyping. If a sporadic chromosomal abnormality is identified, no further investigation is required. However, if a possible inherited abnormality is identified, such as a translocation, the parents' blood can also be taken to look for a balanced translocation in one of the partners.

The options of treatment for a genetic cause need to be discussed on an individualised basis with couples, usually by a geneticist. The options broadly are to try for spontaneous pregnancy, *in vitro* fertilisation (IVF) pregnancy with pre-implantation genetic diagnosis (PIGD) or IVF with donor gametes. PIGD involves IVF with one or two cells removed from the developing embryos to analyse for genetic abnormality, and then implanting normal embryos in the uterus.

For a couple where the female is over the age of 45, any subsequent spontaneous pregnancy has a very high chance of lethal chromosomal abnormalities. The most appropriate option for this couple if pregnancy is desired may be IVF with donor eggs, but IVF with PIGD could also be considered. It is important to remember that IVF has strict criteria for National Health Service (NHS) funding, and patients not eligible for funding may not be able to afford private treatment.

[See 'Infertility' page 35.]

ANTIPHOSPHOLIPID SYNDROME

Antiphospholipid syndrome is the most common non-genetic cause of miscarriage, identified in 15% of females with recurrent miscarriage. It leads to miscarriage by causing inflammation and activating complement proteins at the placental bed, resulting in poor placental development and thrombosis of the vasculature. Blood tests are performed for lupus anticoagulant and anticardiolipin antibodies. If either is positive, the tests are repeated 12 weeks later. Two positive samples

Table **3.8** Maternal Age and Risk of Miscarriage	
MATERNAL AGE (YEARS)	**MISCARRIAGE RISK**
16–34	12%
35–39	25%
40–44	50%
More than 45	More than 90%

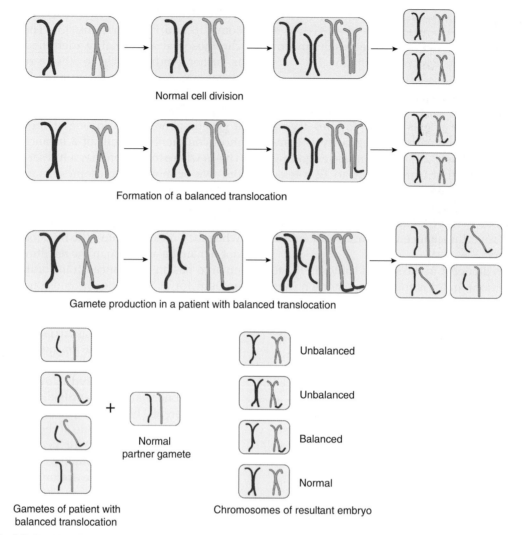

Fig. 3.7 Simplified Example of Balanced and Unbalanced Translocations. The vast majority of pregnancies from a patient with a balanced translocation are unbalanced.

separated by 12 weeks are diagnostic. It is also advisable not to test in pregnancy, or for the first 12 weeks after a pregnancy, due to a significant false positive rate.

Treatment of antiphospholipid syndrome in a subsequent pregnancy involves administration of low molecular weight heparin (LMWH) from the time when pregnancy is diagnosed, and low dose aspirin (75–150 mg) from 12 weeks onwards. These have been shown to improve pregnancy outcome, with a mechanism of action of reducing thrombosis of the placental vasculature and improving trophoblastic differentiation.

Aspirin is regarded as safe in pregnancy from the second trimester. LMWH does not cross the placenta, but maternal risks are the same for any person given LMWH: an increased propensity to bleed and, very rarely, heparin-induced thrombocytopaenia.

THROMBOPHILIAS

Thrombophilias have the greatest adverse effect on the fetus in the second and third trimester, where thrombosis of uteroplacental vessels cause placental

insufficiency and result in intrauterine growth restriction and/or stillbirth. For this reason, thrombophilia testing is usually reserved for investigation following a second trimester miscarriage. However, thrombophilias may also have an effect on early miscarriages, so some clinicians do test for them as part of recurrent first trimester miscarriage investigation. Thrombophilias can be inherited or acquired. The most common thrombophilias investigated for (by maternal blood tests) are:

- Factor V Leiden.
- Factor II (prothrombin gene mutation).
- Protein S deficiency.
- Protein C deficiency.
- Antithrombin III deficiency.

Protein S causes a 14-fold increase in miscarriage rates, whereas the other thrombophilias increase the risk by around five times. The most common thrombophilia identified is factor V Leiden; up to 5% of Caucasians are heterozygous for the mutation and 1% are homozygous. If any of these thrombophilias are identified, management of a subsequent pregnancy is with LMWH. Warfarin is teratogenic, so it is not considered as a management option.

ENDOCRINE

Uncontrolled DM, hyperthyroidism and hypothyroidism all increase the risk of miscarriage and stillbirth. However, if these conditions are well controlled, there is no increased miscarriage risk. Testing for these conditions in recurrent miscarriage should be reserved for patients who are symptomatic of disease. The blood tests are TSH, free thyroxine (T_4), and fasting blood glucose. The management of these conditions in the context of pregnancy is covered in more detail in separate chapters.

[See 'Thyroid Disease in Pregnancy' page 239.]
[See 'Diabetes in Pregnancy' page 228.]

UTERINE MALFORMATIONS

Both an arcuate and a septate uterus are associated with miscarriage. These are identified on a pelvic ultrasound scan. If an abnormality is seen, it can be further imaged with a hysteroscopy or hysterosalpingogram (HSG). An HSG requires the injection of a radio-opaque dye into the uterus through the cervix while x-rays are taken; this identifies the shape of the uterine cavity. To correct a uterine malformation, operative hysteroscopy or laparoscopy may be performed. Uterine surgery has a risk of causing scarring. Scar tissues can reduce fertility and can cause uterine weakness, increasing the risk of uterine rupture in pregnancy and during labour.

Research is ongoing into the histological features of the endometrium which may prevent implantation in some patients. Some centres are trialling 'scratching' of the endometrium during hysteroscopy in an attempt to increase the chances of successful implantation.

LIFESTYLE FACTORS

Obesity, smoking and moderate alcohol intake (more than five units per week) may all increase the rates of miscarriage and decrease fertility rates. To increase the chances of a successful pregnancy, patients are advised to achieve a healthy BMI, stop smoking, stop alcohol intake, stop any unnecessary medications prior to pregnancy and during pregnancy, eat a healthy diet and take regular exercise. Pre-pregnancy vitamins, in particular folic acid and vitamin D, are also advised (as they would be in any pregnancy).

PROGESTERONE

High levels of progesterone maintain the uterine environment to support a healthy ongoing pregnancy. It is believed that low progesterone levels in early pregnancy contribute to miscarriages in some women, with evidence that the more unexplained miscarriages a woman has the more likely it is that progesterone deficiency may be a causative factor.

In the UK progesterone testing in pregnancy is not currently undertaken. If a woman with at least one previous miscarriage develops vaginal bleeding (threatened miscarriage) in the first trimester of a current pregnancy, they are advised to take progesterone (given as vaginal pessaries) up to 16 weeks gestation to support the ongoing pregnancy to reduce the risk of miscarriage.

INVESTIGATIONS IN A SUBSEQUENT PREGNANCY FOLLOWING A SECOND TRIMESTER MISCARRIAGE

Cervix

Some second trimester miscarriages can occur due to cervical incompetence—a weak cervix that dilates and causes a miscarriage. Risk factors for this include previous cervical surgery, such as a LLETZ, and uterine malformations.

There is no investigation to test for cervical incompetence. If a previous second trimester miscarriage is thought to have been caused by cervical incompetence, then in subsequent pregnancies serial cervical length scans are offered, usually every 2 weeks from 16 to 24 weeks. If the length shortens to less than 2.5 cm, then progesterone pessaries or cervical cerclage may be offered. Cerclage is a 'purse string' stitch used to hold the cervix closed. A cerclage is usually inserted in theatre under local, regional or general anaesthesia. A speculum is inserted into the vagina to view the cervix, and a stitch is then tied around the cervix as proximal to the uterus as safely possible. If successful, the stitch is taken out around 36 weeks to allow for labour. If labour commences before this time, the stitch is removed as an emergency to prevent the cervix from tearing as it tries to dilate with the stitch in place.

Infection

Any large systemic infection can cause miscarriage. The cause for this is not clear but may be related to inflammation and the maternal immune response.

There is also an association with bacterial vaginosis (BV) and second trimester miscarriage. BV is normally asymptomatic, but can present as a fishy-smelling, white-coloured vaginal discharge. It is caused by an overgrowth of normal bacterial flora of the vagina, often resulting in a reduced number of lactobacilli and increased numbers of bacteria like *Gardnerella vaginalis*.

In a subsequent pregnancy, some obstetricians advise taking low vaginal swabs in the first and second trimesters, and if BV is diagnosed, treating with a course of antibiotics, such as clindamycin or metronidazole.

[See 'Sexually Transmitted Infections' page 124.]

PROGNOSIS

If a cause for recurrent miscarriage is identified, appropriate treatment should improve the chance of a successful

Table 3.9 Summary of Management of Recurrent Miscarriage

CAUSE	INVESTIGATION	TREATMENT
Genetics: parental age, parental genetic abnormality	Fetal karyotyping +/– parental karyotyping	Pre-implantation genetic diagnosis or donor gametes
Antiphospholipid syndrome	Serum lupus anticoagulant anticardio-lipin antibodies	Aspirin and LMWH
Thrombophilia	Protein S, protein C, antithrombin III, factor V Leiden, prothrombin gene mutation	LMWH
Thyroid dysfunction (test if symptomatic)	Serum TSH and T_4	Hypothyroid: levothyroxine Hyperthyroid: propylthiouracil
Diabetes (test if symptomatic)	Serum glucose	Diet, metformin, insulin
Uterine abnormality	Pelvic ultrasound scan +/– hysterosal-pingogram or MRI	Operative laparoscopy or hysteroscopy
Lifestyle factors	Obtained from history taking	Optimise BMI, stop smoking and alcohol, stop unnecessary medications, advise folic acid and vitamin D
Additional Investigations in Subsequent Pregnancy for Second Trimester Miscarriages		
Infection	Low vaginal swabs for bacterial vaginosis in first and second trimester	Antibiotic treatment
Cervical incompetence (previous loss 16–24 weeks)	Cervical length scans every 2 weeks from 16 to 24 weeks gestation	Cervical cerclage or progesterone pessaries if scan suggests shortening cervix

BMI, Body mass index; *LMWH*, low molecular weight heparin; T_4, thyroxine; *TSH*, thyroid-stimulating hormone.

pregnancy (Table 3.9). If the cause of miscarriage is not found after investigations, this is actually quite reassuring. In a future pregnancy if any of these women develop bleeding in the first trimester they will also be offered progesterone pessaries to reduce the risk of miscarriage.

Overall, 75% of patients with recurrent miscarriage (under the age of 40) will go on to have a successful subsequent pregnancy.

❓ QUESTIONS

Mrs Thompson has recently had her fourth miscarriage in the last 2 years. She has never had a live birth. Her primary care physician has referred her to the gynaecology team to advise her on how to maximise her chance of a successful pregnancy.

Q1   Which statement is correct regarding miscarriage?
  A First trimester pregnancies end in miscarriage in 50% of cases.
  B Miscarriage is defined as a pregnancy loss up to 12 weeks' gestation.
  C Miscarriage is defined as pregnancy loss up to 16 weeks' gestation.
  D Miscarriage is defined as pregnancy loss up to 24 weeks' gestation.
  E Recurrent miscarriage investigations are advised if a patient has two or more consecutive first trimester miscarriages.

Q2   Answer true or false: Which of these factors is associated with recurrent miscarriage?
  A Cocaine use.
  B Haemophilia.

  C Hyperthyroidism.
  D Maternal age more than 40.
  E Vigorous exercise.

Q3   No cause for recurrent miscarriages is found in Mrs Thompson. Which of the following medications would you advise her to take, either before or during a subsequent pregnancy?
  A Aspirin.
  B Carbimazole.
  C Folic acid.
  D LMWH.
  E None of the above.

[Answers on page 183.]

TERMINATION OF PREGNANCY

Termination of pregnancy is the process of intentionally ending a pregnancy so that it does not result in the birth of a baby. Another term used interchangeably with termination is abortion.

EPIDEMIOLOGY

- There are approximately 1 million pregnancies in the United Kingdom each year.
- Twenty percent of these pregnancies will end in a miscarriage.
- Twenty percent of these pregnancies will end by termination.

- Ninety-eight percent of terminations are performed for what are commonly referred to as 'social indications'.
- One percent of terminations are performed for severe fetal abnormality.
- Less than 1% of terminations are performed where continuing the pregnancy would risk severe harm or death of the mother.
- Ninety percent of terminations are performed before 12 weeks, with less than 1% performed after 20 weeks.

The term social termination is used throughout this section. This refers to any legal termination where the indication is not either risk of death or severe injury to the pregnant woman or risk of a child born severely handicapped.

UK LAW

The Abortion Act 1967 was originally enacted to put an end to the high number of dangerous, unregulated, illegal terminations being carried out, which caused serious morbidity and mortality in the women that sought them. The result of this law is that termination of pregnancy is now a very safe medical procedure, but the legalisation has also increased the number of terminations carried out.

The key points of the Abortion Act 1967:
- Terminations can only be carried out in a hospital or a specialist licensed clinic.
- Two doctors must agree on the indication for the termination and both must sign a certificate.
- Doctors with a moral objection to termination do not have to certify a termination but they must recommend a doctor who will.
- There are four indications for a termination listed in the act, of which one must be fulfilled for a termination to be legally certified:

A The pregnancy has not exceeded the 24th week of gestation and that the continuance of the pregnancy would involve risk, greater than if the pregnancy were terminated, of either:
  - Injury to the physical or mental health of the pregnant women.
  - Injury to the physical or mental health of any existing children of the family of the pregnant woman.

B Termination is necessary to prevent grave permanent injury to the physical or mental health of the pregnant woman.

C Continuing the pregnancy would risk the life of the pregnant woman.

D There is substantial risk that if the child were born, it would suffer physical or mental abnormalities that would render it seriously handicapped.

Terminations for indications B, C and D can be carried out at any gestation. Terminations for indication A cannot be carried out beyond 24 weeks' gestation. Indication A is the indication fulfilled when terminations are carried out for 'social indications'.

Termination of Pregnancy Around the World

The law on abortion varies greatly in different countries and can even vary between different states within a country.
Europe
- Republic of Ireland – termination is permitted unconditionally up to 12 weeks of pregnancy. Termination of pregnancy after 12 weeks is only permitted where there is significant threat to the life of the mother or there is a fatal fetal abnormality.
- Poland – termination is legal in cases of threat to the life of the mother, severe fetal abnormality and cases of rape. Poland has the lowest recorded rates of abortion in Europe, with only around 0.1% of pregnancies ending in termination.
- Russia – unconditional termination before 12 weeks of gestation. Russia has the highest termination rate in Europe, with approximately 40% pregnancies being terminated.
- Netherlands – The legal time limit for termination is 24 weeks but late abortion after the 24th week is possible for serious medical reasons only.
- Others – most other European countries allow terminations with few restrictions up to around 12 weeks' gestation, with terminations legal at later gestations in specific situations.

Africa, South America and the Middle East
- In most countries, termination is either illegal or only permitted in select situations, such as severe threat to the life of the mother.
- South Africa, Turkey, Cuba and Uruguay are less restrictive, with termination legal in the first trimester and later in specific instances.

Asia and Indonesia
- In most countries, termination is either illegal or only permitted in select situations, such as rape or incest, and often needs consent of the parents or spouse.
- Termination is broadly permitted in the first trimester in China, Cambodia and Nepal.

USA, Canada, Australia
- Federal systems have different rules for different states/territories, but termination is commonly permitted in the first trimester, and later for specific indications.
- As of 2023, a few US states had made terminations illegal, with many other states increasing the number of specific restrictions regarding abortion.

PRESENTATION

Women requesting a social termination most commonly present to their primary care physician or family planning clinic, or they may directly refer themselves to a termination service. Women meeting the criteria for a termination for severe maternal or fetal health reasons will almost always be under the care of a specialist obstetric team.

The reasons a woman is requesting a social termination should be sought, but the clinician completing the termination certificate should be adequately trained to understand the vast number of reasons and the varying degrees these reasons effect a patient. An example of some potential reasons include:

- Religious reasons.
- Social situation that present major challenges with bringing up a child.
- Family already complete.
- Timing not suitable.
- Pregnant as a result of rape.

CONSENT

The earlier an abortion is carried out, the easier and safer the procedure is to perform. However, the patient must be given sufficient time to consider all her options so that she is as comfortable as possible with her decision.

The consent process for a termination is the same as for any other medical procedure. However, it is particularly important that alternatives to termination are fully explored. These include:

- Keeping the baby.
- Adoption.
- For a fetus with a severe handicap, palliative care following birth.

Discussion with health professionals, counsellors and, where appropriate, family members, friends and the partner may help the woman decide on her care. It is important, where possible, to identify and prevent external influences, coercion or any pressure that may affect a patient's decision.

 Under the Age of 16

If a child under 16 years of age requests a termination, as with any procedure she can do so without informing her parents as long as the clinicians believe the procedure is in her best interests and she demonstrates Gillick competence (in line with the Fraser guidelines). Of course, clinicians should encourage parental involvement in the decision. A clinician will also have to consider breaking confidentiality on the grounds of safeguarding the child, depending on the circumstances of the pregnancy.

[See 'Contraception' page 71.]

INVESTIGATIONS

- Confirming gestation – LMP and ultrasound.
- Offer screening for STIs.
- Other tests dependent on gestation and mode of termination:
  - Full blood count.
  - Group and save – collected in case of haemorrhage. Rhesus status can also be obtained; if Rhesus negative, the patient should be offered anti-D after termination.

MANAGEMENT

The management options are similar to the options for miscarriage. Roughly 50% of patients opt for medical termination and 50% choose surgical termination.

MEDICAL TERMINATION

Mifepristone is given as a tablet. It is an anti-progestogen which counters the supportive effect of progesterone on the uterus, resulting in endometrial shedding and a loss of blood supply to the developing fetus, resulting in pregnancy loss. After 36 to 48 hours, one or more courses (depending on gestation) of a prostaglandin (usually misoprostol) are given. This causes cervical dilatation and uterine contractions, which expel the pregnancy. Medical termination can be used at any gestation. The earlier the gestation, the less pain and bleeding occurs, and there is less likely to be retained products.

For late terminations (beyond 20 weeks), feticide (injection of potassium chloride into the fetal heart to cause a fatal arrhythmia) will be offered prior to the rest of the medical management to improve the success rate of the termination. The fetal tissues are also softened after death, making the fetus easier to expel. Performing feticide will also prevent the delivered fetus from showing signs of life, which could understandably be very distressing.

SURGICAL TERMINATION

A plastic tube with a blunt scraper is inserted through the cervix into the uterine cavity. Scraping of the tube against the walls of the uterus whilst suction is attached to the end of the tube pulls away the pregnancy, completing the termination. The procedure can be done with a local anaesthetic block on the cervix or under general anaesthetic. Misoprostol is often given vaginally before the procedure to soften the cervix, making it easier to pass the tube into the uterus.

Surgical termination may not be appropriate before 7 weeks' gestation, as the uterus is very small before this point, and there is an increased risk of perforation. After 15 weeks' gestation, the bones begin to harden, which means that surgical termination may require the surgeon to break the bones of the fetus inside the uterus in order to remove it. For this reason, at later gestations, surgical termination is associated with higher rates of retained products of conception. Strong consideration should be given to medical management beyond 15 weeks.

COMPLICATIONS

- Intrauterine infection.
  - Complicates 10% of terminations.
  - Presents with pain, fever and vaginal discharge.
  - A course of antibiotics may be all that is required.
- Retained products of conception.
  - Occurs in 5% of terminations.

- Presents either as an infection despite antibiotics or as ongoing pain and bleeding.
- Identified with an ultrasound to confirm retained products.
- Repeat medical or surgical management is offered to empty the uterus.

RARE COMPLICATIONS

- Haemorrhage – everyone will have some bleeding after a termination, which reduces gradually over a couple of weeks. 1:1000 will have a severe haemorrhage. They will require fluid resuscitation and blood products, and if not settling, an examination under general anaesthetic to control the bleeding.
- Failed termination – occurs in 3:1000 cases; if this occurs, the termination can be repeated.

PROGNOSIS

PSYCHOLOGICAL IMPACT

Women vary greatly in their emotional responses to having a termination. Termination most commonly does not lead to long-term mental health problems, but a patient may require short-term support, so they should have access to a counselling service. Women often describe emotions including feelings of guilt, sadness and disappointment. Partners are often neglected in these situations, but they should also be included as they often also suffer temporary distress, with feelings of guilt, apprehension and a sense of loss of control.

CONTRACEPTION

It is essential to discuss, and where possible start, contraception following a termination to prevent a repeat unwanted pregnancy. In many cases, a long-term contraception, such as a Mirena, copper coil or implant, may be inserted at the same as undergoing the termination.

[See 'Contraception' page 71.]

FUTURE PREGNANCIES

A single termination is not associated with any significant increase in complications in future pregnancies. However, recurrent surgical terminations or complications associated with termination may reduce future fertility.

❓ QUESTIONS

Elizabeth is an 18-year-old girl who is medically well. She has a regular boyfriend and uses condoms and the combined oral contraceptive pill. Her period is 6 weeks late and she has just undertaken a urinary pregnancy test, confirming she is pregnant. She visits her primary care physician requesting a termination.

Q1 What is the maximum gestation at which most terminations can be legally performed in the United Kingdom?
- **A** 12 weeks.
- **B** 16 weeks.
- **C** 20 weeks.
- **D** 24 weeks.
- **E** There is no limit; any termination can be carried out at any gestation.

Q2 Answer true or false: The following statements could be valid reasons for a doctor to support the above patient's request for a termination of pregnancy.
- **A** She is very worried about a change in her body shape as a result of pregnancy.
- **B** She is currently a regular smoker and would like to quit smoking before having a baby.
- **C** She thinks the unborn child may not be her boyfriend's.
- **D** She wants to go to university before starting a family.
- **E** She has fallen pregnant following a sexual assault.

Q3 After careful consideration, Elizabeth decides to continue the pregnancy. The 20-week anomaly scan shows significant fetal abnormalities. An amniocentesis confirms the fetus has Down syndrome. Elizabeth is now 28 weeks pregnant. Which of the following statements is correct?
- **A** If Elizabeth decides to terminate this pregnancy, she must do so by 34 weeks' gestation.
- **B** Surgical termination would be the most appropriate method of termination at this gestation.
- **C** If Elizabeth decides to terminate the pregnancy, performing a feticide could be considered.
- **D** Three doctors are required to certify a termination at this gestation.
- **E** The child could not be offered for adoption after birth.

[Answers on page 184.]

KEY REFERENCES

HYPEREMESIS GRAVIDARUM

National Institute for Health and Clinical Excellence, 2021. Antenatal care. NICE Clinical Guideline (NG201).

Qureshi, Z., Maxwell, S., 2014. Unofficial Guide to Prescribing. Churchill Livingstone, London.

Royal College of Obstetricians and Gynaecologists, 2016. The management of nausea and vomiting in pregnancy, and hyperemesis gravidarum. RCOG Green Top Guideline (GTG 69).

MOLAR PREGNANCY

National Institute for Health and Clinical Excellence, 2022. Ectopic pregnancy and miscarriage: diagnosis and initial management. NICE Clinical guideline (NG126).

Royal College of Obstetricians and Gynaecologists, 2020. Gestational trophoblastic disease. RCOG Green Top Guideline (GTG 38).

ECTOPIC PREGNANCY

National Institute for Health and Clinical Excellence, 2022. Ectopic pregnancy and miscarriage: diagnosis and initial management. NICE Clinical guideline (NG126).

Royal College of Obstetricians and Gynaecologists, 2016. Diagnosis and management of ectopic pregnancy. RCOG Green Top Guideline (GTG 21).

MISCARRIAGE

National Institute for Health and Clinical Excellence, 2019. Ectopic pregnancy and miscarriage: diagnosis and initial management. NICE Clinical Guideline (CG 129).

RECURRENT MISCARRIAGE

Royal College of Obstetricians and Gynaecologists, 2022. Cervical cerclage. RCOG Green Top Guideline (GTG 75).

Royal College of Obstetricians and Gynaecologists, 2022. The investigation and treatment of couples with recurrent miscarriage. RCOG Green Top Guideline (GTG 17).

TERMINATION OF PREGNANCY

Centre for reproductive rights: The world's abortion laws, Cited 10 January 2022. Available from: http://worldabortionlaws.com

National Institute for Health and Clinical Excellence, 2019. Abortion care. NICE Clinical Guideline (NG140).

Royal College of Obstetricians and Gynaecologists, 2011. The care of women requesting induced abortion. Evidence Based Clinical Guideline No.7.

United Kingdom Government, 2012. Abortion Act 1967.

World Health Organization, 2022. Global Abortion Policies Database.

Benign Gynaecology

CONTRACEPTION

Contraception involves the use of methods or techniques to prevent pregnancy. A wide variety of contraceptive methods are available (see Tables 4.1–4.3) with individual choice based on weighing up the risks, benefits, cautions, contraindications and practicalities for each patient. Aside from the barrier methods of contraception, none of the other methods described protect against STIs.

COMBINED OESTROGEN AND PROGESTERONE CONTRACEPTION

All combined forms of contraception contain both a form of oestrogen and progesterone; therefore, the user experiences the risks and benefits of each hormone. The underlying principle of any combined contraception is that oestrogen, and to a lesser extent progesterone, inhibits the HPO axis at the hypothalamus and pituitary. This results in decreased FSH and LH release, which prevents oestrogen production and folliculogenesis in the ovaries, resulting in anovulation. Decreased oestrogen production reduces the amount of endometrial proliferation, thereby also reducing menstruation volume and pain. The cervical mucus is also thickened by combined forms of contraception, reducing the ability of sperm to enter the uterine cavity. However, it is anovulation that has the main contraceptive action.

PROGESTOGEN-ONLY CONTRACEPTION

All progestogen-only contraceptives thicken the cervical mucus to act as a physical barrier to sperm, and they also thin the endometrium so that implantation is less likely. Thinning the endometrium reduces the blood volume lost during menstruation, so these medications can be used to treat menorrhagia. Many progestogens also inhibit ovulation (the Desogestrel pill and medroxyprogesterone intramuscular (IM) injection, in particular). Compared to the combined contraceptives, there are fewer risks, as the disadvantages associated with oestrogen are lost. All contraceptives, except the combined contraceptives, can be used while breastfeeding.

NON-HORMONAL CONTRACEPTION

Many women prefer to use non-hormonal contraception because of the perceived or experienced risks and side effects of contraceptives involving hormones. Condoms and diaphragms, however, are prone to user error. The copper intrauterine device (IUD), in comparison, is fitted by a health professional but has contraindications that should be considered. Female condoms also exist as a non-hormonal contraception but are not included here as they have a failure rate of around 20% so are not recommended as an effective form of contraception.

Table 4.1 Combined Forms of Contraception

TYPE OF CONTRACEPTION	BRIEF DESCRIPTION	ADVANTAGES	DISADVANTAGES	PRACTICAL ADVICE	CAUTIONS	CONTRAINDICATIONS
Combined oral contraceptive pill (COCP)	• Contains an oestrogen and a progestogen. • Different regimens exist but users typically take a tablet once daily for 21 days and then have a 7-day break for a withdrawal bleed. • To reduce menstruation frequency, another option is tricycling the COCP. After 21 days of pill use, rather than having a break, a new pack is started for a further 21 days. This can be done again at the end of that pack. After three packets (63 days), a pill free week will then allow menstruation.	• 99% effective if used properly. • Reversible, easy to take. • Lightens the period, reduces dysmenorrhoea and premenstrual symptoms. • Reduces the risk of ovarian and endometrial cancer, ovarian cysts and benign breast disease.	• Needs to be taken regularly – user dependent. • Unsuitable if a patient has two cautions, for example, being a smoker and aged over 35, or one contraindication. • Side effects include nausea, vomiting, abdominal cramps, fluid retention, breast tenderness and spotting in early cycles. • Increased risk of venous thromboembolism (VTE). • Cannot be used while breastfeeding. • Small increased risk of breast cand cervical cancer.	• Detailed explanation on page 77.	• Age over 35 years. • BMI more than 30 kg/m². • Family history of VTE, arterial disease or breast cancer. • Migraines without focal aura. • Hypertension and diabetes. • Smoker. • Long term. immobility.	• Age over 50 years. • BMI more than 35 kg/m². • Venous thrombosis or arterial disease. • Breast cancer history. • Severe migraine with associated aura. • Hypertension or diabetes with associated complications. • Undiagnosed vaginal bleeding. • Prothrombotic blood disorders. • Taking liver enzyme-inducing drugs. • Hepatic impairment. • Gallstones. • Breastfeeding.
Contraceptive patch.	• A 5 cm × 5 cm patch that sticks to the skin. • Contains an oestrogen and progestogen.	• Over 99% effective. • Applied once a week. • Unaffected by diarrhoea and vomiting. • Bleeding usually becomes more regular, lighter and less painful. • It may help with premenstrual symptoms. • May improve acne.	• It can be seen. • Occasionally causes skin irritation. • Side effects include nausea, headaches, breast tenderness and mood changes. • Breakthrough bleeding and spotting are also common in the first few months of use. • Increased risk of VTE.	• Patches are used like the pill with three patches used for a week each, then a patch free week which allows menstruation. • Women should be advised to change the area where they put the patch and not to put the patch on their breasts. • If the patch falls off or stays on for <48 hours stick it back on with a plaster or take it off as necessary, if more than 48 hours has elapsed then a new patch cycle will need to be commenced.	Same as COCP	Same as COCP

Table 4.1 Combined Forms of Contraception—Cont'd

TYPE OF CONTRACEPTION	BRIEF DESCRIPTION	ADVANTAGES	DISADVANTAGES	PRACTICAL ADVICE	CAUTIONS	CONTRAINDICATIONS
Contraceptive ring.	• A flexible, transparent, plastic ring that is placed in the vagina, releasing both oestrogen and a progestogen.	• Over 99% effective. • Not affected by diarrhoea and vomiting. • Not user dependent. • Otherwise same advantages as the COCP.	• Some women may not feel comfortable inserting it. • Sometimes partners may be able to feel it during intercourse which some people find a disadvantage; however, it cannot affect or harm a partner in any way. • Increased risk of VTE. • Otherwise, same disadvantages as COCP.	• The ring should be left in the vagina for 21 days. After that, it should be removed and there should be a ring-free interval of 7 days where a withdrawal bleed occurs. • To insert, squeeze the ring between your thumb and finger and insert into the vagina until it feels comfortable. It does not need to be in an exact position. • Most women cannot feel the ring, but if they can, they need to push it further into the vagina. • To remove the ring, grasp it and gently pull it out.	Same as COCP	Same as COCP

Table 4.2 Forms of Contraception Containing Progestogens Only

TYPE OF CONTRACEPTION	BRIEF DESCRIPTION	ADVANTAGES	DISADVANTAGES	PRACTICAL ADVICE	CAUTIONS	CONTRAINDICATIONS
Progestogen-only pill (POP).	• Progestogens thicken the cervical mucus. • Some of the POPs also cause anovulation, for example Desogestrel. • Pills are taken every day without a break.	• 99% effective if used correctly. • It can be used whilst breastfeeding. • Useful in patients who are not suitable for the COCP, for example a smoker aged over 35. • May help with premenstrual symptoms and painful periods, particularly if they induce anovulation.	• Can cause irregular, light, or more frequent periods or periods may stop altogether. • The patient must remember to take the pill every day. • Temporary side effects, including spotty skin, breast tenderness, weight change and headaches. • Progesterone is the likely cause of premenstrual disorder (PMD). Therefore, progestogens can worsen PMD symptoms.	• It can be started on any day of the cycle and gives immediate protection. • The POP must be taken at the same time every day. • If it is taken later than 3 hours after the time when the pill should have been taken, follow the same advice as the COCP. • Many of the same guidance regarding the COCP should also be given to women on the POP; in particular, guidance on diarrhoea and vomiting, or medications that reduce the effectiveness of the POP for contraceptive purposes.	• Cardiovascular disease or a stroke. • Liver disease. • Systemic lupus erythematosus. • Current breast cancer or breast cancer within the last 5 years. • Deep vein thrombosis (DVT) or pulmonary embolism (PE), particularly if using high dose preparation.	• Taking liver enzyme-inducing drugs.
Intrauterine system (IUS) (contain Levonorgestrel, also called LNG-IUS).	• T-shaped plastic frame that releases progestogen. • Inserted into the uterus through the cervix. • Two strings are left hanging out of the cervix which can be felt to check the IUS remains in place.	• Over 99% effective. • Reduces menstrual blood loss. • Up to 40% of patients have anovulation and amenorrhoea. • Reduces dysmenorrhoea. • Long acting. • 52 mg IUS licensed for 5 years in UK, the 13.5 mg IUS licensed for 3 years. • Not user dependent.	• Can cause irregular bleeding in the first 3–6 months. • Can occasionally be expelled. • Requires special training for insertion and removal. • Rare complications; for example, perforation of the uterus (very unlikely). • Can be uncomfortable to insert and cervical dilatation may be required. • Side effects can include abdominal and pelvic pain and dysfunctional menstrual bleeding.	See notes on IUS below, page 77.	• Severe primary dysmenorrhoea. • Adenomyosis.	• Recent STI. • Distorted or small uterine cavity. • Active PID. • Severe anaemia.

Table 4.2 Forms of Contraception Containing Progestogens Only—Cont'd

TYPE OF CONTRACEPTION	BRIEF DESCRIPTION	ADVANTAGES	DISADVANTAGES	PRACTICAL ADVICE	CAUTIONS	CONTRAINDICATIONS
Intramuscular (IM) injection.	• The IM injection is injected into the upper thigh or buttock. • Unlike the POP, it always inhibits ovulation.	• Over 99% effective – safe and not user dependent. • One injection lasts for 8–12 weeks (depending on type). • Improves premenstrual symptoms and dysmenorrhoea. • Efficacy not reduced by diarrhoea, vomiting, antibiotics or liver enzyme-inducing drugs.	• Menstrual disturbances – bleeding may be frequent, irregular or absent. • Weight gain. • Long delay in return to fertility when stopped; for example, up to a year with the commonly used medroxyprogesterone injection. • Cannot be withdrawn once injected. • May be associated with osteoporosis with long term use. • Same side effects as POPs.	• Injections should only be used on a short-term basis, as use for 5 years or more is associated with loss of bone density. • Should avoid use in adolescents as their bones are growing and increasing in density. Use can reduce final bone density, increasing the risk of early osteoporosis.	• DVT or PE. • Should only be used in adolescents if other forms are inappropriate.	• Same contraindications as for implants.
Implant.	• Small flexible plastic rod containing a form of progesterone. • Using local anaesthetic to numb the skin, a small cut is made in the upper arm and the rod is inserted here.	• Over 99% effective. It is the most effective contraceptive with a 1:300 failure rate. • One implant is effective for 3 years. • Requires little medical attention.	• Requires a minor operative procedure and those inserting implants need to be specially trained in insertion and removal. • Irregular menstrual bleeding may occur. • Same side effects as POPs.	• If implants are inserted within the first days of the menstrual cycle, then no additional contraception is required. If inserted after this, another contraceptive method is required for the first 7 days.	• Raised BMI – it is suggested that these women need to have the implants replaced more regularly.	• Multiple risk factors for cardiovascular disease. • Age more than 50 years. • Risk factors for osteoporosis. • History of breast cancer. • Taking liver enzyme-inducing drugs.

Table 4.3 Non-Hormonal Forms of Contraception

TYPE OF CONTRACEPTION	BRIEF DESCRIPTION	ADVANTAGES	DISADVANTAGES	PRACTICAL ADVICE	CAUTIONS	CONTRAINDICATIONS
Male condoms	• A latex sheath that fits onto the erect penis to act as a barrier to sperm entering the vagina.	• 85%–98% efficacy, variation because it is user dependent. • Under the control of the man and woman. • Convenient and easily accessible. • No systemic effects. • Protection against STIs.	• May interrupt sexual encounter. • Perceived as messy. • Requires forward planning. • Loss of sensitivity.	• Come in a variety of sizes and with different features. • Should only be used once and then disposed of. • Should not be used with oil-based lubricants.	• None.	• If either partner has an allergy to the constituents, usually made of latex, and some contain a chemical spermicide. • Erectile problems.
Diaphragm.	• Diaphragms and caps are latex rubber domes that fit into the vagina and cover the cervix to provide a physical barrier to sperm. • It is held in place by the tension of the ring, the pelvic bones and the muscles of the vagina.	• 92%–96% effective when used correctly with spermicide. • Few systemic side effects. • Can be put in at any convenient time before having sex and under direct control of the woman. • May protect against cervical cancer, some STIs (not HIV) and PID but should be used alongside condoms.	• Not many women are confident fitting them and they have potential for user error. • Requires forward planning. • Must be used with spermicides. • Women have to be fitted initially to know their correct size. • An increased incidence of UTIs in some women with diaphragms. • Can cause vaginal irritation.	• The diaphragm must not be removed until 6 hours after last ejaculation. • Diaphragms should be replaced annually. • Diaphragms come in three main types: flat spring, coiled spring and arching spring diaphragm.	• Aversion to touching genitalia or inserting a device into the vagina. • Recurrent UTIs.	• Uterovaginal prolapse. • Poor vaginal tone. • Latex allergy. • Acute vaginitis.
Copper IUD	• Copper containing plastic T-shaped device that is inserted into the uterus via the cervix. • Two strings are left in place in the vagina and should be checked to ensure the IUD remains *in situ*. • Copper is toxic to sperm.	• Over 99% effective. • Lasts for up to 10 years. • Can be inserted for emergency contraception and then remains in situ, giving ongoing contraceptive cover. • Fertility returns soon after the IUD is removed.	• Risk of perforation. • Risk of expulsion. • Periods may be heavier, longer or more painful although this should improve after the copper IUD has been in situ for several months. • Increased risk of ectopic pregnancy in women who fall pregnant when using the copper IUD.	• It can be uncomfortable for some women to have inserted, especially if they are nulliparous. • The strings will need to be checked after insertion usually once by a health professional and then by the user to ensure it remains in place.	• Cervical or uterine anatomical abnormalities. • Unexplained intermenstrual or postcoital bleeding.	• Untreated STI or active PID. • Wilson disease.

COMBINED ORAL CONTRACEPTIVE PILL

Patients must be made aware of important information required to take the combined oral contraceptive pill (COCP) safely and efficaciously.

WHEN TO SEEK MEDICAL ADVICE

- Hypertension – advise the patient that they will need blood pressure checks at 3 months and annually thereafter, as the COCP can raise patient's blood pressure and should not be taken by women with pre-existing hypertension.
- Migraines – any increase in headache frequency should be reported to a doctor and any development of focal neurological signs (an aura) require discontinuation of the pill.
- Deep vein thrombosis (DVT) and pulmonary embolism (PE)
  - The increased risk of venous thromboembolism (VTE) when taking the COCP is primarily due to the oestrogen, although the type of progestogen also affects the risk, see Table 4.4.
  - Although the COCP increases the relative risk of VTE, overall incidence remains extremely low.
  - The risk of VTE is greatest in the first year of use and on recommencement if stopped for over 4 weeks.
  - The patient should be advised to seek urgent medical help if they develop symptoms of DVT (calf pain, leg swelling) or PE (chest pain, shortness of breath). If the patient has periods of immobility, for example, long haul flights, emphasise the importance of ensuring good hydration and mobilisation.

REASONS TO BE CONCERNED ABOUT CONTRACEPTIVE COVER

- Diarrhoea and vomiting – require an additional method of contraception, as gastrointestinal absorption of the pill may not have occurred.

Table 4.4	VTE Risk for Healthy Women Under 35 Years of Age With a Normal BMI	
RISK FACTOR	**INCIDENCE OF VTE PER YEAR PER 100,000 WOMEN**	
Not pregnant, not on contraception	1	
Levonorgestrel intrauterine system	1	
Progesterone injection or high dose POP	3	
Combined oral contraceptive (containing norethisterone or levonorgestrel)	6	
Combined oral contraceptive (containing desogestrel or drospirenone)	12	
Pregnancy	60	

With other risk factors, VTE risk may be substantially higher.

- Commencement of enzyme-inducing medications – these will increase the metabolism of oestrogen, reducing the contraceptive effect. Alternative contraception should be used if these medications are commenced.
  - Antibiotics – rifampicin, rifabutin.
  - Antiepileptics – carbamazepine, phenytoin.
  - St John's wort.

ADVICE FOR MISSED COCPS

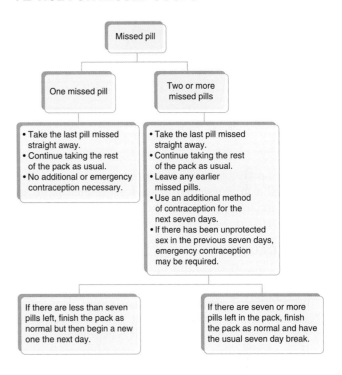

INTRAUTERINE SYSTEM

The 52 mg intrauterine system (IUS) is licensed for contraception for 5 years, while the newer 13.5 mg IUS is licensed for 3 years. The 52 mg IUS is also licensed for management of heavy menstrual bleeding, endometrial hyperplasia and can be used as the progesterone component of HRT. The most common 52 mg IUS used in the UK is the Mirena®.

DYSMENORRHOEA

The IUS decreases endometrial proliferation. Therefore, in cases of menorrhagia associated with dysmenorrhea, the IUS can be helpful. This is due to the theory that menstrual pains are caused by the physical contraction of the uterus and the inflammation and necrosis of the endometrium. By reducing the amount of endometrial lining present, the degree of inflammation and necrosis is reduced and there is also less lining for the uterus to expel during a period. In cases of dysmenorrhoea without menorrhagia, there is more likely to be an element of adenomyosis or endometriosis causing the pain. In these cases, the IUS may improve the symptoms if it causes anovulation because it will reduce the oestrogen levels which often drives the

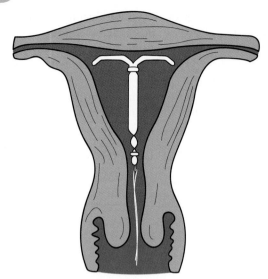

Fig. 4.1 An IUS In Situ Within the Uterus.

growth of endometriosis. However, in some cases, the IUS could also worsen endometriosis-related pain, so the decision to use an IUS in these patients needs additional discussion with the patient.

PRACTICALITIES

- Ideally, the IUS should be fitted (Fig. 4.1) within the first 7 days of menstruation as this would mean no additional contraception is required. However, avoid inserting on the heaviest days of a woman's period to minimise the risk of IUS expulsion.
- If fitted after this, another contraceptive method is required for the first 7 days.
- The IUS may be fitted immediately after a first-trimester termination or miscarriage.
- Coil check 6 weeks after insertion by the woman or primary care physician – this is to check the threads to confirm correct placement (not perforated or expulsed).

Management of erratic bleeding in the first few months after insertion:
- Reassurance.
- Tranexamic or mefenamic acid.
- Tricyclic COCP for 3 months.
- Oral progestogen (such as norethisterone) for 3 months.

ADDITIONAL INFORMATION FOR ALL INTRAUTERINE CONTRACEPTIVE METHODS

- It is important to test all patients at risk of an STI prior to insertion as any pelvic infection is a contraindication for any of these forms of contraception.
- If a copper IUD is inserted for emergency contraception, consider the need for prophylactic antibiotics (such as doxycycline to cover chlamydia).
- If an individual becomes pregnant while using an IUD or IUS, it is recommended that they have this device removed in the first trimester. If the device

is not removed, there is an increased risk of miscarriage, preterm labour and intrauterine infection. There may be a small risk of miscarriage around the time of removal, but this is smaller than the risk of leaving it *in situ*.

OTHER METHODS

A number of methods are used globally as contraception, but are not recommended medically due to their low efficacy:
- Breastfeeding – also known as the lactational amenorrhoea method, it may be used postnatally when a woman is breastfeeding and not menstruating, as she is temporarily infertile for approximately the first 6 months after giving birth. However, this is only the case if she is fully or nearly fully breastfeeding. This method is also difficult because of the narrow time window. The woman also needs to be completely amenorrhoeic.
- Coitus interruptus – also known as the withdrawal method. This is when a couple not using any other form of contraception have sexual intercourse and the male withdraws before ejaculating. However, there is evidence of semen in the female genital tract during intercourse even without ejaculation. Coitus interruptus is one of the least effective methods of contraception.
- Family planning or timing of sexual intercourse – this involves timing sexual intercourse around the non-fertile times of a female's menstrual cycle, using daily body temperature, monitoring cervical secretions and cycle lengths. Used correctly, advocates of this method report up to 99% effectiveness. However, due to difficulties with effective training with this method, mistakes made and variability of a woman's' menstrual cycle, the average effectiveness is around 75%.
- Abstinence – although 100% abstinence is the only way to ensure absolutely no risk of pregnancy, this is difficult for many people to practice and often not a realistic long-term option.

STERILISATION

Sterilisation is a surgical procedure available for men and women who do not want to have any children now or in the future. They are permanent methods of contraception and are regarded as irreversible. Patients should be counselled that some people feel regret after being sterilised. Sterilisation is not immediately effective, taking between 4 weeks and 3 months to be effective. There is no protection from STIs.

Female sterilisation, or tubal occlusion, involves ligation or clipping the fallopian tubes, often with a surgical clip at laparoscopy. After sterilisation, periods will continue for women with the same regularity and volume as they had been before. Failure rate of female sterilisation is 1:200, and if a woman does become pregnant, the chance of it being an ectopic pregnancy is increased.

Male sterilisation, or vasectomy, is when the vas deferens is cut or sealed, often by tying it off. This can be done under local anaesthetic. Vasectomy is the safest sterilisation method, and the most effective form of contraception, with a failure rate of 1:2000. Around 12 weeks after a male sterilisation, a semen analysis is carried out to ensure the procedure has been successful.

CONCLUSION

The majority of contraceptive methods are at least 99% effective when used correctly. The particular choice of contraceptive should take into account the risks and benefits of the method for the individual user.

❓ QUESTIONS

Lucy, an 18-year-old, attends the sexual health clinic to enquire about contraception. She has been with her current boyfriend, who is her only sexual partner, for 6 months. She does not want children in the near future and has no other significant past medical history. She is on no medication and has no allergies. She is currently using the COCP but thinks that she may like to change to a longer-acting form.

Q1 What advice should you give if a patient misses one COCP?
   A To stop taking the pill for a week, as the patient will have to have a withdrawal bleed. To abstain from sexual intercourse during this time.
   B To not take the missed pill, but carry on with the pill from the following day. To also use an alternative method of contraception for the next week, in addition to the pill.
   C To take the missed pill and that day's pill at the same time; no additional contraception is required.
   D To take the missed pill and that day's pill at the same time and to also use an alternative form of contraception for the next week.
   E To seek advice regarding emergency contraception.

Q2 Answer true or false: For which of the following does the COCP have a protective effect?
   A Breast cancer.
   B Cervical cancer.
   C Colorectal cancer.
   D Endometrial cancer.
   E Ovarian cancer.

Q3 Answer true or false: Which of the following are contraindications for COCP use?
   A Age more than 50 years.
   B BMI more than 35 kg/m².
   C Migraine sufferer without aura.
   D Renal impairment.
   E Smoker.

Q4 Which one of the following is an advantage of the 52 mg IUS?
   A Ensures regular menstrual cycles.
   B Lasts 10 years after insertion.
   C Protects against STIs.
   D Reduces dysmenorrhoea.
   E Reduces PID.

Q5 Answer true or false: Which of the following are contraindications for an IUS?
   A Endometriosis.
   B Heavy periods.
   C Nulliparity.
   D Pregnancy.
   E Uterine distortion.

Q6 What is the rate of spontaneous expulsion of an IUS?
   A 1 in 10.
   B 1 in 20.
   C 1 in 100.
   D 1 in 200.
   E 1 in 1000.

A COCP.	**G** Implant.
B Copper coil.	**H** IUS.
C Desogestrel.	**I** Levonorgestrel.
D Diaphragm.	**J** Male condom.
E Female condom.	**K** Sterilisation.
F IM injection.	**L** Vaginal ring.

Q7 Which is the only long-acting reversible contraception available that does not involve hormones?

Q8 Which form of contraception is likely to need altering following pregnancy?

Q9 Which form of contraception is usually inserted into the upper limb?

Q10 Which female form of contraception has the lowest percentage efficacy?

Q11 After use, which form of reversible contraception has the longest time period until optimum fertility is returned?

[Answers on page 185.]

EMERGENCY CONTRACEPTION

Emergency contraception is taken by women after unprotected sexual intercourse as a means of preventing unintended pregnancy. Other terms include "the morning-after pill" or "postcoital contraception".

Three methods are available (Table 4.5).

Table **4.5** **Emergency Contraceptives**

METHOD	CLASS	INDICATIONS
Copper intrauterine device (IUD)	Intrauterine contraceptive method	Within 120 hours of unprotected sex or contraceptive failure, or within 5 days of the estimated date of ovulation
Levonorgestrel	Progestogen hormone	Within 72 hours of unprotected sex or contraceptive failure
Ulipristal acetate	Progesterone receptor modulator	Within 120 hours of unprotected sex or contraceptive failure

Table 4.6 Properties of Post Coital Contraception

METHOD	MECHANISM OF ACTION	ADVANTAGES	DISADVANTAGES
Copper intrauterine device (IUD)	• Copper is toxic to the ovum and sperm therefore copper IUDs are immediately effective after insertion at preventing fertilisation. • If fertilisation has already occurred, then the copper has an anti-implantation effect.	• Failure rate less than 1%, most effective form of emergency contraception. • Unaffected by concomitant drug use. • Provides ongoing contraception for up to 10 years.	• Pain on insertion. • More likely to cause menorrhagia or dysmenorrhoea than other contraceptive alternatives. • Should not be used in a patient with an active STI, and testing should be offered at the time of insertion with antibiotic cover for at least chlamydia. • Avoid in Wilson disease (as it contains copper).
Levonorgestrel (progestogen)	• High levels of progestogen inhibit ovulation. • This method is less effective close to the time of ovulation or if ovulation has already occurred. • It is not effective after fertilisation.	• Failure rate of less than 3%. • Highly effective up to 72 hours after intercourse. • Can be used multiple times in the same cycle.	• Side effects of headache, nausea and altered bleeding patterns, abdominal pain, dysmenorrhea and dizziness. • Cannot be used in patients with current breast cancer.
Ulipristal acetate (progesterone receptor antagonist)	• It inhibits ovulation by blocking progesterone receptors. • If given before ovulation, it is likely to delay ovulation by 5 days, allowing any sperm present to die before ovulation occurs. • Administration after ovulation may be ineffective.	• Failure rate of less than 2%. • Efficacy does not appear to fall until 5 days after intercourse.	• Similar side effects to levonorgestrel. • Should not be used with levonorgestrel – one is a progesterone and the other is a progesterone antagonist. • Cannot be used if breastfeeding, or patient has severe asthma.

INDICATION

Determining whether emergency contraception is required entails taking a history that should include questions regarding:
• LMP and regularity of cycles.
  • To determine when ovulation is likely to occur. If it is not likely to occur within 5 to 7 days of unprotected intercourse, pregnancy is unlikely. However, guidelines state that women who have had unprotected sexual intercourse that has taken place on any day of a natural menstrual cycle should be offered emergency contraception.
  • In addition, irregular cycles and a poor historian can make this information unreliable.
• Fertility of both partners.
• What contraception has or has not been used and whether this was used correctly.
• Pregnancy tests should be used if there is any doubt regarding pregnancy, as emergency contraception cannot be given if the patient is already pregnant.

However, in practice, emergency contraception will often be prescribed without an in-depth consultation or even if pregnancy is deemed to be very unlikely to occur because the side effects of the drugs are relatively

minimal. It is very difficult to determine the risk of pregnancy accurately and the consequences of unintended pregnancy are great.

In determining the most appropriate emergency contraception (Table 4.6) the clinician should consider:
• Medical contraindications.
• Efficacy of each method.
• Number and timing of episodes of unprotected sexual intercourse.
• Previous emergency contraception use within the cycle.
• Need for additional precautions or ongoing contraception.
• Patient choice.

DETERMINING WHICH FORM OF EMERGENCY CONTRACEPTION SHOULD BE USED

Additional information
• Guidelines state that the copper IUD should be offered as the first-line option in all women, this is because it is the most effective and enables ongoing contraceptive cover.
• Women should be advised to seek medical advice if they vomit within 2 hours of taking

levonorgestrel or 3 hours of ulipristal acetate – a repeated dose of the same method or a copper IUD can be offered.

- Liver impairment, or use of liver enzyme-inducing medications, will reduce the efficacy of the oral emergency contraceptives. Therefore, consider the IUD instead.
- Patients should be advised that oral emergency contraceptives may cause menstrual disturbance. If they have concerns regarding their next period, they should have a low threshold for taking a pregnancy test 3 weeks after treatment.
- Ulipristal blocks the action of progesterone and could therefore interfere with progestogen-containing contraceptives. Patients using hormonal contraceptives should use additional precautions for 14 days following administration.
- Levonorgestrel and ulipristal acetate do not provide contraceptive cover for subsequent acts of unprotected sexual intercourse. Further contraception should be advised.

Women presenting for emergency contraception may also be at risk of STIs; therefore, STI testing, including HIV testing, should be offered. Women should however be made aware that recently acquired STIs may not be detected; therefore, they may need to be retested in the future. Follow-up tests are usually arranged for approximately 12 weeks later. In women at risk of STIs, prophylactic antibiotics should be offered before the insertion of an emergency IUD to cover at least *Chlamydia trachomatis*.

MANAGEMENT

- History to determine the requirements for emergency contraception.
- Pregnancy test – emergency contraception cannot be given if the patient is already pregnant.
- Counsel the woman on the different forms of emergency contraception and make an appropriate choice individualised for that patient.
- STI tests as appropriate, and follow-up tests arranged approximately 12 weeks later.
- Discussion regarding ongoing contraception with all women.
  - Women starting contraception may want to wait until pregnancy is definitely excluded before starting a hormonal form of contraception.
  - With women already using contraception it should be discussed whether an alternative would be better suited for them.

Patients who frequently require emergency contraception are not being appropriately engaged by healthcare professionals. They are also at an increased risk of pregnancy and STIs.

PROGNOSIS

Emergency contraception is effective at preventing an unwanted pregnancy. There are no long-term physical effects on the patient or their fertility. If pregnancy does occur following emergency contraception, there are no additional risks for that pregnancy and it can be managed no differently from any other pregnancy (if a copper coil has been used this should be removed in the first trimester). If the patient still does not want the pregnancy, she can be referred for a termination or other alternatives.

[See 'Termination of Pregnancy' page 66.]

❓ QUESTIONS

Holly is a 15-year-old who has presented to her primary care physician asking for emergency contraception because she had unprotected sex with her boyfriend last night. Holly is extremely worried that her mother will find out. Holly is otherwise fit and healthy and is on no other medication.

Q1 As this patient is 15 years old, decide whether the following statements are true or false regarding prescribing her contraception.
  A Emergency contraception can be provided to a competent young person aged under 16 years without parental consent or knowledge using the Fraser criteria.
  B Emergency contraception can be provided to a competent young person aged under 16 years without parental consent or knowledge using the Gillick criteria.
  C Emergency contraception can be provided without parental consent; however, a termination requires a parent or carer to be informed.
  D Emergency contraception may only be prescribed by a doctor or nurse for patients under 16.
  E Copper intrauterine devices cannot be fitted in patients under the age of 16.

Q2 How many days after unprotected sex can emergency contraception be prescribed?
  A One day.
  B Three days.
  C Four days.
  D Five days.
  E One week.

Q3 Which of the following statements regarding emergency contraception are true?
  A Emergency contraception causes abortion of the embryo.
  B Ulipristal acetate inhibits ovulation by blocking progesterone receptors.
  C Women who take rifampicin should be advised that the copper IUD is the only method of emergency contraception that can reliably prevent pregnancy.

D All three forms of emergency contraception give ongoing contraceptive efficacy for future acts of unprotected sexual intercourse in the next 72 hours.

E If the reason for taking levonorgestrel was two missed COCPs and the patient continues to take her COCP, then no extra precautions are required after taking this form of emergency contraception.

A Carbamazepine.	**H** Progesterone.
B Ciprofloxacin.	**I** Progestogen.
C Copper IUD.	**J** Renal failure.
D Levonorgestrel.	**K** Sexually transmitted
E Luteinising hormone.	infection.
F Penicillin.	**L** Uliipristal acetate.
G Pregnancy.	

From the options above, select the most appropriate answer to the following questions:

Q4 What is an absolute contraindication for the hormonal forms of emergency contraception?

Q5 What necessitates the dose of levonorgestrel to be doubled?

Q6 Which form of contraception is most likely to disrupt the next menstruation from its expected day?

Q7 Which oral form of emergency contraception can be offered if unprotected sexual intercourse has occurred and levonorgestrel was taken as emergency contraception 4 days ago?

Q8 Which form of emergency contraception is contraindicated in Wilson's disease?

[Answers on page 188.]

MENORRHAGIA AND OTHER MENSTRUAL BLEEDING DISORDERS

For research purposes, heavy menstrual bleeding (HMB), or menorrhagia, is defined as menstrual blood loss of more than 80 mL per menstrual cycle. A more useful clinical definition is excessive menstrual blood loss which causes impairment to a patient's quality of life.

AETIOLOGY

Around 30% of the female population will suffer from menorrhagia at some point during their lives.

PATHOPHYSIOLOGY

There is no identified cause of menorrhagia in most patients, and in most cases, initial management does not require identification of a cause.

Known causes of menorrhagia:

- Endocrine – endometrium stimulated to proliferate excessively.
  - Disturbance of the HPO axis – classically at menarche, around menopause or after pregnancy.
  - Thyroid dysfunction – hyperthyroid and to a lesser extent hypothyroid.
- Excessive or unopposed oestrogen – obesity and liver failure.
- Structural – increased surface area of endometrium.
  - Fibroids.
  - Polyps.
- Other:
  - Clotting disorder – suspect if there is a family history or if menorrhagia has occurred since menarche.
  - Pelvic inflammatory disease (PID).
  - Endometrial cancer or precancerous changes – these are rare pre-menopause although cases are increasing with increasing rates of obesity.

CLINICAL FEATURES

HISTORY

- Assessment of menorrhagia – days of bleeding, number of tampons or pads used, flooding.
- Assessment of effect on quality of life – symptoms of anaemia, effect on work, school or social life.
- A discussion should be had regarding normal menstruation, as a patient describing symptoms of normal menstruation may simply need reassurance.

ASSOCIATED SYMPTOMS WHICH MAY WARRANT FURTHER INVESTIGATION

- Recurrent intermenstrual bleeding (IMB).
- Postcoital bleeding (PCB) – cervical cause, for example, ectropion or cancer.
- Dyspareunia, vaginal discharge, pelvic pain – PID.
- Pressure symptoms – fibroids (see page 86).
- Additional symptoms suggestive of an underlying systemic disorder, for example, clotting or thyroid disorders.
- Patients aged 45 and over with HMB need a biopsy of the endometrium – increased risk of endometrial dysplasia or neoplasia.

SIGNS

Examination is not required prior to first-line therapy unless a possible cause has been identified during the history.

- Signs of anaemia – pale conjunctiva, pale mucous membranes, or nail signs such as koilonychia.
- Abdominal exam – to assess for an enlarged palpable uterus suggestive of fibroids.
- Pelvic exam to assess for cervical cause, enlarged uterus or PID.

INVESTIGATIONS

- Full blood count – all patients with menorrhagia should be assessed for anaemia, and this is the only investigation initially required for most patients. Microcytic, hypochromic anaemia indicating iron deficiency anaemia is most commonly seen.

Other potential investigations to consider if suggested from the history:

- Clotting screen – menorrhagia from menarche, known family history of clotting disorder such as von Willebrand disease.
- Thyroid function – hyperthyroidism and to a lesser extent hypothyroidism can cause HMB.
- Ultrasound scan – structural abnormality, for example, fibroids.
- Hysteroscopy and endometrial biopsy – concern regarding uterine dysplasia or neoplasia, or to assess the endometrium for structural abnormality, for example, polyps.

If initial treatments fail to control symptoms, an ultrasound scan and hysteroscopy are usually offered to rule out underlying pathology.

COMPLICATIONS

- Symptoms of anaemia – iron deficiency anaemia (microcytic) is common in patients with severe menorrhagia. Usually, oral iron supplementation alongside menorrhagia treatments is all that is required to correct anaemia. However, in rare cases, parenteral iron can be used and even blood transfusion.
- Detrimental impact on quality of life – it is important to address the psychological and social impact menorrhagia has on a patient.

MANAGEMENT

NICE have produced guidelines for management of menorrhagia. Pharmaceutical options should be tried first, followed by surgical intervention, but only if the pharmaceutical options fail, are contraindicated or declined by the patient. Many of the treatment options have either a temporary or permanent effect on fertility, so the patient's current and future desire for conception will also affect treatment. Treatment options for menorrhagia should be offered in the order set out below.

FIRST-LINE TREATMENT

- Levonorgestrel (progestogen) releasing IUS (52 mg LNG-IUS)
  - This is the most effective medical management of menorrhagia.
  - The 52 mg IUS can be used for up to 5 years before needing to be changed.
  - It is effective in up to 70% of patients, with 30% of patients becoming amenorrhoeic at 1 year. It is important to inform patients that for the first 3 to 6 months, the IUS may cause erratic bleeding, but that this will settle.

SECOND-LINE TREATMENT

- Tranexamic acid.
  - This is an antifibrinolytic that naturally occurs in the body as part of the antifibrinolytic pathway. It is the only treatment option for patients currently trying to conceive.
  - It can be used for 5 days around the time of menstruation to reduce clot breakdown and fibrinolysis and therefore reduce bleeding.
  - It can be used in conjunction with any of the other treatments discussed in this section.
- Non-steroidal anti-inflammatory drugs.
  - These medications work well in dysmenorrhoea but also have an effect on menorrhagia. The mechanism of action is by antagonism of prostaglandin receptors.
  - They are not as effective as tranexamic acid but can be used in conjunction.
- Combined oral contraceptives.
  - The continued release of oestrogen from the combined pill stops the HPO axis which, as well as stopping ovulation, reduces endometrial proliferation due to reduced ovarian oestrogen production. This results in lighter menstruation.
  - The progesterone component prevents the pill's oestrogen having an unopposed effect on the endometrium, which would cause proliferation and potential dysplasia.
  - The pill is usually used for 21 days, with a 7-day break to allow menstruation. However, the pill may be used without the 7-day break for 3 to 6 months before allowing a break and a withdrawal bleed. The COCP may also be used in this manner for 3 months to treat erratic bleeding caused by a recently inserted IUS.

THIRD-LINE TREATMENTS – SYSTEMIC PROGESTOGEN-ONLY TREATMENTS

These frequently induce amenorrhoea by inhibition of the HPO axis. Progestogen also maintains the endometrium, preventing menstruation.

- Oral progestogen, for example, norethisterone or desogestrel.
  - Can be used long term, often used in addition to a newly inserted IUS to control erratic bleeding.
  - Progestogens are also commonly prescribed short term to induce amenorrhoea for social reasons where women need to ensure they will not menstruate, for example, when running a marathon.
  - It is important to tell patients that when a progestogen is stopped, there is usually a heavy but short-lasting progesterone withdrawal bleed.
- Injected progestogen or the implant – may also be used to treat menorrhagia, but are not as effective as other treatments.

SURGICAL TREATMENT

Subsequent treatments are used by gynaecologists when the above treatment options either are ineffective or contraindicated in a patient.

- Endometrial ablation.
  - This is a quick surgical procedure whereby instruments are inserted into the uterus through the cervix and the endometrium is destroyed either by diathermy, microwaves or direct heat, depending on the technique used. It is now routinely done in the outpatient setting under local anaesthetic.
  - This technique is successful in controlling symptoms in over 70% of cases.
  - As the effects can be permanent, this procedure should only be carried out on women with no intention of having further pregnancies.
  - It is not an effective contraceptive option, so patients at risk of pregnancy should also use appropriate contraception. If someone does become pregnant after having had this procedure, there is a high risk of multiple complications, including miscarriage, haemorrhage and placenta accreta.
- Hysterectomy – ultimately, this is the definitive management for ongoing menorrhagia when all other options have been exhausted. It is major surgery, with the risk of serious complications and a protracted postoperative recovery period.

OTHER TREATMENTS

- Myomectomy or polypectomy – if submucosal fibroids or polyps have been identified, they can be removed to reduce the surface area of the endometrium. These are usually removed with a hysteroscope and surgical device, which is inserted into the uterine cavity through the cervix. The device used resects the unwanted tissue and simultaneously removes it from the uterine cavity using suction.
- Transcervical resection of endometrium (TCRE) – using a resection hysteroscope, the entire lining of the endometrium can be resected, which prevents regrowth of the endometrium. This procedure has been largely replaced by endometrial ablation, as TCRE is associated with similar success rates but has a higher risk of complications, including uterine perforation and hyponatraemia. It does have a role in cases where the uterine cavity is distorted and endometrial ablation is contraindicated.
- Uterine artery embolisation (UAE) – treatment for symptoms caused by large fibroids only. Catheters are passed through the femoral arteries into the internal iliac arteries. The uterine arteries are then embolised, which dramatically reduces blood flow to the uterus. However, the uterus still has collateral blood supply from the ovarian vessels and vessels ascending from the cervix and vagina. The reduction in blood flow causes fibroid necrosis. The long-term effect of this procedure on fertility is unknown.
- Gonadotropin-releasing hormone (GnRH) analogues – these are subcuticular injections given usually every 12 weeks. GnRH is usually released in a pulsatile fashion by the hypothalamus to regulate the HPO axis. The injection provides a continual presence of GnRH, which results in the pituitary no longer responding to GnRH. Therefore, the HPO axis is stopped and the end result is essentially a medically induced menopausal state. Menstruation stops, but menopausal symptoms frequently occur. These analogues are only licensed for 6 months' use, but they may be used to manage symptoms while awaiting further definitive management. Often, they are used alongside hormone replacement therapy (HRT) to reduce menopausal symptoms.

PROGNOSIS

In most cases, menorrhagia can be adequately controlled with simple measures that do not require referral to specialist gynaecology clinics.

INTERMENSTRUAL AND POSTCOITAL BLEEDING

IMB is bleeding at any time during the menstrual cycle which is not at the time of menstruation. PCB is bleeding after intercourse. Usually, IMB and PCB are both associated with only small amounts of blood loss, often referred to as spotting. However, in some women, the bleeding can be heavier. IMB and PCB are common and are rarely due to a sinister pathology, but it is important to investigate to exclude this.

PATHOPHYSIOLOGY

Physiological or Benign Causes of Intermenstrual Bleeding

- Ovulation bleed – oestrogen is at its peak level at the time of ovulation. It is not uncommon for this to cause a small IMB. If the IMB occurs approximately 14 days prior to menstruation each cycle, this is likely to be the diagnosis, particularly in young women where the symptom has been present from menarche. In older women, it is imperative to investigate for other causes.
- Hormonal contraceptives – for the first 6 months after starting a hormonal contraceptive, erratic IMB is common, and if there are no other worrying features, this does not need to be investigated unless it persists beyond 6 months. If the patient has been prescribed the COCP and has developed IMB, using a pill with a higher oestrogen dose may settle the IMB. If IMB does not settle, a different contraceptive can be tried. If IMB persists, investigations should then be carried out to rule out sinister causes.
- Perimenopause – alterations in hormone levels around the time of the menopause often cause erratic bleeding. However, as these patients are older, they have an increased risk of endometrial pathology, so it is prudent to investigate for this.

[See 'Contraception' page 71.]

Physiological or Benign Cause of PCB

Ectropion – in teenagers, women in their 20s and women on the COCP, the most likely cause of PCB is an ectropion. This is the presence of delicate columnar epithelium protruding from the cervical canal onto the ectocervix, which bleed on contact. The ectropion is caused by high oestrogen levels in these patients. Ectropions can be diagnosed on speculum examination. They can be easily treated with cryotherapy, which destroys the top layer of cervical cells by freezing them. It can be performed in minutes as an outpatient. A biopsy is often taken prior to cryotherapy to rule out any other pathology.

[See 'Cervical Screening' page 150.]

Pathological Causes of Intermenstrual Bleeding and Postcoital Bleeding

- STIs – swabs should be taken to exclude any infections.
- Uterine bleeding – the causes can all present as IMB, PCB or menorrhagia.
  - Polyps and fibroids – an ultrasound scan will assess the structure of the uterus. If found they can be further investigated and removed by performing a hysteroscopy.
  - Endometrial hyperplasia and neoplasia – an endometrial biopsy will assess for endometrial abnormality.
- Cervical bleeding – pre-cancerous and cancerous cervical changes. Having regular cervical smears dramatically reduces the chance of developing cervical cancer. If a patient is overdue for a smear, one can be taken during a speculum examination. If the cervix looks abnormal, the patient should be referred urgently for a colposcopy (if seen in a gynaecology clinic a cervical biopsy can also be taken).
- Vaginal bleeding – rarely trauma or neoplasia of the vagina can cause bleeding. This should be visible on the speculum examination.

[See 'Cervical Cancer' page 156.] [See 'Endometrial Cancer' page 146.]

INVESTIGATIONS

It is very easy to fully investigate IMB and PCB:
- Speculum examination.
  - View cervix and vagina.
  - Swabs for STI screen.
  - Cervical smear if not up to date.
  - Endometrial biopsy if persistent IMB.
- Ultrasound scan if palpable mass identified, for example, fibroids.
- Hysteroscopy.

PROGNOSIS

If a cause is found, then this can be treated. However, it is common for no cause of bleeding to be found after investigation, so the patient can be reassured there is no sinister cause for her symptoms, and it is likely to settle spontaneously. If the symptoms are affecting her quality of life, then treatment should be considered usually in the form of a hormonal contraceptive. If the patient does not wish to have treatment, she should be advised to come back for repeat investigations if the IMB or PCB persists beyond a year.

? QUESTIONS

Jennifer, a 19-year-old with no significant past medical history, presents to her primary care physician. She presents with heavy periods, which she says have been a significant problem for her over the last 4 years. She has been very nervous about discussing this with anyone but has presented now because her grandmother has recently been diagnosed with endometrial cancer.

Q1 What is the single most important investigation when managing menorrhagia in this patient?
  A Menstrual calendar.
  B Pad weights to estimate menstrual loss.
  C Pipelle endometrial biopsy.
  D Serum haemoglobin concentration.
  E Ultrasound scan.

A Clotting screen.	H Serum chlamydial antibodies.
B Colposcopy.	
C Day 21 serum progesterone.	I Serum ferritin.
D Endometrial pipelle biopsy.	J Thyroid stimulating hormone.
E Glucose tolerance test.	K Ultrasound scan.
F Liver function tests.	L Vaginal swab for chlamydia.
G No investigation necessary.	

Select the most appropriate investigation from the list above, for a patient presenting with menorrhagia and each of the following symptoms:

Q2 Constipation.

Q3 Recurrent postcoital bleeding.

Q4 History of heavy menstrual bleeding since menarche.

Q5 Uterus palpable abdominally.

Q6 Vaginal discharge.

Q7 Answer true or false regarding the following statements about menorrhagia.
  A The history of endometrial cancer in the family is likely to affect the clinical management of this patient.
  B The levonorgestrel-releasing intrauterine system is the first-line treatment for menorrhagia.
  C The progestogen-containing implant is an alternative to other progestogen-containing contraceptive treatments and has the added benefit of decreased serum concentrations of progestogen compared to the other treatments.
  D Mefenamic acid is a suitable treatment for a patient with menorrhagia and severe asthma.

E A hysterectomy is not offered as first-line treatment for menorrhagia because other treatments are more effective and are cheaper.

[Answers on page 191.]

FIBROIDS

Uterine fibroids are also known as uterine leiomyomas or leiomyomata. They are benign tumours of the uterine myometrium and consist of uterine muscle cells and connective tissue.

RISK FACTORS

- Black ethnicity.
- Obesity.
- Early menarche (before 10 years old).
- Late menopause.
- Increasing adult age (until menopause).
- Nulliparity – increasing number of pregnancies progressively reduces the risk of fibroids.

AETIOLOGY

Fibroids are very common. However, as fibroids are usually asymptomatic, the true incidence and prevalence is not known. It is estimated 70% of women have uterine fibroids by age 45, and the lifetime prevalence of symptomatic fibroids is 25% of White Northern European and 50% of African women.

PATHOPHYSIOLOGY

Uterine fibroids are thought to be a monoclonal tumour of a single mutated uterine smooth muscle cell. Fibroids originate in the uterine myometrium. They are classified by their anatomical location on the uterus (Fig. 4.2), and can grow towards or project away

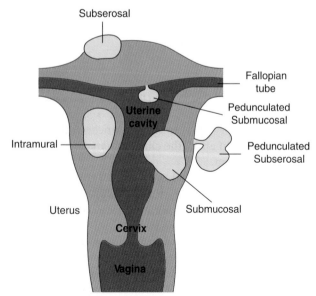

Fig. 4.2 Fibroid Types.

from the uterine cavity. It is common for a woman to have multiple fibroids.

The proliferation and maintenance of uterine fibroids is likely to be due to oestrogen and progesterone; hence, almost all the risk factors are related to increased levels of these hormones. Fibroids can develop at any time in women of reproductive age. Fibroids are more likely to enlarge during times of high hormone levels, such as pregnancy, and usually shrink after menopause, when low hormone levels are present.

CLINICAL FEATURES

The symptoms and signs depend on the size, number and position of the uterine fibroids.

SYMPTOMS

- Asymptomatic:
  - Fibroids are commonly (approximately 50%) asymptomatic.
  - Often detected incidentally on abdominal examination or on imaging.
- Menstrual irregularities:
  - Menstruation disorders are the most common symptomatic presentation of fibroids:
    - Menorrhagia.
    - IMB.
    - Dysmenorrhoea.

The exact mechanism for these symptoms is unknown but may be due to a fibroid directly pressing on the endometrial cavity, increasing the surface area of the endometrium, which increases blood loss. There may also be a local immunological or inflammatory reaction within the uterus in response to a fibroid, disturbing the endometrial haemostasis.

- Symptoms related to effect of a mass in the pelvis:
  - Abdominal bloating, pelvic fullness or pelvic pressure. Rarely, some patients also describe this as chronic pain.
  - Occasionally, pressure exerted by the fibroid on adjacent structures can cause constipation and urinary frequency or retention.
  - Dyspareunia if the fibroid is low in the pelvis.
- Acute pain presentations:
  - Fibroid torsion – a pedunculated fibroid can twist on its pedicle, which causes the blood supply to become occluded. If sustained, this leads to fibroid ischaemia and necrosis. This can present as an acute abdomen. A torted fibroid may require surgical intervention.
  - Red degeneration – this occurs when fibroid growth exceeds its blood supply. This again causes ischaemia and necrosis and therefore pain. The red degeneration is so called because the tissue appears red on histology. It often occurs in pregnancy, as the high hormone levels promote rapid fibroid growth. Red degeneration presents with vomiting, acute pain and fever. It is treated symptomatically with analgesia; therefore, it is important to rule out

all other causes of acute abdomen first, especially placental abruption in pregnant women, as this also presents with acute pain.

- Torsion and red degeneration can also occur intermittently, causing a more chronic pain presentation.
- Identified as part of investigations for infertility, recurrent miscarriage or complications in pregnancy.

SIGNS

- Palpable mass originating from the pelvis on abdominal examination.
- Firm, irregularly enlarged uterus noted on bimanual pelvic examination.

INVESTIGATIONS

PELVIC ULTRASOUND SCAN

- Usually, transabdominal and transvaginal scanning is performed. Transvaginal often provides the best imaging for smaller fibroids and for alternative causes of symptoms, whereas larger fibroids extending into the abdomen are better viewed transabdominally.
- Fibroids are easy to identify on an ultrasound scan.
- Most differentials of presenting symptoms can be excluded on an ultrasound scan:
  - Irregular bleeding – uterine polyps or endometrial cancer.
  - Pelvic mass – ovarian cysts and masses arising from other organs.

Usually, an ultrasound scan is the only investigation required to diagnose fibroids. However, depending on the clinical presentation, other investigations may be required to guide management:

- Urine pregnancy test in anyone of childbearing age with abnormal bleeding or a pelvic mass.
- Full blood count if irregular bleeding is a symptom, to assess for anaemia.
- Endometrial biopsy can be used in the investigation of abnormal vaginal bleeding and is especially important in postmenopausal bleeding.
- Hysteroscopy to further assess the uterine cavity. Submucosal fibroids can also be resected at hysteroscopy.
- Laparoscopy if chronic pelvic pain is the predominant symptom.
- MRI if images are not clear on ultrasound or there is concern that the mass is a sarcoma. MRI is also usually performed prior to treatment of fibroids using UAE.

The pelvic ultrasound scan can be organised routinely for a woman with no signs or symptoms of cancer and classic history and examination findings for fibroids. However, urgent referral and investigation is required if red flags, such as weight loss and unexplained bleeding, are detected during the history taking, as these may indicate a possible malignancy.

DIFFERENTIAL DIAGNOSIS

Fibroids are a very common and benign condition; however, fibroid symptoms overlap with symptoms produced by more serious pathologies. Also, as fibroids are so prevalent, an asymptomatic fibroid can coexist with a more serious pathology. It is therefore always essential to perform a full history and examination to exclude alternative pathologies. The differential diagnosis depends on the presenting symptoms.

ABNORMAL VAGINAL BLEEDING

- Endometrial polyp.
- Endometrial cancer.
- Cervical cancer.
- For other differentials, *see menorrhagia page 82*.

PELVIC MASS

- Ovarian cancer.
- Benign ovarian mass, for example, dermoid cyst, haemorrhagic cyst, or endometrioma.
- Endometrial cancer.
- Tubo-ovarian inflammatory abscess.
- Pregnancy.
- Adenomyosis.
- Non-gynaecology mass.
- Uterine sarcoma (leiomyosarcoma) – this is a rare group of cancers that develop from the uterine corpus, equating to the neoplastic form of a fibroid. Like fibroids, they present with abnormal uterine bleeding or a pelvic mass, but unlike fibroids, they may have rapid growth.

PELVIC PAIN

- Endometriosis.
- Adenomyosis.
- PID.
- Adhesions.
- Non-gynaecology causes, for example, genitourinary or bowel cause.

COMPLICATIONS

- Pain – torsion or red degeneration.
- Infertility complications – submucosal fibroids negatively affect fertility, but this effect can be reduced by removing the fibroid. The relationship between intramural fibroids and infertility is unclear, and it is unlikely that subserosal fibroids affect fertility. Unfortunately, treating fibroid-associated infertility is a balance of risks, as the surgical treatments for fibroids can themselves reduce fertility. For example, myomectomy increases the risk of uterine rupture in subsequent pregnancies, and UAE may reduce successful pregnancy rates due to reduced uterine blood supply.
- Pregnancy complications – fibroids, especially submucosal, are associated with obstetric complications. However, fortunately, the majority (70% to 90%) of women with fibroids have no associated complications during pregnancy. The mechanism

for obstetric complications is unclear, although thought to be related to mechanical obstruction and decreased uterine distension.

- Fibroids increase the risk of:
  - Bleeding in early pregnancy – especially if the placenta implants close to the fibroid.
  - Spontaneous miscarriage – unknown mechanism.
  - Preterm labour.
  - Malpresentation and/or obstructed labour – can act as a mechanical obstruction to the fetus entering the pelvis for vaginal birth.
  - Caesarean birth.
  - Postpartum haemorrhage – fibroids may prevent uterine contraction after birth.

MANAGEMENT

Fibroids, in themselves, are not a sinister pathology that require treatment. Treating fibroids should be aimed at improving a patient's quality of life by improving her symptoms. Asymptomatic fibroids do not need any treatment or follow-up.

The treatment options available for symptomatic fibroids depend on which symptoms the patient is suffering. Other key factors include whether the patient has a desire to maintain fertility and/or preserve her uterus.

MENORRHAGIA

If menorrhagia is the presenting symptom, investigate with a full blood count to rule out iron deficiency anaemia and then manage as with any cause of menorrhagia. These treatments include the 52 mg IUS, tranexamic acid, mefenamic acid, combined oral contraceptive pill and progesterone-based contraceptives. All these treatments reduce blood loss by their own specific actions. The treatments which also cause anovulation may also reduce fibroid size, as anovulation reduces the amount of oestrogen and progesterone produced.

[See 'Menorrhagia and Other Menstrual Bleeding Disorders' page 82.]

If the medical treatments do not control symptoms adequately, a referral should be made for specialist management. The following procedures are usually offered in the order below, with increasing invasiveness.

SURGICAL TREATMENT
Endometrial Ablation
- A process of destroying the endometrial lining of the uterus by either diathermy (electric current producing heat), laser (light), radiofrequency waves, microwaves or heated water. It is usually a day case procedure and can be done under local or general anaesthetic. It can significantly improve menorrhagia symptoms in up to 80% of patients.
- It cannot be used if the cavity is severely distorted by the fibroid. It is not suitable for women who may get pregnant in the future, as destroying the endometrium negatively affects fertility, as well as creating a high risk of miscarriage.

- The risks include uterine perforation, cervical laceration (as the procedure instruments reach the uterus via the cervix), infection, bleeding and burns to the uterus or surrounding structures.

Hysteroscopic Resection of a Fibroid
- Hysteroscopic resection of a fibroid is removing the part of the fibroid that projects into the uterine cavity using a resectoscope. The resectoscope is inserted through the cervical os and an electrical current is passed through a cutting loop to remove the fibroid. It is usually a day case procedure and can be done under local or general anaesthetic.
- As this procedure only removes the part of the fibroid that projects into the cavity, it is only suitable for submucosal and intracavity fibroids. The fibroid can be cut and removed in pieces. Removing the intracavity portion of a fibroid may improve fertility.
- The risks include uterine perforation, cervical laceration, infection, bleeding and rarely pulmonary oedema and hyponatraemia. During the procedure, the uterine cavity is filled with hypotonic fluid which can be absorbed into the circulation through the blood vessels as the fibroid is cut away. If a significant amount of fluid is absorbed, this can cause profound hyponatraemia which, in rare cases, can be life threatening.

Uterine Artery Embolisation (UAE)
- UAE is an interventional radiological procedure that involves injecting an embolic agent into the uterine arteries to reduce the blood supply to the uterus and fibroid. As the fibroid requires a higher blood supply than its surrounding myometrium, the fibroid is preferentially affected. The fibroid size depends on its blood supply, so with the blood supply reduced, the fibroid atrophies.
- This procedure induces fibroid necrosis, which is painful, often causing protracted period-like pains that require simple analgesia for a couple of weeks. This needs to be included in the consent for this procedure.
- UAE is particularly useful in those patients who are at high surgical risk, as well as those who have symptoms from the fibroid compressing adjacent structures.
- UAE has an unknown effect on fertility; fibroid removal increases fertility, but the reduced blood flow has a detrimental effect on fertility.
- The risks include infection, haemorrhage, incomplete uterine artery occlusion, unintended embolisation of other organs and femoral artery puncture site haematomas.

Myomectomy
- Myomectomy is a surgical procedure to remove a fibroid either via a laparoscopic or an open abdominal incision. The aim of the procedure is to remove the fibroid while maintaining fertility.
- The risks of myomectomy include haemorrhage, adjacent organ injury and infection. There is a small risk

of uncontrolled heavy bleeding at the time of surgery, which may require a hysterectomy to save the patient's life. This, of course, would be devastating for a patient being treated for infertility. The reoccurrence rate of fibroids post-procedure varies between 10% and 50%.

- A subsequent pregnancy following a myomectomy carries a small risk of uterine rupture during labour, as the uterus will not be as strong in the scarred area following the surgery. If, during the myomectomy, the uterus was opened fully (serosa, muscle, and mucosa), the risk of rupture in labour is even higher, so the patient may be advised to have an elective caesarean rather than go into labour.

Hysterectomy

- Hysterectomy is the removal of the uterus. It is a definitive treatment for fibroids that prevents recurrence of symptoms and new fibroid growth; it also provides permanent contraception. The uterus can be removed via an abdominal incision (open abdominal hysterectomy), vaginal incision (vaginal hysterectomy or laparoscopic-assisted vaginal hysterectomy) or a total laparoscopic hysterectomy. The route of the hysterectomy will depend on uterine size, uterine descent, patient co-morbidities and patient choice.
- The risks of a hysterectomy include bleeding, infection, vaginal vault prolapse and damage to surrounding structures, including the urinary tract and bowel.

Hysteroscopic resection, myomectomy and hysterectomy can be preceded by short-term medical therapy with GnRH agonists. These treatments temporarily reduce the fibroid size by up to 50%, which reduces intraoperative blood loss and can improve surgical operability. The medications are usually prescribed for three to 6 months prior to the surgery. However, if the fibroids shrink significantly in that time and relieve symptoms, then surgery may not be necessary. The medications cannot be used long term due to their side effects.

GnRH Agonists, for Example, Leuprorelin and Goserelin

- These medications are generally given as injections.
- They inhibit the HPO axis, causing a temporary medically induced menopause. This results in low oestrogen and progesterone levels. These hormones are believed to promote and maintain fibroid growth; therefore, lowering these hormone concentrations causes fibroid shrinkage.
- The treatment causes menopausal symptoms; for example, night sweats, hot flushes and irritability. If a patient is symptomatic, HRT can be given as an "add back" therapy. GnRH analogues are not licensed for long-term use, and prolonged use leads to osteoporosis.

Antiprogesterones, for Example, Ulipristal

- Progesterone antagonists block the uterine progesterone receptors. Progesterone is thought to

stimulate fibroid growth, so blocking the receptors on the uterus causes the fibroids to shrink.
- These medications were intended to be used as long-term medical options to reduce the need for surgery, or to shrink the fibroid to make surgery easier. However, they are now very rarely used due to the rare but life-threatening complication of liver failure. Where they are used every other management option must have been excluded, they are only used intermittently, and close liver function monitoring is required.

PAIN OR PELVIC FULLNESS

If pain or pelvic fullness is the presenting symptom, then the management options are:
- Analgesia following the WHO pain ladder.
- UAE, myomectomy or hysterectomy.

PROGNOSIS

It is impossible to predict the course of a fibroid in an individual patient. Usually, fibroids shrink and therefore symptoms resolve with menopause, due to the effects of reduced oestrogen and progesterone.

❓ QUESTIONS

Danica, a 38-year-old non-smoking woman, visits her primary care physician as she has been trying to conceive for a year. She also describes a long history of menorrhagia. On direct questioning, she also admits bloating and urinary frequency, and she has been treated recently for recurrent UTIs. An abdominal exam reveals increased body habitus and an irregularly enlarged, tender uterus. Her conjunctiva is pale. A pregnancy test is negative, and a transvaginal scan shows a large intramural fibroid.

Q1 Which is the most common type of uterine fibroid?
  A Cervical.
  B Intraligamentous.
  C Intramural.
  D Submucosal.
  E Subserosal.

Q2 Which of these presenting complaints is not an indication for surgery?
  A Failure of conservative medical management.
  B Fibroid torsion.
  C Heavy menstrual bleeding.
  D Red degeneration.
  E Very large fibroids causing pressure symptoms.

Q3 The patient above states these symptoms are having a significant impact on her quality of life, and she wishes to discuss a long-term solution. Which of the treatments below would you recommend to this patient?
  A Combined oral contraceptive.
  B Goserelin.
  C Hysterectomy.
  D Myomectomy.
  E Naproxen.

[Answers on page 193.]

PREMENSTRUAL DISORDER

Premenstrual disorder (PMD), also called premenstrual syndrome (PMS), is characterised by physical, behavioural or psychological symptoms which are severe enough to affect a woman's quality of life, that occur regularly during the luteal phase of a woman's menstrual cycle, which then resolve after menstruation.

Physiological premenstrual symptoms (mild PMD) are the same symptoms as those of PMD but do not have an impact on a woman's quality of life. Severe PMD is also sometimes referred to as Premenstrual dysphoric disorder (PMDD).

AETIOLOGY

Premenstrual symptoms occur in 95% of women at some time in their lives, with around 5% experiencing symptoms severe enough to be diagnosed as PMD. PMD occurs during the luteal phase of the menstrual cycle, meaning that women who are prepubescent, postmenopausal or pregnant will not be affected. Hormonal contraceptives, which inhibit ovulation, also decrease the incidence of PMD.

PATHOPHYSIOLOGY

The precise pathophysiology is unknown. Given that symptoms (Table 4.7) appear to occur after ovulation and resolve at the end of the luteal phase, the current theory is that increased production of progesterone during this time of the menstrual cycle may be an important factor. There is evidence that progesterone and its metabolites have an effect on the production and receptors of certain neurotransmitters, in particular serotonin and gamma-aminobutyric acid (GABA). As progesterone is implicated as a cause of PMD, progesterone-containing contraceptives may also cause PMD (even the preparations which inhibit ovulation).

RISK FACTORS

- Family history.
- Poor diet, lack of exercise and raised BMI.
- Smoking.
- Lack of support network.

CLINICAL FEATURES

It is important to note the significant crossover of premenstrual symptoms and symptoms associated with depression and other psychiatric disorders. Depression would be expected to affect someone most of the time, whereas PMD symptoms should resolve for at least a week during the follicular phase of the menstrual cycle.

INVESTIGATIONS

With a clear-cut history, the only investigation usually required is a symptom diary. The most commonly used diary is the 'daily record of severity of problems in PMD.' This is a diary which is used every day over a menstrual cycle. The patient records which symptoms from the above bullet point list affect her, and how severely. The diary also asks the woman to record if any symptom affects her ability to function at work, social activities or relationships with others, and to what extent. The patient is also asked to record dates of menstruation. The diary should be completed over three menstrual cycles.

The diary is used to confirm or refute the diagnosis. Symptoms occurring in a cyclical pattern in the luteal phase of the menstrual cycle, which improve with menstruation, with at least one symptom-free week is diagnostic of PMD. Conversely, if symptoms are demonstrated to not be cyclical, or continuous without a symptom-free week, this suggests another diagnosis.

The diary also helps decide on appropriate management by demonstrating whether symptoms are severe enough to affect a woman's quality of life, and if so, which symptoms are the most severe.

DIFFERENTIAL DIAGNOSIS

Psychiatric conditions:
- Depression.
- Hypomania.
- Bipolar disorder.
- Borderline personality disorder.

Medical conditions which may present with some similar symptoms:
- Hypothyroidism.
- Phaeochromocytoma.
- Irritable bowel syndrome.

Table 4.7 Premenstrual Disorder Symptoms

PSYCHOLOGICAL SYMPTOMS	BEHAVIOURAL SYMPTOMS	PHYSICAL SYMPTOMS
• Low mood, hopelessness, worthlessness, feelings of guilt. • Anhedonia – loss of interest in usual activities. • Anergia – abnormal lack of energy. • Anxiety. • Emotional lability – Mood swings, overly sensitive. • Irritability, anger. • Inability to cope.	• Change in appetite or food cravings. • Change in sleep pattern. • Change in concentration, cognition, and visuospatial awareness. • Changes in libido.	• Breast tenderness and swelling. • Abdominal bloating. • Headaches. • Joint or muscle pains. • Swelling of hands or feet.

It is important to emphasise that PMD will resolve around menstruation, with at least 1 week symptom-free (follicular phase) each menstrual cycle. Other differential diagnoses may still have exacerbations during the luteal phase like PMD, but they will not fully resolve at menstruation.

Sometimes complicating the diagnosis is an underlying psychological condition with an element of PMD which may exacerbate one or both conditions. This is called premenstrual exacerbation. In this situation, both conditions may need to be treated, but a clinician should monitor the patient cautiously to confirm that an accurate diagnosis has been made.

COMPLICATIONS

PMD has no significant medical complications. However, the quality of life is often reduced due to the effect on work, hobbies, daily activities, social life and personal interactions.

MANAGEMENT

LIFESTYLE MODIFICATIONS

- Maintaining a healthy BMI.
- Exercise.
- Healthy diet.
- Smoking cessation.
- Alcohol reduction.
- Stress reduction.

PAIN MANAGEMENT

- Paracetamol.
- Ibuprofen or mefenamic acid.
- Codeine.

VITAMIN SUPPLEMENTATION

- Vitamin B6 (pyridoxine) 10 mg once daily is recommended as a first-line treatment of PMD.
- Vitamin D and calcium – appears effective for PMD and has a good safety profile

PSYCHOLOGICAL MANAGEMENT

- Cognitive behavioural therapy (CBT) – has been shown to reduce the severity of PMD.
- Selective serotonin reuptake inhibitors (SSRIs) – have been shown to be as effective when used just in the luteal phase or continuously, with less side effects reported when used only in the luteal phase. The proposed mechanism of action is countering the effect of progesterone on serotonin in the central nervous system, so reducing symptom severity. A common starting dose would be citalopram oral 10 mg once daily. Doses can be increased to 40 mg if needed.
- Women with underlying mental health problems should be referred for psychiatric assessment.

COMBINED ORAL CONTRACEPTIVE

- Oestrogen inhibits FSH and LH release from the anterior pituitary by negative feedback on the HPO axis. Ovulation does not occur, so the luteal phase with progesterone rise does not occur.
- A third-generation COCP should be used as these contain a progestogen (drospirenone) which is not associated with causing PMD. These can be used cyclically with the normal pill-free week or can be used continuously without having a regular pill-free week. Continuous use is more likely to improve symptoms but is more likely to cause IMB.
- Older COCPs and progesterone-only contraceptives can worsen, or even be the cause, of PMD due to the progestogen they contain. If a patient is on one of these it should be stopped or changed to a third-generation COCP.

SPECIALIST REFERRAL

If symptoms have not improved satisfactorily with the above measures, a primary care physician should refer to a gynaecologist for more specialised treatments.

HIGH-DOSE OESTROGEN TREATMENT

- High-dose oestrogen works by negative feedback in the same way as the lower dose in the combined pill but is more likely to be successful in preventing ovulation and therefore progesterone production.
- Usually given as oestradiol by percutaneous patch (100 to 200 mcg twice a week). This treatment is not licensed as contraception, so if required, barrier or intrauterine methods should be used.
- The long-term effect of this treatment is unknown, but theoretically, it may increase the risk of oestrogen-dependent cancers of the breast and endometrium.
- A progestogen should be given to protect against the negative effects of the oestrogen. To reduce the chances of the progestogen causing PMD it is advised that micronised progesterone (given either orally or per vagina) is given for 10 days in the luteal phase. Alternatively, a 52 mg IUS can be inserted. Both of these options can still cause premenstrual symptoms in a few cases.

GONADOTROPIN-RELEASING HORMONE ANALOGUE

- As well as a treatment for severe PMD, it can also be used as a diagnostic tool in difficult-to-diagnose cases, as giving a 3-month course should improve PMD symptoms significantly.
- Given as a subcutaneous injection which releases the GnRH analogue. Depending on the preparation each injection lasts for one or 3 months.
- Normally, GnRH is released by the hypothalamus in a pulsatile fashion. Giving the GnRH analogue continuously actually causes downregulation of the receptors, resulting in complete inhibition of the HPO axis.

- The patient is effectively in a medically induced menopausal state.
- This treatment completely stops ovulation and significantly lowers oestrogen and progesterone levels. It is usually highly effective. Therefore, if symptoms of PMD persist despite GnRH treatment, another diagnosis should be considered for the patient's symptoms.
- It is advisable to give the patient HRT along with this treatment, as they will otherwise develop symptoms of the menopause.
- GnRH analogues are not licenced for longer than 6 months as they increase the risk of developing osteoporosis due to the low levels of oestrogen caused by the treatment. If longer-term treatment is considered the patient should certainly be given add-back HRT and have a yearly bone mineral density scan (dual-energy x-ray absorptiometry (DEXA)) with a view to stop treatment if density declines. To reduce the chance of the HRT causing PMD symptoms, it is advised to use a continuous combined regime of a low-dose oestradiol patch and micronised progesterone, or to use tibolone.

BILATERAL OOPHORECTOMY

- Very rarely, if symptoms of PMD are severe and uncontrolled by other treatment, then a definitive treatment would be to remove the ovaries.
- It is advisable for the patient to try GnRH analogues first, to confirm that menopause will resolve symptoms.
- Hysterectomy is offered at the same time. With the uterus removed, treatment of menopausal symptoms can consist of oestrogen HRT alone, whereas if a patient has a uterus, progesterone must be given as well to prevent endometrial cancer. However, the progestogen may provoke premenstrual symptoms.
- Sometimes testosterone replacement is considered, as the ovaries are responsible for 50% production in the female, and low levels may decrease libido.

PROGNOSIS

Overall, 5% of women will develop severe premenstrual symptoms. Correct diagnosis of the condition is important so the correct treatment can be instigated. Relatively simple treatments can have a significant impact on a woman's quality of life.

❓ QUESTIONS

Kelly is a 40-year-old who has had two previous vaginal births. She has regular 28-day menstrual cycles. For the past 4 years, from days 16–28 of her cycles, she gets very low in mood, is irritable, has no energy and gets a feeling of abdominal distension. These symptoms frequently require Kelly to take time off work, which is causing her significant conflict with her boss.

A Adrenocorticotrophic hormone.	**F** Human placental lactogen.
B Beta human chorionic gonadotropin.	**G** Luteinising hormone.
C Cortisol.	**H** Oestradiol.
D Follicle stimulating hormone.	**I** Oestrone.
	J Somatostatin.
E Gonadotropin releasing hormone.	**K** Testosterone.
	L Progesterone.

Select the most appropriate hormone from the above list that corresponds to the following statements.

Q1   Steroid hormone, which causes negative feedback on the hypothalamus and pituitary during the follicular phase of the menstrual cycle.

Q2   Hormone likely to be responsible for the symptoms of premenstrual disorder.

Q3   The hormone responsible for inhibiting ovulation in the combined oral contraceptive.

Q4   The hormone released in a pulsatile manner from the hypothalamus.

Q5   The hormone which is in peak concentration just before ovulation.

Q6   Which patient is the most likely to suffer from premenstrual disorder?
     A A 60-year-old woman with angina.
     B A 29-year-old woman who is 4 months pregnant.
     C A 27-year-old woman who is fit and well.
     D A 24-year-old man with gynaecomastia.
     E A 16-year-old girl who has not had any pubertal changes.

Q7   Answer true or false: These treatments may be of use in the treatment of premenstrual disorder.
     A Selective serotonin reuptake inhibitors.
     B Electroconvulsive therapy.
     C Progestogen-only pill.
     D Third-generation combined oral contraceptive.
     E Nicotine patch.

[Answers on page 194.]

MENOPAUSE

Menopause has occurred after a woman has not menstruated for 1 year (when not on hormonal contraception).

However, periods normally do not suddenly stop; they usually become more irregular and infrequent over a number of months to years before they finally stop completely. This time is referred to as perimenopause. Women often develop menopausal symptoms during this time.

AETIOLOGY

The average age of menopause in the UK is 51.

Premature menopause is said to have occurred if it happens before 40 years of age. This occurs in approximately 1% of women. There are a number of causes for premature menopause:

- Primary premature ovarian insufficiency (POI) – no cause found.
- Family history of premature menopause – daughters of women with idiopathic POI have a 10% risk of premature menopause.
- Chromosomal abnormality in 10% of cases, of which Turner syndrome and fragile X gene mutation are commonly identified.
- Autoimmune – associations with hypothyroidism and Addison disease.
- Iatrogenic – surgical removal of the ovaries or damage by chemotherapy or radiotherapy.
- Systemic infection (rare).
- Other causes of secondary amenorrhoea.

[See 'Secondary Amenorrhoea' page 26.]

PATHOPHYSIOLOGY

After fetal development *in utero,* there is no further increase in the number of oocytes and the number then decreases throughout life. A typical female newborn has around one million primordial follicles. At the age of menarche, 400,000 remain; by 40 years old, a few thousand remain; and at menopause, none remain.

During reproductive life, oocytes are used up during the menstrual cycle. Stimulation of oocytes by FSH results in around 20 primordial follicles developing and maturing each cycle, with one becoming the dominant follicle for ovulation.

[See 'The Menstrual Cycle and Physiology of the HPO Axis' page 8.]

As the number of oocytes falls to very low levels towards the end of reproductive life, it takes a larger concentration of FSH to stimulate oocyte maturation. This results in irregular and infrequent menstrual cycles. Once all the oocytes have been used, there are no more menstrual cycles.

The symptoms of menopause arise as a result of a lack of oestrogen. Prior to menopause, oestradiol is produced by the dominant ovarian follicle during each menstrual cycle. This causes endometrial proliferation and acts by negative feedback on FSH to prevent the development of other follicles. After menopause, there are no oocytes to produce oestradiol.

The predominant oestrogen in the postmenopausal female is oestrone, which is predominantly synthesised by adipose tissue. The serum concentration and biological effect of oestrone is much less than that of oestradiol.

SIGNS AND SYMPTOMS

Overall, 80% of women will develop menopausal symptoms. However, only 10% have symptoms severe enough for them to consult healthcare providers.

Symptom duration varies from around 6 months to 10 years for most women (median duration of 7 years), but over 10% will have symptoms lasting longer than 10 years.

SYMPTOMS

- May be asymptomatic.
- Hot flushes – last a couple of minutes, with a sensation of feeling hot in the upper body and face. They can be associated with sweating and dizziness and can occur multiple times a day.
- Night sweats (nocturnal hyperhidrosis) – can cause the woman to wake multiple times per night, which can have a massive effect on their psychological state. Can require frequent changing of drenched night clothing and bedsheets.
- Vaginal dryness – if sexually active, this can cause dyspareunia. It can also cause pruritus (atrophic vaginitis).
- Loss of sexual desire (libido) – related to low androgen levels. About 50% of female androgens are made in ovarian follicles.
- Other associated symptoms – muscle aches, joint pains, difficulty concentrating, low mood or other depressive symptoms.

SIGNS

- Hair thinning.
- Dry skin.
- Atrophic vagina.

INVESTIGATIONS

- Rarely necessary as usually menopause or perimenopause can be diagnosed from a history of amenorrhea or symptoms.
- In premature menopause, or where there is doubt as to the cause of symptoms, a raised serum FSH level suggests a perimenopausal state. Two raised FSH levels at least 4 weeks apart are required to make a diagnosis of ovarian insufficiency. FSH should not be used as a diagnostic tool in women over the age of 45 years, as FSH levels can be high or low in the perimenopausal patients in this age group, so this is unreliable for diagnostic purposes. Clinical features should be used to make the diagnosis in this age group.

DIFFERENTIAL DIAGNOSIS

- Any cause of secondary amenorrhoea.
- Rare conditions can give symptoms of night sweats and or hot flushes. If these symptoms are associated with other systemic symptoms, consider alternative causes:
  - Phaeochromocytoma.
  - Renal cell carcinoma.
  - Leukaemia.

- Sarcoidosis.
- Tuberculosis.
- Symptoms of low mood, loss of libido and memory changes could be associated with depression.
- Joint pains and muscle aches may be caused by arthritis, osteoporosis, fibromyalgia and other musculoskeletal conditions which are more common with advancing age.

COMPLICATIONS

- Psychological effect of the symptoms – they can have a significant detrimental effect on quality of life.
- Recurrent UTIs – more common after menopause due to the change in vaginal mucosa and bacterial flora as a result of the lack of oestrogen.
- Osteoporosis – oestrogen has a role in maintaining the balance of osteoblast and osteoclast activity. After the menopause, oestrogen levels fall, resulting in demineralisation of bone and osteoporosis over time, increasing the risk of fracture. HRT is protective against osteoporosis, reducing the risk in postmenopausal women on HRT by 20%. Women who undergo premature menopause are advised to use HRT until the time of the natural menopause (around the age of 51), regardless of whether they have menopausal symptoms, as they would otherwise be at an increased risk of osteoporosis.
- Unexpected pregnancy – it is important to advise patients that in the perimenopausal time there can still be some residual ovarian function and the possibility of ovulation and therefore pregnancy. This may present late if the amenorrhoea is assumed to be menopause rather than pregnancy. Advise women to continue contraception until 1 year after their last menstrual period.

MANAGEMENT

CONSERVATIVE MEASURES

Diet and lifestyle should be optimised in order to promote general health and well-being. In particular, weight, alcohol consumption, smoking cessation and exercise should be discussed.

HORMONE REPLACEMENT THERAPY

Menopause is a physiological process which will occur in all females who live long enough. HRT should be offered as first-line treatment to a woman whose menopausal symptoms are having a detrimental effect on her life.

HRT should not be offered to women without symptoms simply to reduce their osteoporosis risk, as other effective treatments are available for this, such as calcium supplementation and alendronic acid. The exception to this is women with premature menopause, where HRT is advised until the average age of menopause.

Symptom relief is achieved by giving oestrogen. Progesterone is given as well (unless the patient has had a hysterectomy) to protect the uterus from the effect of unopposed oestrogen on the endometrium, as this would otherwise result in endometrial hyperplasia and increase the risk of endometrial cancer. HRT was traditionally prescribed as tablets, but other preparations, such as transdermal patches, gels, nasal spray or implants, are available and have better safety profiles.

HRT reduces symptom severity and frequency by 80% to 90%. It takes a couple of weeks for symptoms such as hot flushes and night sweats to start to improve and a couple of months for vaginal symptoms to improve.

Systemic HRT has risks which must be explained to the patient so that she can assess whether the benefit to her in terms of symptom reduction warrants the increased risk.

Table 4.8 shows that although the relative risk can be significantly increased when using HRT, due to the relatively low incidence of these events occurring in the 50 to 70 age group, the absolute risk difference is small. For example, the 2% risk of breast cancers in non-HRT users is increased to 3% with HRT use. The main contraindication to HRT use is a current or personal history of breast cancer.

To minimise the risks:
- The lowest dose of oestrogen required for adequate reduction in symptoms should be used. After commencing HRT the woman should be reviewed 3 months later to assess efficacy.
- HRT should only be used while needed to control symptoms. Women should be reviewed yearly, and considered for discontinuing HRT after 2 years to see if symptoms are manageable without treatment.
- Parenteral preparations should be offered first line, as they do not appear to increase the VTE risk.
- Similarly to hormonal contraception, there should be consideration to stopping oral HRT 4 weeks prior to any planned surgery to limit the risk of postoperative VTE.

Table 4.8 | Risks Associated With Hormone Replacement Therapy Use

RISK	BASELINE INCIDENCE PER 1000 OVER 7 YEARS IN FEMALES AGE 50-70	APPROXIMATE RELATIVE INCREASED RISK USING HRT
VTE (oral HRT preparations only)	5	100%
Stroke	10	50%
Breast cancer	20	50%
Ovarian cancer	5	20%

- HRT is not a form of contraception. Although the risk of conception over the age of 45 is low, perimenopausal women should be advised to use additional contraception. An IUS can be used to provide the progesterone component of combined HRT, whilst providing contraceptive cover.

VAGINAL BLEEDING ON HRT

Unscheduled bleeding in the first 3 months of commencing HRT is common due to the stimulatory effect of oestrogen on the endometrium. If the bleeding begins or persists beyond 3 months, women should be referred for investigation of postmenopausal bleeding.

[See 'Endometrial Cancer' page 146.]

Two types of combined HRT are available: continuous combined and sequential release. In women who have stopped having periods, the continuous combined HRT should be used, as it provides a continuous dose of oestrogen and progestogen. Women who are still having periods but are being treated with HRT for symptom relief should use sequential HRT, which provides a continuous dose of oestrogen to manage symptoms but the progesterone is stopped every 3 weeks, like in the combined oral contraceptive, to allow for a withdrawal bleed. If a continuous regime is used in these patients, they often get recurrent IMB.

NON-HORMONE TREATMENTS FOR SYSTEMIC SYMPTOMS

Non-hormone treatments are available and can be used in conjunction with HRT or alone. They are not as effective as HRT.

- Cognitive behaviour therapy (CBT) – may improve coping mechanisms for all symptoms and may improve mood symptoms, in particular.
- Clonidine – A$_2$ receptor agonist which improves vasomotor symptoms.
- Selective noradrenaline reuptake inhibitors (SNRIs) and SSRIs; for example, venlafaxine or fluoxetine – limited evidence of improvement in menopausal symptoms, and no evidence of improving menopausal mood symptoms that are not formally diagnosed depression.
- GABA analogues; for example, gabapentin – may improve vasomotor and other symptoms.
- There is limited evidence that alternative therapies, such as soy extract, yam extracts, black cohosh and St John's wort, may improve vasomotor symptoms, but their preparations are unlicensed and long-term safety is unknown.

VAGINAL SYMPTOMS

- Local vaginal oestrogen creams or pessaries – there is little systemic absorption from these preparations so they can be used long-term, without a progestogen, and often even in patients where systemic HRT is contraindicated.
- Topical lubricants (oil and water-based) can aid sexual intercourse.
- Topical moisturisers for dry skin.

LOSS OF LIBIDO

- Testosterone supplements can be given if HRT alone is ineffective.
- Tibolone is a synthetic steroidal medication which has oestrogen, progesterone and androgen agonist properties. It is a type of HRT with mild androgen properties, so it can improve libido. It is also commonly used in younger patients who are being treated with GnRH analogues to reduce the associated menopausal symptoms.

PROGNOSIS

Menopause and its associated symptoms are a self-limiting event but can last for many years, It is the role of the clinician to guide the woman through this time with as little detriment as possible to her short-term quality of life and long-term health.

❓ QUESTIONS

Mrs Robinson visits her primary care physician. She is a 46-year-old with no previous significant medical history. She attends because she thinks she is menopausal and would like your opinion on what she should now do. She has stopped having periods for the last 10 months and is getting frequent 'hot flushes' while at work.

A Anti-diuretic hormone.	**G** Gonadotropin-releasing hormone.
B Anti-Mullerian hormone.	**H** Inhibin.
C Atrial natriuretic hormone.	**I** Insulin.
D Cortisol.	**J** Oestrogen.
E Follicle stimulating hormone.	**K** Oxytocin.
F Glucagon.	**L** Progesterone.

From the options above, select the most appropriate hormone that matches the following descriptions.

Q1 The hormone raised during the perimenopause.

Q2 The hormone replaced to reduce menopausal symptoms.

Q3 The hormone given as part of hormone replacement therapy to reduce the risk of endometrial cancer.

Q4 The hormone released by the anterior pituitary.

Q5 The hormone which, if pathologically raised, is commonly associated with amenorrhoea and weight gain.

Q6 What is the average age women go through the menopause in the UK?

A 41.

B 44.

C 49.

D 51.

E 55.

Q7   Answer true or false to the following statements regarding menopause and HRT.

  A The above woman is now postmenopausal because she has now stopped having periods for 10 months.

  B The progestogen part of combined HRT treatment reduces the menopausal symptoms.

  C A recent deep vein thrombosis is a contraindication for oral HRT use.

  D It is reasonable to make the diagnosis of the menopause on history alone.

  E Women with premature menopause but no symptoms may benefit from HRT.

[Answers on page 196.]

VULVAL DISORDERS

LICHEN SCLEROSUS

Lichen sclerosus is an autoimmune, inflammatory skin condition which predominantly affects the genital areas. Histology reveals thickening and excessive keratinisation of the epidermis, with inflammatory cell infiltration in the dermal layers. Classically, lichen sclerosus appears as well-defined and hard white patches on the vulva. Over time, the skin lesions cause destruction and adhesions of the normal anatomy of the vulva.

AETIOLOGY

The true incidence of lichen sclerosus is unknown, as it can be treated by many different specialities. Additionally, many women will not present with the condition as it can be asymptomatic.

  Lichen sclerosus is an autoimmune condition that typically affects postmenopausal women, although there is also a peak in incidence in prepubertal girls and it can rarely affect males. Of the women with lichen sclerosus, 40% have an additional autoimmune condition. The most commonly associated conditions are autoimmune diseases of the thyroid gland.

SIGNS AND SYMPTOMS

Lichen sclerosus (Fig. 4.3) typically affects a 'figure of eight shaped' region (see Fig. 4.4) within the vulval and anal regions. It may affect only one small, isolated area or the entire region.

Symptoms
- May be asymptomatic.
- Pruritus – most common symptom, often worse at night.
- Generalised vulva pain.
- Dyspareunia – pain on intercourse. This is often due to a combination of tender tissues, and due to introital narrowing from adhesions, preventing the stretch needed to allow for penetrative intercourse.

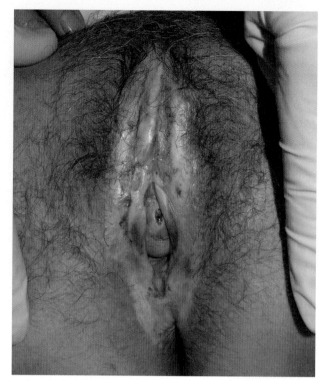

Fig. 4.3 Lichen Sclerosus.

- Urinary and bowel symptoms – constipation can occur if there are perianal lesions, and urination can be obstructed by adhesions.

Signs
- White plaques.
- Hyperkeratosis.
- Ecchymoses (discolouration of the skin caused by bleeding underneath).
- Erosions.
- Fissures.
- Excoriation marks.
- Abnormal architecture of the vulva.
  - Adhesions.
  - Destruction of the labia minora, or midline fusion of the labia minora.
  - Fusion of the clitoral hood, or burying of the clitoris by overlying adhesions.
  - Narrowing of the vaginal opening (introitus) due to adhesions.
- Lichen sclerosus does not affect the vagina, so the vaginal tissue should appear normal on examination.

INVESTIGATIONS

The diagnosis of lichen sclerosus is largely clinical, as the characteristic white plaques alongside a typical history are extremely suggestive of the condition. However, if there are any atypical features or if cancer is suspected, then a biopsy must be performed. Additionally, if the patient's condition does not respond to treatment, then a biopsy should be taken.

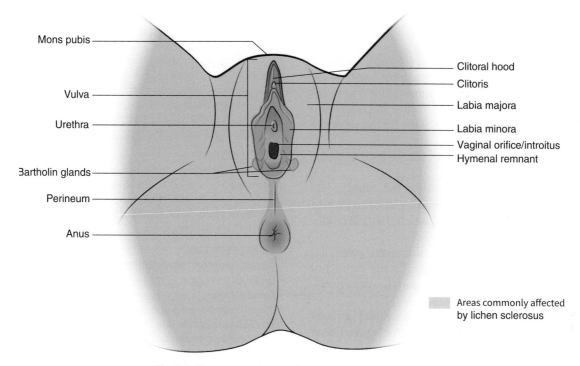

Mons pubis
Vulva
Urethra
Bartholin glands
Perineum
Anus

Clitoral hood
Clitoris
Labia majora
Labia minora
Vaginal orifice/introitus
Hymenal remnant

Areas commonly affected
by lichen sclerosus

Fig. 4.4 Diagram showing the distribution of Lichen Sclerosus.

As lichen sclerosus is an autoimmune disease, an autoantibody screen may be necessary if there are any clinical signs of other autoimmune conditions. As thyroid disease is the most commonly related of these conditions, thyroid function tests are frequently performed. This is particularly important as many patients will be asymptomatic from their thyroid disease.

Lichen sclerosus is usually not associated with infectious processes. However, in cases where the skin is broken (such as fissures or erosions), secondary infections may be present. If this is suspected, then swabs of the lesion should be taken and sent to microbiology for analysis.

DIFFERENTIAL DIAGNOSIS

Vulval skin conditions often present with similar symptoms such as itching, pain and fissuring of the skin. The following conditions should be considered in the differential diagnosis of lichen sclerosus.
- Lichen planus.
- Lichen simplex.
- Vulval eczema.
- Vulval psoriasis.
- Vulval intraepithelial neoplasia (VIN).
- Vulvodynia.

COMPLICATIONS

Dysaesthesia or chronic pain syndromes, including vulvodynia (vulval pain), may also result from the inflammation in lichen sclerosus. Treatments can include topical local anaesthetics, painkillers targeted at neuropathic pain and sometimes surgery.

Patients who suffer from lichen sclerosus may experience psychosexual dysfunction as a result of the condition, leading them to lose interest in sex. Psychosexual counselling may be required in cases where sexual function does not improve upon treating the physical disease.

The most severe physical complication of lichen sclerosus is squamous cell carcinoma (SCC) of the anogenital region. Around 60% of SCCs within the vulva are found to occur following a background of lichen sclerosus. However, the risk of developing SCC as a result of lichen sclerosus is less than 5%, so this is a relatively rare complication. A multidisciplinary team is required to treat vulval SCCs as both surgical and medical approaches are likely to be necessary. Lichen sclerosus can cause SCCs directly, or precancerous epithelial cell changes (VIN) can occur first, which may then progress to an SCC.

MANAGEMENT

Conservative

Patients should always be given written information about their condition and be advised to self-examine regularly in case of any cancerous changes. They should be advised to seek medical help if they experience any change in appearance of the lesion, such as ulceration, lumps, skin thickening or bleeding. Patients should be reviewed yearly by a doctor to look for cancerous changes requiring further investigation.

In order to help manage their condition, patients should also be advised to use emollients, avoid scratching where possible, avoid tight-fitting underwear and avoid soaps and other chemicals when bathing to prevent further irritation to the area.

Medical

Initial medical treatment for uncomplicated lichen sclerosus should be topical ultra-potent steroid agents; for example, clobetasol propionate ointment for 3 months:

- Ointment applied every night for the first 4 weeks.
- Ointment applied every other night for the second 4 weeks.
- Ointment applied twice a week for the final 4 weeks.

If a secondary infection is suspected, then ultra-potent steroid preparations containing antifungal and antibiotic agents may be used as an alternative to clobetasol propionate.

The patient should then be reviewed after the 3-month course of steroids. If symptoms have not resolved, a biopsy should also be taken to confirm the diagnosis and rule out cancer.

Patients with steroid-resistant disease should be managed jointly by dermatologists and gynaecologists. Other medical treatments, such as topical calcineurin inhibitors, oral retinoids and phototherapy, have shown some success in clinical trials, so these are occasionally used.

Surgical

Surgery is usually reserved for complicated cases of lichen sclerosus where adhesions need to be removed in order to improve the patient's function. It is also used in cases of malignancy in order to excise tumours.

PROGNOSIS

Around 50% of patients' symptoms fully resolve after treatment for the first episode of lichen sclerosus, and subsequently only require annual review by their primary care physician. The patients should also regularly self-examine and report changes in order to promote early cancer diagnosis. For the remaining 50%, lichen sclerosus is a lifelong condition which either does not fully resolve or often reoccurs. However, most of these patients will respond to repeated courses of steroid treatment, optimising their quality of life.

 Other Vulval Skin Conditions

All can present with vulval pain, itching, dyspareunia, and urinary and bowel symptoms.

LICHEN PLANUS

Autoimmune inflammatory condition most commonly appears as erythema and erosions of skin and mucosal surfaces, commonly affecting the vulva, vagina and sometimes the mouth (Fig. 4.5). By contrast, lichen sclerosus does not affect the vagina or other mucosal areas. In lichen planus, pale lines can be seen at the edges of the lesions, called Wickham striae. Scarring is frequently seen. The diagnosis is clinical, but where doubt exists, a biopsy will show saw tooth acanthosis. Treatment is with conservative measures and potent steroids, like in lichen sclerosus.

LICHEN SIMPLEX

Lichenification and excoriations caused primarily by excessive scratching, so most often occurs on the side opposite the dominant hand (Fig. 4.6). Most commonly associated with medical conditions that cause pruritus, such as obstructive liver diseases, kidney failure, and lymphoma. It is also strongly linked with psychiatric disorders, such as anxiety and obsessive-compulsive disorders. Treatment includes emollients, steroids, antihistamines to decrease the pruritus sensation and psychiatric treatments such as CBT.

VULVAL ECZEMA

Atopy, with allergic or irritant causes, is similar to eczema anywhere else on the body (Fig. 4.7). In most cases, there will be a history of eczema in other body areas. Patch testing can help identify an allergic stimulus. Treatment consists of emollients and steroids, and the patient should avoid any known trigger factors.

VULVAL PSORIASIS

Usually presents along with plaque psoriasis affecting other areas of the body. Erythematous plaques and fissuring are usually present, but the classical scaling seen in other areas of the body is usually absent (Fig. 4.8). Treatment is with emollients, steroids and coal tar, like the treatment of psoriasis elsewhere on the body.

VULVAL INTRAEPITHELIAL NEOPLASIA

Vulval epithelial skin changes in response to the human papilloma virus (HPV). This is a precancerous condition which can lead to SCC in 20% of cases. HPV can also cause cancer in the vagina and cervix, so regular follow-up is required to monitor for this. Vulval lesions are often painful, raised papules, with a wart-like appearance and surrounding erythema. Biopsy confirms the diagnosis. Treatments include surgical destruction or excision, or topical medical treatments such as imiquimod or fluorouracil. Both the disease itself and the treatments can cause significant pain, scarring and psychosexual problems.

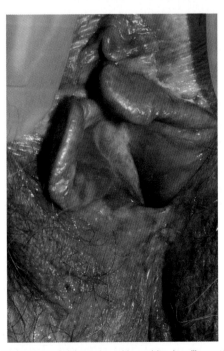

Fig. 4.5 Lichen planus of the vulva with a white, lacelike pattern and erythema. (Source: From Crum CP et al: Diagnostic gynecologic and obstetric pathology, ed 3, Philadelphia, 2018, Elsevier.)

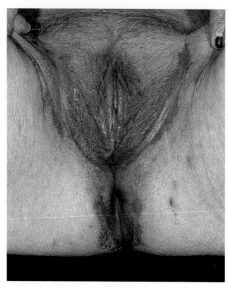

Fig. 4.8 Psoriasis, red scale involving the vulva, perineum and gluteal cleft. (Source: Habif, Thomas P., et al. Skin disease e-book: diagnosis and treatment. Elsevier, 2018.)

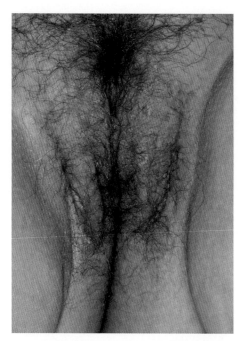

Fig. 4.6 Lichen simplex chronicus of the vulva. (Source: Micheletti, Robert G., et al. Andrews' Diseases of the Skin Clinical Atlas. Elsevier, 2023.)

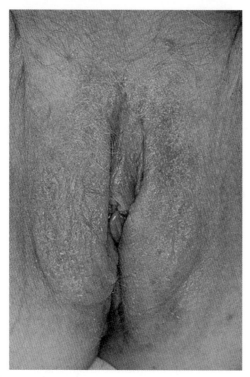

Fig. 4.7 Eczema involving the vulva. (Source: From Simpson R, Nunns D: Skin diseases affecting the vulva. Obstetrics, Gynaecology, and Reproductive Medicine 27(3): 77–85, 2017. Fig. 2.)

BARTHOLIN CYST

Bartholin glands, also called the greater vestibular glands, are two glands approximately 1 cm in diameter situated laterally at the 5 and 7 o'clock positions at the entrance of the vagina, lying distal to the hymen (Fig. 4.9). The ducts of these glands enter the vagina at the introitus, secreting fluid in order to provide lubrication of the vulva and vagina for sexual intercourse.

A Bartholin cyst occurs when there is an occlusion of this duct and fluid builds up in the gland and duct. If the static fluid becomes infected, then the cyst will develop into an abscess (Fig. 4.10).

AETIOLOGY

Bartholin cysts are present in around 3% of women, but only around two-thirds of these patients will develop pain and seek medical help.

Most cases occur between the ages of 20 and 40 years, with 70% of cases occurring before the age of 30. During periods of high sexual activity, Bartholin cysts become larger, so are more commonly seen in women who are sexually active. These cysts are rare in patients over the age of 40, so in these patients presenting with a possible Bartholin cyst, malignancy should be excluded.

SIGNS AND SYMPTOMS

Some patients will not complain of any symptoms and the finding may be incidental, such as on palpation during clinical examination or when imaging the pelvis.

If the patient does have symptoms, these are likely to be:
- Awareness of a lump.
- Pain, which can be severe, worse upon walking or sitting.
- Dyspareunia.
- Feelings of fullness in the vulva.
- The patient may feel systemically unwell and have a raised temperature in the case of an abscess.

On examination, the lump may be visible or only detected by palpation. It should be around the expected anatomical site of the Bartholin gland, medial to the labia minora. There may also be some surrounding erythema and warmth if an infection is present.

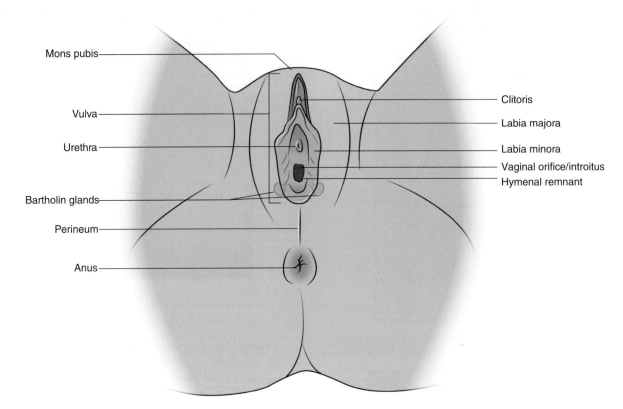

Fig. 4.9 Anatomy of the Vulva including Bartholin Glands.

Labels (top to bottom, left): Mons pubis, Vulva, Urethra, Bartholin glands, Perineum, Anus

Labels (top to bottom, right): Clitoris, Labia majora, Labia minora, Vaginal orifice/introitus, Hymenal remnant

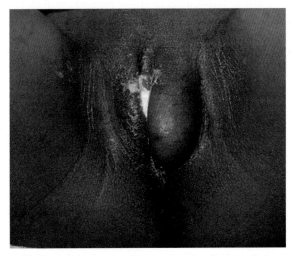

Fig. 4.10 Bartholin's abscess. (Source: Douglas, Graham, Fiona Nicol, and Colin Robertson, eds. Macleod's Clinical Examination. Elsevier, 2013.)

INVESTIGATIONS

Diagnosis of a Bartholin cyst is usually clinical, based on the history and examination findings. Cysts can be seen on MRI, but this is not necessary for diagnosis. If an infection is suspected, then swabs should be taken and sent for microscopy and culture. This may help in the choice of antibiotics for treatment of an abscess. In women over 40, or those with suspected malignancy, a biopsy of the lesion should be taken and sent for histological examination.

DIFFERENTIAL DIAGNOSIS

Due to its superficial location, the differential diagnoses for a Bartholin cyst are similar to those for any skin lump. These include:

- Sebaceous cyst.
- Lipoma.
- Tumour – malignant or fibroma.

COMPLICATIONS

Persistent dyspareunia can occur following treatment of a Bartholin cyst. This may occur as a result of scar tissue or due to vulval dryness if the gland is removed. This may subsequently have psychological sequelae.

The most severe complication is a Bartholin-rectal fistula. Although this is rare, it should be suspected in any patient who has experienced many infections and extreme discomfort around the anogenital region.

MANAGEMENT

Conservative

An asymptomatic cyst may need no treatment at all, as it may spontaneously resolve. A symptomatic cyst can be managed conservatively using warm compresses, baths, and the patient can be directed to squeeze the area to help the fluid drain from the cyst through the duct. Abscesses may also be treated in a similar way, especially if they have ruptured naturally and are spontaneously draining, although drainage may be required if symptoms fail to improve.

In patients with a cyst or abscess where the opening or punctum is visible, it is possible to squeeze the cyst, opening the occluded duct and pushing the fluid out. This has the advantage of easing the pressure and pain without requiring surgery. It is important to explain to the patient before doing this that it will hurt and offer appropriate analgesia.

Medical

The main aim of medication in the management of Bartholin cysts is to prevent or treat infection. Broad-spectrum antibiotics, such as amoxicillin with clavulanic acid, are used in the first instance. If analgesia is required, simple agents such as paracetamol are often sufficient.

Surgical

Needle aspiration of the cyst contents is effective in decompression of the lesion. However, these cysts have a high level of recurrence, so this is now rarely the surgical method of choice. The following options may be used for the surgical treatment of a Bartholin cyst:

- Marsupialisation – this is where a permanent opening from the cyst to the vagina is surgically formed by creating a new mucocutaneous junction. The procedure can be done using several different methods, including temporary packing of the cyst after drainage or excision of an oval-shaped portion of the cyst wall (the 'window operation'). This allows the gland to drain freely and should allow it to maintain a normal function, thus preventing vaginal dryness.
- Fistulisation with catheter insertion – a catheter is inserted into the cyst and allowed to remain *in situ* for 4 to 6 weeks. This allows an epithelialised tract to form around the catheter, permitting free flow of fluid from the gland into the vagina.
- Excision of Bartholin gland and/or duct – recurrence rates are low, but because of the high risk of vaginal dryness, this is usually reserved for recurrent cysts.

PROGNOSIS

Treatment is successful in 85% of women, although cysts can reoccur regardless of treatment offered. The least successful form of treatment is needle aspiration, as cysts recur in 40% of women.

CHRONIC VULVAL PAIN DISORDERS

Vulval pain disorders are characterised by vulval discomfort, most often described as burning pain, occurring in the absence of relevant visible findings or a specific, clinically identifiable, neurologic disorder. Vulvodynia can be categorised into different conditions depending on whether or not the pain is provoked. The diagnosis also depends on whether the pain is localised to a particular area or generalised around the vulva.

Provoked vulvodynia is a condition of provoked pain within the vestibular area of the vulva. The provocational stimulus is usually penetrative sexual intercourse, insertion of tampons into the vagina or touching an area of the vulva. Other names previously used for this condition are vestibulodynia and vestibulitis.

Unprovoked vulvodynia is pain within the vulva that is not precipitated by an external stimulus to the area.

Vaginismus is pain caused by involuntary contractions or spasms of the pelvic floor muscles when anything is inserted into the vagina. It is increasingly being diagnosed in isolation and alongside vulvodynia. The most commonly implicated muscles are the bulbospongiosus, pubococcygeus and puborectalis.

AETIOLOGY

The aetiology of vulvodynia is unknown in most cases, but like many chronic pain conditions, it is likely to be multifactorial. Some theories hold that vulvodynia may be preceded by physical trauma, inflammation or an infective process such as candidiasis within the lower genital tract. Vulvodynia and vaginismus may also be caused by a psychologically traumatic experience, such as traumatic intercourse or sexual assault. Whatever the cause, significant psychological and psychosexual dysfunction often occur as a result of vulvodynia.

SIGNS AND SYMPTOMS

Patients with vulvodynia will often have a long history of pain for which an organic cause has never been found. A full sexual and pain history should be taken in order to ascertain the cause of the pain. If pain occurs during intercourse (dyspareunia), it is essential to establish whether the pain occurs on initial insertion (superficial dyspareunia), which is associated with vulval dysfunction. If pain occurs deeper within the vagina (deep dyspareunia), this is associated with other causes, such as endometriosis and sexually transmitted infections (STIs).

Typical symptoms of provoked vulvodynia include pain at the vaginal introitus upon penetrative intercourse and pain at the same location when inserting tampons. Patients with vaginismus sometimes report feeling a tightening within their vagina on initiation of intercourse. Patients with unprovoked vulvodynia will often not attribute the pain to an external stimulus, but an external stimulus may worsen the symptoms.

Examination must be conducted with particular care, as the examination is likely to elicit pain, and the patient may have psychological sequelae associated with genital examination.

- Provoked vulvodynia pain can be reproduced by applying pressure to a specific affected area, usually with a cotton bud ('Q-tip test'). This test is helpful in differentiating local from generalised vulvodynia.

- In cases of unprovoked vulvodynia, the patient is likely to experience pain prior to examination, which then may or may not be exacerbated by the exam.
- If vaginismus is present, the examiner can identify strong contractions of muscles of the pelvic floor (often pubococcygeus and puborectalis) on digital vaginal examination.
- The absence of visible signs of inflammation or vulval skin changes is important to rule out other causes of the symptoms.

INVESTIGATIONS

Diagnosis of vulvodynia should be based on the patient's history and examination. Usually, vaginal swabs are taken to rule out easily treatable infections as the cause. A biopsy is not required to diagnose vulvodynia, but one may be considered if the appearance of the vulval epithelium suggests an inflammatory skin condition.

DIFFERENTIAL DIAGNOSIS

As the vulva can often appear normal on examination, it is important to consider all conditions which may cause vulval pain when formulating a differential diagnosis:

- Provoked vulvodynia.
- Unprovoked vulvodynia.
- Vaginismus.
- Infective process – candida.
- Inflammatory dermatoses – lichen sclerosus.
- Neuropathic pain – herpes neuralgia.
- Pudendal neuralgia.
- Malignancy.

COMPLICATIONS

Vulvodynia can have a significant impact on a patient's quality of life. It is associated with chronic pain, sexual dysfunction and psychological disease. There is a high incidence of both anxiety and depression associated with vulvodynia. Pain from vulvodynia will make intercourse painful and, in many cases, penetration is not achievable. Over time, this can lead to a decreased interest in sexual activities, which can put relationships under strain.

MANAGEMENT

Vulvodynia is a chronic condition, and expectations of treatment should be counselled as such. The aim of management is to improve a patient's quality of life by improving their pain and restoring sexual function, but not necessarily fully resolving their symptoms. The patient should be offered a full explanation of their condition and should understand that the treatments take time to become effective. Treatment approaches should be conducted with a multifaceted approach including conservative, medical, physical and psychological

therapies, requiring the involvement of multiple members of the multidisciplinary team.

Conservative Measures for All Causes

- Avoid known skin irritating factors, such as chemicals in bathing products. Patients should be advised to wear loose-fitting cotton underwear and to use emollients instead of soap.
- Vaginal transcutaneous electrical nerve stimulation (TENS) may provide effective pain relief for some women.

Psychological Approaches for All Causes

- CBT and biofeedback training.
- Relaxation techniques.
- Specialist psychiatric services may be required in cases with previous traumatic experience.
- Psychosexual counsellors may be of help where intercourse is the predominant concern.

Directed Treatments

Provoked vulvodynia

First-line simple medical treatments should be tried first to make penetrative intercourse tolerable:

- Lubricants.
- Topical local anaesthetic gel – applied to the area 20 minutes prior to intercourse.
- Vaginal dilators (also called vaginal trainers) – if a patient has not had penetrative intercourse either ever or for a long time due to the pain. Using lubricant, and if required, an anaesthetic they are advised to insert a small-diameter dilator themselves every day. Over time the idea is to gradually increase dilator size, which will increase the acceptance of intercourse when it is attempted.

Second-line medications:

- If simple measures are not sufficient, then treatments can be started to treat a neuropathic element to the pain. Amitriptyline is usually the initial medication used, although pregabalin or gabapentin are also effective options. The starting dose of amitriptyline is 10 mg, but over many weeks may be titrated up to 100 mg/day depending on the patient's response to treatment.
- If the above measures are not sufficient, subcutaneous infiltration of steroid agents with local anaesthetic into the area of provoked vulvodynia may be tried. Alternatively, support from the chronic pain team may be required.

Surgery:

- If other treatments are unsuccessful, surgery for provoked vulvodynia may be considered. This would be the form of a partial or complete vestibulectomy. The area of the vestibule causing pain is removed, and the posterior wall of the vagina is advanced to close the incision. Patient selection is essential when offering surgery, as only the patients where topical local anaesthetic was effective are likely to benefit from surgery.

Vaginismus

- Vaginal dilators – insertion of a small dilator with lubricant, and then gradually increasing the size of dilator used over several weeks can help the patient desensitise to vaginal penetration which aims to prevent muscle contraction and allow sexual intercourse. Patients may also be more comfortable with using vibrators/dildos as they may feel they are more socially acceptable.
- Perineal and pelvic floor massage – physical techniques can be taught to encourage muscle relaxation. Specialist physiotherapists can support this training.
- Botulinum toxin – in refractory cases Botox injections into the muscles of the pelvic floor can stop the muscles contracting. The effect is only temporary so repeat injections may be required. However, a single dose may allow for successful intercourse which breaks the psychological fear allowing successful intercourse long after the physical effects of the botulinum have ceased.

There is a significant psychological aspect to all the pain conditions. Psychological therapies treat one aspect of this, while the physical therapies such as vaginal dilators in the case of provoked vulvodynia and vaginismus attempt to break the psychological association of vaginal penetration with pain.

Unprovoked Vulvodynia

- Neuropathic pain medication improves symptoms in 80% of cases of unprovoked vulvodynia. Amitriptyline is used first line (pregabalin or gabapentin are alternatives).
- Occasionally local anaesthetic gel may be tried, but irritation is a common side effect.
- Other treatments used for provoked vulvodynia or vaginismus, including surgery, are ineffective.
- If medication fails, referral to a specialist chronic pain clinic is advised. Specialist clinics have had some success using diverse treatments such as acupuncture and sacral nerve stimulation.

PROGNOSIS

The multistage multidisciplinary approach to treatment is a protracted process and requires a significant amount of patient motivation. There are physical, psychological and social factors which need to be explored and optimised. Therefore, it may take a long time for treatment to successfully improve a patient's symptoms adequately. Women who have suffered psychological sequelae as a result of the disease may need to be followed up for several years after the physical condition has been resolved.

❓ QUESTIONS

Janet is a 48-year-old who has noticed intense itching within her vulva over the past 2 months. The itching gets worse in the evenings and often keeps her awake at night. She tries to avoid scratching, as when she does she often finds that her vulva becomes painful afterwards. She is also worried about whether or not sex will be painful as she has recently met a new partner.

A	Amitriptyline.	G	Excision of Bartholin gland.
B	Amoxicillin and clavulanic acid.	H	Fistulisation.
C	Calcineurin inhibitors.	I	Loop diathermy.
D	Clobetasol propionate ointment.	J	Marsupialisation.
E	Cognitive behavioural therapy.	K	Modified vestibulectomy.
F	Combined oral contraceptive pill.	L	Topical local anaesthetic agent.

Select the most appropriate treatment from the above list that corresponds to the following statements.

Q1 The first-line medication for unprovoked vulvodynia.

Q2 A treatment for Bartholin cysts which may be performed by a 'window operation'.

Q3 This may cause vulval dryness and is reserved for recurrent Bartholin cysts.

Q4 The initial treatment of choice for uncomplicated lichen sclerosus.

Q5 Beneficial in the context of vulvodynia if used prior to sexual intercourse.

Q6 Answer true or false: Which of the following associated features would support a diagnosis of lichen sclerosus in Janet?
A Type 1 diabetes mellitus.
B Purpura.
C Premenopause.
D Postmenopause.
E Recurrent vaginal fungal infections.

Q7 Which symptom would most suggest a diagnosis of provoked vulvodynia?
A Constant widespread pain in the vulva.
B Deep pelvic pain during intercourse.
C Pain upon touching the entrance to the vagina.
D Vulval itching.
E A feeling of fullness in the vagina.

[Answers on page 197.]

KEY REFERENCES

CONTRACEPTION

Faculty of Sexual & Reproductive Healthcare, 2022. Drug Interactions with Hormonal Contraception. FSRH Clinical Guidance.

Faculty of Sexual and Reproductive Healthcare, 2016. UK Medical eligibility criteria for contraceptive use. Clinical guidance (UKMEC 2016, amended 2019).

Joint Formulary Committee, 2022. British National London, 83rd ed. BMJ Group and Pharmaceutical Press, London.

National Institute for Health and Clinical Excellence, 2005, updated 2019. Long-acting reversible contraception. NICE guideline (CG 50).

NHS, 2021. Your contraception guide. https://www.nhs.uk/conditions/contraception/

EMERGENCY CONTRACEPTION

Faculty of Sexual and Reproductive Healthcare, 2017, amended 2020. Emergency Contraception. FSRH Clinical Guidance.

MENORRHAGIA AND OTHER MENSTRUAL BLEEDING DISORDERS

National Institute for Health and Clinical Excellence, 2018. Heavy Menstrual Bleeding: Assessment and Management. NICE Clinical Guideline (CG 44).

FIBROIDS

National Institute for Health and Clinical Excellence, 2007. updated 2016. Heavy Menstrual Bleeding. NICE Clinical Guideline (CG 44).

National Institute for Health and Clinical Excellence, 2010. Uterine Artery Embolisation for Fibroids. Interventional Procedures Guidance (IPG367).

Younas, K., Hadoura, E., Majoko, F., Bunkheia., A., 2016. A review of evidence-based management of uterine fibroids. TOG 18 (1), 33–42. https://obgyn.onlinelibrary.wiley.com/doi/abs/10.1111/tog.12223

PREMENSTRUAL DISORDER

Royal College of Obstetricians and Gynaecologists, 2016. Premenstrual Syndrome, Management. RCOG Green Top Guideline (GTG 48).

MENOPAUSE

Joint Formulary Committee, 2022. British National Formulary, 83rd ed. BMJ Group and Pharmaceutical Press, London.

National Institute for Health and Care Excellence, 2019. Menopause: Diagnosis and Management. NICE Clinical Guideline (CG 23).

Royal College of Obstetricians and Gynaecologists, 2010. RCOG. Alternatives to HRT for the Management of Symptoms of the Menopause. RCOG Scientific Impact Paper (SIP 6).

The British Menopause Society. NICE: Menopause, Diagnosis and Management – from Guideline to Practice Guideline Summary. Tools for clinicians. https://thebms.org.uk/wp-content/uploads/2019/04/09-BMS-TfC-NICE-Menopause-Diagnosis-and-Management-from-Guideline-to-Practice-Guideline-Summary-01-April2019.pdf

VULVAL DISORDERS

British Association for Sexual Health and HIV, 2014. Management of Vulval Conditions. BASHH UK Guideline.

Lewis, F., Tatnall, F., Velangi, S., 2018. British Association of Dermatologists Guidelines for the Management of Lichen Sclerosus. Br. J. Dermatol. 178, 839–853.

Mandal, D., Mandal, D., Byrne, M., McLelland, J., Rani, R., Cullimore, J., et al., 2010. Guidelines for the management of vulvodynia. Br. J. Dermatol. 162, 1180–1185.

Urogynaecology

PELVIC ORGAN PROLAPSE

Pelvic organ prolapse is the protrusion of one or more pelvic organs (Fig. 5.1) through the supporting fascia of the vagina, leading to downward displacement of the associated vaginal wall. These protruding structures can include the urethra, bladder, rectum, uterus or vaginal vault. The herniation of these structures causes indentation of the vaginal wall, with the appearance of a lump or bulge at the introitus (opening of the vagina).

There are different methods to stage and size a prolapse. A prolapse can be small, causing no symptoms and only identified on examination, up to the prolapsed tissue protruding through the introitus.

TYPES OF PROLAPSE

ANTERIOR WALL PROLAPSE

- Cystocoele – prolapse of the bladder (upper anterior vaginal wall) (Fig. 5.2).
- Urethrocoele – prolapse of the urethra (lower anterior vaginal wall).

POSTERIOR WALL PROLAPSE

- Rectocoele – prolapse of rectum (lower posterior vaginal wall) (Fig. 5.3).
- Enterocoele – prolapse of pouch of Douglas (upper posterior vaginal wall); this often contains small bowel.

UTERINE PROLAPSE

Prolapse of the uterus into the vaginal canal. In severe cases, the uterus can prolapse through the introitus and become external. This is called a procidentia (Fig. 5.4).

VAULT PROLAPSE

A prolapse of the vault (top) of the vagina. This can occur after someone has had a hysterectomy, as the supporting ligaments to the vault are cut during the operation to allow removal of the uterus (Fig. 5.5).

AETIOLOGY

Pelvic organ prolapse is common and seen to some degree in 50% of parous women. There is a 7% lifetime risk of requiring surgery for prolapse.

RISK FACTORS

The vagina is a hollow tube. A combination of the pelvic floor muscles, pelvic ligaments and the strong vaginal connective tissue 'hold up' the pelvic organs, preventing them from protruding into the vagina and causing a prolapse. Consequently, if any of these structures are damaged, a prolapse is more likely to occur. Also, if increased force is applied to these support structures, they are more likely to fail and result in prolapse.

Risk factors for prolapse can be categorised into factors that damage the pelvic floor anatomy and factors that increase the abdominal pressure. The biggest risk factors are parity and age.

DAMAGE TO THE PELVIC FLOOR

- Parity – the greater the number of children a woman has, the greater her risk of developing a prolapse later in life. Vaginal births, and in particular difficult deliveries (such as those with a long second stage of labour or those requiring forceps), increase the risk. Caesarean birth does not completely negate the risk of prolapse; pregnancy itself puts stress on ligaments and vaginal fascia, regardless of the mode of birth.
- Post-menopause – oestrogen supports the formation of vaginal connective tissue (fascia). After menopause, the oestrogen levels drop significantly, so the amount of fascia declines and the remaining fascia weakens, increasing the risk of prolapse.
- Age – the risk of anatomical damage and loss of function of supporting muscles, ligaments and fascia is generally higher in elderly patients.
- Smoking – reduces the quality of connective tissue repair.

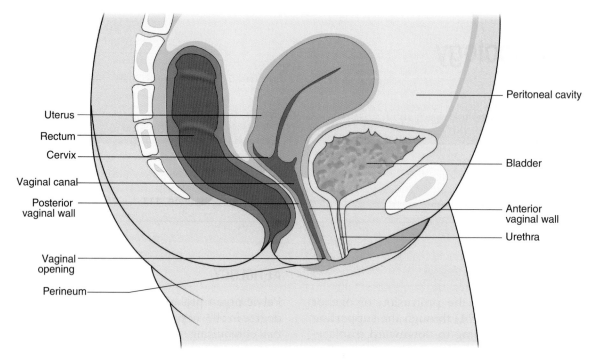

Fig. 5.1 Normal Pelvic Anatomy.

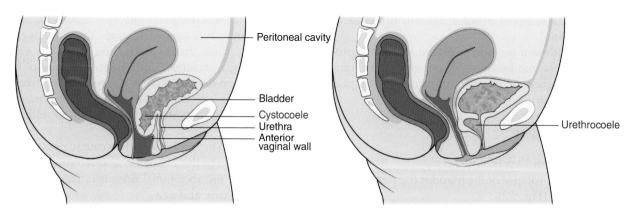

Fig. 5.2 Anterior Wall Prolapses: Cystocoele and Ureterocoele.

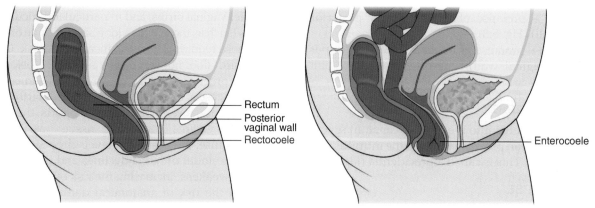

Fig. 5.3 Posterior Wall Prolapses: Rectocoele and Enterocoele.

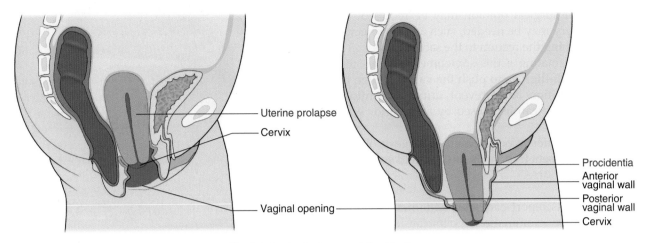

Fig. 5.4 Uterine Prolapse and Procidentia.

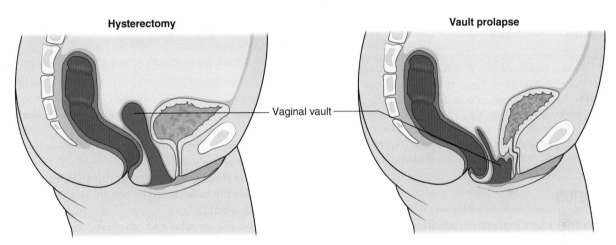

Fig. 5.5 Normal Anatomy After a Hysterectomy, and Vault Prolapse.

- Pelvic surgery – during hysterectomy, the ligaments which support the uterus and the upper vagina are cut to remove the uterus, leaving the vaginal vault with less support.
- Connective tissue disorders – conditions such as Ehlers-Danlos syndrome can lead to abnormal collagen metabolism and lead to weakness of the connective tissue that support the vaginal walls

INCREASED ABDOMINAL PRESSURE

- Obesity – results in a constant increase in force on the vaginal support structures due to increased weight of adipose tissue.
- Abdominal mass – fibroids, tumours and ascites.
- Valsalva manoeuvre – constipation, chronic cough and heavy lifting.

PREVENTING PROLAPSE

Pregnant women should be advised that vaginal birth is a risk factor for development of prolapse and urinary incontinence in later life. To reduce the risk, they should be taught how to do pelvic floor exercises and should be encouraged to do these every day for the rest of their lives. Other healthy lifestyle advice includes smoking cessation, maintaining a healthy BMI and avoiding constipation.

SYMPTOMS

COMMON

- Feeling a 'dragging sensation', 'vaginal fullness' or pressure in the pelvis or vagina.
- Feeling 'something coming down' in the vagina.
- Feeling or seeing a bulge or lump in the vagina.

Prolonged standing or exercise often worsens symptoms due to the effect of gravity. Symptoms then often improve upon lying flat.

LESS COMMON

- Difficulty defecating – this sometimes requires the patient to self-digitate to push a bulge in the vagina back to allow stool to pass. A posterior vaginal wall prolapse may cause this, by allowing the rectum to kink. However, if this is the predominant symptom, a colorectal surgical opinion may be required, as rectal surgery may be needed, such as a sacrorecto-pexy (attaching the rectum to the sacrum).

- Difficulty urinating – this sometimes requires the patient to self-digitate to push the vaginal bulge to allow micturition and prevent urinary retention. This is rare but can be caused by an anterior wall prolapse.
- Coital difficulties – occasionally, a large prolapse may prevent penetration or cause an odd sensation during intercourse.

Some patients report backache, abdominal pain or dyspareunia. On examination, a clinician identifies a prolapse. It is rare and well-debated that a prolapse could cause these symptoms. Therefore, if these are the predominant symptoms, a clinician should consider other causes, rather than treating an otherwise asymptomatic prolapse unnecessarily.

 Vaginal Birth Trauma

A major cause of vaginal prolapse is damage at the time of childbirth. Stress incontinence is also caused by trauma in childbirth, so the two may present simultaneously. Sometimes, an anterior prolapse causes a kink to the urethra that actually prevents stress incontinence, but when the prolapse is repaired, stress incontinence occurs.

EXAMINATION

An abdominal examination is required to assess for a mass. An abdominal ultrasound should be considered if there are concerns. Any stress incontinence or anal pathology should also be identified. A speculum examination is required to assess for vaginal prolapse. This examination is carried out with a C-Shaped speculum*, with the patient lying in the left lateral position.

USING A C-SHAPED SPECULUM

1. As with a Cusco speculum examination, prepare your equipment, introduce yourself, explain what you are going to do and get informed consent from the patient. Always have a chaperone for pelvic examinations. Lubricate the speculum before use.

[See 'Introduction to Gynaecology' page 1.]

2. Lay the patient in the left lateral position – on the left side with knees slightly curled.
3. Ask the patient to lift her upper leg using her hand.
4. Inspect the vulva. Ask the patient to bear down or cough, as this may elicit a prolapse protruding through the introitus.

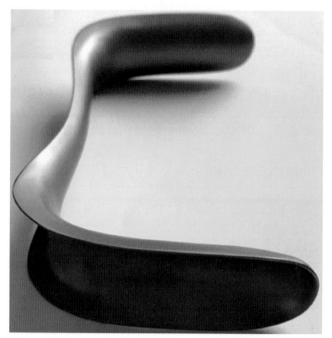

Fig. 5.6 C-shaped Vaginal speculum (formally called a Sims speculum*).

5. Insert the speculum (Fig. 5.6) into the vagina with the end of the speculum against the posterior wall of the vagina. This will allow you to assess the anterior wall of the vagina.
6. If there is no obvious bulge in the anterior wall, ask the patient to bear down or cough, as this may demonstrate a bulge.
7. Look at the cervix and vaginal vault and again ask the patient to bear down or cough to look for descent or prolapse of these structures.
8. Repeat the examination with the end of the speculum against the anterior vaginal wall so you can assess the posterior wall. The uterus and vault can be viewed again in this position.
9. If no prolapse is identified with the above examination, but the history is strongly supportive, some clinicians ask the patient to either sit on the edge of the examination couch or to stand, and then undertake a digital vaginal exam to feel for any descent while the patient bears down with the addition of gravity.

STAGING A PROLAPSE

- Stage 0 – no prolapse.
- Stage 1 – lowest part of a prolapse is more than 1 cm higher than the hymenal remnant.
- Stage 2 – lowest part of a prolapse extends between −1 cm and +1 cm in relation to the hymen.
- Stage 3 – lowest part of the prolapse protrudes outwards of the vagina, more than 1 cm beyond the hymenal remnant (Fig. 5.7).

The assessment of prolapse descent is performed at the time of maximal Valsalva effort by the patient.

*Whilst Sims developed this speculum and other methodologies, it is important to acknowledge that much of his work was founded on exploitation and abuse of Black women.

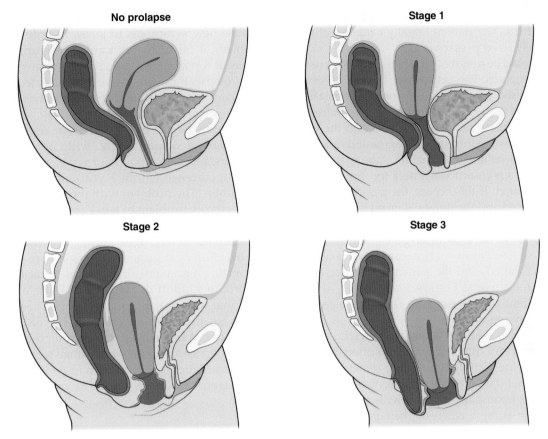

No prolapse   **Stage 1**

Stage 2   **Stage 3**

Fig. 5.7 Example of Stages of Prolapse: Uterine Prolapse.

MANAGEMENT

The management options for prolapse are no treatment, conservative, vaginal pessaries or surgery.

NO TREATMENT

Pelvic organ prolapse is not a condition which will affect patient mortality. Therefore, no treatment is a reasonable management option. The aim of management is to improve symptoms. If the patient is asymptomatic and the prolapse has been identified incidentally, this would certainly be the most sensible management, along with general healthy lifestyle advice. Early surgical intervention does not improve either the initial outcome or long-term recurrence risk.

CONSERVATIVE

- Lifestyle advice.
  - Maintain a healthy weight.
  - Smoking cessation.
  - Treat chronic conditions, such as constipation and a long-term cough.
- Pelvic floor exercises.
  - Patients can be advised to undertake regular pelvic floor muscle exercises to improve muscle strength and reduce the prolapse size and symptoms.
  - Referral to specialist physiotherapists can be useful to teach effective pelvic floor exercises.

- Topical oestrogen – for post-menopausal women clinicians may prescribe topical oestrogen to be used in the vagina. It is available as a cream, pessary or a ring. This may improve the integrity of the fascia which, when combined with other conservative treatments, may improve symptoms. This can also be prescribed prior to surgery to improve the quality of the fascia being repaired.

VAGINAL PESSARIES

- A vaginal pessary is a plastic or silicone device that fits into the vagina and pushes on the vaginal walls to support the walls and pelvic organs. There are many types available (Fig. 5.8); the most commonly used is a ring pessary.
- The correct size pessary needs to be used. If a pessary is too small, it can fall out, and if it is too big, it can cause discomfort. Finding the right size for the patient may take a few of attempts. Clinicians should advise the patient to walk around immediately after

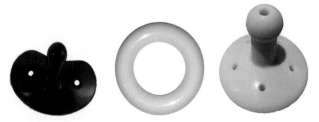

Fig. 5.8 Shelf, Ring and Gellhorn Pessaries.

insertion and to come back if the pessary does not suit the patient. The patient usually cannot feel an appropriately sized pessary *in situ*.

- Pessaries should be removed, washed and re-inserted every 4 to 6 months. This is to reduce the risk of complications caused by the pessary applying constant pressure to the tissues. These include vaginal ulcers, incarceration (where the pessary embeds in the tissues) or even eroding through the vagina and causing a fistula. A speculum examination should be performed prior to re-insertion to check for vaginal erosion or ulceration. If this occurs, the pessary should not be reinserted and the tissues allowed time to heal (often aided by a prescription for topical oestrogen) prior to further pessary use or surgery.
- A pessary is a good option where conservative management has failed, and the patient either declines or is unfit for surgery. Pessaries can also be used while a patient awaits surgery. They can also be used during pregnancy.
- Pessaries are also useful in young women who wish to have further children. Surgery is not offered until their families are complete, as future deliveries are likely to further damage the pelvic floor.
- Intercourse is potentially possible with a pessary *in situ*, although some women or their partners find it uncomfortable. There are some newer pessaries which can easily be removed and reinserted by the patient, which may help in this situation.

SURGICAL

There are different surgical options depending on patient age, fertility status, severity and type of prolapse. Surgery could involve repair of the anterior vaginal wall, posterior vaginal wall, the vaginal vault, removal of the uterus or a combination.

Complications of surgery depend on which procedure is carried out. The surgical risks for all the procedures are bleeding, infection, venous thromboembolic (VTE), injury to adjacent organs (bowel, bladder, ureters), pain, dyspareunia and failure of the procedure to improve symptoms.

Anterior and Posterior Colporrhaphy

These are commonly called anterior and posterior vaginal wall repairs. They are the surgical treatments of cystocoeles, rectocoeles and enterocoeles.

Colporrhaphy involves making a sagittal incision in the vaginal wall at the site of the prolapse to identify the vaginal fascia. The lateral edges of the fascia are stitched together to tighten the fascia, thereby supporting the deeper pelvic organs and closing the prolapse. The vaginal epithelium is then re-sutured.

Specific complications:
- Sexual function – if the vaginal tissues are pulled too tight, the vagina can be narrowed leading to dyspareunia.

- Urination – repair of a cystocoele can worsen or cause new symptoms of stress incontinence. Conversely, it can also very rarely cause urinary retention. If a patient has urinary symptoms as well as a prolapse, these are usually investigated with urodynamics and treatment optimised prior to surgical management of prolapse.
- Symptom recurrence – there is a significant failure rate of colporrhaphy, with 20% of anterior repairs and 5% of posterior repairs having symptom recurrence within 5 years. Repeat surgery is common. The problem with the surgery is that the underlying problem of weak fascia is not resolved. The fascia that has been tightened is still weak, so it can stretch over time and allow prolapse recurrence. At repeat surgery, surgeons were previously, inserting a non-absorbable surgical mesh onto the fascia to support it. However, the use of mesh for vaginal wall prolapse in the UK has been stopped because it can erode into the vagina and cause pain, or can erode deeper into either the bladder or bowel, causing fistulae and other serious complications. Patients with recurrent prolapse must be managed through a specialist multi-disciplinary team.

Uterine Prolapse Repair

Uterine prolapse is treated by hysterectomy (often vaginally). If the hysterectomy is being performed for a procidentia, it is common for the patient to be treated with pessaries and vaginal oestrogens first. Procidentias often have a very ulcerated tissue due to exposure to external trauma, such as rubbing on clothes. If this is not treated prior to surgery, there is a high risk of infection and wound breakdown. Hysterectomy is effective in the majority of patients, however, the support to the remaining vaginal vault can become deficient over time, with about 10% of these women going on to develop a vaginal vault prolapse.

For women who wish to preserve their uterus, there are uterus-sparing surgical procedures:
- Hysterosacropexy – this involves attaching the uterus to the sacrum using mesh. This procedure can be carried out via an open or laparoscopic approach. The permanent nature of the procedure and the potential mesh complications must be explained to patients.
- Manchester repair – this involves shortening the cervix and securing ligaments to the remaining uterus.

Vaginal Vault Prolapse Repair
- Sacrocolpopexy – this involves attaching the apex of the vagina to the sacrum using mesh, completed in a similar way to a hysterosacropexy with similar risks.
- Sacrospinous fixation – this procedure involves making an incision in the vaginal wall and suturing the vaginal vault to one of the sacrospinous ligaments (a pelvic ligament lateral to the vagina connecting the sacrum to the ischial spine). A complication of

this procedure is dyspareunia, which is caused by the axis of the vagina being pulled laterally. Buttock pain after the procedure is also common. It is generally less effective than sacrocolpopexy; however the post-operative morbidity is lower.

- Colpocleisis – this procedure is simple and effective at treating vault prolapse or any other form of vaginal prolapse. However, penetrative sexual intercourse will not be possible afterwards, so it is often reserved for elderly patients who no longer wish to be sexually active. The procedure involves making incisions in the anterior and posterior walls of the vagina, and then stitching the margins of the incisions to each other, in order to close the anterior and posterior walls together, thereby closing the vagina.

PROGNOSIS

Whilst pelvic organ prolapse is not a life-threatening condition, it can have a serious effect on quality of life by causing symptoms of pressure and discomfort. It also has an impact on urinary, bowel and sexual function. Recurrence can occur following surgical treatment; recurrence rates depend on the type of procedure conducted. Approximately one-third of all prolapse surgery is for recurrent defects.

❓ QUESTIONS

Karen, a 67-year-old retired estate agent, presents to her primary care physician describing a 'dragging sensation down below'. This sensation is made worse after being on her feet all day, and she can sometimes feel a lump in her vagina when she is trying to defecate. She has two children, aged 40 and 43. Both were vaginal births, although the first birth was a forceps delivery and she suffered a second-degree perineal tear. She is overweight and smokes five cigarettes a day. She takes amlodipine for hypertension but has no other past medical history.

Q1 Which of the following is not a risk factor for pelvic organ prolapse?
  A Childbirth.
  B Chronic obstructive pulmonary disease (COPD).
  C Congestive cardiac failure.
  D Menopause.
  E Obesity.

Q2 What is the correct description of a cystocoele?
  A Prolapse of the urethra.
  B Prolapse of the bladder.
  C Prolapse of the rectum.
  D Prolapse of the pouch of Douglas.
  E Prolapse of the vaginal vault.

Q3 Answer true or false: The following are treatment options for pelvic organ prolapse.
  A Weight loss.
  B Pelvic floor exercises.
  C Mid-urethral sling.
  D Vaginal ring pessary.
  E Laxatives.

Q4 Which surgical procedure would be a treatment option for a cystocoele?
  A Anterior repair.
  B Hysterectomy.
  C Manchester repair.
  D Posterior repair.
  E Sacrocolpopexy.

[Answers on page 199.]

URINARY INCONTINENCE

Urinary incontinence is defined as any involuntary urinary leakage.

Urinary incontinence is sub-classified depending on the situations when urine is leaked.

- Stress incontinence – involuntary urine leakage on effort or exertion; for example, sneezing, coughing or during exercise. Urine loss occurs when the pressure within the bladder (usually created externally to the bladder from increased intra-abdominal pressure) exceeds the pressure at which the urethral sphincter can remain closed. Therefore, a defect of the urethra or urethral sphincter is the usual cause of stress incontinence.
- Urge incontinence – involuntary urine leakage accompanied by, or immediately preceded by, urgency (sudden desire to urinate). This is usually caused by an increase in pressure within the bladder caused by the bladder detrusor muscle contracting inappropriately. The increased pressure gives the symptom of urgency, and if the pressure is great enough to overcome the urethral sphincter pressure, incontinence occurs.
- Mixed urinary incontinence – involuntary urine leak associated with symptoms of both urgency and stress incontinence.

Other important definitions to be aware of are:
- Urinary frequency – urinating more than eight times in 24 hours. Most people urinate, on average, six to eight times in 24 hours.
- Nocturia – being woken from sleep with the need to urinate. Getting up to urinate once a night is considered normal. Two or more urination episodes per night is abnormal.

AETIOLOGY

The prevalence of urinary incontinence increases with age. Approximately 45% of women and 30% of men will suffer from urinary incontinence. It is thought that many people do not admit or seek advice for their symptoms.

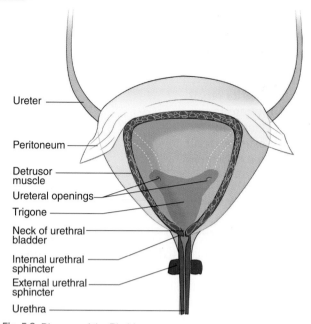

Ureter

Peritoneum

Detrusor muscle

Ureteral openings

Trigone

Neck of urethral bladder

Internal urethral sphincter

External urethral sphincter

Urethra

Fig. 5.9 Diagram of the Bladder.

PHYSIOLOGY

STRUCTURES

- The bladder wall is made up of smooth muscle known as the detrusor muscle. Contraction of the detrusor muscle squeezes urine into the bladder neck, and then through the urethra during normal urination.
- There are three orifices at the base of the bladder, so this area is named the trigone. These orifices are the insertion points of both ureters and the urethra (Fig. 5.9).
- At the base of the bladder, surrounding the urethra, is the internal urethral sphincter, which is made of smooth muscle.
- Below the internal urethral sphincter is the external urethral sphincter, a ring of skeletal muscle. This is under somatic control.

INNERVATION

- The detrusor muscle is innervated by the parasympathetic nervous system, which causes the detrusor muscle to contract, allowing urination in normal circumstances. Acetylcholine is the predominant neurotransmitter of the parasympathetic nervous system and acts on muscarinic receptors in the bladder.
- The internal urethral sphincter is innervated by the sympathetic nervous system, which releases the neurotransmitter norepinephrine, which acts on adrenergic receptors, causing contraction of the sphincter and preventing urine leakage.
- The external urethral sphincter is innervated by the somatic motor neurons that cause contraction. This is under voluntary control via the pudendal nerve. The muscle can be consciously contracted to actively

try to prevent urination when the urge to pass urine is felt.

BLADDER FILLING

- During the filling stage, the sympathetic nervous system stimulates the internal urethral sphincter and the somatic motor neurons signal to the external urethral sphincter to contract. Therefore, the sphincters are closed, preventing urine leakage.
- There is also little parasympathetic input to the detrusor muscle during filling, ensuring it remains relaxed. This means that the bladder wall provides very little resistance to stretching, so as the bladder fills, the pressure within the bladder remains low throughout the early stages of filling.

SENSATION TO VOID

- As the bladder continues to fill, stretch receptors in the bladder wall send signals through afferent fibres to the higher centres, giving the sensation of a partially full bladder. These sensations begin after filling to around 200 to 250 mL in a healthy individual.
- As the bladder fills further, it begins to reach its maximal size and becomes less able to stretch. The feeling of fullness increases and stretch receptors send afferent signals to the spinal cord, stimulating parasympathetic neurones. This causes the detrusor to contract, giving the sensation of urgency. This is the micturition reflex. The capacity of the female bladder where these strong urges to urinate occurs is approximately 500 mL.
- Impulses from the parasympathetic component of the pelvic nerve keep the detrusor muscle contracted. As the bladder continues to fill, the micturition reflex becomes more frequent and more powerful, increasing the sensation of urgency and increasing the desire to micturate.

MICTURITION

- With the desire to void, a person can then micturate. The process is a conscious one, whereby the person relaxes their external urethral sphincter. This then causes inhibition of the sympathetic fibres to the internal sphincter, leading to relaxation, and there is simultaneous contraction of the detrusor muscle (Table 5.1).
- If it is not appropriate to urinate, this can be voluntarily prevented. However, over time, if voiding does not occur, there will be increasing pressure within the bladder and increasing activation of stretch receptors stimulating the micturition reflex. Stretch receptors also cause signals to inhibit the sympathetic and somatic nerves of the sphincters, causing relaxation. This causes involuntary voiding, which is essentially when someone is unable to overcome their micturition reflex.

Table 5.1 Summary of Detrusor and Sphincter Control

MUSCLE	TYPE	INNERVATION	
		DURING FILLING	DURING MICTURITION
Detrusor – smooth muscle	Parasympathetic – causes contraction	Inhibited	Stimulated
Internal urethral sphincter – smooth muscle	Sympathetic – causes contraction	Stimulated	Inhibited
External urethral sphincter – skeletal muscle	Somatic motor – causes contraction	Stimulated	Inhibited

PATHOPHYSIOLOGY

STRESS INCONTINENCE

The problem in stress incontinence is the inability of the urethral sphincters to hold urine in the bladder during the filling phase. This occurs either because there is damage to the sphincter or the pressure upon the sphincters is increased, or a combination of both. Causes include:

- Increased abdominal pressure – anything which increases the pressure within the abdomen increases pressure upon the bladder, which in turn increases pressure upon the sphincters. Causes include obesity, pregnancy, a job or hobby requiring repetitive heavy lifting or a chronic cough. If the pressure exceeds a level that the sphincters can maintain, incontinence occurs.
- Sphincter tone failure – if the urethral sphincter is unable to contract efficiently, urine leaks. This sphincter can be damaged during vaginal birth, particularly prolonged second stage and assisted vaginal birth. Ageing can also lead to reduced sphincter tone. Medications blocking sympathetic activity or conditions which damage autonomic neurons can also contribute to sphincter failure.
- Urethral hypermobility – the urethra is integral to continence. The pelvic floor muscles contract, supporting the position of the urethra and maintaining continence. When a defect exists within these muscles, the urethra can move, leading to hypermobility of the urethra and incontinence. This urethral support can be reduced due to postmenopausal oestrogen loss, childbirth or pelvic surgery. Mid-urethral sling surgery is a treatment which acts upon this pathology.

URGE INCONTINENCE

The problem in urge incontinence is usually inappropriate contraction of the muscular wall of the bladder, the detrusor muscle.

- Detrusor overactivity – this is the name given when the detrusor muscle contracts inappropriately, usually when the bladder is only partly filled. This increases the pressure within the bladder, giving the sensation of urgency, and if the pressure is great enough to overcome the urethral sphincters, incontinence occurs. Detrusor muscle overactivity is a urodynamic finding; therefore, it cannot be diagnosed from symptoms alone.

RISK FACTORS

STRESS INCONTINENCE

- Increasing age.
- Obesity.
- Smoking.
- Pregnancy and childbirth.
- Previous pelvic surgery.
- Chronic cough.

Stress incontinence often coexists with uterovaginal prolapse, as many of the risk factors are the same.

[See 'Pelvic Organ Prolapse' page 105.]

 Pelvic Floor Exercises

The risk of developing stress incontinence can be reduced by encouraging a pregnant woman to follow a pelvic floor muscle training program following the birth and to continue the exercises for the rest of her life.

URGE INCONTINENCE

- Alcohol or caffeine intake – can be an irritant causing detrusor contractions.
- Excessive fluid intake.
- Urinary tract infections – infections cause detrusor contractions.
- Neurological conditions such as Parkinson disease or multiple sclerosis.
- Bladder tumours.

SIGNS AND SYMPTOMS

HISTORY

Incontinence is primarily diagnosed from the history. It is important to ask about:

- Overactive bladder symptoms – frequency, urgency and/or nocturia.
- Stress incontinence triggers – coughing, sneezing and/or exercise.
- Incontinence episodes – timing, volume, effect on quality of life and/or whether incontinence pads need to be worn.
- Obstructive symptoms – hesitancy, dribbling, poor urine flow and the feeling of incomplete emptying.
- Pain – dysuria may suggest UTI; pain on filling may suggest interstitial cystitis.

A thorough medical history can also help to highlight conditions that can exacerbate urinary incontinence, such as UTIs, uncontrolled diabetes mellitus and chronic coughs. Certain medications, such as diuretics, can exacerbate urinary incontinence.

EXAMINATION

Abdominal and pelvic examinations are vital to exclude a pelvic mass or severe prolapse, both of which would require specialist referral. During a vaginal examination, the clinician can also ask the patient to contract her pelvic floor muscles to assess their strength, as pelvic floor exercises form part of the management of incontinence. The patient can also be asked to cough to see if there is any leakage of urine.

INVESTIGATIONS

INITIAL INVESTIGATIONS FOR ALL PATIENTS

Urinalysis

Obtaining a sample of urine for bedside dipstick testing is a simple way of identifying other pathologies. Presence of:

- Leucocytes and nitrites – if the patient is symptomatic and has a positive urine dip for both leucocytes and nitrites, then a mid-stream urine sample (MSU) should be sent for culture, and antibiotics prescribed. If the dipstick is positive for just one of these variables, then antibiotics should only be started if the culture is positive.
- Glycosuria – glucose in the urine may indicate a new diagnosis of diabetes, which can cause polyuria and recurrent UTIs.
- Haematuria – in the absence of infection, identification of haematuria requires further investigation:
  - Urgent specialist referral, renal tract ultrasound scan and cystoscopy are usually required to exclude urological cancer.
  - Intermittent loin to groin pain may suggest renal calculi, which can be identified on a plain abdominal radiograph or non-contrast computerised tomography (CT).
  - Referral to a renal physician may be required where nephritic syndrome or other primary kidney disease is considered.

Bladder Diary

- The patient should be given a diary to record fluid input and output, including incontinence episodes and symptoms at the time of the episode. This should be done for a minimum of 3 days, although not necessarily consecutive, covering both work and leisure days. A measuring jug should be used for accurate urine measurement.
- Bladder diaries are very useful for demonstrating the frequency and severity of a patient's symptoms. It also helps identify the timing and volume of fluid intake in relation to symptoms. This information

aids greatly when forming an appropriate management strategy (Fig. 5.10).

Post-Void Residual Volume

This is checked via a bladder scanner (a handheld ultrasound probe) after a patient has passed urine to provide a sample for urinalysis. This should be performed if there are any symptoms of obstructed micturition.

- After a patient has passed urine, there should be less than 50 ml left in the bladder.
- A high post-void residual volume (PVR) (more than 100 mL) indicates a poor voiding ability or bladder outlet obstruction, increasing the risk of a UTI.
- A very high PVR is seen in neurological conditions due to a loss of the sensation of bladder filling. This causes high pressure within the bladder, which can lead to upper urinary tract damage and overflow incontinence.

URODYNAMICS

Urodynamics do not usually form part of the initial investigations. They are usually performed when the diagnosis after initial investigations is unclear, there are symptoms of obstruction, or if initial management has not improved symptoms. Urodynamics is the umbrella term for a variety of different tests. They are conducted in a hospital clinic setting. The most common tests are:

Cystometry

- A catheter, which contains a pressure sensor, is placed in the bladder, and another pressure sensor, which measures the abdominal pressure, is placed in the rectum. The bladder is then filled with water using the catheter, and the pressures monitored during filling, storing and voiding.
- A computer subtracts the rectal pressure from the intravesical pressure (which should be equivocal). Any remaining pressure rise has to be caused by contraction of the detrusor muscle of the bladder. This urodynamic finding is diagnostic of detrusor muscle overactivity, confirming the cause of urge incontinence.
- Normal maximum bladder capacity is about 500 mL and should fill at low pressure. If the filling causes pain at a smaller volume, it suggests a lower-capacity bladder. If the pressure spontaneously increases during filling, it suggests detrusor overactivity.
- Once the bladder is full, the patient is asked to stand, cough and jump, to see if stress incontinence occurs.

Uroflowmetry

On voiding, a sensor measures how fast a patient is able to empty her bladder. This helps to diagnose causes of voiding problems, such as bladder muscle weakness or bladder outflow obstruction.

Patient name:

Date:

Time	Fluid in		Urination		Leaks			
	Type	Volume	Number of times	Volume	Number of times	Amount	Urge to urinate?	What were you doing?
Example	Tea	250 mL	1	120 mL	1	Medium	No	Walking
0600 - 0700								
0700 - 0800								
0800 - 0900								
0900 - 1000								
1000 - 1100								
1100 - 1200								
1200 - 1300								
1300 - 1400								
1400 - 1500								
1500 - 1600								
1600 - 1700								
1700 - 1800								
1800 - 1900								
1900 - 2000								
2000 - 2100								
2100 - 2200								
2200 - 2300								
2300 - 0000								
0000 - 0100								
0100 - 0200								
0200 - 0300								
0300 - 0400								
0400 - 0500								
0500 - 0600								

Approximate sizes: Mug - 300 mL Cup - 200 mL Pint - 550 mL	Describing leak amounts: Small - few drops Medium - damp underwear or liner Large - clothes or pad soaked

Fig. 5.10 Example of a bladder diary.

DIFFERENTIAL DIAGNOSIS

CAUSES OF EXCESSIVE URINE PRODUCTION

- Diabetes mellitus.
- Diabetes insipidus.
- Excess fluid intake.

OVERFLOW INCONTINENCE

Overflow incontinence can occur from bladder over-distension which eventually can lead to overflow. Detrusor inactivity caused by autonomic neuropathies allows the bladder to overfill and the pressure increases until it overcomes the sphincters. It is characterised by frequent, involuntary dribbling of urine in the absence of an urge to urinate. On examination, patients have a distended non-tender bladder. Whatever the underlying pathology, this is often difficult to cure. Patients are either required to learn how to pass a catheter regularly to empty their bladder (intermittent self-catheterisation), or they require a long-term indwelling catheter. This is usually inserted suprapubically to reduce the incidence of urinary infections.

Causes of overflow incontinence:
- Multiple sclerosis.
- Spinal cord injury.
- Spina bifida.

- Nerve damage after trauma giving birth.
- Recent spinal or epidural anaesthesia.
- Fowler syndrome – the urethral sphincter fails to relax normally. This most commonly affects young women.

CAUSES OF PAIN AND INCONTINENCE

- Recurrent urinary tract infections.
- Bladder pain syndrome (previously called interstitial cystitis).
- Small capacity bladder.

OTHER

- Nocturnal enuresis – this is commonly known as nighttime bed wetting. This is common in children and young adults, is usually transient and is related to psychological conditions.
- Pelvic mass or haematuria – neoplasm.

 Overactive Bladder (OAB) Syndrome

This is the very common clinical diagnosis given to a patient with symptoms of urinary urgency, with or without urge incontinence. Usually, frequency and nocturia are associated symptoms. If these symptoms are further investigated, urodynamic studies usually reveal the diagnosis of detrusor overactivity as the cause of the symptoms.

Bladder Pain Syndrome

A chronic pain condition of unknown pathology, characterised by suprapubic pain (usually sharp or burning in nature), which is worse on bladder filling and relieved on bladder emptying. This is frequently accompanied by other bladder symptoms such as urgency, frequency and nocturia, which are themselves a result of an early desire to void on filling and a low-capacity bladder. Unlike in OAB, detrusor contractions are uncommon. Diagnosis is one of exclusion, ruling out infection, endometriosis, bladder cancer, bladder stones and bladder outlet obstruction. Urine culture, urodynamics, cytology and cystoscopy are common investigations. Initial treatments are simple analgesia and lifestyle modifications, with supporting psychological therapies. Additional treatments include tricyclic antidepressants, and a variety of medications injected into the bladder including heparin, Botox or local anaesthetic. For severe cases, bladder surgery may be considered.

 Primary Nocturia

This is a condition where the main complaint is frequent urination at night, without associated day symptoms. It is most common in the elderly, caused by the body's decreased response to antidiuretic hormone (ADH). In the young, ADH acts increasingly at night to decrease urine production compared to in the day, so there is diurnal variation in urine production. In the elderly, this diurnal variation is lost, increasing night production and the need to urinate. Altering timing of fluid intake can improve symptoms. A synthetic ADH (desmopressin) can be given, but it should be used with caution in the elderly as it can cause heart failure and hyponatraemia as a result of fluid retention.

MANAGEMENT

CONSERVATIVE

Conservative management is important in both stress and urge incontinence.
- Treat constipation.
- Aim for adequate fluid intake, approximately 2000 mL a day.
- Optimise treatment of comorbidities, such as chronic cough and diabetes.
- Avoid substances that irritate the bladder such as caffeine, alcohol, carbonated drinks, acidic drinks such as citrus fruit juices, and smoking.
- Weight loss to achieve a healthy body mass index (BMI).
- Absorbent pads, padded undergarments or portable commodes can significantly improve quality of life especially if patients have reduced mobility.

When there is mixed incontinence, treatment for the most predominant symptom should be tried initially. If this fails, urodynamics should be considered to guide management

STRESS INCONTINENCE MANAGEMENT

Pelvic Floor Muscle Training +/– Biofeedback

The aim of pelvic floor muscle training is to increase the strength and durability of contraction of the pelvic floor muscles. This increases the urethral closure pressure and stabilises the urethra. Biofeedback refers to the use of a vaginal probe to capture the electrical activity of the pelvic floor muscles, which can then be displayed on a screen. Biofeedback helps teach the correct contraction technique. It also allows patients to see the activity of their pelvic floor during activity which may increase motivation and compliance with prescribed exercises.

A trial of supervised pelvic floor muscle training (usually with a physiotherapist to ensure the correct muscle groups are strengthened) is advised for a minimum of 3 months as first-line treatment for stress or mixed urinary incontinence. A patient should be taught to perform a set of eight pelvic floor contractions at least three times a day. These are also referred to as Kegel exercises. Vaginal 'cones' of increasing weights can be used to increase the effects of pelvic floor muscle training. The 'cones' are inserted and then held in position by voluntary muscle contraction.

Surgical

There are different surgical options that are available for the management of stress incontinence including mid-urethral slings, autologous fascial slings and colposuspension. The effectiveness to treat stress incontinence is comparable between these procedures.

Mid-Urethral Sling
- Mid-urethral sling (MUS) includes tension-free vaginal tape (TVT) and transobturator tape (TOT).
- Sling operations aim to stabilise the urethra which increases the bladder outlet resistance during episodes of increased intra-abdominal pressure.
- These operations are considered if conservative measures have failed.
- Urodynamics is often performed to confirm the diagnosis prior to surgery.
- The surgery can be performed under local or general anaesthetic.
- Sling material is guided under the urethra to support it, with the ends of the sling being placed either retropubically in the TVT (preferred option) or through the obturator foramen in the TOT.

  Risks of MUS include:
- Bladder perforation – rarely occurs with TOT as the needle does not enter the retropubic space. The risk of bladder injury is much higher with TVT hence cystoscopy is performed to check for this after the sling has been placed.

- Urinary retention if the sling is too tight – can require catheterisation in around 15% of cases, although often this is only temporary.
- Failure of the procedure if the sling is too loose.
- New OAB symptoms in about 15% of cases.
- Mesh erosion – the synthetic material used to make the sling, over time, can erode either into the vagina and cause pain, or into the bladder and cause a fistula. This occurs in around 1% of patients.

Autologous Fascial Sling

This involves the use of native fascia, rather than synthetic mesh, to create a sling with the same function as MUS. The fascia is most commonly harvested from the rectus sheath to create the sling however the fascia lata can also be used.

Colposuspension

Sutures are used to approximate the paravaginal tissues of the lateral vaginal fornix to the ipsilateral iliopectineal ligament. This elevates the bladder neck and will repair any associated cystocoele (prolapse of the bladder into the vagina). This procedure can be done via a suprapubic incision open approach or laparoscopically. It has a longer operative time and a higher risk of patients requiring further surgery compared to MUS.

 Synthetic Mesh

Since its introduction, polypropylene synthetic mesh for MUS insertion had been the gold standard surgical treatment for stress incontinence in many countries as it has cure rates of up to 90%. However, reports of serious life changing adverse events such as mesh erosion, chronic pelvic pain and dyspareunia following mesh use for vaginal prolapse surgery and to a lesser extent MUS has led to a significant controversy about the use of synthetic mesh. Public concerns have led to a reduction in MUS procedures worldwide and increased use of other surgical procedures such as autologous fascial slings and colposuspension. However, there is increased morbidity, resources and recovery times with autologous fascial slings and colposuspension compared with TVT or TOT. These alternative surgical procedures are also considered more invasive and technically challenging compared to MUS.

Duloxetine

This is a medical therapy for stress incontinence which can be used if surgery is contraindicated or for patient choice. Duloxetine is a serotonin and noradrenaline reuptake inhibitor which inhibits the presynaptic re-uptake of the neurotransmitters, causing an increased concentration of neurotransmitters in the synaptic cleft. The resting tone of the internal urethral sphincter is maintained by the sympathetic nervous system, so an increase in the stimulation of the serotonin and noradrenaline receptors on these sympathetic neurones increases the resting tone and contraction of the urethral sphincter. Side effects include nausea, dry mouth, constipation, fatigue, insomnia and vomiting.

Other Treatments of Stress Incontinence

- Periurethral bulking agents – silicone, collagen or other materials can be injected into the urethral wall. These agents augment the urethra and increase resistance to leakage of urine. The procedure is less invasive compared to other surgical options and the injections can be performed under local anaesthesia. The effect diminishes with time, so repeat procedures may be necessary. These agents are not as effective as MUS surgery but the morbidity is lower.
- Artificial sphincter – rare complex surgery.
- Urethral plugs – not routinely advised. These are small plugs which the patient can insert into the urethra to prevent leaking. They are not a long-term solution and increase the risk of UTI but may be of use in a small subset of younger women who are troubled by stress incontinence purely during exercise.

URGE INCONTINENCE MANAGEMENT

Bladder Training

This is a treatment programme where patients void at increasingly longer time intervals, rather than voiding immediately following the desire to pass urine. It is therefore aimed at retraining the conscious minds of patients so they do not need to pass urine at every bladder sensation. This, in turn, retrains the unconscious neurological activity that urination and detrusor contraction is not needed at early filling volumes. This programme can be used in conjunction with simple lifestyle measures, and a trial of at least 6 weeks should be advised as first-line management. If this initially fails, it is recommended to continue with a programme in combination with an antimuscarinic. However, bladder training can take months and needs to be continued long term, as its effectiveness decreases once the programme is stopped. This form of management requires high levels of motivation.

Medications

- Anti-muscarinics – the detrusor muscle is controlled by the parasympathetic nervous system, which causes contractions. Therefore, blocking the acetylcholine receptors of the bladder reduces the bladder's ability to contract and also alters the sensation. Oxybutynin is one of the first-line treatments in overactive bladder and urge incontinence if bladder training has been ineffective. Since oxybutynin is a non-selective anti-muscarinic, the side effects (dry mouth, constipation, blurred vision, fatigue, cognitive dysfunction) are sometimes poorly tolerated. Due to the risk of severe side effects, oxybutynin is contraindicated in elderly and frail patients. If oxybutynin is not tolerated or is contraindicated, other anti-muscarinics should be considered (which are more selective for bladder muscarinic receptors), including solifenacin and tolterodine. From commencement, each medication can take up to 4 weeks to reach its maximal effect.

- Beta agonists – sympathetic nerve stimulation causes relaxation of the detrusor muscle. Mirabegron is a medication that is selective for bladder adrenergic receptors which limits its side effects. It can be used in combination with, or instead of, antimuscarinics.
- Vaginal oestrogen – symptoms of urge incontinence, urgency, frequency and nocturia can be improved with topical vaginal oestrogen in postmenopausal women with vaginal atrophy.

Invasive Treatments

If the non-invasive treatments above are unsuccessful, urodynamic studies are performed prior to invasive treatments. Cystoscopy may also be considered to look for interstitial cystitis.

- Botulinum toxin (Botox) – this is a neurotoxin derived from the bacterium *Clostridium botulinum.* It is used to block the release of acetylcholine, and it temporarily paralyses muscles where it is injected. It is injected directly into the bladder wall via a flexible cystoscope under local or general anaesthesia, as a day-case procedure. It should only be used in the treatment of idiopathic detrusor overactivity when conservative management has been unsuccessful. Women must be able and willing to self-catheterise, as there is a risk of bladder paralysis resulting in urinary retention. If the treatment is effective, repeat courses may be necessary every 6 to 12 months as the effect wanes.
- Posterior tibial nerve stimulation (PTNS) – this is reserved for patients who have not responded to the treatments above. The posterior tibial nerve is electrically stimulated via a needle inserted percutaneously, just above the ankle. Stimulation of this nerve stimulates the sacral micturition centre via S2 to S4 of the sacral nerve plexus, since the posterior tibial nerve and nerves supplying the bladder and pelvic floor originate from the same spinal segments. The exact mechanism of PTNS is unclear, but the current theory is that by continuously stimulating nerves, the brain's response to the stimulation is down-regulated. Therefore, by overstimulating the nerves involved in voiding, the brain will eventually down-regulate its response, making voiding less frequent.
- Sacral nerve stimulation (SNS) – a permanently implanted sacral root stimulator is surgically placed, which provides chronic stimulation to S3 nerve roots in order to inhibit the reflex behaviour of the bladder. This treatment option is recommended in urge incontinence caused by detrusor overactivity if there has been no response to non-invasive methods or botulinum toxin.
- Bladder augmentation – this is reconstructive surgery to increase the functional capacity of the bladder. A section of ileum is used to increase the capacity. This procedure is restricted to women with severe symptoms who have not responded to other treatments. Patients need to be counselled on the serious potential complications which include; bowel disturbance, metabolic acidosis, mucus production into the bladder from the inserted bowel, urinary retention, UTIs and a small risk of malignancy occurring in the inserted bowel.

COMPLICATIONS

The main problem with urinary incontinence is the impact it has on people's lives. Poorly managed incontinence can lead to depression and social isolation. Other complications are secondary to prolonged contact of urine on the skin, leading to dermatitis, candida infections and cellulitis.

PROGNOSIS

Urinary incontinence can be treated, and a number of different management options are available. It is important to manage patient expectations. A successful outcome of treatment is to improve the patient's symptoms and quality of life. However, it is rare for treatment to completely resolve all symptoms.

❓ QUESTIONS

Marlena, a 61-year-old retired primary school teacher, presents to the outpatient clinic complaining of leaking small amounts of urine when she coughs or lifts her shopping bags. This has been progressively worsening over 12 months, but following three recent accidents when out with friends, she feels her social life is now being affected. There is no pain on passing urine, but she occasionally has a strong desire to go to the toilet. She has three grown-up children, all vaginal births and normal birth weights. She has had a previous cholecystectomy, has a BMI of 35 kg/m², smokes 15 cigarettes a day and drinks two glasses of wine a night.

Q1 Answer true or false: When initially assessing the urinary incontinence in this lady, which of the following would you carry out as a primary investigation?
  A Bladder diary.
  B Post-void residual volume.
  C Renal ultrasound.
  D Urinalysis.
  E Urodynamics.

Q2 Which of the following is not a risk factor for stress incontinence in this lady?
  A Alcohol.
  B Chronic cough.
  C Lack of oestrogen.
  D Obesity.
  E Vaginal birth.

Q3 Some presentations of urinary incontinence require referral immediately to secondary care, without first trying conservative management. Which of the following situations could be managed initially in primary care?

A Haematuria.

B Mixed incontinence picture.

C Previous surgery for urinary incontinence.

D Recurrent UTIs.

E Symptomatic pelvic organ prolapse.

Q4 Answer true or false: Which of the following are treatment options for stress incontinence?

A Botulinum toxin.

B Duloxetine.

C Oxybutynin.

D Pelvic floor muscle training.

E Colposuspension

[Answers on page 200.]

KEY REFERENCES

PELVIC ORGAN PROLAPSE

National Institute for Health and Clinical Excellence, 2019. Urinary Incontinence and Pelvic Organ Prolapse in Women: Management. NICE Interventional Procedure Guidance (NG123).

National Institute for Health and Clinical Excellence, 2019. Transvaginal Mesh Repair of Anterior or Posterior Vaginal Wall Prolapse. NICE Interventional Procedure Guidance (IPG 599).

Royal College of Obstetricians and Gynaecologists, 2015. Post-Hysterectomy Vaginal Vault Prolapse. Green Top Guideline (GTG 46).

URINARY INCONTINENCE

European Association of Urology, 2020. Urinary Incontinence in Adults. Clinical Guideline.

National Institute for Health and Care Excellence, 2019. Urinary Incontinence and Pelvic Organ Prolapse in Women: Management. NICE Interventional Procedure Guidance (NG 123).

Royal College of Obstetricians and Gynaecologists, 2016. Painful Bladder Syndrome. RCOG Green Top Guideline (GTG 70).

Outline

ENDOMETRIOSIS

Endometriosis is the presence of endometrial-like tissue outside of the uterus.

AETIOLOGY

Chronic pelvic pain affects up to 20% of women at some point in their lives. There are many causes for this, but one of the commonest causes is endometriosis, which may be present in up to 50% of female patients with chronic pelvic pain.

RISK FACTORS

The main risk factor for endometriosis is menstrual cycles – the more cycles, the more likely endometriosis is to occur:
- Early menarche.
- Short menstrual cycle.
- Nulliparity.
- Family history.
- Age – being of reproductive age increases the risk. Symptoms usually settle after the menopause as oestrogen levels (which drive endometrial cell production) drop after the menopause.

PATHOPHYSIOLOGY

How endometrial tissue can exist outside the uterus is not understood. The two most popular theories are:
1 Retrograde menstruation – cells from the endometrium pass through the fallopian tubes and implant in the abdominal and pelvic cavity.
2 Metaplasia or neoplasia of cells, resulting in endometriosis wherever the cell changes occur.

The most common sites of endometriosis are the ovaries, uterosacral ligaments and the peritoneum of the pouch of Douglas. Less commonly, it is found in other local structures, such as the fallopian tubes, the uterus, bladder and rectum. Endometriosis has been reported, although rarely, in almost every site in the body, including the lungs, brain and skin. It is unknown whether endometriosis arrives at these distant sites by lymphatic or haematological spread, or whether there is a metaplastic process.

The endometrium in the normal menstrual cycle proliferates under the influence of oestrogen produced by the dominant follicle of the ovary. In a similar way, endometriosis proliferates in response to oestrogen. This fact is important because it explains:
- Why endometriosis does not occur before menarche and is rare after the menopause.
- Why the pain and other symptoms are often cyclical in nature.
- How the medical treatments of endometriosis work.

The most common locations for endometriosis are shown in Fig. 6.1.

SIGNS AND SYMPTOMS

COMMON SYMPTOMS

Pain – thought to be caused by inflammatory responses triggered by endometriosis.
- Chronic pelvic pain.
  - May show a regular pattern that follows the cyclic proliferation of the endometriosis in response to oestrogen produced in the menstrual cycle.
  - May be constant due to larger lesions, such as ovarian endometriomas, which cause persistent inflammation.
- Dysmenorrhoea.
  - Endometriosis can invade the muscle of the uterus and cause inflammation. This condition is called adenomyosis.
- Deep dyspareunia.
  - Commonly due to endometriosis in the pouch of Douglas, which is irritated during intercourse.
  - Rarely can be due to endometriosis in the vagina or cervix.

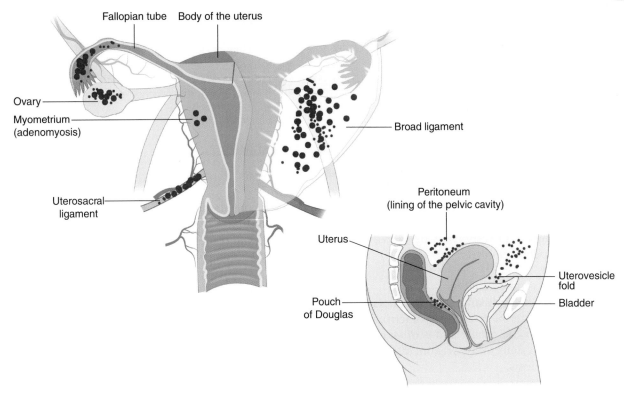

Fig. 6.1 Common Sites of Endometriosis.

OTHER PRESENTATIONS

- Infiltration into other organs:
  - Dysuria or haematuria due to bladder endometriosis.
  - Rectal bleeding or dyschezia (pain on defecation) due to rectal endometriosis.
- Rarely, other organs may be affected, presenting with haematemesis or pneumothorax with lung involvement, or local pain and bleeding from skin involvement.
- Subfertility – endometriosis may be diagnosed during investigation for subfertility.
- Asymptomatic – endometriosis is commonly identified during laparoscopy being performed for another cause. These asymptomatic findings have demonstrated that the degree of endometriosis does not often correlate with the severity of the symptoms a patient experiences.

Some clinicians advise patients to keep a pain and symptom diary to aid with diagnosis.

EXAMINATION

Examination may be completely normal.
- Abdominal examination may reveal deep tenderness around sites of endometriosis, especially if a cyst has formed.
- Bimanual examination may reveal a retroverted, tender uterus, and areas of tenderness at the top of the vagina (fornices).

- Large areas of endometriosis may be palpated as firm masses or nodules.
- Speculum examination may demonstrate red, hypertrophic lesions, most commonly seen in the posterior fornix.

INVESTIGATIONS

INITIAL INVESTIGATIONS

- Ultrasound, if acceptable transvaginal.
  - Assess for pelvic masses, particularly endometriomas.
  - Ultrasound is not very effective for identifying peritoneal disease.
- Diagnostic laparoscopy +/– biopsy
  - The best investigation for identifying peritoneal disease.
  - A biopsy should be taken for histological confirmation of the diagnosis.
  - At the time of laparoscopy, surgical treatment can also be initiated.

OTHER INVESTIGATIONS

- MRI – not as effective as laparoscopy for identifying peritoneal disease but is of use when deep endometriosis is suspected; for example, infiltration of the bladder, bowel or vagina. Endometriosis in these areas may be poorly identified on routine laparoscopy.
- Tests to investigate for other differential diagnoses:
  - FBC and CRP – infection.

- Vaginal and endocervical swabs – infection.
- Urinalysis – infection.
- Cystoscopy – interstitial cystitis, infiltrating endometriosis.
- Colonoscopy – Inflammatory bowel disease (IBD), infiltrating endometriosis.

DIFFERENTIAL DIAGNOSIS

Chronic pelvic pain often presents with features of many differential diagnoses. Often, after the initial history, examination and investigations, a diagnosis may not be clear. Clinicians will then treat the most likely cause and subsequently investigate and treat other causes, depending on the response. Common differentials for chronic pelvic pain are:

- Endometriosis.
- Irritable bowel syndrome (IBS).
- Adenomyosis – glandular tissue (often endometrial) within the uterine muscle (myometrium). This is hard to diagnose clinically and is often only confirmed after a hysterectomy. Treatment is the same as for endometriosis.
- Dense adhesions.
- Non-endometrial pelvic masses – for example, large ovarian cysts and fibroids.
- Interstitial cystitis.
- PID – usually infection is acute, but chronic effects include hydrosalpinx and adhesions.
- Primary dysmenorrhoea – painful periods are common in the teenage years, without an underlying pathology.
- Musculoskeletal pain.
- Neuropathic pain.
- Psychogenic pain.

Two or more causes of chronic pain may occur at once. Neuropathic pain or psychogenic pain may be the primary cause of symptoms. The pain may also be caused by another underlying condition:

- Nerve remodelling following persistent pain can cause ongoing chronic pain, even if the initial insult has resolved.
- Chronic pain can cause depression and social isolation. However, depression and social isolation cause a patient to be less able to tolerate pain, and so the patient is more likely to present with chronic pain.

Irritable Bowel Syndrome

Patients are regularly referred with symptoms suggestive of IBS rather than endometriosis-like symptoms. The diagnostic criteria for IBS are at least a 6 months history of abdominal pain or discomfort, occurring at least 3 days a month for 3 months, and associated with at least two of:

- Pain improves with defecation.
- Onset associated with change in bowel frequency.
- Onset associated with a change in the form of stool (consistency, presence of mucus).

Treatment

- Dietary advice – increase fibre intake, avoid food types which trigger symptoms.
- Laxatives for constipation.
- Antispasmodics; for example, mebeverine.
- Antidepressants and psychological therapy may also improve symptoms.

MANAGEMENT

Making the diagnosis of endometriosis can be difficult. There are no pathognomonic symptoms or signs and there is considerable presentation overlap with multiple other causes of chronic pelvic pain. It is also important to give patients realistic expectations for their care. The aim of treatment will be to lessen their pain and improve their quality of life. It is unlikely that treatment will entirely resolve their symptoms. It may also take some time and a review by many specialists to fully explore all aspects of the causes of their symptoms.

Endometriosis is the key diagnosis to exclude from the gynaecology side of chronic pain management. However, infections and adhesions may also be treatable by the gynaecology team. Treatment regimens should be decided after a full discussion of all possible options with the patient, with management directed to symptom control and based on fertility wishes. The initial treatments for all patients are to provide access to general measures (as described below) and optimise analgesia.

Patients then usually choose between hormonal contraceptives or laparoscopy as their next choice of treatment. The benefit of laparoscopy is that diagnosis can be confirmed with a biopsy and the endometriosis can be physically treated during the laparoscopy. The benefit of trying medical treatments first is that if symptoms are sufficiently improved then surgery (and the risks of surgery) have been avoided. The downside is that a definitive diagnosis has not been made in this instance.

If after medical treatment symptoms have not sufficiently improved, then a laparoscopy may still be required. Similarly, if laparoscopy was the first-choice treatment, hormonal contraceptives are then advised to reduce the risk of recurrence of symptoms. In women whom the above treatments have not been successful, more complex or definitive surgery can be considered.

TREATMENTS
General Measures
- Education and psychological support.
- Patient support groups.

Pain Management
- Simple analgesia, including paracetamol, non-steroidal anti-inflammatory drugs (NSAIDs) with escalation to opioid medications.
- Complementary therapies; for example, transcutaneous electrical nerve stimulation (TENS) machines.

Hormonal Contraceptives

All these treatments act by inhibiting the HPO axis to prevent follicular development, oestrogen production by the ovaries and ovulation. Oestrogen is the main stimulus for endometrial proliferation, so inhibition of oestrogen production should cause endometriosis to regress. Progestogens may also have a direct inhibitive effect on endometrial proliferation.

Once a treatment has been started, the patient should be advised to use the medication for at least 3 to 6 months before reviewing symptoms. If the treatments are effective, they can be used long term. Options include:

- Levonorgestrel intrauterine system.
  - Progesterone inhibits endometrial growth.
  - Causes anovulation in some women.
  - Has a variable effect when adenomyosis is present. Some patients find their symptoms improve; others find their symptoms deteriorate.
- Combined oral contraceptives.
  - Very effective treatment for endometriosis as it causes complete anovulation in most patients.
  - Can be used continuously (not taking a break every 21 days), classically having a 1-week break every 63 days. In patients where menstruation is very painful, the patient could use the pill for longer without stopping, but with no breaks, they are likely to develop breakthrough bleeding. If this occurs the advice is to have a break and recommence, and then plan some breaks (which can be planned around the patient's lifestyle) to prevent further breakthrough intermenstrual bleeding.
- Progestogen-only contraceptives.
  - Examples include desogestrel and medroxyprogesterone acetate.
  - Patients can be treated with pills, injections or the implant. The injection provides the highest dose of progesterone and is the most likely to cause anovulation.

Other Hormonal Therapies

- GnRH analogues.
  - GnRH is normally released in a pulsatile manner by the hypothalamus to stimulate the rest of the HPO axis. Giving it continuously downregulates GnRH receptors, completely inhibiting the HPO axis and effectively inducing a menopause-like state. This causes very low oestrogen levels, so removing the stimulus for endometriosis proliferation.
  - Side effects include symptoms experienced in menopause, such as hot flushes, vaginal dryness and loss of libido. HRT should be prescribed along with the GnRH to avoid these symptoms (which in some women can be as bad or worse than the presenting symptoms) and to avoid the risk of osteoporosis associated with long-term GnRH use. While HRT contains oestrogen this is at a much lower dose than what is produced naturally by the body during the menstrual cycle so does not appear to cause endometriosis proliferation. The progesterone component of HRT may also have an inhibitory effect on endometriosis.
  - GnRH analogues are only licensed for 6 months' use, as prolonged use causes osteoporosis (especially without HRT). With concurrent HRT some clinicians will offer GnRH use for longer periods, particularly when surgery and other treatments are not available or have been ineffective.
  - These analogues are best used for definitive assessment of whether a patient's pain improves with complete loss of HPO axis stimulation. If this is the case, then definitive surgery may be offered in the form of a bilateral oophorectomy +/− hysterectomy, which removes the oestrogen stimulation of endometriosis and the uterus where endometrium is made.
- Danazol and gestrinone are derivatives of testosterone which are sometimes used. They lower oestrogen levels, which can improve endometriosis, but they are associated with significant side effects, so they are no longer routinely used.

Surgical Therapies

- Laparoscopy.
  - Used to diagnose endometriosis.
  - Treatment can also be performed at the same time. Laparoscopic procedures for endometriosis include:
- Ablation – destroy the endometriosis areas with heat.
- Resection – cut out the endometriosis. This can then be sent for histology to confirm the diagnosis. This is generally regarded as a more effective treatment than ablation.
- Adhesiolysis – break down dense adhesions caused by endometriosis, infection or previous surgery; this will also improve pain.
- Remove endometriomas (ovarian cysts of endometriosis), which often cause pain.

If not imminently planning pregnancy after surgery, a patient should be advised to commence hormonal therapy after surgery to reduce the risk of recurrence.

Deep Infiltrating/Complex Endometriosis Surgery

In cases where endometriosis has infiltrated into pelvic organs such as the bowel, bladder or pelvic nerves, symptoms can be severe and surgical excision very difficult with a high risk of organ injury. In the UK there are a number of specialist endometriosis centres where they specialise in this complex surgery. Gynaecologists often operate jointly with bowel surgeons and urologists to remove this deep endometriosis (usually laparoscopically). These operations while improving pain can have significant complications such as temporary or permanent colostomy (stoma) formation and bladder dysfunction.

Definitive Operations

These operations are irreversible, will remove fertility and are major operations with associated risks. The patient must be aware of all these points before opting for surgery:

- Hysterectomy and removal of all visible endometrial tissues.
  - The removal of all endometrial tissue can drastically improve symptoms.
  - However, without removal of the ovaries, the condition can recur, so it is rarely performed in isolation. In cases where adenomyosis is suspected to be the main cause of symptoms, a hysterectomy alone may be considered in a patient who wishes to preserve her ovaries.
- Bilateral salpingo-oophorectomy.
  - Without ovaries, the oestrogen levels fall to a menopausal level. Endometriosis will resolve and symptoms will improve. However, as with a hysterectomy, this is a large operation and is irreversible.
  - HRT is advised in all patients below the age of 50 to reduce the chance of developing osteoporosis. There is only a very small chance that the small concentrations of oestrogen in HRT will stimulate any remaining endometriosis.

Fertility Support in Endometriosis

- Laparoscopic surgery to remove endometriosis, endometriomas and adhesions. In severe disease, this has been shown to improve fertility rates.
- Intrauterine insemination (IUI) with ovarian stimulation in mild to moderate disease with patent fallopian tubes.
- *In vitro* fertilisation (IVF).

[See 'Infertility' page 35.]

PROGNOSIS

It is important when treating patients with chronic pain that a multidisciplinary team is employed in the care, and that realistic expectations are discussed with the patient. It is rare to be able to cure chronic pain, so the aim should be to improve symptoms and improve quality of life.

If, after laparoscopy and/or a course of hormonal treatment, the symptoms have not improved and the cause not identified, it would be prudent to consider another diagnosis. A referral to a specialist pain team is appropriate at this stage, as chronic pain teams can provide specialist analgesia for pain when the diagnosis is not evident. They also have access to specialist psychologists and psychiatrists. Their input is helpful because chronic pain can affect a patient's quality of life to such an extent that a mental health disorder can be caused by the pain, or alternatively, a mental health disorder can initially present with physical symptoms.

Women with endometriosis have an approximately 3.5% risk of ovarian cancer (background population lifetime risk 2%). This is considered a small absolute risk increase, so at present, there is no additional management in the UK for this risk. There is possibly a genetic link to the development of endometriosis and ovarian cancer, but research is ongoing in this field.

❓ QUESTIONS

Shikha, a 32-year-old woman, presents to her primary care physician stating she is 'fed up' with her body. Just before menstruation, she experiences cramping pelvic pain that radiates into her back and has the feeling of pressure in her bowels. Her periods are very painful, as is intercourse, and despite years of trying, she has failed to become pregnant.

Q1 What is the best investigation for diagnosing endometriosis?
- A CA-125.
- B History and examination alone.
- C Laparoscopy.
- D MRI.
- E Transvaginal ultrasound.

Q2 Answer true or false: Which of these non-surgical treatment options are recommended for endometriosis?
- A Combined oral contraceptives.
- B Levonorgestrel intrauterine system.
- C NSAIDs.
- D Patient support groups.
- E Statins.

Q3 Answer true or false: If the patient would like to become pregnant, which of the following are appropriate options to offer?
- A Hormonal therapies.
- B IUI.
- C IVF.
- D Laparoscopic ablation and adhesiolysis.
- E Tubal flushing.

[Answers on page 202.]

SEXUALLY TRANSMITTED INFECTIONS

Sexually transmitted infections (STIs) are infections passed through vaginal, anal or oral sex, or by genital contact. The risk of STIs being transmitted are increased in people who have unprotected sex; that is, sex without barrier contraception. Specific STIs are discussed below, but there are some useful principles that apply to most infections.

SEXUAL HISTORY

With all STIs, a thorough sexual health history is key. Important factors include the 5Ps:

- Partners – particularly within the last 12 months.
- Practices – with every partner, ask about vaginal, anal and oral sex. It is also important to ask about high risk activities such as being paid or paying for sex and any use of intravenous drugs. If known, it is also useful to ask about their partners' sexual histories.
- Protection from STIs – use of barrier protection.
- Past history of STIs – any previous diagnoses and what treatment and follow-up has occurred.

- Prevention of pregnancy – it may be important to determine if there is a risk of pregnancy and to determine if the contraception used is appropriate.

However, a full sexual history includes everything in a routine medical clerking, with weighting on particular questions, such as date of last sexual contact, partner's gender (never make assumptions), infection risk or symptoms in the partner, previous sexual partners' details and a gynaecological history. It is also important to be aware of the possibility of sexual abuse, particularly in those under 18. Symptoms related to an STI maybe the first opportunity to identify a vulnerable woman/girl.

RISK FACTORS

These risk factors apply to most STIs; however, the importance of each factor varies with each disease:
- Not using barrier contraception.
- Higher number of sexual partners.
- A recent change in a sexual partner.
- Recent sexual activity. In a country or area of a country with a high STD incidence.
- Men who have sex with men (MSM), and female partners of these men.
- Commercial sex work.
- Coexisting and previous STIs.
- Age less than 25.
- Immunocompromised individuals; for example, those with HIV, diabetes and steroid users.
- Use of intravenous drugs such as heroin, particularly if sharing needles.

PRINCIPLES OF MANAGEMENT OF STIS

DIAGNOSIS AND TESTS FOR OTHER DISEASES

History, examination and investigations are required to diagnose an STI. When an STI is suspected from the clinical history, the patient is offered testing not just for the most likely presenting infection, but for a range of the common STIs (chlamydia, gonorrhoea, syphilis, HIV and hepatitis B), as transmission of multiple infections is possible from the same sexual encounter.

COUNSELLING

The diagnosis must be explained and information given, including:
- What the infection is.
- How it was caught.
- Possible short- and long-term consequences of the disease.
- The intended treatment and follow-up.
- Practices to reduce the risk of further infection.

TREATMENT

Essential advice to be given regarding treatment:
- The medication type, and how and when it should be taken.

- The importance of complying with the treatment.
- To abstain from sexual intercourse, even with barrier contraception, for 7 days after a single dose treatment or until completion of a 7 day, or longer, therapy. It is particularly important that a couple, where both members may be infected, abstain from sexual contact until both have been treated fully to prevent re-infection.
- Follow-up plans:
  - To return if symptoms persist after treatment.
  - For some STIs, a test of cure should be offered 3 months after initial therapy to confirm the treatment was successful.

CONTACT TRACING

The majority of STIs will require contacting recent sexual partners of the patient to offer them investigation and treatment. The patient can contact partners themselves, but most genitourinary medicine (GUM) clinics will ask the patient for the contact details of their sexual partners. The clinic will then contact the partners to inform them that they are at risk of an STI and advise they should be tested while maintaining anonymity for the initial patient.

Contact tracing is important because it:
- Prevents disease progression in others.
- Can reduce the spread of disease in society.
- Prevents reinfection after the initial patient has been treated by having their current sexual partners also tested and treated.

DIFFERENTIAL DIAGNOSIS

The most common presenting symptoms are pain, discharge or intermenstrual bleeding. Patients can also present with a genital lump or ulcer. The differentials are discussed below. These symptoms can occur in isolation or together. A patient may also have an infection and be completely asymptomatic.

DIFFERENTIAL DIAGNOSIS FOR PAIN

- Chlamydia.
- Gonorrhoea.
- Pelvic inflammatory disease (PID).
- Urinary tract infection (UTI).
- Urethral or vaginal foreign body.
- Endometriosis.
- Ectopic pregnancy.
- Most gastrointestinal causes of abdominal pain may be referred or occur in the pelvic region, for example, appendicitis or diverticulitis.

DIFFERENTIAL FOR A CHANGE IN DISCHARGE

- Bacterial vaginosis (BV).
- *Trichomonas vaginalis* (TV) infection.
- Vulvovaginal candidiasis.
- Chlamydia.
- Gonorrhoea.
- Physiological changes.
- Pregnancy.

DIFFERENTIAL FOR LUMPS, BUMPS AND ULCERS (TABLE 6.1)

Table 6.1 Differential Diagnosis for a Lump or Ulcer

LUMPS	ULCERS
Anogenital warts	Herpes
Pearly penile papules (men)	Syphilis
Molluscum contagiosum	Squamous cell carcinoma C
Bartholin's cyst or abscess	Chancroid
	Lymphogranuloma venereum (LGV)
	Donovanosis

NORMALISING GUM CLINIC USE

Many people may have an asymptomatic infection. If they are identified and treated long-term complications may be avoided. It is therefore advised that anyone who has had a sexual encounter which increases their risk of catching an STI should attend a GUM clinic.

PRESENTATION IN MEN

The most common STIs in men are chlamydia and gonorrhoea. They may present with penile discharge, testicular pain (epididymo-orchitis) or may be asymptomatic. Urine culture and urethral swabs are commonly used for diagnosis. Long-term infection can cause male infertility and prostatitis. Other infections, such as warts, herpes and syphilis, present similarly in women.

CHLAMYDIA

Chlamydial infections are caused by the bacterium *Chlamydia trachomatis*. This is found in the semen or vaginal fluids of infected men and women. It is one of the most common STIs, affecting 10% of sexually active young people. The incubation period is approximately 21 days, as the organism is relatively slow to replicate, so symptoms can take several weeks to develop.

SYMPTOMS

Chlamydia is asymptomatic in 70% of women and 50% of men. However, the symptoms that women commonly experience are:
- Lower abdominal pain.
- Changes in vaginal discharge.
- Dyspareunia.
- Dysuria.
- Intermenstrual bleeding.
- Postcoital bleeding.

If the infection is in the rectum, this will often be asymptomatic, but discomfort or discharge may occur. Conjunctivitis due to *Chlamydia trachomatis* can occur if there is contact to the eye with infected genital secretions. Chlamydia does not tend to cause infections or symptoms in the throat.

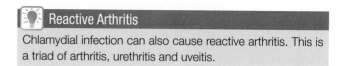

Chlamydial infection can also cause reactive arthritis. This is a triad of arthritis, urethritis and uveitis.

INVESTIGATION

Internal and speculum examinations are often used to elicit symptoms such as pelvic pain and also to observe cervical discharge or any cervicitis. During the speculum examination, swabs can be obtained.

Specific investigations should be undertaken in anyone who has symptoms or has been referred to the GUM clinic because of an infected partner. However, chlamydial tests are often offered to asymptomatic young people under the age of 25 since it is common in this age group and is often asymptomatic. This is primarily a nucleic acid amplification test (NAAT) from vaginal swabs, collected either by the clinician or by a patient, or from a urine sample. If self-collected, these will be vaginal swabs, whereas clinicians can also take endocervical and urethral swabs. Rectal, throat and conjunctival swabs may also be taken if indicated.

TREATMENT

Treatment is very successful with antibiotics. Always check local policy, but current guidelines advocate either 7 days of doxycycline twice daily or a single higher dose of azithromycin if there is likely to be an issue with compliance. Longer treatment regimens may be given if the infection has ascended.

COMPLICATIONS

- PID.
- Infertility.
- Ectopic pregnancy.
- Reactive arthritis.
- Perihepatitis as part of Fitz-Hugh Curtis syndrome – a rare complication of PID causing liver capsule inflammation and adhesions.

PROGNOSIS

The treatment of chlamydia is relatively simple and very effective. Therefore, in individuals treated soon after infection, the prognosis is very good. However, those with asymptomatic, untreated chlamydia can go on to develop long-term complications, including pain and subfertility.

GONORRHOEA

Gonorrhoea is caused by the bacteria *Neisseria gonorrhoeae*, which is found in the semen and vaginal fluids of infected individuals. The incubation period is 2 to 7 days. Infection is usually symptomatic.

SYMPTOMS

- Lower abdominal pain.
- Change in vaginal discharge – thin, watery, yellow or green.
- Dysuria.
- Intermenstrual or postcoital bleeding.

Rectal infection is usually asymptomatic but can cause discomfort or discharge. Conjunctivitis can be caused by gonorrhoea, but it rarely causes pharyngitis or symptoms in the throat.

INVESTIGATION

- NAAT testing with swabs or urine.
- Microscopy of genital specimens to look for gram-negative diplococci.
- Culture for antimicrobial sensitivity testing.
- Rectal or pharyngeal swabs, if indicated by the sexual history.

TREATMENT

Treatment is with antibiotics, following local guidelines as strains and antibiotic resistance vary by area. Example treatments are ceftriaxone or ciprofloxacin given IM can both be given as a single dose if the infection is uncomplicated. These can be given empirically while awaiting investigation results if there is strong clinical suspicion of gonorrhoea. Unfortunately, the number of antibiotic-resistant strains of gonorrhoea is increasing, so these infections may require more aggressive antimicrobial treatments. A test of cure is important in gonorrhoea infections.

COMPLICATIONS

- PID.
- Infertility.
- Conjunctivitis.
- Rarely, haematogenous spread can occur causing skin lesions and arthritis.

PROGNOSIS

Treatment is relatively simple with uncomplicated gonorrhoea. However, with resistant strains of *Neisseria gonorrhoeae*, finding curative treatments is becoming increasingly difficult. Inadequately treated infection can cause long-term complications.

PELVIC INFLAMMATORY DISEASE

PID is the broad term for infection of the female reproductive tract, including the uterus, fallopian tubes, ovaries and the peritoneal cavity. It is most commonly caused by chlamydia or gonorrhoea, but it can be caused by other organisms.

PID is more likely to occur if an infection is not treated, if the patient has an immunodeficiency, and after gynaecological procedures that can help the infection ascend through the genital tract, such as insertion of an intrauterine device or surgical termination.

SYMPTOMS AND SIGNS

- Lower abdominal pain – usually bilateral.
- Fever and additional signs of sepsis.
- Deep dyspareunia.
- Mucopurulent vaginal or cervical discharge.

Cervicitis and purulent cervical discharge may be seen on speculum examination. Cervical excitation and adnexal tenderness may also be elicited on bimanual examination.

INVESTIGATION

- FBC and CRP – raised inflammatory markers support the diagnosis of infection.
- Lactate – should be measured in all cases of significant sepsis as a guide to the severity of systemic compromise.
- Blood cultures – as per investigation of any significant sepsis.
- Cervical and endocervical swabs – for STIs, particularly chlamydia and gonorrhoea. A referral to GUM should be considered for more extensive STI testing.
- Urinalysis, urine culture and urine βhCG – important to rule out UTI or ectopic pregnancy.
- Ultrasound – pelvic collections and tubo-ovarian abscesses can be identified.

TREATMENT

Treatment is with antibiotics, according to local policy. Mild or moderate disease can be managed using oral antibiotics and remain an outpatient with regular follow-up. Severe cases should be treated with IV antibiotics and require hospital admission. Appropriate pain relief should also be given. If there is an IUD *in situ*, the long-term benefits and risks associated with removal should be considered particularly considering recent intercourse and risk of pregnancy if removed. If disease is mild or moderate and the IUD is not removed, it should be reviewed after 72 hours and if there is no clinical improvement then the IUD should be removed.

In severe cases, where intravenous antibiotics have not improved the clinical condition, further investigation and treatment may be considered:

- CT or MRI – abscesses can be identified. Imaging-guided percutaneous drainage may be considered.
- Laparoscopy – allows direct visualisation of the pelvis but is invasive. Abscesses can be drained surgically.

COMPLICATIONS

All the complications are caused by inflammatory damage to the pelvis:

- Adhesions – chronic pelvic pain.
- Infertility.
- Increased risk of ectopic pregnancies – due to tubal damage.

- Fitz-Hugh Curtis syndrome.
- Chronic tubo-ovarian abscess.

PROGNOSIS

PID has a spectrum of severity; however, it is a disease that causes a lot of emotional and physical difficulties for patients due to its association with chronic debilitating pain and infertility.

HERPES

Traditionally, herpes simplex virus type 1 (HSV 1) caused 'cold sores' around the mouth and herpes simplex virus type 2 (HSV 2) was responsible for genital herpes. However, with changes in common sexual practices, both viruses can cause herpetic lesions in either location. The incubation period typically is 2 to 7 days; however, there are reports of patients acquiring the virus several years before symptoms develop. Patients are infectious when they are symptomatic, typically for 7 to 12 days.

SYMPTOMS

Symptoms of the first outbreak of genital herpes usually follow a pattern involving:
- Malaise – flu-like symptoms of fever, fatigue, lymphadenopathy and myalgia.
- Stinging, tingling or itching in the genital area.
- Small, fluid-filled vesicles developing near or on the genitals.
- Bursting of vesicles, leaving red sores which can be acutely painful.
- Dysuria occurs, which, if severe enough can lead to retention.

Symptoms of recurrent herpes are similar to the first outbreak but usually are much milder and quicker to resolve.

INVESTIGATION

Examination may allow strong clinical suspicion of herpes, but the diagnosis should be confirmed with investigations. Local policies differ, but investigations that are available for HSV include:
- DNA detection using polymerase chain reaction (PCR) from a swab of the fluid in the ulcers.
- Viral culture from a swab.
- Blood tests for HSV serology can detect asymptomatic infections but may be falsely negative if taken in the first 12 weeks of the primary infection.

TREATMENT

Supportive treatment for pain.
- Saline bathing, simple analgesia and topical lidocaine 5% gel.
- Advise if there is severe dysuria, to micturate in a bath as this will reduce the pain (the pain is caused by the urine running over the open sores).

Antiviral therapy – oral antiviral treatment; for example, aciclovir, if used within 5 days of onset, reduces the severity and duration of the symptoms. A typical treatment course is 5 days.

Arrange follow-up for 2 to 3 weeks' time to ensure resolution and give the patient education on the infection. Recurrent attacks.
- Antiviral treatment can be started as soon as symptoms occur.
- If a patient has more than six attacks a year, suppressive treatment with antivirals may be offered.

Contact tracing is also offered; however, testing is only suggested in partners who are symptomatic. Condoms reduce the risk of herpes transmission but do not completely prevent it.

COMPLICATIONS

- Urinary retention.
- Autonomic neuropathy.
- Secondary bacterial infection in the lesions.
- Spread to extra-genital areas.
- Psychological problems.

PROGNOSIS

Antiviral treatment does not eradicate HSV, and the virus remains dormant. Therefore, the majority of people will have a recurrence of symptoms after their first outbreak.

SYPHILIS

Syphilis is an STI caused by the spirochaete bacterium *Treponema pallidum*. Individuals are most contagious in the primary and secondary stages of the disease. The prevalence of syphilis is increasing, particularly among MSM.

SYMPTOMS

There are five stages of syphilis infection:
1 Primary – characterised by a painless ulcer, called a chancre (Fig. 6.2), typically on the genitals, with associated localised lymphadenopathy. The ulcer will have a sharply marginated border with a clean base.
2 Secondary – multisystem involvement, which may present with lymphadenopathy, malaise, a generalised non-pruritic maculopapular rash typically on the palms and soles, moist wart-like lesions called *condylomata lata* at sites of skin friction, and patchy lesions on the oral mucosa. Other less common presentations may include uveitis, meningitis, hepatitis and glomerulonephritis.
3 Early latent – positive syphilis serology within the first 2 years of infection, but without any symptoms or signs.
4 Late latent – positive syphilis serology after 2 years of infection, but without any symptoms or signs.

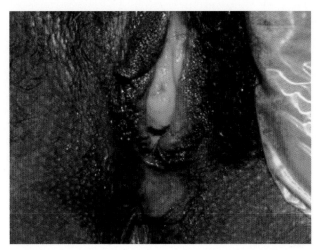

Fig. 6.2 Chancre in syphilis. (Source: Kumar, Sunesh, V. G. Padubidri, and Shirish N. Daftary, eds. Howkins & Bourne: Shaw's Textbook of Gynaecology. Elsevier India, 2022.)

5 Tertiary – now rare because of the antibiotic treatments available. Clinical presentations are caused by neurosyphilis, cardiovascular syphilis or gummatous syphilis.

INVESTIGATIONS

Blood tests.

- Syphilis serology – IgM is usually positive 2 weeks after infection, IgG after 5 weeks. Serology is the most sensitive test for the presence of syphilis, but not the stage of disease. IgG may remain positive in patients who have cleared the infection.
- Venereal Disease Research Laboratory (VDRL) test – an old test, which detects anti-cardiolipin antibodies produced in response to syphilis infection. The level of antibody can be quantified and is used to gauge activity of the bacteria, stage of disease and response to treatment.

    Virology swab of any active lesions.
- Direct microscopy.
- PCR.

    False-negative results are possible, so tests should be repeated at 6 and 12 weeks, especially if clinical suspicion remains.

TREATMENT

Treatment is with penicillin antibiotics, unless patients are allergic, and the exact form and dose depends on the stage of syphilis infection. The Jarisch-Herxheimer reaction is a reaction to the treatment caused by the release of endotoxins from the dead bacteria. It typically causes headaches, myalgia, chills, rigors, pyrexia and tachycardia. It resembles sepsis but is usually self-limiting, lasting for approximately 24 hours. It can be treated with non-steroidal anti-inflammatory medications.

COMPLICATIONS

People infected with HIV are more likely to develop complications of syphilis which include:

- Neurosyphilis – meningitis, cerebrovascular dementia due to meningovascular syphilis, dementia-like symptoms due to parenchymatous syphilis and sensory ataxia and weakness due to tabes dorsalis (demyelination of the dorsal columns of the spinal cord).
- Cardiovascular syphilis – aneurysms, coronary artery stenosis, aortic regurgitation and aortitis (can be remembered as the 4 As).
- Gummatous syphilis – granulomatous masses may cause localised tissue destruction, forming ulcers that occur mainly in skin, bone and liver.
- Complications of secondary syphilis, as listed above.

PROGNOSIS

The prognosis for syphilis is good if treated early. However, if untreated, one-third of people will go on to develop tertiary syphilis, which has a poor prognosis.

ANOGENITAL WARTS

Anogenital warts are benign epithelial skin tumours caused by the human papillomavirus (HPV) types 6 and 11 (Fig. 6.3). HPV can be acquired sexually; however, it can also be transmitted by routes other than sexual contact. The incubation period can be from 2 weeks to 8 months.

SYMPTOMS

Warts may be broad-based or pedunculated lesions that may be skin coloured or pigmented. Keratinisation depends on the skin the warts are present on, with those on warm, moist, non-hair bearing skin being non-keratinised and warts on dry, hairy skin often being firm and keratinised. Warts may be single or multiple, occurring at any site, including the vulva, within the vagina, anorectal region, or anywhere else on the body. Perianal warts can occur in anyone but are more commonly seen in men who have sex with men.

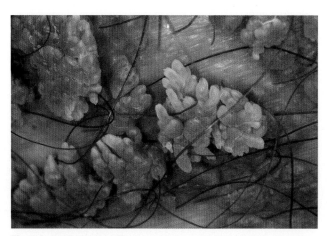

Fig. 6.3 **Genital warts.** (Source: Dinulos, James G. Habif's Clinical Dermatology. Elsevier, 2021.)

INVESTIGATION

The diagnosis is often clinical after seeing the warts on examination. However, if there is any doubt, a biopsy should be taken. Examination should also include the entire anogenital region and surrounding skin. A speculum examination should be performed in females and proctoscopy can be performed in both sexes if there is a history of anal receptive sex. Further examination, such as urethroscopy or examination of extragenital sites, should be led by the clinical history.

TREATMENT

Treatment choice depends on multiple factors, such as anatomical location, number and distribution of the warts, morphology and patient preference. It is also important to consider that all treatments have a significant failure rate, with subsequent relapse. Treatments also often have multiple side effects, and this all needs to be discussed in depth with the patient (Table 6.2).

COMPLICATIONS

Other strains of HPV cause cervical cancer; therefore, a vaccination exists against four types of HPV. HPV has also been associated with some penile, oral and anal cancers. Warts themselves, however, have minimal complications except for the psychosexual impact.

[See 'Cervical Cancer' page 156.]

PROGNOSIS

Anogenital warts themselves are physically harmless, so they can be left untreated if the patient is not concerned by them. Over time, they can resolve spontaneously. Treatment failure is common, due to recurrence. The aesthetic effect of warts can cause significant psychosexual problems.

BACTERIAL VAGINOSIS

Normally, the vaginal pH is approximately 4.5, kept at this level by the presence of lactobacilli as the prominent bacilli (Fig. 6.4). However, in BV the pH is elevated up to 6. The vaginal bacterial flora becomes dominated by anaerobic organisms, such as *Gardnerella vaginalis*.

Risk factors include vaginal douching or other hygiene methods that alter the pH of the vagina, recent change of sexual partner, presence of other STIs, antibiotic use and smoking. Therefore, there is a debate as to whether BV has an element of sexual transmission or if it is simply a response to changes in vaginal flora by other mechanisms. However, it is an important differential for any changes in vaginal discharge.

SYMPTOMS

The predominant symptom is a change in vaginal discharge, usually thin and white with a fishy offensive smell. However, many women can also be asymptomatic. Inflammation and vaginal irritation are not common, and another diagnosis should be considered if these symptoms are present.

INVESTIGATION

The British Association of Sexual Health and HIV (BASHH) recommend diagnosis in GUM clinics using a Gram-stained vaginal smear and then evaluating on microscopy:
- Normal – lactobacilli predominate.
- Intermediate – mixed vaginal flow with some lactobacilli present.
- BV – predominantly *Gardnerella* or *Mobiluncus*.

Finding *Gardnerella vaginalis* in a patient is not diagnostic in itself unless associated with a relative decline in lactobacilli.

Table 6.2 Treatment Options for Anogenital Warts

TREATMENT OPTION	ADVANTAGES	DISADVANTAGES
Cryotherapy	Used in localised areas of small numbers of warts	Health and safety issues with liquid nitrogen
Excision	Used in localised areas of small numbers of warts	Risk of haemorrhage and local anaesthetic
Electrosurgery	Used in localised areas of small numbers of warts	As with all ablative therapies, scarring can develop
Podophyllotoxin	• Cytotoxic topical solution to which soft, non-keratinised warts respond well • Not as aggressive as ablative methods • Suitable for home treatment	• May not be effective for keratinised warts • Side effects include soreness and ulceration
Trichloroacetic acid	Can be used at most anatomical sites	• Can only be applied in a specialist clinic setting • Can cause significant discomfort soon after application, as it is corrosive • Ulceration can occur, therefore should only be used for low volume warts
Imiquimod	• Immune response modifier suitable for keratinised and non-keratinised warts • Suitable for home treatment	• Can weaken latex condoms after contact • Can be an irritant for sexual partners

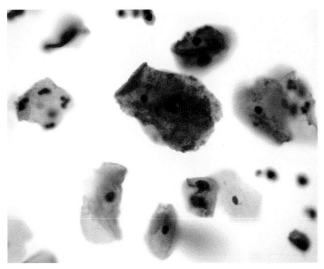

Fig. 6.4 Clue cells present in a swab with a woman affected by bacterial vaginosis. (Source: Nucci, Marisa R. and Carlos Parra-Herran. Gynecologic pathology. Elsevier Inc, 2020.)

TREATMENT

General advice should be given to all women to avoid the use of any chemicals in the vagina and to avoid any form of vaginal douching.

Further treatment is then indicated only for women who are symptomatic. Local guidance should be sought for antibiotic choice, but metronidazole is often used.

COMPLICATIONS

There are no systemic complications of BV. In pregnancy, there is some evidence that may link BV to preterm labour and late miscarriage.

PROGNOSIS

The prognosis for BV alone is good, as it is a benign condition. However, if left untreated, the vaginal discharge and strong odour may cause psychosexual problems.

TRICHOMONAS VAGINALIS

TV is a sexually acquired anaerobic flagellated protozoan found in the urethral area in men and women (Fig. 6.5). The incubation period is around 28 days.

SYMPTOMS

- Vaginal discharge – classically a frothy yellow discharge but can vary significantly.
- Vulval pruritus – vulvitis and vaginitis can occur.
- Dysuria.
- Offensive smelling urine.
- Occasionally, lower abdominal discomfort or vulval ulceration can occur.

Many women are asymptomatic with TV. Men can also be asymptomatic but may develop urethral discharge, urethral irritation, increased urinary frequency and dysuria.

INVESTIGATION

Examination may reveal erythema due to the associated vaginitis or vulvitis. The cervix may also be inflamed and a 'strawberry cervix' may be seen.

Vaginal swabs should be taken. NAAT is a gold standard diagnostic tool, but cultures could also be carried out. If the facilities exist, light field microscopy can be performed, where motile trichomonads will be seen in vaginal discharge.

In men, a urethral swab and first void urine are cultured to make the diagnosis.

TREATMENT

Systemic antibiotics should be given orally according to local policy. Metronidazole is often used either as a high single dose or a 5- to 7-day course.

COMPLICATIONS

TV is associated with HIV, as there is a higher prevalence of TV in the HIV-positive community. Having TV is also thought to increase the risk of HIV transmission. In non-pregnant women, the complications associated with TV are minimal. In pregnancy, TV may be associated with preterm birth.

PROGNOSIS

The prognosis of TV is good due to the effective treatments available and because TV infection leads to minimal complications.

VULVOVAGINAL CANDIDIASIS

The majority of vulvovaginal candidiasis is caused by the fungus *Candida albicans*, but occasionally it can be caused by another *Candida* species. The incubation period is 1 to 5 days. *Candida albicans* can cause opportunistic oral and genital infections. It is not typically an STI, but the fungus can be transmitted during sexual contact. Recurrent vulvovaginal candidiasis is defined as four or more episodes in a single year.

SYMPTOMS AND SIGNS

- Non-offensive vaginal discharge that is typically described as curdy.
- Vulval pruritus, soreness and swelling.
- Superficial dyspareunia.
- Vulval pain on urination or external dysuria.

Examination may reveal erythema, fissuring, excoriation and satellite lesions, as well as discharge on speculum examination.

INVESTIGATION

To diagnose, microscopy and culture should be performed on vaginal swabs.

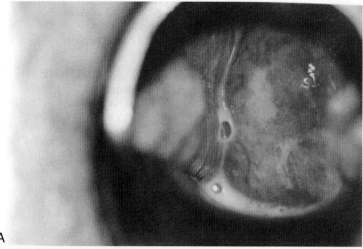

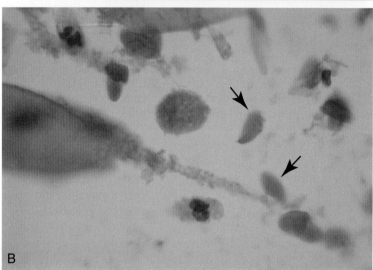

Fig. 6.5 Trichomonas vaginalis. A. Trichomonas vaginalis discharge. B. Trichomonas vaginalis under a microscope. (Source: A, Oats, Jeremy JN, and Jacqueline Boyle. Llewellyn-Jones Fundamentals of Obstetrics and Gynaecology. Elsevier Ltd, 2023. B, Shiland, Betsy J. Medical Assisting Module F. Elsevier Inc, 2050.)

TREATMENT

Lifestyle advice should be given: to avoid tight-fitting clothing, avoid irritants and use soap substitutes. Anti-fungal treatment, for example, clotrimazole, should be given as an oral medication, as a topical cream or as a pessary.

COMPLICATIONS

Complications are uncommon, but the main complication is that the candidiasis is recurrent. It is likely to be more severe in immunocompromised patients.

PROGNOSIS

The prognosis for vulvovaginal candidiasis is good.

HIV AND HEPATITIS

HIV and hepatitis are also STIs that often have significant impact on the severity and treatment of other STIs. It is therefore important that blood samples are taken to test for these diseases when another STI is diagnosed. These are covered in more depth in the obstetric chapter.

[See 'HIV in Pregnancy' page 244.]

[See 'Hepatitis B in Pregnancy' page 242.]

PREGNANCY

Investigating and treating (Table 6.3) an STI in pregnancy is similar to the steps used outside of pregnancy. The chosen antimicrobial may differ, to avoid fetal side effects. Chlamydia and gonorrhoea are less likely to be contracted during pregnancy due to the thickening of the cervical mucus plug.

If an STI is diagnosed in pregnancy, an obstetrician should be involved in the ongoing care of the patient, as antenatal, intrapartum and neonatal management need alteration to reduce the chance of fetal infection. Further information is available in the obstetric section.

[See 'Congenital Intrauterine Infections' page 325.]

Table 6.3	Treatment of Sexually Transmitted Infection in Pregnancy

SEXUALLY TRANSMITTED INFECTION	SPECIFIC OBSTETRIC MANAGEMENT
Chlamydia	Monitor neonate for signs of chlamydial eye disease and pneumonia.
Herpes	Consider planned caesarean if primary infection <6 weeks before birth to avoid neonatal infection.
Syphilis	Increased antenatal monitoring including ultrasound scans to monitor for growth restriction.
	Antibiotics may be given to the neonate and regular follow-up for the first year of life.
Hepatitis B	Fetal blood sampling, fetal scalp electrode use, and difficult assisted vaginal births increase the risk of fetal scalp laceration and transmission of hepatitis B infection; these should therefore be avoided in labour for hepatitis B positive mothers.
	Neonatal treatment with immunoglobulin therapy and or vaccination.
HIV	Close monitoring of viral load in pregnancy.
	• <50 HIV RNA copies/mL at 36 weeks – vaginal birth if no obstetric contraindications • ≥400 HIV RNA copies/mL at 36 weeks – planned caesarean is recommended to reduce risk of transmission. • 50–399 HIV RNA copies/mL at 36 weeks – planned caesarean should be considered after full review of individual case.
BV and TV	Consideration of treatment of asymptomatic cases to reduce the risk of preterm birth.

❓ QUESTIONS

You have been called to help in a busy GUM clinic. The waiting room is full of patients, and the clinic is running behind. Many patients are becoming angry at the delay in being seen.

A Anogenital warts.
B Bacterial vaginosis.
C Candidiasis.
D Chlamydia.
E Gonorrhoea.
F Hepatitis.
G Herpes.
H HIV.
I PID.
J Syphilis.
K Trichomonas vaginalis.
L Urinary tract infection.

Choose one of the above options for each question: which is the most likely diagnosis?

Q1 A 22-year-old female presents with a known history of recurrent chlamydia. She has now developed pelvic pain ongoing for the last 2 months and has a temperature of 39.5°C.

Q2 A 35-year-old female who is a commercial sex worker develops a painless ulcer on her vulva. She has no other symptoms.

Q3 A 25-year-old female has had a change in her discharge over the past 3 weeks; it has an offensive smell and on microscopy, mobile organisms are seen.

Q4 A 27-year-old female returns after having cryotherapy treatment 2 months ago; her STI has reoccurred.

Q5 A 12-year-old female has a vaccine called Gardasil administered. Which STI is she protected against?

Q6 Answer true or false to the following statements regarding contact tracing.
A Patients should be encouraged to contact people possibly at risk of having an STI themselves.
B As long as both partners are undergoing treatment, they can engage in sexual intercourse.
C Many GUM clinics offer a service to contact people who could be at risk of having an STI.
D With all STIs, individuals should only consider contacting those with whom they have had sexual intercourse within the last 6 months.
E Only those who have engaged in vaginal and anal sexual intercourse need to be contacted.

Q7 Which of the following is the triad of symptoms in reactive arthritis?
A Arthritis, gingivitis and urethritis.
B Arthritis, myositis and uveitis.
C Arthritis, urethritis and uveitis.
D Gingivitis, myositis and urethritis.
E Gingivitis, myositis and uveitis.

Q8 Which of the following statements describes Fitz-Hugh Curtis syndrome?
A Areas of endometrial tissue outside of the uterus in the pelvic cavity.
B Atony of the bladder resulting from autonomic neuropathy following PID.
C Infertility developing due to tubal scarring following PID.
D Liver capsule inflammation and adhesions following PID.
E Renal failure developing due to ascending infection following PID.

[Answers on page 204.]

BENIGN OVARIAN CYSTS

An ovarian cyst is defined as a fluid-filled sac arising from, or within, an ovary. With the increasing use of ultrasound for the assessment of abdominal pain, pelvic pain, and other symptoms in females, ovarian cysts are commonly being seen. It is important to understand the different types of cysts (Fig. 6.6), so the patient can be managed correctly. Clinicians with inadequate knowledge commonly attribute the cause of a patient's pain to cysts which do not cause pain, or they send patients for unnecessary further investigations

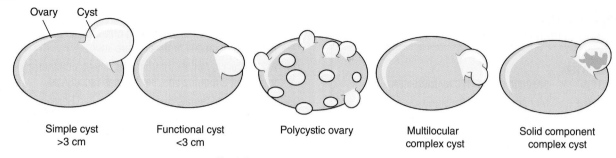

Fig. 6.6 Different Forms of Cysts on an Ovary.

when the patient could have been safely discharged with no follow-up.

Ovarian cysts are very common, with the vast majority requiring no intervention. However, women have approximately a one in ten lifetime risk of requiring surgery for an ovarian mass. Most ovarian cysts which arise prior to the menopause are benign.

SIMPLE CYSTS

SIMPLE OVARIAN CYST

- Fluid-filled, unilocular cyst with a diameter greater than 3 cm.
- These cysts form from a developing follicle during the menstrual cycle. Usually, once the oocyte has been released from the dominant follicle, the cyst should regress over the next couple of menstrual cycles. Occasionally, however, these cysts can continue to enlarge.
- For treatment purposes, they are classified by size; small (<5 cm), medium (5 to 7 cm) and large (more than 7 cm).

FUNCTIONAL CYST

- Fluid-filled, unilocular cyst with a diameter of less than 3 cm.
- These are the physiological cysts that form from the dominant follicle as part of a normal menstrual cycle. They are differentiated from simple ovarian cysts only because these are physiological cysts and will be seen in every ovulating woman during her menstrual cycle. They will regress spontaneously.
- They do not cause pain, do not require any treatment and are at no risk of ovarian torsion.

POLYCYSTIC OVARIES

- Characterised by multiple small functional cysts on the ovaries (typically each <10 mm diameter).
- This finding on ultrasound may form part of the diagnosis of polycystic ovarian syndrome (PCOS) but is not a diagnosis by itself.
- Cysts in polycystic ovaries do not cause pain.

[See 'Polycystic Ovarian Syndrome' page 31.]

COMPLEX CYSTS

- Any ovarian cyst which is not simple in nature. It may be:
  - Multi-locular.
  - Contain solid components.
  - Contain blood – blood clots can be difficult to differentiate from solid components.

HAEMORRHAGIC CYST

- A simple cyst can bleed into itself, giving it a complex appearance on ultrasound.
- It should regress naturally without treatment.

CORPUS LUTEAL CYST

- The corpus luteum is a normal part of the menstrual cycle. However, on ultrasound, it can sometimes be difficult to differentiate from a complex cyst as it may contain small solid areas and bleeding.
- Usually, these cysts do not become larger than 2 cm.
- Should regress without treatment.

ENDOMETRIOMA

- Endometriosis forming on the ovary forms a cyst with a complex appearance, typically having a ground-glass appearance on ultrasound.
- Often present with pain and may be associated with infertility.
- Not likely to resolve spontaneously and often requires surgical management.
- Endometriomas are also referred to as 'chocolate cysts' due to the brown liquid drained from them during surgery.

DERMOID CYST

- Benign growth of germ cell origin, also called a mature teratoma.
- Can form into any type of mature tissue. Typically, cysts contain hair, sebum, fat, teeth and cartilage.
- Malignant transformation is extremely rare.
- Often slow growing (1 to 2 mm per year).
- Very unlikely to resolve spontaneously. Often require surgery.

CYST ACCIDENT

Cyst accident is a provisional diagnosis often used by clinicians to describe acute pain attributed to a cyst. This can be due to cyst rupture, cyst haemorrhage or ovarian torsion. Cyst rupture and cyst haemorrhage are self-limiting and only require analgesia. However, ovarian torsion needs to be quickly identified and operated on to prevent necrosis of the ovary.

SYMPTOMS AND SIGNS

Commonly, benign ovarian cysts are asymptomatic and are only identified on an ultrasound requested for an alternate reason. Persistent ovarian cysts can cause symptoms:
- Pain.
  - Persistent lower abdominal or pelvic pain.
  - Dysmenorrhoea.
  - Dyspareunia.
- Mass effect
  - Increased urgency and frequency of urine.
  - Early satiety.
  - Abdominal distension – may be palpable abdominally or on bimanual examination.
- Infertility – endometriomas and PCOS.

Benign ovarian cysts can also present with acute pain following a cyst accident.

INVESTIGATIONS

ULTRASOUND

This is the gold standard investigation of a benign ovarian cyst. It allows the assessment of cyst size, location and consistency, all of which will guide the management plan. Transvaginal ultrasound is preferable to a transabdominal approach due to the increased sensitivity.

A key role of the investigation is to assess the likelihood of an ovarian cyst being benign or malignant. The following features are reassuring for a benign cyst (International Ovarian Tumour Analysis (IOTA) criteria):
- Unilocular cyst.
- Acoustic shadow.
- No blood flow.
- If the cyst is multilocular, it must be smooth and less than 10 cm in diameter.
- If there are solid components, the largest component must be less than 7 mm.

Occasionally a cyst may be difficult to confidently characterise on ultrasound, especially if it is a very large cyst. In these situations, an MRI scan may also be requested to support the ultrasound findings.

BLOOD TESTS (TUMOUR MARKERS)

- CA-125
  - In postmenopausal patients, CA-125 should be requested for any ovarian cyst.
  - In premenopausal patients, it should be requested for all complex ovarian cysts to rule out ovarian adenocarcinoma, although the risk in this patient group is very small. An elevated result must be interpreted with caution in premenopausal women due to its low specificity in this patient group, as endometriosis, infection, and menstruation can all increase CA-125 levels. These factors are far more likely than malignancy to be the cause of an abnormal result.
- If an ovarian cyst is deemed to be complex on ultrasound, and the patient is less than 40 years old, the risk of a germ cell tumour is increased. The following blood tests should also be undertaken:
  - Lactate dehydrogenase.
  - Alpha-fetoprotein.
  - Human chorionic gonadotropin.

The risk of malignancy index (RMI) is a scoring system that helps to estimate the malignancy risk, based on the ultrasound findings, the CA-125 level and the patient's menopausal status. If these investigations suggest the possibility of malignancy, the patient should urgently be referred to an onco-gynaecology team for further assessment and management. See ovarian malignancy for more information on calculating the RMI.

[See 'Ovarian Cancer' page 142.]

MANAGEMENT

The management of a benign ovarian cyst in premenopausal women depends on the size, the presence of symptoms, results of blood tests and the classification of the cyst.

SIMPLE CYSTS

- Small cysts (<5 cm) and functional cysts (<3 cm).
  - No treatment, no follow-up scans.
  - These cysts are usually physiological and likely to remit within a couple of months.
  - They are very unlikely to cause pain or any other symptom.
- Medium cyst (5 to 7 cm).
  - Watchful waiting is recommended, with repeat ultrasound 1 year later.
  - Small risk of torsion with cysts of this size.
- Large cyst (more than 7 cm).
  - Surgery offered to remove cyst.
  - The larger the cyst, the more likely it is to cause pain and pressure symptoms, and the risk of ovarian torsion increases.

- Further imaging, such as MRI, may be considered prior to surgery, as it is difficult to assess large cysts fully on ultrasound.
- Polycystic ovaries.
  - Do not cause pain; no follow-up if found incidentally.
  - If identified while investigating infertility or PCOS, then treatment is for those conditions.

[See 'Polycystic Ovarian Syndrome' page 31.]
[See 'Infertility' page 35.]

COMPLEX CYSTS

- Small complex cysts of less than 3 cm.
  - Likely to resolve spontaneously, particularly if they appear as haemorrhagic cysts or corpus luteum cysts on ultrasound.
  - Repeat ultrasound after 8 weeks.
  - If the cyst has resolved, no further management.
  - If the cyst is enlarging, consider checking tumour markers and consider surgical removal.

DERMOID CYST

- Unlikely to resolve and likely to enlarge over time. As they enlarge, the risk of pain and ovarian torsion increases.
- Surgical management is recommended.
- Conservative management with ultrasounds 2 or 3 times a year may be considered where the cyst is less than 5 cm.

ENDOMETRIOMA

- Unlikely to resolve.
- Other areas of endometriosis are likely within the pelvis. If pain is suspected due to endometriosis, laparoscopy and excision is advised.
- Small asymptomatic endometriomas can be managed conservatively with ultrasound follow-up.
- Cysts more than 5 cm should be considered for surgery in view of the risk of ovarian torsion.
- For patients presenting with subfertility the decision to treat an endometrioma is complex. If pain is preventing intercourse, then surgery could be considered. However, surgery can potentially damage oocytes potentially reducing fertility potential, so if treatments such as IVF are planned it would be better to defer any surgery until after pregnancy.

SURGERY

Surgery is recommended where cysts are not resolving or are increasing in size, complex in nature, or causing persistent pain. The options available are cystectomy, which involves removing the cyst and leaving the ovary in place, or oophorectomy, where the entire ovary is removed along with the cyst. Laparoscopy is the preferred surgical option, due to faster patient recovery time. However, laparotomy may be required if a cyst is very large.

Cysts can also be aspirated using an ultrasound-guided needle through the abdomen or vagina. This is not the preferred treatment, as the cyst recurrence rate is at least 50%. It is occasionally performed for patients with a symptomatic cyst in pregnancy where, ideally, abdominal surgery should be avoided.

MANAGEMENT OF POSTMENOPAUSAL PATIENTS

- A simple ovarian cyst less than 5 cm diameter with a normal CA-125 may be managed with watchful waiting, with a repeat ultrasound and repeat CA-125 carried out every 4 months for 1 year. If the cyst enlarges or its features change, surgery should be offered. If the cyst resolves or remains unchanged, the patient can be reassured and discharged from follow-up.
- For all other cysts, surgical removal should be offered, with bilateral oophorectomy and salpingectomy offered rather than simple cystectomy, as the risk of cancer is higher in this set of patients.
- To assess the risk of cancer, an RMI should be calculated and the patient should be referred to the onco-gynaecology multidisciplinary team for a decision on the appropriate surgical management.

COMPLICATIONS

ACUTE PAIN

Patients can present with acute abdominal or pelvic pain associated with ovarian cysts. Clinicians diagnose these events as cyst accidents. The pain can be caused by either:

- Cyst rupture or haemorrhage – both of which are self-limiting.
- Ovarian torsion – a medical emergency where urgent surgery is required to save the affected ovary.

CYST RUPTURE

An ovarian cyst can burst before it then regresses. The fluid which leaks from the cyst can irritate the peritoneum and cause pain. It is self-limiting and is treated with simple analgesia.

MID-OVULATORY PAIN (MITTELSCHMERZ)

This occurs when the dominant follicle ruptures during the menstrual cycle at the time of ovulation to release the egg. The fluid is released from the follicle in exactly the same way as a cyst rupture, irritating the peritoneum and causing pain. This again is a self-limiting pain, treated with analgesia, if required. If this is a recurrent pain every cycle and is affecting a patient's quality of life, then a contraceptive such as the combined pill can be used to inhibit ovulation, thereby preventing this pain.

HAEMORRHAGIC CYST

A simple cyst can bleed into itself, which can cause pain from increased pressure in the cyst. The cyst can also burst and then leak. The leaked blood irritates the peritoneum, causing pain. Again, this is self-limiting and usually only requires simple analgesia. If this haemorrhagic cyst has been identified on an ultrasound scan, it is important to arrange a repeat scan in 8 weeks to check for cyst resolution.

OVARIAN TORSION

The ovary can rotate upon its axis and cut off its own blood supply in exactly the same manner as testicular torsion. It can happen to any ovary but is more likely to occur when a cyst of 5 cm or larger is on the ovary. Similarly to testicular torsion, this is also a medical emergency requiring urgent surgery to correct the torsion to prevent necrosis and death of the ovary. Unfortunately, unlike testicular torsion, ovarian torsion presents with a vague presentation of acute onset of pelvic pain. The pain localises late in the clinical course, as significant oedema is required to irritate the parietal peritoneum.

When assessing a female with acute pelvic pain, it is therefore imperative to be vigilant regarding the possibility of ovarian torsion to make an early diagnosis. The patient should be assessed as for any patient with acute abdominal pain, by taking a history and examination, including a bimanual vaginal exam. Classically, the pain is sharp, more to one side of the abdomen and associated with nausea and vomiting. A patient with a previous history of an ovarian cyst, an acutely tender abdomen and tenderness in the adnexa on bimanual examination should prompt the clinician to place ovarian torsion as the top diagnosis to be excluded.

Initial investigations are the same as for any acute pelvic pain presentation, which should include FBC, CRP, U&Es, LFTs, lactate, G&S, pregnancy test and urinalysis. Vaginal swabs for pelvic infection may also be considered. Ovarian torsion causes inflammation, resulting in a raised white cell count and CRP, and raised lactate as necrosis of the ovary occurs.

If pelvic ultrasound can be quickly arranged, it may show absent blood flow through the ovary, as well as oedema. However, if there is likely to be a delay in obtaining imaging or any other investigation result, this should not delay treatment. If ovarian torsion is strongly suspected, the patient should be taken for emergency laparoscopy to untwist the ovary. The surgeon may stitch the ovary to the pelvic wall to prevent it from torsioning again. If possible, the surgeon will try not to remove the ovary, as even a necrotic appearing ovary may have some functional tissue remaining; the necrotic areas of the ovary will be reabsorbed by the body over time. Some surgeons may also stitch the unaffected ovary to the pelvic wall in an attempt to prevent future torsion in the unaffected ovary.

Unfortunately, due to delayed diagnosis and treatment, around 80% of torsioned ovaries have infarcted at the time of surgery, and the surgeon may not be able to remove the associated cyst causing the torsion without also removing the ovary. Fortunately, there is not a significant reduction in these patients' fertility rates after removal of one ovary. The recurrence risk for ovarian torsion is around 10%.

PROGNOSIS

Most ovarian cysts are benign, with no long-term adverse outcome, and many, after initial identification, do not even require follow-up. If surgical intervention is undertaken, it is unlikely that the cyst will recur. However, avoiding unnecessary surgical intervention is important, as premature ovarian failure occurs in over 2% of patients following cystectomies on both ovaries.

Ovarian cysts rarely cause significant acute pain, and acute pain is usually self-limiting. It is essential to consider the diagnosis and treat ovarian torsion quickly to prevent irretrievable damage to the ovary.

LONG-TERM PREVENTION

The COCP has been shown to prevent the development of simple cysts, and it also reduces the progression of endometriosis. It is likely that other contraceptives that cause anovulation, like the COCP, will also reduce the development of cysts and endometriosis.

? QUESTIONS

Joanne is a 30-year-old who was found to have an ovarian cyst on routine ultrasound. It was identified as a simple cyst of approximately 8 cm in diameter. No solid areas were observed, and there was no blood flow through the cyst.

Q1 Answer true or false to the following statements with regards to benign ovarian cysts.

A A benign ovarian cyst is a fluid-filled sac with a diameter of more than 5 cm, arising on, or within, an ovary.

B The gold standard investigation is a transvaginal ultrasound of the ovaries.

C A unilocular cyst with no blood flow is indicative of a benign cyst.

D CA-125, lactate dehydrogenase, alpha-fetoprotein and human chorionic gonadotropin should be measured in all patients with an ovarian cyst seen on ultrasound.

E Transvaginal aspiration of a benign ovarian cyst is a common treatment of choice.

Select the most appropriate choice of treatment for each of the cysts below. Each treatment option can be used once, more than once or not at all.

A	Antiandrogens.	G	Mirena®.
B	Chemotherapy.	H	No treatment.
C	COCP.	I	Oophorectomy.
D	Laparoscopic aspiration.	J	Total abdominal hysterectomy.
E	Laparoscopic cystectomy.	K	Transvaginal aspiration.
F	Laparotomy and cystectomy.	L	Watchful waiting.

Q2   Simple cyst less than 5 cm.

Q3   Simple cyst 5–7 cm.

Q4   Simple cyst more than 7 cm.

Q5   Dermoid cyst.

Q6   Haemorrhagic cyst, 3 cm diameter.

Q7   Answer true or false: Which of the following are complications of benign ovarian cysts?

   A Cyst rupture.

   B PCOS.

   C Cervical cancer.

   D Ovarian torsion.

   E Cyst haemorrhage.

[Answers on page 206.]

KEY REFERENCES

ENDOMETRIOSIS

European Society of Human Reproduction and Embryology, 2022. Endometriosis. European Guideline.

National Institute of Health and Care Excellence, 2013. (Updated in 2020). Neuropathic Pain in Adults: Pharmacological Management in Nonspecialist Settings. NICE Clinical Guidance (CG 173).

National Institute of Health and Care Excellence, 2017. Endometriosis: Diagnosis and Management. NICE Guideline (NG 73).

Royal College of Obstetricians and Gynaecologists, 2012. The Initial Management of Chronic Pelvic Pain. RCOG Green Top Guideline (GTG 41).

SEXUALLY TRANSMITTED INFECTIONS

British Association for Sexual Health and HIV, 2012. The Management of Bacterial Vaginosis. BASHH UK National Guideline.

British Association for Sexual Health and HIV, 2015. The Management of Anogenital Warts. BASHH UK National Guideline.

British Association for Sexual Health and HIV, 2018. The Management of Genital Tract Infection with Chlamydia Trachomatis. BASHH UK National Guideline.

British Association for Sexual Health and HIV, 2018. The Management of Gonorrhoea in Adults. BASHH UK National Guideline.

British Association for Sexual Health and HIV, 2018. The Management of Pelvic Inflammatory Disease. BASHH UK National Guideline.

British Association for Sexual Health and HIV, 2019. The Management of Vulvovaginal Candidiasis. BASHH UK National Guideline.

Gilleece, D.Y., Tariq, D.S., Bamford, D.A., Bhagani, D.S., Byrne, D.L., Clarke, D.E., et al., 2019. British HIV Association guidelines for the management of HIV in pregnancy and postpartum 2018. HIV Med 20, s2–s85.

BENIGN OVARIAN CYSTS

European Society of Human Reproduction and Embryology, 2022. Endometriosis. European Guideline.

Royal College of Obstetricians and Gynaecologists, 2011. Management of Suspected Ovarian Masses in Premenopausal Women. RCOG Green Top Guideline (GTG 62).

Royal College of Obstetricians and Gynaecologists, 2016. The Management of Ovarian Cysts in Postmenopausal Women. RCOG Green Top Guideline (GTG 34).

Onco-Gynaecology

Outline

PRINCIPLES OF GYNAECOLOGICAL CANCER MANAGEMENT

The options available for treating gynaecological cancer vary depending on the type, stage and grade of the cancer. The chosen management of each patient is individualised to optimise the care for that person. However, there are some general principles for the management of gynaecological cancer which we will discuss in this opening section.

MULTIDISCIPLINARY APPROACH TO CARE

A multidisciplinary team (MDT) should be involved in the care of all patients who are diagnosed with cancer. Gynaecologists, oncologists, pathologists and radiologists review the patient's history and investigations collectively, in order to decide what forms of treatment are appropriate to offer the patient. Specialist cancer nurses should also be involved to act as a regular point of contact for the patient and to help answer any questions that the patient and their families may have in between hospital appointments. There is good evidence that specialist nurse involvement significantly improves patient satisfaction with the overall care provided during this difficult time. In certain cases, particularly those where radical surgery has been performed, other healthcare professionals such as dieticians and physiotherapists may be involved.

The MDT will offer appropriate management options dependent on the likely stage and grade of the cancer, which will be based on available imaging and histology. The general health of the patient and their wishes will also determine management. Treatment can include surgery, radiotherapy, chemotherapy and palliative approaches.

GRADE

The grade of a cancer is how malignant the tumour appears on histology (when viewed under a microscope). If a biopsy has been taken, this can be assessed prior to surgery; otherwise, the grade can be determined from specimens removed at surgery.

- 0 – non-invasive (this is how borderline tumours are graded).
- 1 – low grade/well differentiated.
- 2 – moderate grade/moderately differentiated.
- 3 – high grade/poorly differentiated.

The lower the grade, the more the cancer resembles the normal cells of the organ of origin, whereas the higher the grade, the more abnormal the cells appear. Higher-grade cancers are likely to be faster replicating and usually hold a worse prognosis than low-grade cancers.

STAGE

Staging is an assessment of how far a cancer has spread within the body.

- Magnetic resonance imaging (MRI) is usually the most appropriate imaging modality to assess the pelvic organs. It is the first-line staging modality for endometrial, cervical, vaginal and vulval cancers. Computed tomography (CT) is used first line for ovarian cancer.
- CT is most useful at assessing the thorax and abdomen for metastatic spread.

The Fédération Internationale des Gynaecologistes et Obstetristes (FIGO) has written criteria to stage each gynaecological cancer (Table 7.1). The specific criteria for each cancer are discussed within the appropriate book subchapter.

Table 7.1   Simplified Version of the FIGO Staging Criteria

STAGE	DESCRIPTION
0	Carcinoma *in situ*
I	Cancer confined to organ of origin
II and III	Cancer dependent, criteria often include one or more of: • Local invasion of tissue adjacent to original organ • Invasion of other pelvic organs • Lymph node involvement
IV	Metastatic spread to distant parts of the body

SURGERY

Traditionally, surgery for gynaecological cancer was an open procedure, usually performed by a midline laparotomy. However, improvements in surgical equipment and techniques are allowing increasing numbers of patients to be treated laparoscopically. Laparoscopic surgery gives similar disease-free survival results with additional benefits, such as shorter hospital stays, swifter recovery, less blood loss and fewer postoperative complications. The organs for removal can be taken out through extensions in the laparoscopic port incisions, or more commonly through the vaginal vault (after the uterus has been removed). Where possible, the surgeon tries to avoid opening the organ containing the tumour while the organ is still in the body, as this can lead to tumour spread and a worse prognosis. Robot assisted laparoscopic surgery is also increasingly being used to undertake complex gynaecological cancer procedures.

At the time of surgery, the abdomen and pelvis are carefully inspected, including the diaphragm, liver, bowel and peritoneal surfaces of the pelvis. Where disease is thought to have advanced beyond the primary organ, removal of the omentum and pelvic and para-aortic lymph nodes for histological assessment is considered. This whole process is surgical staging, which corroborates staging based on previous imaging.

CURATIVE SURGERY

Where possible (low-stage disease), surgery will aim to be a curative procedure, removing the entire tumour. Depending on the stage, this may involve removal of just the single organ affected, but more commonly all of the uterus, cervix, ovaries and fallopian tubes are removed. Pelvic and para-aortic lymph nodes may also be removed, the omentum may be biopsied or removed entirely, and fluid from the pelvis sent for cytology. Recovery from this level of surgery is usually good, with few long-term sequelae.

SALVAGE SURGERY

In cases of either recurrent cancer or cancer that has spread locally within the pelvis at presentation, extensive surgery is required if the intent is curative. Salvage surgery can be performed, which typically involves pelvic exenteration (the removal of all organs from the pelvis) and subsequent reconstruction. The removal of the organs from the pelvis has significant consequences for the patient. As the patient will no longer have a rectum, she will require a colostomy or ileostomy. The removal of the bladder means that urine must also be diverted, either through a urostomy or ileal conduit. The vagina may also be removed, meaning that the woman will no longer be able to have penetrative sexual intercourse. The recovery from this type of operation is protracted, with a multitude of potential complications. The patient, her partner and family are likely to undergo significant psychological distress, so they should be counselled appropriately prior to consent for the procedure.

PALLIATIVE SURGERY

In high-stage disease, where there is metastatic spread, complete resection is rarely possible. Although not curative, palliative surgery can be offered, where as much of the tumour is removed as is safely possible (debulking procedure), with the aim of improving the quality and duration of life. Surgery may be able to improve specific problems, such as bowel obstruction, where a colostomy can be formed using bowel from above the area where cancer is causing an obstruction.

RADIOTHERAPY

Ionising radiation in high concentration causes DNA damage and cell death (Table 7.2). This is traditionally delivered with external beam radiotherapy (EBRT), where radiation is aimed into the body from various directions and meets at a single point where the cancer is situated, providing maximal energy and therefore damage to that specific area. In some cancers, such as vaginal or cervical cancer, the radiation source can be placed next to the cancer in the vagina (brachytherapy),

Table 7.2   Uses of Radiotherapy for the Treatment of Cancer

REGIMEN	DESCRIPTION
Adjuvant	Commonly used after curative surgery has been attempted, to destroy any remaining cancer in the local area of the surgery.
Neo-adjuvant	Occasionally, radiotherapy is used to shrink a cancer prior to surgical intervention.
Radical	Used when surgery is not an option, often still with a curative intent. If cure is not achieved, radiotherapy may still have reduced tumour bulk, symptoms of the cancer, and delay progression of disease.
Palliative	Used to relieve symptoms such as vaginal bleeding or bone pain from metastatic spread.

which reduces the amount of radiation exposure experienced by the rest of the body.

The dose of radiotherapy is limited by the side effects. The bowel and bladder are sensitive to radiotherapy and are invariably close to the cancer where the area of the maximum dose of radiotherapy is targeted. The oncology team has to balance the dose of radiotherapy given to maximise effect on the cancer against the long-term damage to adjacent organs. The common acute side effects of radiotherapy include nausea and vomiting, skin irritation, local swelling, diarrhoea and pain. Long-term effects include:
- Tissue fibrosis causing pain.
- Vaginal stenosis, dryness and dyspareunia. Lubricants and dilators can improve sexual function.
- Radiation colitis – diarrhoea, defecation frequency, rectal urgency, incontinence, malabsorption and weight loss.
- Bladder urgency, pain and reduced capacity.
- Lymphoedema - leg swelling due to damage of the lymphatic system preventing return of interstitial fluid from the lower limbs.

CHEMOTHERAPY

Women who are at high risk of recurrent disease following surgery may be offered adjuvant chemotherapy. In very advanced disease, where palliation is the only treatment option, chemotherapy can be used for symptomatic relief. Platinum-based treatments, such as carboplatin and paclitaxel, are commonly used for gynaecological malignancy.

PALLIATION

Securing the involvement of a palliative care team early in the process allows for proactive management of the patient's problems. Pain relief and symptom control are essential parts of management. Mental health is also important, as very high rates of depression are reported in patients with cancer, so counsellors and psychologists are also available. Similarly, many patients need support at home due to increasing disability; some may need financial or legal advice or may need to speak to a spiritual advisor. These are just a few examples where the palliative care team can provide excellent holistic patient support.

COMPLICATIONS OF CANCER

Complications of cancer typically occur during the later stages of the disease, since this is when other tissues and organ systems become involved. Complications may also occur as a result of treatment for the cancer.
Local tumour invasion:
- Pain.
- Vaginal symptoms – bleeding, discharge, malodour and sexual dysfunction.
- Bowel obstruction.
- Ureteric obstruction and renal failure.
- Bladder or bowel fistula and infections.
- Lymphoedema – caused either by metastatic spread to the lymph nodes or following surgical removal of the lymph nodes.

Systemic cancer complications:
- Cachexia, anorexia and fatigue.
- Organ failure from metastatic spread – commonly the lung and liver.
- Venous thromboembolism.
- Death.

Complications associated with cancer treatment:
- Menopause symptoms after removal of the ovaries in premenopausal women.
- Depression following diagnosis.
- Anxiety about recurrence.
- Altered body image due to scarring.
- Feeling a loss of womanhood after removal of reproductive organs.
- Altered sexual function after surgery or radiotherapy.
- Effect on work, finances, relatives, friends and social interactions.

FOLLOW-UP

Patients undergoing treatment with curative intent are followed up to assess for recurrence for 5 years. The typical follow-up regimen for cancer in the UK is outpatient review 3 to 4 times a year for the first couple of years, followed by one to two reviews a year to complete 5 years. However, there is increasing evidence that patient-initiated follow-up when they experience symptoms is as effective as planned follow-up for a number of cancers.

At follow-up, the patient is asked about symptoms which may suggest recurrence, such as:
- Pain, abdominal distension or bloating.
- Bleeding or other vaginal discharge.
- Anorexia.
- Weight loss.
- Change in bowel or urinary symptoms.

The patients usually also undergo:
- Abdominal examination for masses and lymphadenopathy.
- Speculum examination to visualise vaginal and vault recurrence.
- Pelvic examination to palpate masses.

Urgent imaging is arranged if there is suspicion of recurrence. This is commonly either a computed tomography (CT) or a positron electron tomography (PET) CT of the chest, abdomen and pelvis.

Treatment will depend on the site of recurrence, previous treatments undertaken and general health of the patient. The management may involve surgery to the local recurrence, radiotherapy, chemotherapy or palliation only. The treatment intent may be to prolong life or to improve symptoms.

Cancer in Women of Childbearing Age

If a woman who is diagnosed with a gynaecological cancer wishes to retain her fertility, this poses a complex challenge. The decision will need to be considered carefully, taking into account the cancer type, grade and stage, as well as the risk of recurrence. If the patient wishes to carry a child herself, this may mean suboptimal surgery is performed with a higher risk of recurrence to allow this. Aggressive follow-up is then required to monitor for early recurrence. If the patient would consider surrogacy, then egg collection could be undertaken prior to definitive treatment. This process can delay treatment significantly while it is completed.

It is essential to remember that both chemotherapy and radiotherapy can result in irreversible ovarian damage causing infertility, so women with non-gynaecological cancer wishing to conserve future fertility should be offered egg collection prior to these treatments.

Unfortunately, some of the women who develop cancer will be pregnant at the time of diagnosis. The most common cancers in women of childbearing age are breast cancer, cervical cancer, lymphomas and melanomas. Both the gestational age of the fetus and the stage of the cancer should be considered when choosing treatment. The woman must make the difficult decision of whether or not to continue the pregnancy as normal and have treatment after the baby has been born naturally. Her other options are a termination of pregnancy, immediate delivery if the baby is viable, or a delayed preterm birth, allowing time for the fetus to mature. Some surgeries can be considered in pregnancy and some chemotherapy regimens are considered safe for the fetus after the first trimester.

OVARIAN CANCER

Ovarian cancer is a malignancy which arises primarily from the ovaries (Fig. 7.1). The malignancy may be solid or cystic. The histological subtypes of ovarian cancer are split into the following subtypes:
- Epithelial tumours – 90% of ovarian cancer.
- Sex cord stromal tumours – 8%.
- Germ cell tumours – 2%.

AETIOLOGY

Ovarian cancer is the fifth most common cancer in females, with a lifetime risk of 2%. It is the leading cause of death from gynaecological cancer, as it often presents late. The peak incidence is in the 60–65 age group, with 90% of all ovarian cancer occurring after the age of 45. Ovarian cancer is rare below the age of 40.

RISK FACTORS

PROLONGED OESTROGEN EXPOSURE
- Increasing age.
- Obesity.
- Hormone replacement therapy.

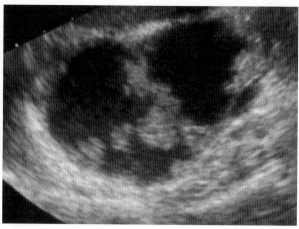
Fig. 7.1 Transvaginal of a complex ovarian mass that was later diagnosed as ovarian cancer. (Source: Meriwether, Kate V., et al. Obstetrics & Gynecology Morning Report: Beyond the Pearls. Elsevier Inc, 2019.)

PROLONGED DURATION OF OVULATION
- Early menarche.
- Late menopause.
- Nulliparity.

Pregnancy, breastfeeding and use of a hormonal contraceptive, which all stop ovulation, are therefore protective.

FAMILY HISTORY
- 10% of ovarian cancer has a genetic predisposition.
- Lynch syndrome:
  - Autosomal dominant condition with an 80% lifetime risk of colorectal cancer and 50% risk of endometrial cancer, but also causes a number of other cancers less commonly. The lifetime ovarian cancer risk is 10%. Previously, when the condition was only known to cause colorectal cancer, it was known as hereditary non-polyposis colorectal cancer (HNPCC).
  - Genetic testing is now offered to all patients diagnosed with colorectal or endometrial cancer in the UK, and if positive, family members are offered screening.
  - If a patient is found positive for a Lynch syndrome mutation, screening with colonoscopies is recommended and prophylactic surgery can be offered to remove the uterus and ovaries once the patient has completed their family.
- Breast cancer gene type 1 (BRCA1) and BRCA2
  - Originally identified in breast cancer. There is an approximately 50% lifetime chance of developing ovarian cancer with the BRCA1 mutation and a 30% chance with BRCA2.
  - Genetic testing is advised if a person has a greater than 10% chance of having the gene variant, such as having a first-degree family history of one person with ovarian cancer and either one person with breast cancer under 40 years old or two people with breast cancer under 50 years old.

- If genetic testing is positive, a patient can be offered screening (pelvic ultrasound and mammography) or prophylactic surgery (bilateral mastectomy and salpingo-oophorectomy).

PATHOLOGY

EPITHELIAL CELL TUMOURS

Epithelial cell tumours represent over 90% of all ovarian cancer. They rarely occur in women under 40 years old, so are predominantly identified in postmenopausal women.

Epithelial cells form the outer lining of the ovary. Every time an egg is released during ovulation, a follicle containing the egg has to form on the surface. The follicle then bursts to release the egg, leaving behind a hole that needs to be repaired. The repair process requires new cell growth, so the greater the number of new cells that have to form, the more likely it is that a cell may form abnormally, causing dysplasia. Therefore, factors that increase the lifetime number of ovulations increase the risk of ovarian cancer.

Recently, it has also been proposed that a significant number of epithelial cancers may originate from, or be caused by, the fallopian tubes. This is supported by evidence showing that patients who have had removal of the tubes, or even just tubal ligation, have a decreased risk of ovarian cancer.

The subtypes of epithelial tumours (Table 7.3) are usually identified on histology after surgery. They are mostly named according to their microscopic appearance. Identifying the type, grade and stage guides ongoing treatment and likely prognosis. CA-125 is the tumour marker used to aid in diagnosis of epithelial tumours in women presenting with complex ovarian cysts.

Table **7.3** Epithelial Tumour Subtypes	
COMMON EPITHELIAL TUMOUR SUBTYPES	**PERCENTAGE OF OVARIAN CANCER BY SUBTYPE**
Papillary serous cystadenocarcinoma	25%
Borderline adenocarcinoma	15%
Endometroid carcinoma	10%
Mucinous cystadenocarcinoma	5%
Clear cell carcinoma	5%

💡 Primary Peritoneal Cancer

Primary peritoneal cancer is cancer found in the peritoneum that, on histology, looks like ovarian cancer but there is no cancer found in the ovaries. Research is ongoing to determine whether this is caused by remnants of ovarian tissue in the peritoneum from the embryological translocation of the ovaries *in utero*, or whether the peritoneum may be a causative organelle in ovarian cancer. Primary peritoneal cancer is treated in the same way as ovarian cancer.

Table **7.4** The Commonest Germ Cell Tumours and Their Tumour Markers	
GERM CELL TUMOUR	**LIKELY TUMOUR MARKER**
Dysgerminoma	Lactate dehydrogenase (LDH)
Teratoma (malignant form of dermoid)	Alpha fetoprotein (AFP)
Endodermal sinus tumour	AFP, β hCG
Choriocarcinoma	β hCG

GERM CELL TUMOURS

Germ cell tumours arise from the precursor cells of gametes (oocytes). They represent 1%–2% of ovarian cancers. They are very rare in women over 40 years of age, so most affect younger women, with 5% diagnosed in prepubertal girls. They are more common in women with gonadal dysgenesis, such as Turner syndrome and androgen insensitivity syndrome.

Germ cell tumours usually make one or more of lactate dehydrogenase (LDH), AFP and β hCG (Table 7.4). These tumour markers should be checked, along with CA-125, in any women under 40 years of age with a complex ovarian cyst to rule out a germ cell tumour.

Extremely rarely, germ cell tumours can present as an endocrinological pathology. Once oocytes combine with spermatozoa to make a baby, every single cell type in the body can be made from them. Therefore, potentially, a germ cell tumour can differentiate into any bodily tissue within the tumour. Sometimes the tumours can make hormone producing endocrine tissue. The most common of these produce TSH so that, in a rare event, a new case of hyperthyroidism may be caused by a germ cell tumour.

SEX CORD (STROMAL) TUMOURS

Stromal tumours account for around 8% of ovarian carcinoma. They are more common in postmenopausal women but are also present in adolescence. They are derived from cells involved in hormone production, primarily theca cells and granulosa cells, which form part of the developing ovarian follicles during the menstrual cycle. They are frequently hormone secreting tumours. The most common are:

- Granulosa (Sertoli) cell tumours – secrete oestrogen and inhibin.
- Theca (Leydig) cell tumours – secrete androgens.
- Gynandroblastoma, Sertoli-Leydig cell tumours – mixed cell types, may secrete both oestrogen and androgens.

Sex cord tumours can present with clinical features secondary to excess hormone production:
- Excess unregulated oestrogens – vaginal bleeding or other menstrual irregularity.
- Excess androgens – hirsutism or virilisation.

SIGNS AND SYMPTOMS

Early-stage ovarian cancer is often asymptomatic. It is frequently only when spread has occurred that symptoms arise, often meaning poor prognosis. Symptoms of ovarian cancer are vague and can easily be attributed to other conditions, with the most common misdiagnosis being irritable bowel syndrome (IBS). Unfortunately, no screening tests are available for ovarian cancer, so clinical vigilance is essential.

- Symptoms caused by local invasion or tense ascites:
  - Abdominal discomfort or pain.
  - Abdominal bloating.
  - Change in bowel habit.
- Non-specific systemic cancer symptoms:
  - Nausea.
  - Early satiety, decreased appetite.
  - Lethargy.
  - Weight loss – significant ascites can also cause unexplained weight gain.
  - Symptoms of metastasis – examples include bone pain, breathlessness and jaundice.

Ascites

There are multiple pathologies that combine to cause ascites in ovarian cancer:
- Exudate ascites (high protein content).
  - Anorexia and a raised metabolism – cause hypoalbuminaemia, resulting in reduced oncotic pressure.
  - Peritoneal metastasis causes local inflammation, increasing vascular permeability.
  - Cancers produce vascular endothelial growth factor (VEGF), which increases vascular permeability.
- Transudate ascites (low protein content).
  - Liver metastasis can cause liver failure, resulting in transudative ascites due to the raised intravascular pressure of portal hypertension.

If a woman presents with any of the above nonspecific symptoms, especially women over 50 years old, or in any woman where symptoms occur more than 12 times a month, a CA-125 should be requested. If this is abnormal (more than 35 IU/mL), an ultrasound scan should be requested. If this is also abnormal, the patient should be referred urgently to secondary care.

Examination should look for ascites, pelvic mass and cachexia. If examination findings suggest ovarian pathology, urgent secondary care referral is required and CA-125 and an ultrasound scan should be requested.

INVESTIGATIONS

- CA-125.
  - Elevated in 80% of ovarian cancers, but less than 50% in stage one disease.
  - Elevated following any cause of peritoneal irritation, so it is frequently elevated, particularly in premenopausal women, for non-malignant causes. Examples include menstruation, endometriosis and pelvic infection. It can also be elevated in other malignancies.
  - In women under 40 years of age, tumour markers for germ cell tumours (AFP, β hCG and LDH) must also be checked.
- Pelvic ultrasound scan – identifies ovarian cysts and masses and characterises their morphology.

The findings on ultrasound scan and the CA-125 level are then used to calculate the likelihood of the cyst being cancerous, and to decide where best to manage a patient. This is done using the risk of malignancy index (RMI).

Calculating the Risk of Malignancy Index

RMI = ultrasound score × menopause score × CA-125 level.
- Menopause score = 1 for premenopausal, 3 for postmenopausal.
  - Postmenopause for RMI is defined as: no periods for 1 year, or over 50 years of age and undergone a hysterectomy.
- Ultrasound score = 0 for no features on ultrasound, 1 for one feature and 3 for two or more features.
  - Ultrasound features: multi-locular cyst, solid areas, bilateral lesions, ascites and metastasis.
- CT thorax, abdomen, pelvis – when the RMI index suggests cancer is likely, a staging CT is obtained to identify local and metastatic spread (Table 7.5).

Table 7.5	How the Risk of Malignancy Index Is Used in Clinical Practice	
RISK OF MALIGNANCY INDEX	**RISK OF CANCER**	**PLACE OF TREATMENT**
Less than 25	Low (less than 3%)	General gynaecologist
25–200	Medium (20%)	Gynaecological oncologist
More than 200	High (75%)	Specialist oncology centre

DIFFERENTIAL DIAGNOSIS

- Benign ovarian cysts – likely benign cysts may be managed conservatively, with ultrasound and CA-125 monitoring.

[See 'Benign Ovarian Cysts' page 133.]

- Other malignancies.
  - CA-125 can be elevated with any peritoneal irritation, so local spread from bowel cancer or metastatic spread to the pelvis from another cancer may cause an elevation.
  - The primary cancer can be difficult to distinguish with advanced disease, as many organs are involved, and certain cancers (such as breast and lymphoma) have metastatic spread to the ovaries.

- Further tumour markers, for example, CEA (bowel) and CA 19-9 (pancreas), can aid diagnosis.
- An ascitic tap (cytology) or tumour biopsy (histology) may confirm cancer origin.
- An MDT discussion between gynaecology, general surgeons, radiology and oncology may be needed to decide on the best management plan.

COMPLICATIONS

Most complications are discussed in the introduction to the management of gynaecological cancer section. A common specific complication of ovarian cancer is ascites. The accumulation of large volumes of this extravascular fluid can cause:

- Abdominal pressure or pain.
- Compressive renal failure.
- Pleural effusion.

Draining the ascites can provide significant symptom relief.

MANAGEMENT

General management, including the MDT, grade, stage and treatment, is covered in the Management of Cancer section.

[See 'Principles of Gynaecological Cancer Management' page 139.]

STAGING AND GRADING OF OVARIAN CANCER

FIGO have produced an international staging regimen for ovarian cancer (Table 7.6).

Unlike in cervical, vulval and endometrial cancer, where a biopsy is easily obtainable, it is rare to biopsy a suspected ovarian cancer which appears confined to the ovary prior to surgery as the act of taking the biopsy can cause disease spread. Therefore, tumour grading is not possible until after surgery, when the removed tumour is sent for histology.

Table 7.6	FIGO Staging Classification for Ovarian Cancer
STAGE	**DESCRIPTION**
I	Cancer confined to the ovaries: • IA – confined within one ovary. • IB – confined within both ovaries. • IC – cyst rupture before or during surgery or malignant cells identified on peritoneal washings.
II	Cancer has spread from the ovary into the pelvis or uterus.
III	Cancer has spread to the peritoneum, surface of the bowel and local lymph nodes.
IV	Cancer has spread to other parts of the body, such as the liver, spleen or lungs.

SURGERY

When attempting curative surgery (low-stage disease), the operation required is a laparotomy, total hysterectomy and bilateral salpingo-oophorectomy (uterus, both ovaries and fallopian tubes). Also at surgery, pelvic fluid will be sent for cytology (to look for disease spread beyond the ovary), and part or all of the omentum is removed. Where possible, the surgeon tries not to burst the ovarian cyst, as the fluid leaking out may contain cancerous cells which can then spread into the pelvic cavity, resulting in an increase in the stage of the disease and a worse prognosis.

Where there is higher-stage disease the operation may also include additional procedures depending on how advanced the cancer is and whether the patient is physically well enough for extensive surgery. Where optimal clearance of the cancer is intended, a full staging laparotomy is performed to fully examine the abdominal and pelvic cavities, removing all visible cancer. In addition to the standard operation this could also involve removal of all pelvic organs (exenteration), excision of pelvic or para-aortic lymph nodes and removal of parts of the liver or other abdominal organs if cancer has spread to them.

A patient who has advanced disease but is not suitable for extensive surgery may be offered debulking surgery, where the same surgery is done as for low-risk disease, plus removal of any other visible tumour which can be removed safely without damaging other organs. The aim of this surgery is to improve the effects of adjuvant treatments to prolong life, and reduce the chance of complications such as bowel obstruction.

CHEMOTHERAPY

Final staging and grading is confirmed after surgery. If the grade is 2 or below and the stage is 1B or below, the procedure is regarded as curative and adjuvant chemotherapy is not required. Unfortunately, as the cancer usually presents in the later stages, adjuvant chemotherapy is often required:

- First line – six cycles of a platinum-based compound, such as cisplatin or carboplatin.
- Second line – platinum-based compound and paclitaxel.

In patients where surgery is not possible, chemotherapy can be used alone for symptomatic relief and prolong life. Most MDTs advise obtaining a tissue biopsy, percutaneously under ultrasound guidance, to confirm the diagnosis before commencing chemotherapy.

Occasionally chemotherapy is offered prior to surgery (neo-adjuvant chemotherapy) for higher stage 3 cancer to reduce the amount of disease, to improve the success of the subsequent operation. Again a biopsy would be obtained before commencing chemotherapy to confirm the diagnosis and then choose the optimal chemotherapy agents.

Table 7.7	Five-Year Relative Survival Rates for Ovarian Cancer
STAGE	**FIVE-YEAR SURVIVAL**
Stage 1 and 2	80%–100%
Stage 3	15%–20%
Stage 4	5%

RADIOTHERAPY

EBRT is most effective when used on a single site. It is rarely used for ovarian cancer because the cancer has usually spread to multiple sites meaning high doses are required, and due to the proximity of the bowel, the side effects outweigh the benefits.

PROGNOSIS

Unfortunately, most postmenopausal women with ovarian cancer present when the disease is at an advanced stage, so 5-year survival rates are low. However, most germ cell and stromal cell tumours that present in women less than 40 have a 5-year survival rate of around 90% (Table 7.7).

FOLLOW-UP

After primary treatment is completed, patients treated are reviewed regularly for 5 years to assess for recurrent disease; an example regimen is every 4 months for 2 years, then every 6 months for 3 years. For ovarian germ cell or sex cord stromal tumours, follow-up may include monitoring of a tumour marker, if one of the markers was raised before treatment.

 Ovarian Cancer in Women of Childbearing Age

To maintain fertility in a young woman with ovarian cancer, a unilateral salpingo-oophorectomy may be considered, keeping one ovary for future conception. However, this decision will need to be considered carefully, taking into account the cancer type, grade, stage, recurrence risk and risk of there being concurrent disease in the remaining ovary. Egg collection, with a view to future IVF with a surrogate, may also be a possibility; however, the collection process may increase the stage of the cancer and delay treatment.

❓ QUESTIONS

Joan, a 60-year-old, presents to their primary care physician with abdominal bloating, lethargy and 'not feeling quite right'. On further questioning, they have unintentionally lost two stone in the last 3 months. Joan has a history of infertility and never managed to become pregnant. They went through menopause at age 56. They have a past medical history of IBS and hypertension. Joan is a non-smoker and occasionally drinks alcohol.

Q1   Answer true or false: Which of the following are risk factors for ovarian cancer?
A Early menopause.
B Infertility.
C Irritable bowel syndrome (IBS).
D Multiparity.
E Use of hormone replacement therapy (HRT).

Q2   Using the history above, which of the following would be the most appropriate course of action?
A Dismiss the symptoms, they are too vague.
B Organise a CA-125 test.
C Organise an urgent CT scan.
D Review the patient in 2 weeks to assess if the symptoms improve.
E Send the patient to the emergency department (ED).

Q3   What is the most common type of ovarian cancer?
A Choriocarcinoma.
B Embryonal carcinoma.
C Epithelial tumour.
D Immature malignant teratoma.
E Stromal tumour.

Q4   What is the optimal first-line treatment option for stage 1 ovarian cancer?
A Chemotherapy and radiotherapy.
B Platinum-based chemotherapy.
C Radiotherapy.
D Total abdominal hysterectomy and bilateral salpingo-oophorectomy.
E Unilateral salpingo-oophorectomy.

[Answers on page 207.]

ENDOMETRIAL CANCER

Endometrial cancer develops from the endometrium, which is the internal lining of the uterus (Fig. 7.2). Endometrial cancer is the most common gynaecological malignancy in the developed world and the fourth most common cancer in the female population in the UK, after breast, lung and colorectal cancer. Survival rates are better than for most other cancers, as women usually develop postmenopausal bleeding (PMB) early in the disease process, leading to early diagnosis and treatment.

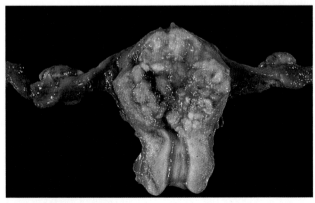

Fig. 7.2 Endometrial cancer. (Source: From Damjanov, I., & Linder, J. [Eds.]. Anderson's pathology [10th ed.]. Mosby, 1996.)

RISK FACTORS

- Age – 90% of endometrial cancer is diagnosed in postmenopausal women, with a mean age of diagnosis of 60 years old. It is extremely rare in women under 40 years of age.
- Unopposed oestrogen – in the normal menstrual cycle, proliferation of the endometrium is caused by oestrogen. Later in the menstrual cycle, progesterone influences the growth of the endometrium so that it becomes secretory, stopping the proliferation. The key cause of endometrial cancer is oestrogen exposure throughout life, specifically unopposed oestrogen (oestrogen not opposed by progesterone) (Table 7.8).

SYMPTOMS AND SIGNS

- The most common symptom of endometrial cancer is PMB. 10% of patients with PMB have endometrial cancer.
- In the perimenopausal patient, the most common symptom is recurrent intermenstrual bleeding, or heavy menstrual bleeding.
- As with other cancers, the symptoms and signs of local spread, metastasis and systemic symptoms may also be present in advanced disease.
- A good history, followed by an examination that includes the abdomen and genital tract, will help to identify other causes of bleeding.

DIFFERENTIAL DIAGNOSIS

Endometrial causes:
- Cancer.
- Hyperplasia.
- Polyps.
- Dysfunctional uterine bleeding.

Cervical causes:
- Cancer.
- Ectropion.
- Polyps.

Vaginal causes:
- Atrophic vaginitis.
- Sexually transmitted infection.

Non-gynaecological bleeding:
- Rectal bleeding.
- Haematuria.

Atrophic vaginitis is the most common cause for PMB. This can be easily treated with local oestrogen therapy. Dysfunctional uterine bleeding is the most common cause of perimenopausal bleeding, which again can be easily treated. However, it is essential to investigate to rule out the serious pathology first.

INVESTIGATIONS

Any woman reporting PMB should be urgently referred to a gynaecologist for investigation. The initial investigation arranged is a pelvic ultrasound scan, which may then be followed by an endometrial biopsy.

Perimenopausal women with either persistent intermenstrual bleeding, or women over 45 years old with heavy menstrual bleeding, should also be referred urgently for both a scan and biopsy. Younger women with heavy menstrual bleeding that is not controlled by medical treatment may also be investigated for endometrial pathology, although the risk is very low below the age of 45.

Table 7.8	Risk Factors Associated With Endometrial Cancer
RISK	**DETAILS**
Age	75% cases occur between ages of 40–75, 25% cases occur over age 75.
Obesity	Fat tissue metabolises androgens to oestrogens. Increased levels of oestrogen increase the risk of endometrial cancer. A BMI of 30 kg/m² doubles the risk, whereas a BMI of 40 kg/m² increases the risk sevenfold.
Menopause	A late menopause demonstrates prolonged exposure to normal oestrogens from the menstrual cycle. Late menopause or early menarche both double the risk.
Hormonal medication	HRT utilising oestrogen combined with progesterone doubles the risk of endometrial cancer after 5 years of use. If oestrogen-only HRT has been given incorrectly to a patient with a uterus, there is a sixfold increased risk. This risk is similar for women being treated following breast cancer with tamoxifen, a selective oestrogen receptor modulator which promotes endometrial proliferation.
Nulliparity	Not having children doubles the lifetime risk of endometrial cancer compared to a multiparous woman. Pregnancy stops the menstrual cycle, so it reduces oestrogen exposure and endometrial proliferation for the duration of the pregnancy. Similarly, contraceptives that cause anovulation, such as the combined oral contraceptive, reduce oestrogen-related endometrial proliferation and are also protective against endometrial cancer.
Genetics	Lynch syndrome is an autosomal dominant genetic mutation associated with a 50% lifetime risk of endometrial cancer.
Others	Polycystic ovarian syndrome
	Oestrogen producing tumours, such as an ovarian granulosa cell tumour
	Hypertension
	Diabetes mellitus
	Previous pelvic radiation
	History of breast cancer

TRANSVAGINAL ULTRASOUND

Transvaginal ultrasound (TVUS) is used to view the uterus and endometrium. Fibroids and polyps can be seen, allowing arrangements to be made for their surgical removal. The endometrial thickness can also be measured on TVUS. Postmenopausal women should have very little oestrogen, meaning growth of the endometrium should be minimal. When measuring the endometrium, the sonographer measures the thickness of the endometrium on both sides of the endometrial cavity. These are added together to give the double layer thickness. If the measurement of the double layer endometrial thickness is 4 mm or more, a biopsy must be arranged. If the thickness is less than 4 mm, this is considered normal and no further investigation is required at this time, as the risk of endometrial cancer is low (less than 1%). However, if recurrent PMB occurs, most gynaecologists then obtain a biopsy, regardless of the scan findings.

If a patient is on HRT, this can cause a degree of benign endometrial proliferation, so 8 mm is used as the cut off in these patients. Similarly, in perimenopausal patients, a thickened endometrium is expected during the normal menstrual cycle, so the measurement is usually unhelpful.

ENDOMETRIAL BIOPSY

Biopsies can be performed in an outpatient clinic. A speculum is used to visualise the cervix, and then a sampler is passed through the cervix and into the cavity. Moving the sampler backwards and forwards and rotating it within the cavity scrapes off a small amount of the endometrium, which can then be sent for review by histopathology.

In some cases, the cervix can be stenosed or the patient can find the examination too uncomfortable, so obtaining a biopsy is not possible. In addition, over 5% of the biopsies are reported as inadequate by the pathologists. In all these cases, the next step would be to undertake a hysteroscopy.

A hysteroscopy can be performed under local or general anaesthetic. A small camera is passed through the cervix, allowing direct visualisation of the endometrial cavity. Biopsies can be taken, and if identified, other abnormalities like polyps or submucosal fibroids can be resected.

PATHOLOGY

The histology result from the biopsy will determine the most appropriate management of the patient (Table 7.9).

ENDOMETRIAL HYPERPLASIA

Endometrial hyperplasia is a pre-malignant growth of the endometrium. It is characterised by a greater gland to stroma ratio than is observed in normal endometrial tissue. If cytological atypia is present, this means the individual cells also look abnormal; for example, they show an increased nuclear to cytoplasm ratio.

Table 7.9 Management of Endometrial Biopsy Results	
BIOPSY RESULT	**MANAGEMENT**
Insufficient sample	Repeat biopsy or perform hysteroscopy to obtain sample
Normal sample	Discharge and treat any benign cause for symptoms
Hyperplasia without atypia	Progestogen and repeat biopsy in 6 months
Atypical hyperplasia	Hysterectomy and bilateral salpingo-oophorectomy
Endometrial carcinoma	Further assessment

Hyperplasia without atypia has less than a 5% 20-year risk of developing into endometrial carcinoma. However, treatment with progestogens, either as oral tablets or preferably by inserting a levonorgestrel intrauterine system (Mirena), can reverse this endometrial hyperplasia in the vast majority of patients. Current practice advises repeating an endometrial biopsy after 6 months and 1 year after treatment, by which time the changes should have resolved. If the hyperplasia has not resolved or has progressed, then a hysterectomy is usually recommended.

Hyperplasia with atypia (atypical hyperplasia) has around a 30% 20-year risk of developing into endometrial cancer. It responds less well to progestogen therapy, so hysterectomy is usually the first-line treatment. However, in patients who are not medically fit for surgery or who decline it, progestogen therapy remains an option. It should also be noted that a significant number (up to 40%) of cases that are classified as atypical hyperplasia who elect for a hysterectomy are found to have concurrent endometrial carcinoma on the histology after surgery, demonstrating the limitations of biopsy.

ENDOMETRIAL CARCINOMA

On histology, endometrial cancer can be divided into two subtypes (Table 7.10). Type 1 is by far the most

Table 7.10 Endometrial Cancer Types and Characteristics	
TYPE 1	**TYPE 2**
Ninety percent of endometrial cancer	Ten percent of endometrial cancer
Endometrioid adenocarcinoma	Uterine (papillary) serous or clear cell carcinoma
Affects perimenopausal or early postmenopausal women	Affects elderly women
Low grade	High grade
Oestrogen dependent	Non-oestrogen dependent
Good prognosis more likely	Poor prognosis (40% of deaths)

common and has the best prognosis. Type 2 causes 10% of cases but accounts for 40% of deaths from endometrial cancer.

MANAGEMENT

General management, including the MDT, grade, stage and treatment, is covered in the Management of Cancer section.

[See 'Principles of Gynaecological Cancer Management' page 139.]

STAGING AND GRADING

- MRI is the best modality for detecting local invasion into the myometrium, cervix or beyond, and for detecting local lymphadenopathy (Table 7.11).
- CT is the best modality for detecting disease spread outside of the pelvis.

Tumour grading will have been assessed by the histology team using the biopsy taken. Grading can be confirmed on the specimens removed at the time of surgery.

SURGERY

The recommended primary treatment for stage 1A endometrial cancer is a total hysterectomy (uterus and cervix) and bilateral salpingo-oophorectomy (BSO) (Table 7.12). For stage II disease, a radical hysterectomy is required, where the uterus, cervix, upper vagina and parametrium are removed. In addition, a BSO, systematic pelvic lymphadenectomy and, if required, para-aortic lymphadenectomy and omentectomy will be performed. Lymphadenectomy is essential to guide surgical staging and adjuvant therapy in stage II disease. Lymphadenectomy is also sometimes considered in stage I disease, depending on the grade.

Table 7.11 FIGO Staging Classification for Endometrial Cancer

STAGE	DESCRIPTION
I	Tumour confined to corpus of the uterus • IA – less than 50% of the myometrium invaded • IB – more than 50% of the myometrium invaded
II	Tumour invades cervical stroma but does not extend beyond uterus
III	Local and/or regional spread of the tumour • III A – uterine serosa invaded • III B – vagina or parametrial invasion • III C – pelvic or para-aortic lymph nodes involved
IV	Cancer is widespread: • IVA – tumour involves adjacent organs such as bowel or bladder • IVB – distant metastases or inguinal lymph node involvement

Table 7.12 Surgical Options for Endometrial Cancer

STAGE		SURGICAL OPTION
Stage I	IA grade 1 or IA grade 2	Hysterectomy with BSO
	IA grade 3 or IB	Hysterectomy with BSO ± bilateral pelvic/para-aortic lymphadenectomy
Stage II		Hysterectomy with BSO + bilateral pelvic/para-aortic lymphadenectomy
Stage III		Maximal surgical cytoreduction with a good performance status
Stage IV	IVA	Pelvic exenteration (complete pelvic clearance)
	IVB	Palliative surgery

Table 7.13 Adjuvant Radiotherapy Treatment for Endometrial Cancer

ADJUVANT TREATMENT OPTIONS IN ENDOMETRIAL CANCER	
Stage IA, IB, grade 1 and 2, POLE genetic mutations	No further treatment
Stage I grade 3, stage II, p53 genetic mutation	Vaginal vault brachytherapy
Stage III and beyond	EBRT + vaginal vault brachytherapy

In advanced stage disease, more invasive surgical procedures are considered, which may improve the survival chances of the patient, but they have an increased risk of causing significant morbidity.

RADIOTHERAPY

Radiotherapy may be used as an adjuvant therapy (after surgery) for advanced disease (Table 7.13). It can also be used as primary treatment when surgery is not possible, and can also provide palliation. Both EBRT and brachytherapy can be used. The decision on whether to give radiotherapy, which radiotherapy regime to use or whether to use both after surgery is dependent on the grade, staging, and any genetic mutations identified on histological and genetic analysis of the tissue removed at surgery. Endometrial cancer with a POLE gene mutation is less likely to recur so adjuvant therapy is not required, whereas p53 mutations increase the risk or recurrence so adjuvant treatment is offered.

CHEMOTHERAPY

Chemotherapy is increasingly used as an adjuvant for high-risk (stages III and IV) disease and has a palliative role for metastatic or recurrent disease. Carboplatin, doxorubicin and paclitaxel are commonly used.

COMPLICATIONS

Most of the complications are discussed in the introduction to the management of gynaecological cancer section. A common specific complication of endometrial cancer is heavy vaginal bleeding, as the cancer sheds from the endometrium. Surgical removal of the uterus will prevent or stop this complication, so surgery may be considered for this reason even in advanced disease.

PROGNOSIS

In general, prognosis depends on the age and health of the patient, in addition to the histological grade and stage of the tumour. The overall survival is affected by the stage at diagnosis.

Five-year survival rates for endometrial cancer:
- Stage I – 85%.
- Stage II – 75%.
- Stage III – 45%.
- Stage IV – 25%.

FOLLOW-UP

Cure is possible, and the overall 5-year survival rate for all stages of endometrial cancer is 80% (as most cases are diagnosed at an early stage). Patients are reviewed regularly for 5 years; a common regimen for patients treated with curative intent is outpatient review every 4 months for 2 years, then every 6 months for 3 years to assess for recurrence.

Endometrial Cancer in Women of Childbearing Age

In these women, surgery would be the advised treatment, with the option of egg collection to allow the possibility of future surrogacy. However, if a woman decides, after careful counselling, to preserve her fertility, she may be treated with progestogens (like the treatment for endometrial hyperplasia). Aggressive monitoring, including hysteroscopy with endometrial sampling every 3 months, is suggested, with surgery being undertaken once childbearing is completed.

QUESTIONS

Mrs Green, a 53-year-old, is referred to the gynaecology clinic with an episode of vaginal bleeding. They had a normal smear 4 years ago. They are postmenopausal and their last period was 2 years ago. Mrs Green has no children and menarche started at age 11. They are a non-smoker and have a BMI of 36 kg/m². Her mother died of bowel cancer and her maternal aunt had endometrial cancer.

Q1   Answer true or false: Which of the following are risk factors for endometrial cancer?
  A Early menopause.
  B Multiparity.
  C Nulliparity.
  D Raised BMI.
  E Smoking.

Q2   Which one of the following options would not be of use to the clinician assessing this patient?
  A Cervical examination.
  B Cervical smear.
  C Hysteroscopy.
  D Pipelle biopsy.
  E Transvaginal ultrasound.

Q3   Answer true or false, considering each of the following statements regarding postmenopausal bleeding (PMB).
  A Endometrial thickness on TVUS of less than 10 mm is considered benign.
  B Approximately 30% of patients presenting with PMB have endometrial cancer.
  C Reinvestigation of recurrent PMB should be considered after 6 months.
  D PMB is defined as an episode of bleeding 6 months or more after the last period.
  E The 5-year survival rate for a patient diagnosed with endometrial cancer after presenting with PMB is 20%.

[Answers on page 209.]

CERVICAL SCREENING

The aim of the cervical screening programme is to detect pre-cancerous changes of the cervix, so that treatment can then be offered to remove or destroy these abnormal areas, preventing the patient from developing cervical cancer in the future. Women should be aware that screening is not designed as a test for cancer. However, some cases of cancer are detected on rare occasions following investigations for an abnormal smear. Cervical screening prevents the development of 75% of cervical cancers.

To undertake cervical screening a brush is used to remove a sample of cells from the cervix. The brush simply rubs the cervix, causing epithelial cells to fall off onto the brush. The brush is then kept in a vial of preservative fluid until the sample is ready to be analysed. The sample is then tested for the presence of the high-risk subtypes of human papillomavirus (HPV). This is called primary HPV screening. The main cause of cervical cancer is persistent infection with HPV.

Samples taken that are negative for HPV are considered low risk. When the primary screening for HPV tests positive the cervical sample is then processed for cytological examination (review of the individual cervical cells using a microscope). Depending on the result of this, further assessment and treatment may be necessary (Fig. 7.3).

The location that the cells for cytological analysis come from is very important, which is why the screening sample must be taken using a speculum to ensure good visualisation of the cervix. The cells should be taken from the transformation zone, which is where the columnar epithelium of the cervical canal undergoes metaplasia to become squamous epithelium on the visible surface of the cervix. Since the cells are already undergoing metaplasia in this area, they are at the highest risk of developing into cancerous cells.

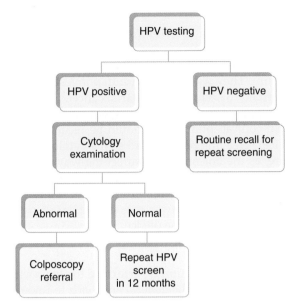

Fig. 7.3 Flow chart of the NHS Cervical Screening Programme (NHSCSP) Using Human Papillomavirus (HPV) as a Primary Test.

PATHOPHYSIOLOGY

Persistent HPV infection is the single biggest risk factor for developing cervical cancer, with HPV present in over 99% of cases. It is this virus which can act on cells within the transformation zone and can cause them to develop abnormally at an increased rate. The normal physiological metaplasia is altered and becomes dysplasia, which initially is precancerous but can progress to become cancer. It is very unlikely that a patient who has never been exposed to HPV will develop cervical cancer. Therefore current screening programme involves testing for presence of HPV on smear samples first, and only if present further cytology examination is carried out. HPV is discussed in more detail on page 156.

[See 'Cervical Cancer' page 156.]

The key concepts to understand with regards to cervical screening and cervical cancer are the transformation zone (TZ) and the squamous columnar junction (SCJ). The diagram in Fig. 7.4 represents the view of a cervix as it may be seen on speculum examination at different times in an individual's life. The middle circle represents the cervical os which is the opening of the cervical canal. The red line represents the squamocolumnar junction. The transformation zone is the area which has undergone metaplastic change from columnar epithelium to squamous epithelium. The SCJ may be the border of the transformation zone, but often it is not. Using the figure below:

A This is the cervix in childhood. The columnar epithelium is within the cervical canal and the squamous epithelium is on the ectocervix. The SCJ cannot be seen, as it most likely lies just inside the cervical canal. There is unlikely to be any significant metaplasia occurring at this time.

B This is the cervix of a person in their late teenage years. High levels of oestrogen shortly after puberty cause the cervix to evert slightly, exposing the columnar epithelium to the acidic vagina. The presence of columnar epithelium on the ectocervix like this is called an ectropion. The columnar epithelia are delicate and are likely to bleed on contact. Therefore, cervical ectropion is a common cause of postcoital bleeding in women in their teens and twenties. Over time, the columnar cells undergo metaplasia to form squamous epithelium, so they are then able to cope with trauma and the acidic conditions of the vagina.

C This is a cervix of a person in her late twenties. Oestrogen levels are now lower than when she was a teenager, and metaplasia has occurred, so the SCJ is now closer to the os than before. The thin black line on this diagram would not be seen on the cervix, but represents where the SCJ was when the woman was younger, as in picture B. The area between the imaginary black line and the area inside the cervical os where the SCJ started in picture A is the transformation zone. This is the whole area that has undergone metaplasia and so is susceptible to neoplastic changes.

D The same person has now become pregnant. The high oestrogen levels have caused further progression of the columnar epithelium, moving the SCJ outwards in a similar way to the teenager in picture B. Women taking the combined oral contraceptive pill are also at risk of developing an ectropion as a result of the exogenous oestrogen present in these pills.

E This same person is now 50 years old and is perimenopausal. The SCJ has retreated right back to the edge of the cervical os. However, in many patients, it may be within the cervical canal. There is no imaginary black line this time, but the TZ is the area that was covered by ectropion in picture D, to where the SCJ was in picture A.

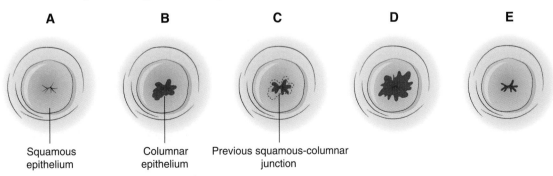

Fig. 7.4 The Cervix at Different Stages in a Woman's Life.

The squamous columnar junction is where the junction between the two epithelial types is at the present time. The transformation zone is the area between the furthest points that the SCJ has ever been. This is the area which has undergone metaplasia and is susceptible to neoplasia, particularly in the presence of HPV. In cervical screening, it is essential to sample the entire TZ, so the collection brush is shaped so that some bristles enter the canal, and other bristles are wide enough to sample the outermost areas.

CERVICAL SCREENING PROGRAMME

Cervical screening is offered to all women in England from the age of 25, initially being invited for screening every 3 years until they reach age 49 and then every 5 years thereafter until they reach age 65. The screening is most often performed by trained nurses in general practices. Unscheduled screening is not recommended in any circumstance, even if the clinician suspects cervical cancer. If this is the case, then the patient should be referred urgently to gynaecology to prevent any delay in treatment.

TAKING A CERVICAL SMEAR

Prior to commencing the examination, explain what you are going to do, and reassure the woman that a smear test should not be painful. The patient should understand that you are performing a screening test for pre-cancerous cells, and that she will receive written results. She should be aware of the next step if the result is abnormal.

The patient should be asked if she is currently menstruating. If she is, the smear should be deferred until menstruation has ceased; this is because menstrual tissue can reduce the sensitivity of the smear. Also, if endometrial cells are seen on a smear, the cytology department might presume that the smear was not taken during menstruation and then conclude that these cells are being abnormally shed from the endometrium. They will then advise that investigations be performed to exclude endometrial cancer.

The patient should be asked about any current hormonal contraception. This should be recorded on the cervical screening request card so the cytology team is aware, as the hormones can affect the way the results are interpreted. There is no problem taking a cervical smear with threads in view from an intrauterine contraceptive device; however, care should be taken not to accidentally pull out the device.

EXAMINATION

A speculum examination is performed to obtain a good view of the cervix. The general approach to undertaking a speculum examination is discussed on page 2.

[See 'Introduction to Gynaecology' page 1.]

Additions to this approach when taking a cervical smear are:

1 Prepare the trolley – appropriate-size speculum, liquid-based cytology kit, lubricating jelly, swabs, tissues and non-latex gloves.
2 Use only a small amount of lubricant on either side of the speculum near to, but not on, the tip. Lubricant affects the smear result so it should not touch the area where the sample will be taken from.
3 Once the speculum is inserted, open it and obtain a good view of the cervix. Note the appearance of the cervix and identify the transformation zone.
4 For liquid-based cytology, insert the broom tip into the external os and turn the broom 360 degrees clockwise five times (Fig. 7.5).

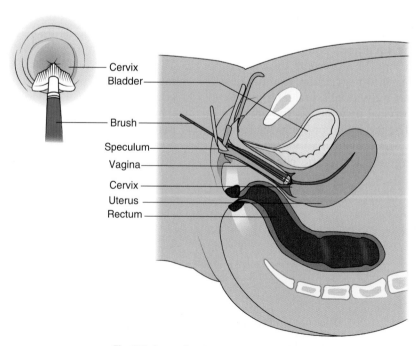

Fig. 7.5 Smear Brush Approaching Cervix.

5 Withdraw the broom and stamp it vigorously in the collecting vial 10 times.

6 Note any contact bleeding on the cervix. Gently remove the speculum.

Once the examination is completed, cover the patient and allow her to get dressed. Complete the request card and label the screening collecting vial, double checking the patient's details with the patient. The patient should be aware that she may have very light vaginal bleeding for a couple of days following the smear, which is entirely normal. Prior to leaving, the patient should be reminded about how she will be informed of the result and any further management required.

SMEAR RESULTS AND DYSKARYOSIS

Patients whose smear test is positive for HPV will have cytological examination of the smear sample. The smear taken will be looked at under the microscope; what can be seen is a collection of individual cells. These cells are observed to look for changes from the normal. The cell nuclei are the main area of focus, looking for hyperchromatism, irregularity, enlargement or an increase in number. The smears are then reported as normal, low-grade dyskaryosis (also referred to as borderline or mild) or high-grade dyskaryosis (also referred to as moderate or severe). This result determines the ongoing management (Fig. 7.6). Around 5% of smears reveal an abnormal cytology result requiring further management.

If women have had a positive colposcopy result, then they are likely to go on to have more regular future smear tests.

INADEQUATE SMEAR

Two percent of smears are reported as inadequate. This usually means insufficient cells from the cervix were obtained. It could also be that the sample was contaminated with blood or mucus or that the wrong cell type was sampled.

If a patient has an inadequate smear, then they should be asked to return for a repeat smear test. This should not be repeated in less than 3 months from the previous test. This is to allow the epithelial covering of

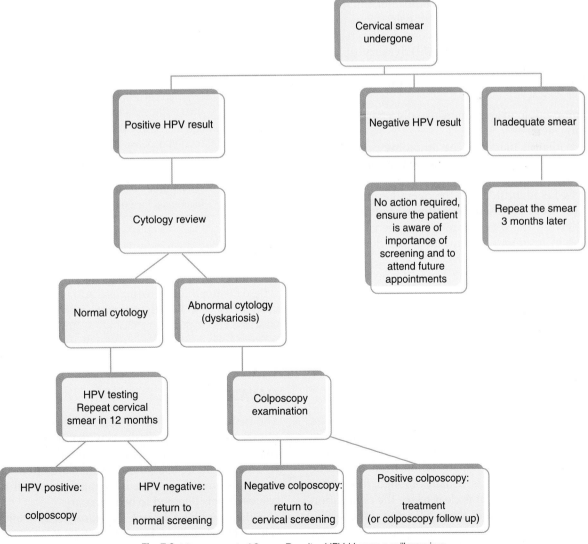

Fig. 7.6 Management of Smear Results. *HPV,* Human papillomavirus.

the cervix to re-grow, as studies have found that if the second smear is performed too soon then some abnormalities are at increased risk of being missed.

Patients who have two consecutive HPV tests unavailable or inadequate cytology results are referred to colposcopy.

DYSKARYOSIS

Patients with smear screening results positive for HPV and cytology reported as borderline or mild dyskaryosis should be referred for colposcopy.

Cytology results reported as moderate or severe dyskaryosis are referred urgently for further assessment in colposcopy. The greater the degree of dyskariosis the more likely it is that treatment will be needed.

COLPOSCOPY

If smear test cytology is abnormal, the patient is referred for colposcopy for further assessment. A colposcopy is usually performed by a gynaecologist or a specialist nurse. It is a detailed examination of the cervix, using a speculum to view the cervix, and then looking at the cervix through a binocular microscope called a colposcope. Indications for colposcopy are:

- High-grade (moderate and severe) dyskaryosis.
- Low-grade (borderline and mild) dyskaryosis.
- Recurrent inadequate smears.
- Follow-up of patients after treatment.

A colposcopic examination usually consists of the following steps:

1 The patient is placed in the lithotomy position and a speculum is inserted to allow visualisation of the cervix.
2 The SCJ is identified and the overall appearance of the cervix is assessed. Sometimes applying saline, or viewing the cervix through a green light filter, can help to identify abnormal vessel development in keeping with neoplasia.
3 Stains are applied to the cervix to help visualise abnormal cell proliferation. Dysplastic cells contain an increased level of protein and lower levels of glycogen in comparison to normal cells. To delineate the types of cells two stains can be applied:
   - Acetic acid – causes protein to coagulate, which causes the dysplastic cells with enlarged nuclei and high protein levels to appear white. This is termed 'aceto-white' staining.
   - Iodine – stains glycogen a dark brown colour. Normal cells contain high levels of glycogen so they stain dark brown, whereas abnormal cells do not stain and remain white from the acetic acid stain, which is usually applied first. After using both stains, it is clear to see the delineation between normal and abnormal areas of the cervix.
4 If any areas of the cervix appear suspicious after staining, then the clinician should take a biopsy of

the areas and send them for histological analysis. Depending on how the cervix appears and what level of dyskaryosis was identified on examination, the clinician will decide how to do a biopsy for a histology assessment:

- Punch biopsy – taking a small sample for histology.
- Cone biopsy – large biopsy, requires local anaesthetic.
- Large loop excision of transformation zone (LLETZ) – requires local anaesthetic. A diathermy loop is used to excise the abnormal looking tissue. The aim is to remove the abnormal area, with free margins, in order to treat at the same time as diagnose any abnormalities.

5 When the examination is complete, the speculum is removed like after a smear test.
6 Once the patient has dressed herself and feels comfortable, the clinician should explain the examination findings to her and tell her what will happen next.

HISTOLOGY

Biopsies are sent for histology. Cervical histology reports describe the severity of neoplasia seen, called cervical intraepithelial neoplasia (CIN) (Table 7.14).

Table 7.14	Cervical Intraepithelial Neoplasia (CIN) Types
CIN	**DESCRIPTION OF HISTOLOGY**
CIN 1	Mildly atypical cellular changes in the lower third of the epithelium.
CIN 2	Moderately atypical cellular changes confined to the basal two thirds of the epithelium, with preservation of epithelial maturation.
CIN 3	Severely atypical cellular changes involving greater than two thirds of the epithelial thickness, including full thickness lesions.

It is important to appreciate the difference between CIN and dyskaryosis (Fig. 7.7). CIN is a histological diagnosis (a piece of tissue taken as a biopsy at colposcopy) where the depth of the neoplasia and type of CIN can be established (Fig. 7.8). By contrast, dyskaryosis is used to describe cervical smear cytology examination, which is reported according to the degree of abnormality of individual cells.

MANAGEMENT

The treatment required for CIN depends on the extent of the abnormal cells. Patients with CIN 1 often do not routinely require treatment, as the condition frequently resolves itself. Instead, these women are offered repeat screening until HPV test is negative, or until further colposcopy is deemed to be necessary.

Patients with CIN 2 or CIN 3 (and occasionally those with CIN 1) should be offered treatment. The most commonly performed procedure is a LLETZ, which

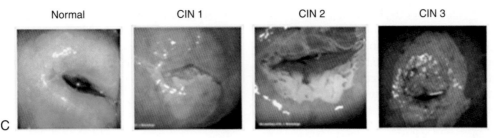

Fig. 7.7 Appearance of the cervix with CIN at colposcopy (acetic acid applied in each photo). (Source: From Huether S, McCance K. Understanding Pathophysiology, ed 5. Elsevier, Mosby, 2012.)

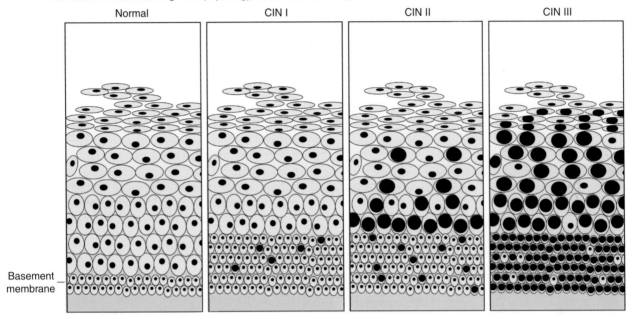

Fig. 7.8 Pictorial Representation of Cervical Histology. *CIN*, Cervical intraepithelial neoplasia.

is usually performed as an outpatient procedure. A colposcopy is performed with staining to identify the abnormality. Local anaesthetic is injected into the cervix, and then the diathermy loop is used to cut the piece of abnormal tissue off the cervix. The benefit of a LLETZ is that the excised tissue can be sent to histology and checked to confirm the abnormal area has been completely removed in the sample, with normal tissue at all margins of the sample. The downside of a LLETZ is that the procedure shortens the cervix, and if a LLETZ procedure needs to be done more than once this can increase the risk of cervical incompetence, causing miscarriage or preterm labour in a future pregnancy. An alternative to LLETZ, where a tissue sample is required, is a cone biopsy (where a conical section of the cervix is removed).

If the transformation zone is clearly visible and there is no evidence of disease spread or glandular abnormality, then ablative methods can be used to treat the abnormality seen. In these treatments, the abnormal cells are destroyed using either heating or freezing methods:

- Heat – laser vaporisation, "cold" coagulation and radical electrodiathermy.
- Freeze – cryocautery.

The damaged areas will heal over with normal cervical tissue. The benefit of these treatments is that very little cervix is removed compared to a LLETZ procedure. However, with these treatments no tissue sample is obtained, so it is not possible to confirm that all diseased tissue has been destroyed.

Whichever treatment is chosen, most patients are able to tolerate the treatment for CIN under local anaesthetic, but if patients experience extreme discomfort during colposcopy, then they may be offered a general anaesthetic.

Glandular Dysplasia

Cervical screening was set up in order to identify and treat squamous epithelial dysplasia. However, glandular dysplasia can also be incidentally identified during cervical smear cytology. Glandular dysplasia has a high risk of transforming into cervical cancer, so any form of glandular dysplasia is referred to colposcopy.

Glandular cells line the cervical canal, so they can be difficult to view adequately during colposcopy. Therefore, clinicians should have a low threshold to perform LLETZ procedures to obtain adequate biopsy for histology and treat at the same time. Abnormal histology is reported as cervical glandular intra-epithelial neoplasia (CGIN). If the LLETZ procedure has completely excised the abnormal cells (evidenced by clear margins on histology), then cervical smear follow-up is required. This is usually undertaken in colposcopy to make sure the smear samples are deep within the cervical canal.

FOLLOW-UP

Any patient that has had CIN, no matter what level of severity and whether they were treated or not, continues to be at risk of developing cervical cancer. This could be due to incomplete treatment of the disease or the development of new disease.

Local protocols vary; however the commonest follow up regime is a repeat smear 6 months after treatment. If this is normal the patient returns to the routine screening programme. If the result is HPV positive the patient returns to colposcopy where further treatment or follow up can be arranged.

❓ QUESTIONS

Kerry is 38 years old. They arrive in clinic for a scheduled cervical smear. Kerry is healthy and only takes omeprazole for gastric reflux due to a known slight hiatus hernia. Kerry has no gynaecological symptoms and attends for cervical smears regularly because their mother had cervical cancer.

Q1 Ideally, when should cervical screenings take place during a typical menstrual cycle?

   A Day 7.
   B Day 14.
   C Day 21.
   D Day 28.
   E It does not matter.

Q2 Answer true or false: In the following situations cervical screening is not required?

   A Over the age of 55.
   B Previous cervical ablation.
   C Sexually inactive lifelong.
   D Three previous negative results.
   E Total hysterectomy.

Q3 If this patient had received only negative results from their previous cervical smears, how often should they be screened?

   A Every year.
   B Once every 2 years.
   C Once every 3 years.
   D Once every 4 years.
   E Once every 5 years.

Q4 Which of the following HPV vaccine and virus pairings are correct?

   A Cervarix® and HPV subtypes 2, 7, 16 and 18.
   B Cervarix® and HPV subtypes 6, 11, 16 and 18.
   C Gardasil® and HPV subtypes 2, 7, 16 and 18.
   D Gardasil® and HPV subtypes 6, 11, 16 and 18.
   E Gardasil® and HPV subtypes 16 and 18.

[Answers on page 211.]

CERVICAL CANCER

Cervical cancer is a malignancy which occurs at the neck of the uterus. The histological subtypes of cervical cancer are:

- Squamous cell carcinoma – the most common subtype, approximately 80% of cases.
- Adenocarcinoma – 10% of cases.
- Poorly specified cervical cancer – 10% of cases.

AETIOLOGY

In the UK, there are approximately 2800 diagnoses of invasive cervical cancer each year, with the highest incidence occurring in women between the ages of 30 and 34. In the UK a woman's risk of developing cervical cancer during their lifetime is 1 in 136. It is the 11th most common cause of cancer in UK women. However, 80% of cervical cancer cases occur in developing countries, where cervical cancer is the second most common cause of cancer in women. This is largely due to a lack of cervical screening in these countries.

The three major risk factors for developing cervical cancer are:

- Infection with the HPV.
- Smoking.
- Inadequate cervical screening – screening leads to early identification and then treatment of precancerous dyskaryosis, preventing cancer developing.

[See 'Cervical Screening' page 150.]

PATHOLOGY

HPV is detected in over 99% of cervical cancer cases. Variants 16 and 18 of HPV cause the majority of the cases, but there are at least 15 variants associated with the disease. The oncogenic forms of the virus have two viral genes, called E6 and E7. If these are expressed, then the regulation of cell proliferation is disturbed and the cells at the transformation zone of the cervix may begin to grow abnormally and divide more rapidly than normal.

Host factors affect the likelihood of women infected with HPV developing cervical cancer. Smoking increases the risk of women developing cervical cancer. It is thought that smoking inhibits the body's immune response, preventing clearance of HPV. Similarly, immunodeficiency, such as HIV, also increases the risk of cervical cancer. Another risk factor for developing cervical cancer is giving birth to five or more children. The use of the oral contraceptive pill for more than 5 years also increases the risk of cervical cancer in HPV positive women.

The area of the cervix which is most at risk of being affected by HPV, and therefore developing cervical cancer, is the transformation zone. The cervical canal is lined with columnar epithelium whereas the vagina and the ectocervix are lined with squamous epithelium. The transformation zone occurs at the junction where these two cell types meet. This is where the cervical canal joins the external (visible) aspect of the cervix. At this zone the columnar epithelial cells undergo metaplasia (a normal healthy process) and develop into squamous epithelial cells. HPV infection increases the risk of physiological metaplasia at the transformation zone becoming neoplasia. This is why cervical smear samples are taken from the transformation zone. Another major risk factor for developing cervical cancer is not attending cervical screening appointments, as screening allows treatment of precancerous changes, preventing the development of cervical cancer.

HUMAN PAPILLOMAVIRUS IMMUNISATION PROGRAMME

A vaccination programme against HPV has now been introduced and is offered to adolescents in the UK with the aim of preventing cervical cancer. The vaccines are currently known to be effective at preventing HPV infection. The vaccination is predicted to result in a 50% decrease in high-grade CIN and a 70% reduction in cervical cancer. In the UK, HPV vaccination of 12- to 13-year-old girls has been implemented since 2008. The programme had also been extended to include boys in England since 2019.

The current vaccine offered (Gardasil®) protects against 4 HPV subtypes which include 6, 11, 16 and 18, hence it also protects against genital warts.

[See 'Cervical Screening' page 150.]

SIGNS AND SYMPTOMS

Cases of cervical cancer are most often detected through the cervical screening programme, so many patients present without any symptoms. In these cases, the cancer is diagnosed by a biopsy taken as a result of the abnormal smear test. Those who do present with symptoms most often present with abnormal vaginal bleeding:

- Postcoital bleeding.
- Intermenstrual bleeding or blood-stained discharge.
- Postmenopausal bleeding.

Less common symptoms may be foul smelling discharge and pelvic pain or dyspareunia. Patients who present with advanced cervical cancer may also have urinary or bowel symptoms, and symptoms related to metastatic spread, which can vary depending on the site of secondary disease.

On examination using a speculum, the cervix may appear visually normal in early-stage disease. In women with symptoms, the cervix may appear inflamed and friable and may bleed on contact. There may also be ulceration of the cervix and an offensive discharge. Again, depending on the stage of the disease, there may be signs of local spread or distant metastases.

INVESTIGATIONS AND STAGING

If a patient is suspected to have cervical cancer, an urgent referral should be made (within 2 weeks) to colposcopy. There, the patient will be assessed by a specialist and undergo colposcopic examination of the cervix. If there is any clinical suspicion of cancer, then a biopsy of the cervix will be taken and sent for histology.

Once histology confirms a diagnosis of cervical cancer, further investigation in the form of imaging is used to assess the stage of the disease. MRI is the most sensitive scan for staging of cervical cancer within the pelvis. A CT chest and abdomen and CT-PET scans are used to assess for distant metastasis.

Other investigations that may be used to aid diagnosis include:

- Vaginal swabs, if infection is suspected.
- Surgical staging with examination under anaesthetics (EUA), which may include hysteroscopy, cystoscopy (used only where there is discrepancy between imaging and clinical assessment).
- Lymph node biopsy.

DIFFERENTIAL DIAGNOSIS

The symptoms of cervical cancer are, like many gynaecological diseases, very non-specific. Differential diagnosis should therefore include:

- Side effects of hormonal contraception – this is the most common cause of intermenstrual bleeding in young women taking hormonal contraception. If examination of the cervix is normal, then changing the type of contraception would be the first-line treatment.
- Cervical ectropion – may present as postcoital bleeding or intermenstrual bleeding. It occurs due to friable columnar epithelial growth on the ectocervix; usually squamous cells are on the ectocervix and columnar cells line the endocervical canal. It occurs in response to high oestrogen levels. The most common causes for this are the combined oral contraceptive pill and pregnancy.
- Cervical polyps – typically present with postcoital bleeding. The polyps should be excised and examined histologically to ensure that they are not malignant. Symptoms should resolve once the lesion has been removed.
- Cervicitis – caused by a sexually transmitted infection. The whole cervix will appear red due to the inflammation, and palpation of the cervix may be painful.
- PID – an infection of the upper genital tract in women. The patient will typically have pelvic pain and may also have intermenstrual or postcoital bleeding.
- Endometrial cancer – this is more likely in postmenopausal women in whom cervical cancer is relatively rare. The cervix should still be examined thoroughly in order to rule out a cervical origin for the patient's symptoms. Women who present with postmenopausal bleeding should be offered an ultrasound

scan and, if the results are suspicious of endometrial cancer, an endometrial biopsy obtained.

COMPLICATIONS

Most of the complications are discussed in the introduction to the management of gynaecological cancer section. Common specific complications of advanced cervical cancer are:

- Worsening of localised symptoms – as the tumour grows, symptoms such as bleeding, pain, malodour and sexual dysfunction may worsen.
- Hydronephrosis and renal failure due to external obstruction of ureters as the cervical tumour grows.
- Fistulae – if the tumour begins to invade the local structures, the patient may develop fistulae originating from the vagina. These may connect to the rectum (a rectovaginal fistula) or the bladder (a vesicovaginal fistula). Due to the nature of the fistulae, the patient will be prone to developing infections, incontinence, and there may be a worsening of any malodour that they are experiencing.

MANAGEMENT

General management, including the MDT, grading, staging and treatment, is covered in the Management of Cancer section.

[See 'Principles of Gynaecological Cancer Management' page 139.]

TREATMENTS OF CERVICAL CANCER

The treatment which can be offered to women with cervical cancer depends on the staging. The FIGO criteria are an international staging regimen used to stage cervical cancer (Table 7.15).

SURGERY

Surgical resection of tumours is the most preferable treatment of choice for early cervical cancer (stages IA1- IB1). In young patients who are keen to preserve their fertility, fertility-conserving surgery may be offered. In patients who have completed their family, the recommended treatment is usually a radical hysterectomy, where the uterus, cervix, parametrial tissues and upper part of the vagina are removed. Lymph nodes should also be removed if the cancer is stage IA2, IB1 or higher. Women who are postmenopausal or certain that their family is complete will also have both ovaries removed. If the cancer is at a more advanced stage, then salvage surgery or palliative surgery may be offered.

RADIOTHERAPY

Radiotherapy can be delivered externally, or via radioactive brachytherapy pessaries which are inserted into the vagina. Women who undergo surgery are often offered adjuvant radiotherapy to reduce recurrence.

Table **7.15**	FIGO Staging Classification for Cervical Cancer
STAGE	**DESCRIPTION**
0	Carcinoma *in situ* (reported in severe cervical intraepithelial neoplasia (CIN) III cases). Cancer is only in the cervical epithelial layers.
I	Cancer localised to cervix and uterus only: • IA – visible only on microscopy and less than or equal to 7 mm extension (IA1 is less than or equal to 3 mm deep, IA2 has a depth more than 3 mm but less than or equal to 5 mm). • IB – visible clinically (IB1 ≤2 cm diameter, IB2 >2cm but <4cm, IB3 ≥4cm diameter.).
II	Cancer has spread to tissues surrounding the cervix: • IIA shows no obvious parametrial (connective tissue) involvement. • IIB shows parametrial involvement.
III	Cancer has spread into the pelvis: • Tumour involves lower third of vagina but not side wall of pelvis. • Tumour involves pelvic side wall, or alters renal function due to ureteric obstruction.
IV	Cancer is widespread: • IVA – tumour involves adjacent organs such as bowel or bladder. • IVB – tumour has spread to distant organs.

Women with more advanced cervical cancer (Stage ≥1B3), are often not suitable for surgery because there is a high risk of not being able to achieve sufficiently cancer-free margins around the tumour. These women may be offered radical radiotherapy combined with chemotherapy as a primary treatment to shrink the tumour with aim to cure in stage IIA or less.

CHEMOTHERAPY

Chemotherapy delivered alongside radical radiotherapy offers a better prognosis than radiotherapy alone. Women who are still at high risk of metastatic disease following surgery may be offered adjuvant chemotherapy. The most effective agents against cervical cancer are platinum-based therapies such as cisplatin. In very advanced disease, where palliation is the only treatment option, platinum-based agents can be used for symptomatic relief.

PROGNOSIS

Around 65% of women who are diagnosed with cervical cancer will survive for more than 5 years. Younger women tend to have a better prognosis, as do those who present with the disease in its early stages. Those who are diagnosed in stage I of the disease have at least an 80% chance of being cured of the disease. This contrasts with the 5-year survival rate for women who present at stage IV, which is 20%.

Adenocarcinoma of the cervix has a worse prognosis than squamous cell carcinoma. This is because adenocarcinoma tumours grow within the cervical canal, so they are harder to identify at cervical screening, and they do not cause symptoms until they are at an advanced stage.

The best management of cervical cancer is to prevent it. The introduction of the HPV vaccine will hopefully help to this end. Additionally, detecting and treating any pre-cancerous changes as early as possible is a very effective way of preventing around 75% of cervical cancer. Women should therefore be encouraged to have their cervical smears when they are invited by the screening programme.

 Cervical Cancer in Women of Childbearing Age

The age group most at risk of developing cervical cancer is 25 to 34-year-olds. These women are of childbearing age, so many of them will want to remain fertile, if possible. If a woman who is diagnosed with cervical cancer wishes to retain her fertility, then she can opt to retain her uterus and ovaries, and undergo a radical trachelectomy. In this procedure, the cervix, upper portion of the vagina and the medial portions of the cardinal and uterosacral ligaments are removed. This type of surgery can be extremely effective, but there is a higher risk of recurrence after radical trachelectomy than after a hysterectomy, as less tissue is removed.

If chemotherapy or radiotherapy is required, egg collection can be offered prior to treatment so that assisted conception or surrogacy is an option for the patient in the event that the treatments damage her ovaries.

❓ QUESTIONS

Kerry had a normal smear test when aged 25, but then does not attend for any further screening appointments. At the age of 40, Kerry begins to experience some pain during sex and abnormal bleeding between periods which seems to be worse after intercourse. Kerry is concerned, so visits the primary care physician. On examination, they note that the cervix appears inflamed, so Kerry is sent for urgent colposcopy. During this appointment, a biopsy is taken, which is later reported as cervical cancer.

Q1 Answer true or false: Which of the following women are at an increased risk of developing cervical cancer?

A A woman who is HIV positive.

B A woman in her 60s who tells you her mother took treatment to increase her oestrogen levels to prevent a miscarriage.

C A woman whose two older sisters have been diagnosed with cervical cancer.

D A woman in her early thirties who has had several sexual partners, she has been using a COCP for 7 years and does not use barrier contraception.

E A woman who has previously tested positive for *Chlamydia trachomatis* antibodies.

Q2 Which of the following characteristics does not increase the risk of psychosocial problems in women diagnosed with cervical cancer?

A Having a child who is under 21 years of age.

B History of psychiatric illness.

C Living alone.

D Lymphoedema.

E Older patient.

Q3 Which of the following surgical treatment options for cervical cancer is the most appropriate for a young woman who wishes to retain her fertility?

A Bilateral salpingo-oophorectomy.

B Mastectomy.

C Pelvic exenteration.

D Radical hysterectomy.

E Radical trachelectomy.

[Answers on page 212.]

VULVAL CANCER

Vulval cancer in the UK is rare, with an incidence of 3 per 100,000. The majority of women who are diagnosed with vulval cancer are over the age of 65, with the disease being extremely rare below the age of 50. There should be a low threshold to biopsy any new vulval skin changes in a postmenopausal woman to exclude malignancy.

The most common form of vulval cancer is squamous cell carcinoma (SCC), although there are other forms, including basal cell carcinomas, melanomas, verrucous carcinomas and Bartholin gland carcinomas.

RISK FACTORS

Vulval lichen sclerosus and HPV infection are the two main risk factors for developing vulval cancer. Both of these conditions can lead to pre-cancerous changes of squamous cells, called vulval intraepithelial neoplasia (VIN) (Fig. 7.9). The percentage of women with VIN who go on to develop an SCC is around 10%–20%.

Paget disease of the vulva (adenocarcinoma *in situ*) and melanoma are less common pre-cancerous conditions than VIN but have a high risk of progressing into invasive cancer.

SIGNS AND SYMPTOMS

Cancer of the vulva and VIN may be detected incidentally during examination in asymptomatic women or during surveillance of a pre-cancerous lesion (most commonly lichen sclerosus). Symptomatic patients with VIN or cancer may present with a lump or swelling, pain, itching or an abnormal discharge, which can sometimes be bloody.

VIN can appear in a single site, in multiple areas or can appear extensively involving the whole vulva and perineum. Its appearance varies, but it often appears as

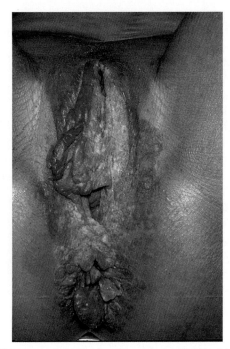

Fig. 7.9 Widespread VIN. (Source: From Black M, McKay M. Obstetrics and Gynaecological Dermatology, ed 2. Mosby, 2002.)

raised, white, erythematous, wart-like papules, which are clustered closely together.

DIFFERENTIAL DIAGNOSIS

- Vulval cancer.
- VIN.
- Lichen sclerosus.
- Lichen simplex.
- Vulval eczema.
- Human herpes virus ulcerations.
- Syphilitic ulcer (chancre).
- Candidal vulvovaginitis.
- Vulvodynia.

INVESTIGATIONS

Women with suspected vulval cancer should have a biopsy taken, which incorporates the margin of the lesion, so that the borders can be assessed accurately. This can often be done as an outpatient under local anaesthetic.

MANAGEMENT

Like any cancer, vulval cancers are graded, staged (using FIGO criteria) and management decided through an MDT. The treatment of vulval cancer is primarily achieved by surgery. If the lesion is localised to one area, then a wide local excision may be sufficient, providing that there are clear margins (usually 1–1.5 cm). In cases of extensive disease, a vulvectomy (surgical excision of all vulval tissue) may be necessary. If there is risk of disease spread to the inguinal lymph

nodes, then a lymphadenectomy may be required, as may chemotherapy and radiotherapy. Obviously, the larger the excision, the greater the risk of effects on the appearance of the vulva and sexual function. Removal of the lymph nodes increases the risk of lower limb lymphoedema.

VULVAL INTRAEPITHELIAL NEOPLASIA

VIN can be treated like vulval cancer with surgery, particularly where there is a small site of disease. However, where there is extensive disease, surgery would likely cause significant psychosexual dysfunction. In younger patients, where this is likely to be a significant concern, other treatments can be considered to preserve anatomical function. Other treatment options include localised destruction techniques, such as cryotherapy and 5-fluorouracil cream. An immune modulator cream, called imiquimod, is also useful for this condition. Regular follow-up is necessary to monitor for recurrence of VIN, and clinicians should have a low threshold for taking a biopsy of any suspicious areas to rule out progression to vulval cancer.

If a patient has VIN due to HPV, she should also undergo colposcopy to exclude any HPV-related cervical pathology. At the same time, the vagina can be assessed to rule out the much rarer HPV-induced vaginal changes. If VIN lesions are in the perianal region, the patient should also be referred for anoscopy.

[See 'Cervical cancer' page 156.]

PROGNOSIS

The 5-year survival for vulval cancer is 80% in cases without lymphatic spread. If the inguinal lymph nodes are affected, then this falls to 50%, with spread beyond the nodes leading to a worse prognosis.

VAGINAL CANCER

Vaginal cancer is even rarer than vulval cancer, with an incidence of less than 1 per 100,000 in the UK. The incidence of vaginal cancer increases with age, with the most commonly affected age group being women over the age of 85.

Cancers of the vagina, like those of the vulva, are most often squamous cell carcinomas. Around 85% of primary vaginal cancers are SCCs, and around 10% are adenocarcinomas, with melanomas and sarcomas accounting for a small number of cases.

RISK FACTORS

The cause of vaginal cancer is unknown in most cases. HPV infection is the most commonly associated risk factor, so women with a history of CIN and VIN are at increased risk of vaginal cancer. HPV can cause pre-cancerous changes of the squamous cells of the vagina called vaginal intraepithelial neoplasia (VAIN). If a patient is diagnosed with VAIN, she should also undergo regular colposcopy to exclude any HPV-induced cervical pathology.

SIGNS AND SYMPTOMS

SCC tumours most commonly arise on the superior third of the posterior wall of the vagina. Women with vaginal cancer typically present with abnormal vaginal bleeding or discharge. It is a rare differential diagnosis for postmenopausal bleeding. Patients may also present with an itch, lump or pain in the vagina, or pain during intercourse. Lesions may appear as a lump or an ulcer and are frequently friable on examination.

DIFFERENTIAL DIAGNOSIS

Causes of bleeding, discharge or lump:
- Endometrial – cancer, hyperplasia, polyps, dysfunctional uterine bleeding.
- Cervical – cancer, ectropion, polyps.
- Vaginal – cancer, VAIN, atrophic vaginitis, sexually transmitted infection, prolapse.
- Vulval – any vulval lesion (see above).
- Non-gynaecological – rectal cancer, haemorrhoids, bladder tumour.

INVESTIGATIONS

Women with suspected vaginal cancer should have a biopsy taken which incorporates the margin of the lesion so that the borders can be assessed accurately.

MANAGEMENT

Vaginal cancer is graded, staged (using FIGO criteria) and management decided through an MDT. The treatment of vaginal cancer is predominantly surgical, with most women requiring a radical hysterectomy and excision of the superior section of the vagina. The removal of part of the vagina can lead to sexual dysfunction, which can be very distressing to patients. Radiotherapy can be used as an adjuvant to surgery or as primary therapy in advanced disease. There is a limited role for chemotherapy.

If the woman only has pre-cancerous changes (VAIN), then a carbon dioxide laser may be used instead of conventional surgery in order to preserve sexual function. Imiquimod may also be used to treat VAIN. Regular follow-up is essential to monitor for recurrence of VAIN and for progression to vaginal cancer.

In women wishing to remain sexually active after treatment of cancerous or pre-cancerous conditions of the vulva or vagina, there is a high risk of sexual dysfunction. Referral to specialist psychosexual counsellors can help patients through these problems.

PROGNOSIS

The prognosis of vaginal cancer worsens with increasing age and the involvement of the middle and inferior thirds of the vaginal walls. The 5-year survival rate for vaginal cancer is approximately 60%.

❓ QUESTIONS

Sally is a 56-year-old who presents with a history of postmenopausal bleeding for the last 2 weeks. Sally has noticed bleeding after intercourse and also some discomfort during intercourse. Sally has previously been diagnosed with lichen sclerosus.

Q1 What is the most likely cause for this patient's symptoms?
   A Atrophic vaginitis.
   B Endometrial cancer.
   C Vaginal cancer.
   D Vaginal intraepithelial neoplasia (VAIN).
   E Vulval intraepithelial neoplasia (VIN).

Q2 A biopsy subsequently taken from a suspicious area of lichen sclerosus on the patient's vulva has been reported as containing VIN. Answer true or false, regarding VIN and the management of this patient.
   A VIN may have been caused by lichen sclerosus.
   B VIN may have been caused by the human herpes virus (HHV).
   C VIN may progress to vulval cancer in around 20% of cases.
   D This patient should be offered a colposcopy.
   E Surgery could be avoided as the patient is sexually active.

Q3 With a diagnosis of VIN, which of the conditions is the patient not at an increased risk of developing?
   A Cervical cancer.
   B Cervical intraepithelial neoplasia (CIN).
   C Endometrial cancer.
   D Vaginal cancer.
   E Vulval cancer.

[Answers on page 214.]

KEY REFERENCES

GENERAL PRINCIPLES OF GYNAECOLOGICAL CANCER MANAGEMENT

International Federation of Gynaecology and Obstetrics, 2018. Staging Classifications of Gynaecological Cancer [Internet]. www.figo.org
National Institute for Health and Care Excellence, 2015. Suspected Cancer, Recognition and Referral. NICE Clinical Guideline (NG 12).

OVARIAN CANCER

British Gynaecological Cancer Society, 2017. Epithelial Ovarian/Fallopian Tube/Primary Peritoneal Cancer Guidelines: Recommendations for Practice. BGCS.
National Institute for Health and Clinical Excellence, 2011. The Recognition and Initial Management of Ovarian Cancer. NICE Clinical Guideline (CG 122).
Royal College of Obstetricians and Gynaecologists, 2016. Ovarian Cysts in Postmenopausal Women. RCOG Green Top Guideline (CG 34).

ENDOMETRIAL CANCER

British Gynaecological Cancer Society, 2021. Uterine Cancer Guidelines: Recommendations for Practice. BGCS.

National Institute for Health and Clinical Excellence, 2018. Heavy Menstrual Bleeding. NICE Clinical Guideline (NG88).

Royal College of Obstetricians and Gynaecologists, 2016. Endometrial Hyperplasia, Management of Green-top Guideline No. 67. RCOG, London.

CERVICAL SCREENING

NHS Cervical Screening Programme, 2020. Colposcopy and Programme Management, third edition. Public Health England (NHSCSP no. 20).

Public Health England Guidance, 2019. Cervical Screening: Implementation Guide for Primary HPV Screening. UK Guideline.

CERVICAL CANCER

Bhatla, N., Berek, J.S., Fredes, M.C., Denny, L.A., Grenman, S., Karunaratne, K, et al., 2019. Revised FIGO staging for carcinoma of the cervix uteri. Int. J. Gynecol. Obstet. 145, 129–135.

HPV Vaccines. Centre for disease control and prevention. https://www.cdc.gov/hpv/hcp/schedules-recommendations.html (last accessed 8/12/2022)

NHS Cervical Screening Programme, 2020. Colposcopy and Programme Management, third edition. Public Health England (NHSCSP no. 20).

VULVAL AND VAGINAL CANCERS

Royal College of Obstetricians and Gynaecologists, 2014. Diagnosis and Management of Vulval Carcinoma. RCOG guideline.

British Association for Sexual Health and HIV, 2014. The Management of Vulval Conditions. BASHH UK Guideline.

British Gynaecological Cancer Society, 2020. Vulval Cancer Guidelines: Recommendations for Practice. BGCS.

1 INTRODUCTION

OVERVIEW

Q1: Answer true or false, regarding the use of chaperones.

Women undergoing an intimate examination should be offered a chaperone and be invited to bring a relative or friend to the consultation. There are some disadvantages to the presence of a chaperone; this may be an opportunity for a patient to confide deeply sensitive information such as sexual abuse, previous termination of pregnancy or domestic violence. The presence of another person may reduce the chance of this. Some patients may also feel more embarrassed having another person in the room; however, the benefits of a chaperone for both the patient and the doctor usually offset the disadvantages.

A The chaperone is present only for the benefit of the patient – **False.** Most commonly the presence of a chaperone acts as a safeguard against a doctor causing unnecessary discomfort, pain, humiliation or intimidation during examination and can help reassure an anxious patient. The chaperone also protects the doctor from any false allegations of sexual misconduct and, more regularly, they can assist the doctor or help calm the patient by maintaining eye contact throughout the examination.

B The chaperone must be a nurse or other qualified doctor – **False.** Ideally, a chaperone would be a qualified healthcare professional, for example, a nurse. However, for financial or logistical reasons, this may not always be possible. Therefore, other staff members may act as chaperones in these situations. Medical students may also fulfil this role. The name and job title of the chaperone should be recorded in the patient record.

C Chaperones should be assumed necessary unless the patient states otherwise – **False.** Chaperones should be offered to the patient. As the chaperone is also present for the protection of the doctor, if a patient declines a chaperone this should be explored further. It may be another chaperone to the one offered may be preferred. If a patient

refuses all chaperones, the General Medical Council (GMC) advises that the doctor does not have to perform an examination. If they are not comfortable in doing so, they should instead consider referral to another colleague. If examination is performed without a chaperone, it should be clearly documented in the record that a chaperone was offered, and where appropriate, an explanation why this was declined.

D In certain situations, a chaperone may be a family member – **False.** A family member or relative can certainly accompany the patient for their comfort, and this should be offered prior to any intimate examination. However, for the clinician, a family member does not offer the same level of protection against accusations of wrongdoing that would be provided by a staff member. In addition, in some circumstances, the presence of a family member may hinder the patient's ability to talk about sensitive topics. Examination of the patient may provide the only opportunity for the patient to be spoken to away from relatives. In this setting, the patient can be asked about any concerns they have that cannot be discussed with family present, such as domestic violence or any other sexual relationships.

E Chaperones are not necessary when the doctor performing the examination is female – **False.** A chaperone should be available to assist with gynaecological examinations irrespective of the gender of the gynaecologist. It is appreciated that a chaperone may be more necessary if the doctor is male; however, female clinicians should still use a chaperone for personal protection against false accusations.

> 💬 **Key Point**
>
> Intimate examinations are not just limited to a pelvic examination; other examinations such as breast and rectal examinations are also invasive examinations and need to be carried out with sensitivity to this. This needs to be considered generally, for example when performing an ECG on a ward as this will require exposing a person's chest.

Q2: If this patient had a body mass index (BMI) of 35 kg/m², which of the following is most correct regarding a discussion of their weight.

The correct answer is C. Due to the potentially sensitive nature of discussing a patient's weight, the doctor should wait until after the examination, when the patient has dressed and is back in the consultation room.

It is very important that no uninvited comments about weight are made during any time that the patient has removed any of their clothing. No comments, except for those regarding the examination itself, should be made during a pelvic examination due to the intimate nature of the examination. Patients can feel very vulnerable; therefore, maintaining an air of professionalism is important. Whilst some doctors may sometimes feel personal comments build rapport, this can be viewed as inappropriate by the patient.

A As a patient's BMI is a clinical matter, this can be discussed at any point in the patient's history or examination – **Incorrect.** As explained, discussion of a patient's weight may be a personal and sensitive matter. Inappropriate comments during the bimanual examination could be distressing for the patient and could reduce the likelihood of them accessing medical care in the future.

B As long as the patient is fully dressed, then comments regarding the patient's weight may be made – **Incorrect.** Although discussing this when the patient is fully dressed is preferable to during the examination, this is not the best answer.

C ✔ **Due to the potentially sensitive nature of discussing a patient's weight, the doctor should wait until after the examination, when the patient has dressed and is back in the consultation room** – **Correct.** At the end of the examination, the patient will be left in privacy to dress and then will be asked to join the doctor to finish the consultation. Therefore, if the doctor is going to broach the subject of the patient's elevated BMI, this would be the best time to do this. Discussing a patient's weight in any situation should be done sensitively, and their weight should be discussed in relation to their medical condition.

D The doctor should discuss the patient's BMI before the examination, as this could be deemed inappropriate if done afterwards – **Incorrect.** Whether the discussion regarding the patient's weight occurs before or after the examination is not strictly crucial. However, it may be worth considering that many women get anxious before a pelvic examination. Therefore, it might be much more appropriate to discuss this matter after the examination, so they are more likely to retain this information.

E The doctor should not comment on the patient's weight, as it is unrelated to the patient's presentation – **Incorrect.** In many gynaecological conditions, a patient's weight is an important clinical consideration that may have an impact on their disease, for example, issues with fertility or development of endometrial cancer. It may also be a factor for any treatments offered, for example, surgery often carries higher risks with increasing BMI, and certain medications (such as the combined oral contraceptive) may be contraindicated due to BMI. Therefore, completely ignoring the patient's BMI, especially if it is related to their presentation of disease, is inappropriate and not part of holistic care.

> **Key Point**
>
> Personal comments may include any remarks regarding the patient, such as their suntan, clothes, underwear, tattoos or, as discussed in this question, weight. These should only be mentioned when clinically relevant and in a sensitive manner.

Q3: If pain is experienced on moderate pressure to the cervix, what does this suggest?

The correct answer is D. Pelvic inflammatory disease (PID).

Cervical excitation, or cervical motion tenderness, is elicited by moving the cervix from side to side. This, therefore, disturbs the adnexal organs and overlying peritoneum. A positive sign is the elicitation of acute sharp pain, which suggests active pelvic inflammation. It has been argued that cervical excitation is not a specific sign, so results obtained on examination should be interpreted with caution. Before determining if cervical excitation is present, warn the patient that your action may feel strange, and then move the cervix from side to side, watching the patient's face for any signs of pain.

A Appendicitis – **Incorrect.** Determining if cervical excitation is present can be a distinguishing feature between PID and appendicitis. Appendicitis should not elicit a positive cervical excitation response, as moving the adnexal organs or overlying peritoneum should not disturb the appendix as it is usually higher in the abdomen.

B Cervical cancer – **Incorrect.** Cervical cancer, similar to fibroids, does not present with cervical excitation during a bimanual examination.

C Fibroids – **Incorrect.** Fibroids are often painless in presentation and any pain is not classically sharp in nature. Therefore, moving the cervix should not elicit acute pain.

D ✔ **Pelvic inflammatory disease** – **Correct.** Classically, cervical excitation is a red flag symptom for PID. Bilateral adnexal tenderness is often also present, suggesting inflammation throughout the pelvis. However, a patient with PID may possibly not have cervical excitation. Other common causes for cervical excitation are ectopic pregnancies and sexually transmitted infections (STIs).

E This is a typical examination finding – **Incorrect.** If the cervical excitation is elicited in the correct manner, by simply moving the cervix gently from side to side, pain should not be a normal examination finding. If, however, the cervix is moved quickly with force, then this will cause pain, irrespective of the presence of pathology.

> **Key Point**
>
> The most common STIs which cause PID are chlamydia and gonorrhoea. Other clinical examination findings which are strongly supportive of PID are visualising an inflamed cervix (cervicitis) and mucopurulent discharge. Other signs which are common but less specific are lower abdominal tenderness, adnexal tenderness on bimanual examination, fever and other additional signs of sepsis.

> **Important Learning Points**
>
> - Pelvic examinations and other intimate examinations are essential diagnostic tools.
> - Developing a professional, but sensitive, approach is the best way to keep patients at ease during examination.
> - A chaperone should be offered for all intimate examinations, offering support and reassurance to both the clinician and the patient.
> - Discussing potentially sensitive information with the patient should generally be avoided when the patient is in an exposed state during examination.

2 HPO AXIS

THE MENSTRUAL CYCLE AND PHYSIOLOGY OF THE HPO AXIS

Q1: Which of the following statements concerning the HPO axis are true or false?

Knowledge of the HPO axis is essential for a deeper understanding of gynaecological pathologies. Gonadotropin-releasing hormone (GnRH) released from the hypothalamus acts on the anterior pituitary to release follicle-stimulating hormone (FSH) and luteinising hormone (LH), which act in turn on the gonads to release oestrogen. Oestrogen completes the cycle, acting on the hypothalamus and anterior pituitary to control hormonal secretion. The HPO axis drives secondary sexual development and follicular development.

A ✔ **The HPO axis acts to bring about secondary sexual changes – True.** The HPO axis is functionally involved with the development of secondary sexual characteristics. Primary sexual characteristics refer to the genetically determined sexual characteristics of reproductive organs. Secondary sexual characteristics refer to the further development of these primary sexual characteristics (e.g. enlargement of breasts, growth of pubic hair and commencement of the menstrual cycle).

B GnRH is released from the anterior pituitary – **False.** Pulsatile GnRH is released from the hypothalamus, from specialised neurones in the arcuate nucleus.

C ✔ **GnRH is released in a pulsatile manner – True.** GnRH is released in a pulsatile manner, approximately every hour, with a short half-life of 2 to 4 minutes. Puberty is the result of an increase in secretion of LH due to a gradual increase in GnRH during pubertal years.

D GnRH causes the releases of FSH alone – **False.** GnRH stimulates the production of both LH and FSH, which act on the female gonads to cause secretion of the female sex steroid hormones, oestrogen and progesterone, as well as morphological changes related to folliculogenesis (development of one dominant mature follicle for ovulation).

E ✔ **Negative feedback from oestrogen occurs in the arcuate nucleus and anterior pituitary – True.** The hypothalamus and pituitary (adenohypophysis) modulate their secretion depending on negative feedback from the ovary; therefore, increased levels of oestrogen from the ovary suppress GnRH release from the hypothalamus and LH and FSH release from the pituitary gland.

> **Key Point**
>
> As FSH and LH levels rise, so do their receptor concentrations in the granulosa cells of the developing follicles. The granulosa cells produce oestrogen and inhibin, which lowers FSH and LH levels. As these levels fall, the follicles with the fewest receptors undergo atresia. Eventually, all but one follicle undergo atresia. This dominant follicle has the highest concentration of FSH and LH receptors.

Q2: Which of the following statements concerning the menstrual cycle are true or false?

Understanding the normal physiology of the normal menstrual cycle is essential to understand the mechanism of action of contraception, and how to manage problems such as infertility and heavy menstrual bleeding.

A The average length of a menstrual cycle is 32 days – **False.** The average length of a menstrual cycle is 28 days. If the length is less than 24 days, it is unusually frequent, or if more than 38 days, it is infrequent. The luteal phase is similar in all women, as this phase is controlled by the life cycle of the corpus luteum. The follicular phase, on the other hand, is variable, and this results in different menstrual cycle lengths between women.

B ✔ **Ovarian follicles mature during the proliferative phase – True.** The proliferative phase (part of the follicular phase) occurs between days 5 and 13 of a 28-day menstrual cycle. In this time, multiple follicles initially mature under the influence of FSH. These follicles produce oestrogen. This has two important hormonal effects:

1 Stimulation of endometrial proliferation in preparation for the implantation of an embryo if fertilisation is successful during the menstrual cycle.

2 Negative feedback on the production of FSH.

C ✔ **Declining FSH levels in the follicular phase can lead to follicular atresia – True.** Approximately 20 primary follicles grow in response to FSH. Follicular atresia is seen in follicles with few receptors to FSH until only the single Graafian (dominant) follicle remains.

D ✔ **The mid cycle LH surge occurs in response to high oestrogen levels – True.** During the proliferative phase, initially, low levels of oestradiol suppress secretion of LH from the anterior pituitary. The maturing follicle releases increasing amounts of oestrogen. Once these high levels of oestrogen exceed a threshold (200 pg/mL for approximately 40 hours), an LH surge occurs, which in turn causes the release of the secondary oocyte.

E ✔ **The follicle which released the egg may later become the corpus albicans – True.** The ruptured follicle initially becomes a corpus haemorrhagium, then a corpus luteum, and subsequently the corpus albicans.

💬 Key Point

Folliculogenesis occurs within the ovarian cortex and comprises four major stages:

- Recruitment – the activation of primordial follicles. Primordial follicles remain dormant, held in prophase of meiosis 1 until menarche.
- Follicle development – mainly in response to FSH, the granulosa and theca cells mature.
- Selection – developing follicles produce oestrogen and inhibin, which negatively feedback on FSH production. Only the follicles with the greatest sensitivity to FSH continue developing.
- Atresia – the follicles without sufficient FSH stimulation undergo apoptosis, leaving the single dominant follicle for ovulation.

Q3: Which of the following statements regarding the luteal phase are correct?

The correct answer is A. The end of the menstrual cycle occurs secondary to regression of the corpus luteum.

The luteal phase begins after ovulation. The phase lasts 14 days and is the same length for all women. The variation in menstrual cycle length depends on the follicular phase.

A ✔ **The end of the menstrual cycle occurs secondary to regression of the corpus luteum – Correct.** Towards the end of the menstrual cycle, the corpus luteum begins to regress if the ovulated egg is not fertilised. The withdrawal of progesterone support from the corpus luteum causes breakdown of the proliferated endometrium. This usually results in a flow of menses and also marks day one of the next menstrual cycle.

B Secretory changes of the endometrium are largely due to LH – **Incorrect.** Proliferative changes of the endometrium are largely due to oestrogen during the proliferative phase, while progesterone is responsible for secretory changes in the endometrium. Progesterone's reproductive effects include:

- Secretory changes in the endometrium during the luteal phase, which optimise the endometrium for implantation.
- Thickening of the consistency of cervical mucus, blocking the cervix, protecting a successful implantation.
- Decreases in the maternal immune response, preventing a response to the foreign body that is the embryo and allowing successful implantation and gestation.
- Decreases in contractility of the uterine smooth muscles, preventing the uterus from expelling the pregnancy.
- Inhibition of lactation.

C Increasing levels of progesterone cause a breakdown of the endometrium at the end of the menstrual cycle – **Incorrect.** Progesterone maintains the endometrium. Endometrial proliferation involves enlargement of the stromal cells, swelling of glands and an increase in the blood supply to the area. Decreasing levels of progesterone cause a breakdown of the endometrium.

D The basal body temperature is lower in the luteal phase – **Incorrect.** The biphasic pattern of the basal body temperature can be used as a component of fertility awareness. The basal body temperature is lower in the proliferative phase due to high levels of oestrogen and rises after ovulation due to the higher levels of progesterone.

E If the egg is fertilised, the endometrium is maintained despite falling progesterone and oestrogen levels – **Incorrect.** If the egg is fertilised, the endometrium is maintained by the corpus luteum until the placenta replaces it at approximately 10 weeks. Human chorionic gonadotropin (hCG) maintains the corpus luteum and ensures continued synthesis of oestrogen and progesterone.

💬 Key Point

The menstrual cycle comprises the cyclical activities of the HPO axis and the uterus during the reproductive years of a woman's life. The menstrual cycle facilitates and prepares for blastocyst implantation or menses every 28 days, on average.

Q4: A 15-year-old presents with cyclical lower abdominal pain for 10 months, denies any history of menstruation. She has normal secondary sexual development.

The correct answer is F. Imperforate hymen.

The presentation is classic for an imperforate hymen; given the cyclical pain at menarche, a history of primary amenorrhea and normal development of secondary sexual characteristics. This should prompt clinicians to examine the perineum and vagina, which may show a blue bulging hymen; a result of haematocolpos (blood accumulating in the vagina). Diagnosis is supported by ultrasound scanning. Here, the patient's HPO axis is functioning normally; however, there is a physical barrier to menses.

Q5: A 28-year-old presents to the emergency department following haemorrhagic shock during a spontaneous vaginal birth at home. Following recovery, the patient is unable to lactate for her child.

The correct answer is K. Sheehan syndrome.

Hypertrophy of prolactin cells in the anterior pituitary during pregnancy, combined with a low-pressure portal venous system, leaves the anterior pituitary susceptible to ischaemia. The delay in adequate resuscitation following obstetric haemorrhage resulted in hypoperfusion, which facilitated postpartum ischaemic necrosis of the pituitary gland. This is a type of hypopituitarism which can affect production of all hormones from the anterior pituitary, including those of the HPO axis. Other symptoms can develop over time and include malaise, oligomenorrhoea, amenorrhoea, loss of pubic and axillary hair, and hypotension.

Q6: A 22-year-old presents with her mother complaining of irregular menstrual cycles. Both the mother and patient are overweight and the girl complains of having to shave very frequently.

The correct answer is H. Polycystic ovarian syndrome.

Polycystic ovarian syndrome (PCOS) risk factors include family history, obesity and insulin resistance. Symptoms can be divided into those related to anovulation (oligomenorrhoea, amenorrhoea and infertility), hyperandrogenism (such as hirsutism, acne and male pattern baldness) and unexplained weight gain. Chronically elevated LH and hyperinsulinaemia are linked to the increased ovarian androgen production. Irregular periods and clinical or biochemical hyperandrogenism can indicate PCOS (when other causes are excluded, check TSH, prolactin and FSH). An ultrasound can support the diagnosis in adults (more than 8 years from menarche), but is not required if they already meet diagnostic criteria of irregular periods and clinical or biochemical hyperandrogenism).

Q7: A nulliparous 35-year-old presents with a 2-year history of mild cyclical pelvic pain with a recent onset of pain and bleeding on defecation commencing before menstruation.

The correct answer is D. Endometriosis.

Endometriosis is the presence of endometrial tissue outside the uterus. The cyclical dysmenorrhoea, rectal bleeding and dyschezia (pain on defecation) indicate endometriosis with involvement of the bowel. Ectopic endometrial tissue can react to the hormones produced in the HPO axis in the same way as non-ectopic tissue, causing chronic inflammation, fibrosis and adhesions. Rarely, involvement of other sites may cause cyclical haematuria, epistaxis and haemoptysis. In this scenario, colorectal causes of pain and bleeding, such as bowel cancer and inflammatory bowel disease, should also be investigated.

Q8: A 51-year-old presents to her primary care physician with a 13-month history of absent periods and palpitations, and she would also like to explore treatment for vaginal dryness.

The correct answer is G. Menopause.

The average age of menopause in the UK is 51. Physiological menopause occurs due to ovarian failure from a decline in functional oocytes and a reduction in gonadotropin effect on ovarian tissue. Decreased follicular activity results in increased levels of FSH and low levels of oestrogen and progesterone. Falling oestrogen levels can lead to the patient experiencing vasomotor symptoms (palpitations, hot flushes and night sweats), urogenital symptoms (vaginal dryness, dyspareunia, dysuria and increased urinary frequency), and osteoporosis, along with varying psychological symptoms (poor concentration, lethargy and irritability).

 Key Point

The climacteric describes the period where follicles fail to develop, representing declining fertility. Menopause is defined as permanent cessation of menstruation for at least 12 months after a period.

Important Learning Points

- The HPO axis involves the hypothalamus, pituitary and ovaries, and the interplay of the hormones GnRH, FSH, LH and oestrogen, as well as progesterone, inhibin and androgens.
- Menarche is the menses from a first menstrual cycle and represents the start of reproductive potential, whilst menopause is the termination of menstrual flow and represents the last menstrual cycle and the loss of reproductive potential.
- The menstrual cycle prepares the endometrium for implantation; if fertilisation does not occur, menses immediately follows.
- The proliferative phase occurs after the menstrual phase and comprises endometrial growth and an increase in spiral arteriole length as a result of oestrogen stimulation.
- The secretory phase follows the proliferative phase and comprises increased growth of endometrial glands and convolution of the spiral arterioles in preparation for implantation, as a result of progesterone stimulation.

PUBERTY

Q1: What is the most likely cause of her precocious puberty?

The correct answer is A. Central idiopathic precocious puberty.

This case highlights the presentation of precocious puberty in a 7-year-old girl with no demonstrable underlying pathology. This girl has some thelarche (development of breast tissue), pubarche (pubic and axillary hair development) and a growth spurt before her eighth birthday.

A ✔ **Central idiopathic precocious puberty – Correct.** Central precocious puberty results from hypothalamic GnRH-stimulated episodic gonadotropin secretion and is idiopathic in 80% of cases. A rise in LH and FSH increases the levels of oestrogen that lead to secondary sexual characteristic development.

B Congenital adrenal hyperplasia (CAH) – **Incorrect.** CAH is an example of peripheral precocious puberty, and whilst it potentially could be the cause, it is not the most likely cause and is therefore incorrect. Here, pubertal development is due to stimulation from a hormone which is not hypothalamic GnRH. The most common form of CAH, 21-alpha-hydroxylase deficiency, more commonly presents with virilisation.

C Head trauma – **Incorrect.** Head trauma is an example of a central nervous system (CNS) pathology related to the development of central precocious puberty.

D McCune-Albright syndrome – **Incorrect.** There were no other significant findings on examination. This syndrome is a genetic condition characterised by café au lait spots (hyperpigmented lesions), precocious puberty (primary ovarian cysts secrete oestradiol), polyostotic fibrous dysplasia (cystic bone growth replacing normal bone) and other endocrine disorders.

E Partial premature thelarche – **Incorrect.** The girl in the case had multiple early secondary sexual changes. There are three categories to early partial sexual development, depending on the development of that particular secondary sexual characteristic; these are premature thelarche, adrenarche and menarche.

Key Point

Other causes of CNS precocious puberty:
- Hypothalamic.
- Hamartoma – most common category of CNS tumour causing precocious puberty.
- Hydrocephalus.
- Haemorrhage.
- Infection.

Hypothyroidism is also a common cause, although technically not a CNS cause.

Complete precocious puberty has several causes. Other causes of endogenous peripheral precocious puberty, aside from CAH, include Cushing disease, testicular or ovarian malignancy. Exogenous oestrogen, for example from oral contraceptive pills, can also cause precocious puberty.

Q2: Which of the following regarding puberty are true or false?

Secondary sexual characteristics appear in 95% of girls between the age of 8.5 and 13 years. The average age for menarche is 12.8 years.

A Precocious puberty is the development of secondary sexual characteristics at less than 8 years old in girls and less than 10 in boys – **False.** Precocious puberty is defined as pubertal changes at less than 8 years in females and pubertal changes at less than 9 years in males.

B ✔ **The first sign of puberty in girls is thelarche – True.** The normal pattern of pubertal changes in females is thelarche, then pubarche, then a growth spurt and then menarche.

C The first sign of puberty in boys is pubarche – **False.** The first sign of puberty in boys is gonadarche. The average age of puberty in boys is 11.5 years and follows the sequence of: gonadarche (testicular enlargement), then pubarche (body hair growth), then adrenarche (facial hair and voice changes) and then a growth spurt. This highlights that girls get their growth spurt in an earlier stage of their pubertal changes, relative to boys.

D Pubic hair extending to the medial surface of the thigh indicates Tanner stage 4 development – **False.** Pubic hair extending to the medial surface of the thigh indicates Tanner stage 5.

E ✔ **One of the first-line investigations in precocious puberty is an x-ray of the wrist – True.** This is to assess the patient's bone age compared to their chronological age. If bone age is two or more years ahead of chronological age, this strongly supports the diagnosis of precocious puberty. Comparison of skeletal maturation with the child's height can be used to predict a final adult height.

Key Point

Puberty is the result of an increase in pulsatile secretion of LH because of an increase in pulsatile GnRH. The amplitude of GnRH pulses gradually increases throughout pubertal years and slowly increases the oestradiol levels.

Q3: Which of the following regarding delayed puberty are true or false?

Delayed puberty is pubertal development at an abnormally late age. The onset of breast development after 13.5 years in girls and increase in testicular volume in boys after 14 years are used as the cut-offs for delayed puberty.

A ✔ **Puberty is delayed if a girl has no breast bud development by 13 years of age – True.**

B Puberty is delayed if a girl has not had her first period by 14 years of age – **False.** If a girl has not had her first period by the age of 15, then puberty is considered to be delayed. Investigations include:
- Bloods – LH, FSH, TSH, androgen and oestrogen levels.
- Karyotype – looking for specific chromosomal abnormalities, most commonly Turner syndrome.
- Radiological – wrist x-ray for bone age and ultrasound scan to assess uterine size and any abnormal thickness.

C The most common cause of delayed puberty is chronic illness – **False**. The most common cause of delayed puberty is constitutional, therefore delayed activation of the HPO axis, which is synchronous for height and age. An important differential to rule out when considering constitutional delay in puberty is chronic illness, for example, cystic fibrosis.

D ✔ **Turner syndrome is a cause of delayed puberty – True**. Turner syndrome and Klinefelter syndrome (47XXY) are congenital causes of unresponsive gonads causing delayed puberty. Steroid hormone therapy and acquired gonadal damage, for example, trauma, chemotherapy and radiotherapy, are also causes of an 'unresponsive gonad' leading to delayed puberty.

E ✔ **Kallmann syndrome is associated with delayed puberty – True**. Kallmann syndrome (LHRH deficiency and anosmia), as well as Prader-Willi syndrome, are causes of delayed puberty because of 'failure of the HPO axis'. Other causes of 'failure of the HPO axis' include panhypopituitarism, hypothyroidism and intracranial tumours.

> 💬 **Key Point**
>
> Constitutional delay is the most common cause of delayed puberty, and measurement of gonadotropins (LH and FSH) helps greatly in classifying whether the aetiology is gonadal/primary hypogonadism (elevated LH and FSH) or hypothalamic/secondary hypogonadism (low or normal LH and FSH).

> 🔍 **Important Learning Points**
>
> * Puberty is the process of secondary sexual development brought forth through an increase in pulsatile secretion of LH, as a result of a gradual increase in pulsatile GnRH.
> * Tanner stages 1 to 5 classify the stage of female pubertal growth based on physical features.
> * In girls, pubertal changes are precocious if occurring before the age of eight or menarche before the age of 10.
> * Precocious puberty can be broadly classified into 'complete' and 'partial'.
> * In girls, pubertal changes are delayed if the onset of thelarche more than 13.5 or menarche more than 15 years of age.
> * Delayed puberty can be broadly classified into two groups depending on gonadotropin levels and the function of the HPO axis and the body's response to it.

DIFFERENCES OF SEXUAL DEVELOPMENT

Q1: The paediatrician suspects that Bethany has congenital adrenal hyperplasia (CAH). Which of the following tests would be most helpful to confirm the diagnosis?

The correct answer is A. 17-Hydroxyprogesterone (17-OHP).

These tests are all useful for diagnosing differences of sex developments (DSDs), although, if CAH is suspected, then the other tests can be used to rule out other conditions.

A ✔ **17-OHP – Correct.** The level of 17-OHP is drastically raised in people with CAH, as they are lacking the enzyme which converts this substrate into mineralocorticoids and glucocorticoids.

B Karyotype – **Incorrect.** People with CAH have 46 chromosomes. The genetic abnormality of the enzyme 21-hydroxylase would not be evident on a karyotype; more detailed genetic evaluation would be necessary to identify the abnormality.

C LH:FSH ratio – **Incorrect.** This ratio is sometimes used in the diagnosis of polycystic ovarian syndrome (PCOS). High levels of LH in these patients leads to a high LH:FSH ratio. A ratio of over three is suggestive, but not diagnostic, of PCOS, as one-third of people with the condition have a normal result. The more reliable test used in PCOS is the free androgen index.

D Thyroid stimulating hormone (TSH) – **Incorrect.** TSH is tested as part of a thyroid function test if hypothyroidism is a suspected cause of a person's abnormal development.

E Ultrasound scan of the pelvic organs – **Incorrect.** The internal pelvic organs are normal in CAH. It is only the external genitalia that are atypical, which can be easily visualised on clinical examination without a need for imaging.

> 💬 **Key Point**
>
> For babies who are more than 24 hours old, a 17-OHP level of 100 ng/dL or less is expected. In babies with CAH, the 17-OHP levels are in the range of 2000 to 40,000 ng/dL.

Q2: Answer true or false: Can surgery form an appropriate part of treatment for these conditions?
Surgery can be used to change the cosmetic appearance of the genitalia. It may also be necessary to allow normal healthy functioning of the reproductive system.

A Coeliac disease – **False.** Coeliac disease is not treated by surgical intervention. If the malnourishment which occurs as a result of coeliac disease is corrected by a gluten-free diet, then the patient's development should return to normal.

B ✔ **CAH – True.** Feminisation surgery can be offered to people who have developed with atypical genitalia. It is important to remember that the person will still have the underlying disease, so they will still need glucocorticoid therapy after the surgery is complete.

C Constitutional delay of growth and puberty – **False.** This is not a disease and should resolve by itself without treatment. The genitalia and reproductive tract are normal in this condition, so there is no place for surgical intervention.

D ✔ **Imperforate hymen – True.** Surgery is extremely important in this condition. If menstrual fluid is not able to flow out of the vagina successfully, the individual may experience severe pain and potentially infections. The operation is usually fairly simple and the standard is a hymenectomy.

E ✔ **Mayer-Rokitansky-Kuster-Hauser syndrome – True.** The vagina is shorter in this condition, meaning that sexual intercourse is usually impossible or very painful. Surgery to increase the size of the vagina may help in this condition but is very rarely used. Many people have success using dilators.

> 💬 **Key Point**
>
> Patients should be notified of the risks and benefits of all surgical treatment prior to obtaining consent. This is particularly important in cases of DSDs, as there are many psychological sequelae to these conditions. The clinician should ensure that the patient has realistic expectations for the results of the surgery.

Q3: Answer true or false: Do these conditions result from genetic abnormalities?

DSDs have many different causes. Identification of treatable causes is important to optimise the patient's treatment.

A Anorexia nervosa – **False.** Anorexia nervosa is an eating disorder in which the individual usually becomes extremely malnourished. This malnourishment can cause delayed pubertal development. Anorexia nervosa does not occur as a result of genetic abnormalities.

B ✔ **CAH – True.** The genetic abnormality here leads to a deficiency in the production of the enzyme 21-hydroxylase.

C Imperforate hymen – **False.** This is simply a structural abnormality. The hymen can form in many different configurations, but normally there is an opening which allows the passage of menses. In some cases, this opening does not form, causing the patient to have an imperforate hymen.

D Polycystic ovarian syndrome – **False.** PCOS is a condition of hormonal imbalance. Although it may appear to run in families, no clear genetic cause has been identified.

E ✔ **Turner syndrome – True.** Turner syndrome is also known as 45XO. It can be easily diagnosed by karyotyping the person, as the absent chromosome will become apparent.

> 💬 **Key Point**
>
> Turner syndrome key clinical features:
> - **C**oarctation of the aorta.
> - **L**ymphoedema.
> - **O**varies under developed.
> - **W**ebbed neck.
> - **N**ipples widely spaced.
> - **S**hort stature.

> 🔍 **Important Learning Points**
>
> - DSDs should be identified as early as possible in childhood.
> - Up to 2% of people have a DSD.
> - A multidisciplinary team (MDT) approach should be involved in the care of all individuals and their families.
> - Medication can be used to treat people with many different forms of DSDs.
> - Surgery may be necessary to improve the functioning as well as the cosmetic appearance of the genitalia.
> - People with a DSD can live very fulfilling lives and should be given as much support as possible to enable them to do so.
> - People with undescended gonads (e.g. CAIS, 5 alpha-reductase deficiency, gonadal dysgenesis, Turner's with Y fragment) carry a risk of malignancy and a gonadectomy is recommended.

SECONDARY AMENORRHOEA

Q1: For how many months would Marlena have to experience cessation of their regular menstruation for secondary amenorrhoea to be diagnosed?
The correct answer is B. Three months.

Secondary amenorrhoea in women who have previously had regular menstrual cycles is diagnosed if they have had no menstruation for 3 months. Six months is incorrect in this scenario, as this patient previously had regular periods. If a patient had previously suffered irregular periods, then a doctor would need to wait for 6 months before diagnosing secondary amenorrhoea.

> **Key Point**
>
> When diagnosing secondary amenorrhoea, it is fundamental to determine whether the patient had regular or irregular menstruation previously.

Q2: Answer true or false: Do causes of secondary amenorrhea include?

Pregnancy and menopause are the physiological causes of secondary amenorrhoea. Pathological causes either disrupt the normal function of the HPO axis or cause a physical obstruction to menstruation.

A ✔ **Anorexia nervosa – True.** Anorexia nervosa can cause hypothalamic dysfunction. Anorexia can cause inhibition of the GnRH pulse frequency and amplitude. High stress levels and exercise can also affect the GnRH pulse.

B ✔ **Asherman syndrome – True.** This is a rare cause of secondary amenorrhoea. It is characterised by intrauterine adhesions, usually caused by uterine surgery or infection, which disrupt normal endometrial function.

C Edward syndrome – **False.** Edward syndrome is also known as trisomy 18. It is a genetic condition with a chromosomal abnormality. Babies with this condition have a low survival rate due to many organ malformations and physical abnormalities.

D ✔ **Polycystic ovarian syndrome – True.** This syndrome is the cause of approximately a third of secondary amenorrhea cases. It is a heterogeneous disorder of hyperandrogenic chronic anovulation. There are strict criteria to diagnose the condition.

E Type 2 diabetes mellitus – **False.** Type 2 diabetes is a metabolic condition that is characterised by hyperglycaemia in the context of insulin resistance and insufficient insulin production. It is not a recognised cause of secondary amenorrhoea.

> **Key Point**
>
> When determining the cause of secondary amenorrhoea, exclude pregnancy or medication before performing investigations.

Q3: Answer true or false: Which factors are associated with a disturbance of ovulation?

Conditions which interact and inhibit the hormonal production of the hypothalamus, pituitary or ovary will potentially prevent ovulation from occurring.

A Asherman syndrome – **False.** This is a rare cause of secondary amenorrhoea. It causes a physical change that impairs menstruation due to intra-uterine adhesions. The syndrome has no effect on ovulation.

B Family history of diabetes mellitus – **False.** Diabetes has no effect on the HPO axis; it is a metabolic condition characterised by hyperglycaemia. The condition can be asymptomatic, but patients may complain of polyuria and polydipsia.

C Hypertension – **False.** When assessing a woman presenting with ovulatory disturbance, it is always important to take a full medical history to elicit risk factors and general health. However, hypertension has no effect on ovulation.

D ✔ **Prolactin secreting pituitary adenoma – True.** Prolactin is a hormone produced in the anterior pituitary gland and has a primary role in lactation. However, hyperprolactinaemia disrupts the menstrual cycle as well as causing galactorrhoea. Hyperprolactinaemia can be physiological in women who are breastfeeding or pregnant.

E ✔ **Turner syndrome – True.** Turner syndrome, or 45XO, is a genetic condition characterised by a chromosomal abnormality. Women with this condition usually experience amenorrhoea and infertility due to ovarian insufficiency. Small ovaries seen on imaging are classically described as streak gonads. Many women with Turner syndrome present with primary amenorrhoea, but some will have some initial ovarian function and then present later with secondary amenorrhoea.

> **Key Point**
>
> Oligomenorrhoea is defined as menstruation occurring at intervals of greater than 35 days, with fewer than nine periods per year. In women with oligomenorrhoea, secondary amenorrhoea is likely to occur due to the hormonal changes that occur. Hormone imbalances can seriously affect ovulation, especially imbalances of hormones from the thyroid, pituitary, adrenals and ovaries.

Q4: A 35-year-old presents with secondary amenorrhoea. Which would be your initial investigation?
The correct answer is H. Serum β hCG.

The commonest cause of secondary amenorrhoea is pregnancy. Any patient who reports secondary amenorrhoea should have a pregnancy test to rule this out as a cause. If the test is negative, then a full history and examination should be undertaken, with further investigations. Usually, a urine pregnancy test is sufficient, but the best option in the set provided is serum β hCG.

Q5: A 29-year-old attends the clinic with secondary amenorrhea. They have recently been experiencing headaches and, after visiting their optician, have been diagnosed with bitemporal hemianopia. On questioning, it is revealed that they have also been experiencing some nipple discharge. What is the most likely cause of the symptoms?
The correct answer is G. Prolactin secreting pituitary adenoma.

This patient has some classical symptoms of a pituitary tumour. Due to the location of the pituitary and the optic chiasm, visual disturbances can occur, commonly blurred vision or visual field defects. The patient is experiencing galactorrhoea due to the high levels of prolactin secreted by the adenoma. It is important with any patient with galactorrhoea to check that she is on no medication that can raise prolactin levels, such as dopamine antagonists, selective serotonin reuptake inhibitors, beta blockers, methyldopa, combined oral contraceptives and spironolactone.

Q6: A 32-year-old woman attends the clinic with secondary amenorrhoea. Four years ago, she had her first pregnancy, which was uneventful. She and her partner are trying for a second child but they have experienced some difficulty. She has not menstruated for 8 months and she has a complex past medical history. She had an incomplete termination when she was 16 years old, which required dilation and curettage. She also underwent a difficult hysteroscopy 3 years ago, which diagnosed uterine fibroids, and surgical management of a miscarriage 1 year ago. She is not breastfeeding her child. What is the most likely diagnosis?

The correct answer is A. Asherman syndrome.

This is a rare cause of secondary amenorrhoea. Uterine procedures, such as dilation and curettage, can predispose to uterine adhesions that interfere with normal uterine functioning, leading to secondary amenorrhoea. In income poor countries, pelvic tuberculosis is also a leading cause of Asherman syndrome.

Q7: An 18-year-old attends the clinic with secondary amenorrhea. They have always had irregular menstruation but noticed that it has ceased over the last year. They report weight gain despite exercising and reportedly eating a healthy diet. They have been diagnosed with type 2 diabetes and there is a family history of obesity, diabetes and hypertension. What is the most likely diagnosis?

The correct answer is F. Polycystic ovarian syndrome.

This patient has all of the characteristic features of PCOS. PCOS is a heterogeneous disorder of secondary amenorrhoea; its incidence in high income countries is increasing.

Key Point

Secondary amenorrhoea has many causes, and systematic investigation is needed. Referral to other specialities for management may be indicated, especially if the cause is endocrine, pituitary or hypothalamic.

Important Learning Points

- Secondary amenorrhoea is characterised depending on whether a patient had previously regular or irregular menstruation.
- Pregnancy and menopause are the commonest causes of secondary amenorrhoea.
- It is vital to determine the specific cause, as some causes can lead to infertility and require specialist management.

POLYCYSTIC OVARIAN SYNDROME

Q1: Answer true or false: Can these conditions be a long-term consequence of PCOS?

There are many long term consequences that are associated with PCOS. The disorder is characterised by hyperandrogenic anovulation.

A ✔ **Dyslipidaemia – True.** Women with PCOS have lifelong lipid metabolic dysfunction. If their diet and exercise regimes are not controlled, there is significant risk of cardiovascular disease. For those women at high risk, lipid-lowering medications can be given to normalise the dyslipidaemia.

B ✔ **Endometrial hyperplasia – True.** Women with PCOS are at an increased risk of developing endometrial hyperplasia and carcinoma. This is because they have high levels of unopposed oestrogen. Prolonged unopposed oestrogen exposure causes endometrial stimulation and leads to abnormal endometrial glandular proliferation and dysplasia.

C Hyperthyroidism – **False.** Hyperthyroidism is not associated with PCOS. Hypothyroidism is, however, a differential that should be considered when diagnosing PCOS.

D Myasthenia gravis – **False.** Myasthenia gravis is an autoimmune neuromuscular disease that leads to muscle weakness and fatigability. It is associated with other autoimmune diseases, such as type 1 DM, rheumatoid arthritis and thyroid disease. It is also associated with premature ovarian failure.

E ✔ **Type 2 DM – True.** PCOS is associated with insulin resistance and high levels of circulating insulin. Women are at high risk of developing impaired glucose tolerance and type 2 DM, particularly those with a family history of these illnesses.

Key Point

There are many long-term consequences related to having PCOS, including diabetes, cardiovascular disease, sleep apnoea and infertility. Patients should be informed of these potential consequences at the time of diagnosis of PCOS, and given management strategies to reduce their individual risk.

Q2: Answer true or false regarding these statements relating to polycystic ovarian syndrome.

The management of PCOS is often multifactorial, with treatment regimens that should be individualised to offer the optimum care to each patient.

A ✔ **PCOS can be diagnosed even in the presence of no ovarian cysts – True.** The criteria for the diagnosis of PCOS require two of the following:
- Oligomenorrhoea or amenorrhoea.
- Clinical and/or biochemical manifestations of hyperandrogenism.
- Polycystic ovaries and/or ovarian enlargement on ultrasound.

B ✔ **Complications include infertility and gestational diabetes mellitus (GDM) – True.** Other complications include psychological effects from acne and hirsutism and endometrial cancer.

C Anti-androgens are a safe treatment for a woman with PCOS-associated hirsutism who is also trying to conceive – **False.** Anti-androgens must be used with extreme caution due to their teratogenicity. Women should be counselled regarding these risks and use contraception during treatment.

D Weight loss has only a small effect on the course of PCOS – **False.** Weight loss is the most effective management for PCOS symptoms (in an overweight patient) and has been shown to improve fertility as well as glucose metabolism.

E In patients with oligomenorrhoea or amenorrhoea, it is recommended that withdrawal bleeds be induced every 3 to 4 months due to the risk of ovarian cancer – **False.** Withdrawal bleeds should be induced to decrease the risk of endometrial cancer.

Key Point

PCOS is characterised by irregular periods with clinical and/or biochemical hyperandrogenism. Management is varied and often involves a combination of treatments according to the patient's prime symptoms.

Q3: Which drug can cause hyperkalaemia, ataxia and renal impairment?

The correct answer is L. Spironolactone.

Spironolactone is a synthetic anti-mineralocorticoid with weak anti-androgen and progestogen properties. It is used primarily as a diuretic and antihypertensive, but it is commonly used in PCOS. It is a treatment primarily for hair growth, not to assist in fertility or to regulate menstruation. Spironolactone is indicated as it effectively treats the symptoms of hyperandrogenism found in PCOS. It has many side effects, including urinary frequency, gynaecomastia, hyperkalaemia, ataxia and menstrual irregularity.

Q4: Which drug offers endometrial protection?

The correct answer is C. Combined oral contraceptive.

Women who use oral contraceptives have been shown to have a reduced risk of endometrial cancer. The protective effect of these drugs increases with time and also provides protection for several years after a woman stops taking the drug. Some of the combined oral contraceptives also have anti-androgen effects, which can improve symptoms of acne and hirsutism.

Q5: Which drug can cause hot flushes, mood disturbance and ovarian enlargement?

The correct answer is B. Clomifene citrate.

Clomifene is a selective oestrogen receptor modulator that increases the production of gonadotropins by inhibiting negative feedback on the hypothalamus. Clomifene is used to induce ovulation. It has several side effects, including vasomotor responses, blurred vision, reversible ovarian enlargement, ovarian hyperstimulation syndrome and abdominal discomfort.

Q6: Which drugs can be used topically to treat hirsutism?

The correct answer is E. Eflornithine.

This medication is a cream indicated for the topical treatment of hirsutism. Studies have demonstrated that when applied twice a day, the drug slows the rate of facial hair growth by interacting with cell division and proliferation in the hair follicle.

 Key Point

Medical management of PCOS can be divided into:
- Medication to improve insulin sensitivity.
- Medication to improve ovulation induction.
- Medication to assist in regular menstruation.
- Medication to treat the effects of hyperandrogenism.

 Important Learning Points

- PCOS, a common endocrine disorder in women, is characterised by hirsutism, menstrual irregularities and infertility.
- Several hormone imbalances are associated with PCOS. High levels of circulating androgens cause many of the signs and symptoms, such as hirsutism and acne.
- PCOS is a diagnosis of exclusion; however, criteria assist with the diagnosis. These are: oligomenorrhoea or amenorrhoea, clinical and/or biochemical manifestations of hyperandrogenism and observation of polycystic ovaries on ultrasound.
- The mainstay of management is achieving a healthy BMI; this not only improves insulin resistance but helps reduce circulating unopposed oestrogen.
- PCOS has numerous long-term consequences, including diabetes and cardiovascular disease.

INFERTILITY

Q1: A 35-year-old woman presents to the infertility clinic. On history taking, she says she has always had irregular periods. She has a BMI of 30 kg/m².

The correct answer is A. Day 21 progesterone levels.

The first-line investigation is day 21 progesterone, especially with irregular periods, to check if the patient is ovulating. Progesterone levels rise following ovulation, preparing the uterus for implantation following fertilisation. Based on the raised BMI and irregular periods, the most likely cause of infertility is PCOS. When ovulation is not confirmed, further investigations include LH, FSH, testosterone, sex hormone binding globulin (SHBG), prolactin, cortisol and TSH to help identify a cause for anovulation.

Q2: A 34-year-old woman is referred by her primary care physician, as she has had difficulty conceiving for the last year. On further questioning of her past obstetric history, she reveals that she has had one successful pregnancy 20 years ago. She has also been previously investigated with laparoscopy for chronic pelvic pain and was given a diagnosis of endometriosis. A test has confirmed she is ovulating.

The correct answer is D. Hysterosalpingo-contrast sonography (HyCoSy).

The previous successful pregnancy and normal day 21 progesterone point to a likely disorder of fertilisation. She has a diagnosis of endometriosis. Chronic inflammation in the pelvis from conditions such as endometriosis or PID can cause adhesions and impair the patency of fallopian tubes. A HyCoSy can demonstrate tubal patency. If occlusion is suspected following this test, a laparoscopy and dye test can be offered to confirm the diagnosis, and where possible, to treat the condition.

Q3: A 30-year-old woman presents with difficulties conceiving. On further consultation, she reports she has regular periods, but has suffered with menorrhagia and dysmenorrhea for many years and is on ferrous sulphate

for anaemia. Tests have confirmed she is ovulating and has patent fallopian tubes, however, there was a possible abnormality identified within the uterine cavity.

The correct answer is C. Hysteroscopy.

The above correlates with a uterine abnormality such as polyps or fibroids, which would be identified with HyCoSy or om transvaginal ultrasound. Depending on their size and site within the uterus, fibroids could affect the process of fertilisation or implantation. Here, the menorrhagia is so significant that it has resulted in anaemia. A hysteroscopy is a camera inserted into the womb. If a polyp or fibroid is identified, it can be removed under direct vision.

Q4: A 28-year-old man and his wife present with difficulty conceiving. His wife has previously conceived; however, he has not. When asking for past genitourinary history, he mentions that he had previously suffered from epididymo-orchitis, which was treated with antibiotics.

The correct answer is G. Semen analysis.

Inflammation from epididymo-orchitis may have caused adhesions that have blocked outflow from the testes or may have damaged sperm production. Semen analysis may show oligospermia or azoospermia. If azoospermia is shown, normal FSH levels will strongly suggest obstructive azoospermia, confirmed by a testicular biopsy showing normal sperm development. If oligospermia is confirmed, rule out a treatable endocrine pathology as a cause.

Q5: A 29-year-old man attends a follow-up appointment for the results of his initial investigation for subfertility. It showed that he has aspermia.

The correct answer is F. Post ejaculatory urinalysis.

This patient's semen analysis result has shown no sperm and no seminal fluid. This indicates a problem at or beyond the prostate. The most common cause for this is retrograde ejaculation, where the ejaculate travels into the bladder rather than being expelled out of the body. Prostate surgery and medications such as tamsulosin are the most common iatrogenic causes for this, but it can also occur with spinal injury and multiple sclerosis.

 Key Point

The key initial first-line investigations for female subfertility are day 21 progesterone, and hysterosalpingo-contrast sonography (HyCoSy). The key investigation for men is semen analysis. Finding abnormal results for these investigations will lead to further investigations to identify and treat any cause of subfertility.

Q6: Answer true or false to the following statements.

Anovulation is the most commonly identified cause of subfertility in females. The most common underlying condition is PCOS. Various treatments are available which improve fertility rates by increasing the likelihood of ovulation.

A Surgical ablation of endometriosis is as effective as IVF in improving fertility rates in woman with endometriosis. – **False.** Treatment to destroy or remove endometrial deposits may improve fertility rates, but this is not as effective as IVF. In severe endometriosis, treatment of the deposits may reduce inflammation within the pelvis and improve IVF treatment success.

B ✔ **Metformin is a first-line medical management for subfertility in woman with PCOS – True.** Metformin can be used as a first-line agent or can be used with clomifene as second-line treatment. Clomifene can also be used first line instead of metformin, or they can both be used together.

C Clomifene is an oestrogen receptor modulator that works by increasing oestrogen levels to increase GnRH levels – **False.** Clomifene works by binding to oestrogen receptors in the hypothalamus. This decreases the negative feedback effect of oestrogen, resulting in increased GnRH and FSH levels, and thereby increasing follicle development.

D ✔ **Ovarian drilling is used in clomifene-resistant PCOS – True.** Drilling aims to reduce the androgen-producing ovarian stroma to restore normal ovarian function in those who are not successful with clomifene; this results in ovulation in 80% of cases.

E Letrozole is a competitive reversible agonist of testosterone – **False.** It is a competitive reversible aromatase inhibitor which blocks the conversion of testosterone to oestrogen. This reduces oestrogen levels, which then leads to less negative feedback by oestrogen on the hypothalamus, thereby increasing FSH stimulation of the ovary. Letrozole is an alternative treatment to clomifene, but it is not commonly used as it is less effective.

 Key Point

Clomifene and metformin are the first-line treatments for anovulation. Surgical treatment for anovulation can be of benefit if these medications fail. Other surgical treatments for infertility are less effective, with IVF often being a better treatment option.

Q7: Answer true or false to the following statements.

IVF is the most commonly performed assisted reproductive technique. Each cycle has a 30% chance of ending with a live baby. It is commonly offered to patients with unexplained infertility, or after treatment has failed where a cause for infertility is known.

A ✔ **For IUI, sperm samples can be obtained from post-ejaculatory urinalysis – True.** Sperm can be extracted from a urinalysis sample and prepared for use in IUI.

B After an IVF cycle, remaining embryos are disposed of – **False.** Remaining viable embryos can be frozen for further IVF attempts.

C ✔ **For egg collection in IVF, ovaries are stimulated with daily FSH injections to produce multiple follicles – True.** This process is done over 12 days and monitored with ultrasound scanning for OHSS.

D After egg collection in IVF, oestrogen pessaries are used to prepare the endometrium for embryo transfer – **False.** Progesterone prepares the endometrium for implantation, and the same applies during IVF, where this is done via artificial means, for example, by progesterone pessaries, gels and injections.

E The success of IVF is not age related – **False.** The success of IVF decreases with female age due to the reduction in the number and quality of the remaining oocytes.

> 💬 **Key Point**
>
> Assisted reproductive techniques are used when conservative, medical and surgical interventions are ineffective, with IVF providing the most successful pregnancy outcome. However, IVF requires a lot of medications to stimulate the ovaries to collect eggs and then maintain the uterus for implantation. It requires motivated patients to attend the frequent hospital visits and to take medications correctly.

Q8: Answer true or false to the following statements.

Ovarian hyperstimulation can occur with any treatment used to stimulate ovulation. It is most likely to occur and most likely to result in a severe case following ovarian stimulation for egg collection for assisted reproductive techniques such as IVF. Ovarian hyperstimulation syndrome (OHSS) requires hospital admission for management in severe cases, which occurs in about 1% of patients undergoing egg collection.

A ✔ **Multiple pregnancy rates are reduced by single embryo transfer – True.** There has been a drive to reduce the risk of twin and higher-order pregnancies as these pregnancies pose more complications than singleton pregnancies. Where possible, clinicians are advised to only transfer one embryo to the uterus each cycle.

B ✔ **OHSS is more common in women with PCOS – True.** Patients with polycystic ovaries (20% to 33% of normal women) are at risk, as well as those with PCOS. Assessing the ovarian size and number of follicles on ultrasound prior to starting ovarian stimulation can help minimise the dose of gonadotropins, thereby limiting the risk of hyperstimulation.

C Tense ascites, reduced haematocrit and bleeding are initial signs of critical OHSS – **False.** Critical OHSS is caused by significant vascular permeability causing third space fluid shifts (tense ascites) and intravascular dehydration (demonstrated by a raised haematocrit). The highly concentrated intravascular blood is in a hypercoagulable state, increasing the risk of thromboembolism, not bleeding.

D Diuretics are key in the management of OHSS – **False.** Avoid diuretics as they may deplete intravascular volume, worsening the clinical situation.

E ✔ **OHSS has a risk of ovarian torsion – True.** Due to ovarian enlargement, the ovary has a risk of twisting around its pedicle, constricting the blood supply. This presents with worsening unilateral pain, nausea and a raised white cell count (WCC). If available, colour Doppler ultrasound may help to diagnose ovarian torsion. However, if there is a delay in arranging the investigation, the patient should be presumed to have torsion and be taken to the theatre urgently to prevent necrosis of the ovary.

> 💬 **Key Point**
>
> OHSS is an important complication of fertility treatment to be aware of, as it results in further complications such as renal failure, thromboembolism and ovarian torsion. Fluid balance is key to management, and escalation to the intensive treatment unit (ITU) should be considered if abnormalities persist.

> 🔍 **Important Learning Points**
>
> - Infertility is defined as a failure to conceive after frequent unprotected intercourse two or three times a week for 12 months. It affects one in seven heterosexual couples.
> - The most common risk factor is maternal age.
> - Ovulatory disorders are the most common cause of female infertility.
> - Clomifene is the most common medical treatment used for anovulation.
> - Surgical management is beneficial in some cases of female infertility, but IVF is usually a better treatment option, with a better pregnancy outcome.
> - Day 21 progesterone and HyCoSy are the key initial investigations of female infertility.
> - Altered spermatogenesis is the most common cause of male infertility. Semen analysis is the gold standard investigation for male infertility.
> - Prognosis depends on patient age, cause of infertility and response to management.

3 EARLY PREGNANCY COMPLICATIONS

HYPEREMESIS GRAVIDARUM

The following medications can be used in the management of hyperemesis gravidarum. To what class of drug do they belong?

Q1: Cyclizine.
The correct answer is D. Histamine H1 receptor antagonist.

Cyclizine acts on the chemoreceptor trigger zone (CTZ) of the brain. It can be given per oral (PO), intramuscular injection (IM) or intravenous (IV). Like other antihistamine medications, the most common side effect is drowsiness. Cyclizine also has some antimuscarinic properties with less common side effects, including dry mouth, constipation and urinary retention.

Q2: Metoclopramide.

The correct answer is B. Dopamine receptor antagonist.

Metoclopramide has its dominant effect on increasing gastric emptying, thereby reducing the volume of food in the stomach and leading to less regurgitation. It also increases the tone of the lower oesophageal sphincter and has some effect on the CTZ. Rare but important side effects of metoclopramide are focal dystonias and oculogyric crisis. These are most common in women under the age of 25, so in this age group, it is sensible to use alternative antiemetics where possible.

Q3: Omeprazole.

The correct answer is H. Irreversible proton pump inhibitor.

Omeprazole inhibits the hydrogen ion (H⁺) active transport mechanism of the H⁺/K⁺ ATPase (proton pump), thereby reducing acid secretion by up to 90%. It is a very well-tolerated medication, with only mild side effects.

Q4: Ondansetron.

The correct answer is L. Serotonin 5-HT3 receptor antagonist.

Ondansetron is highly selective for the 5-HT3 receptors. As a result, there are few side effects associated with it, the most common being constipation and headaches. Its mechanism of action in hyperemesis is primarily on the serotonin receptors of the CTZ. In response to the ingestion of toxic substances, the small intestine releases serotonin, which activates the afferent nerve fibres of the vomiting reflex. Ondansetron also blocks these peripheral receptors, and it is thought these may play a key role in its mechanism of action in controlling vomiting following chemotherapy.

Q5: Prochlorperazine.

The correct answer is B. Dopamine receptor antagonist.

Prochlorperazine is a centrally acting dopamine receptor antagonist that primarily reduces nausea and vomiting by acting on the CTZ. It is also commonly used as a treatment of vertigo in labyrinthitis, and can also be used as an antipsychotic. Dopamine antagonists can worsen Parkinson's symptoms and rarely can cause pseudoparkinsonism and other extrapyramidal side effects in healthy individuals. Dopamine receptor antagonists can also raise prolactin levels and rarely induce lactation by blocking the normal inhibition of dopamine on the anterior pituitary.

Q6: Promethazine.

The correct answer is D. Histamine H1 receptor antagonist.

Promethazine has a similar mechanism of action to cyclizine. It also has some anticholinergic effects and has some antagonist effect on dopamine receptors. It has similar side effects to cyclizine but is more likely to cause confusion in an elderly patient and sedation. In pregnancy, NICE also support its use as a sedative for short-term use for patients with difficulty sleeping.

 Key Point

It is important to be familiar with common medications used in the management of hyperemesis. By understanding their mechanisms of action, it is much easier to recall their common side effects and interactions. When one medication is not adequately controlling a symptom, with good pharmaceutical knowledge it is easy to select multiple medications to treat the same symptom by different mechanisms.

Q7: Which of the following is the major cause of hyperemesis gravidarum?

The correct answer is B. β hCG.

Hyperemesis is a common early pregnancy complication. Nausea and vomiting are common symptoms which need treating in all areas of medicine besides O&G, so a thorough understanding of the medications discussed here, and the receptors they act on is important for any clinician.

A Mass effect of the uterus pressing on the bowel and stomach. – **Incorrect.** Hyperemesis occurs in the first trimester. At 12 weeks, the uterus is usually only just palpable above the pubic symphysis and so is not large enough to cause compression of the intestine and stomach to cause vomiting. Later in pregnancy, the enlarging uterus can have an effect on respiration due to increased pressure abdominally, which pushes up on the diaphragm.

B ✔ **β hCG affecting the vomiting centres of the brain. – Correct.** β hCG is produced by the placenta. It is at its highest concentration in maternal blood in the first trimester, between weeks 8 and 12 gestation, when most cases of hyperemesis present. It is thought to have a direct effect on the CTZ and vomiting centres of the midbrain, resulting in nausea and vomiting. Cyclizine, promethazine and prochlorperazine predominantly have their effects on these central nervous system areas.

C Progesterone relaxing the lower oesophageal sphincter – **Incorrect.** This is likely to have an effect on acid reflux and thereby contribute to hyperemesis but is not the most prominent cause. Omeprazole can reduce acid production and therefore decrease acid reflux symptoms.

D Oestrogen delaying gastric emptying – **Incorrect.** Like progesterone, this is likely to have an effect but is not the prominent cause. Metoclopramide is a dopamine antagonist which increases gastric emptying, so it may improve this aspect of hyperemesis.

E Insulin-like growth factor (IGF1) causing insulin resistance and ketoacidosis – **Incorrect.** There is no evidence IGF has any effect on hyperemesis. It is, however, very important in fetal growth.

Key Point

Hyperemesis gravidarum is likely to have multifactorial causation, including genetic, physical, biochemical, hormonal and psychological elements. However, high levels of hCG are thought to be the most important cause of symptoms.

Q8: Answer true or false to these statements regarding hyperemesis gravidarum.

Simple investigations including urinalysis. FBC and U&Es can help a clinician to easily differentiate patients with hyperemesis gravidarum with significant dehydration requiring intensive management from those with emesis of pregnancy.

A ✓ Ketonuria supports the diagnosis of hyperemesis – True. Recurrent nausea and vomiting cause a patient to lose her appetite and stop eating as ingestion of food and drink can increase the frequency of vomiting. Lack of nutrients, in particular glucose, causes the body's metabolic pathways to change adenosine triphosphate (ATP) production from glycolysis to gluconeogenesis and ketogenesis. The resultant ketone bodies are excreted in the urine. A common misunderstanding, even among practising clinicians, is that rehydration corrects ketonuria. However, this is not the case. Once the patient restarts eating, ketogenesis and gluconeogenesis stop and glycolysis restarts. Ketones are no longer produced, so they are no longer excreted in the urine.

B ✓ A raised haematocrit is a common investigation result in hyperemesis gravidarum – True. The haematocrit is the concentration of red blood cells in a blood sample. Dehydration results in decreased water in the intravascular space, so the concentration of cells increases, resulting in a raised haematocrit. In pregnancy, plasma expansion occurs naturally and decreases the concentration of red cells, causing a physiological anaemia and decreased haematocrit. It is important to remember that both dehydration and pregnancy are independent risk factors for venous thromboembolism (VTE), so patients with hyperemesis should have thromboprophylaxis as part of their management.

C ✓ Ultrasound scanning should form part of first-line investigations in hyperemesis to diagnose molar pregnancies – True. Hyperemesis is caused by raised β hCG levels. B hCG is made by the placenta; therefore, a large placenta produces high concentrations of β hCG and can cause severe symptoms. The two conditions identified on early ultrasound scans that can cause elevated β hCG levels are molar pregnancy and twin pregnancy. Twin pregnancy results in a physiologically enlarged amount of placental tissue. The diagnosis of twin pregnancy is not essential before the routine 12-week gestation examination, but it can occasionally be helpful in identifying whether the pregnancy is monoamniotic or diamniotic. It is

important, however, to diagnose and treat molar pregnancy as quickly as possible to improve the patient's survival rate.

D Pregnancies troubled by hyperemesis are more likely to end in miscarriage – False. Actually, hyperemesis appears to be associated with fewer miscarriages than occur in the general population. It is thought that hyperemesis is a sign of high β hCG levels and good placental function.

E Hyperemesis commonly presents in the second trimester – False. Hyperemesis usually presents in the first trimester. The β hCG levels are highest around 8 to 12 weeks' gestation and they drop in the second trimester, so most patients' symptoms resolve by 16 weeks' gestation.

Key Point

The investigation results of a patient with hyperemesis will show biochemical investigation results similar to any patient undergoing starvation. Knowledge of the likely abnormalities for these investigations will help when treating patients with starvation in other specialities. Understanding the process of ketone formation will also be of particular use in managing diabetic ketoacidosis.

Important Learning Points

- Hyperemesis gravidarum is a common early pregnancy complication, which is often self-limiting and resolves by around 16 weeks' gestation.
- Treatment is simple, with most cases improving with a single antiemetic. Knowledge of the different antiemetics and their mechanism of action are essential when prescribing multiple medications to optimise patient condition.
- As well as antiemetic treatment, rehydration, thiamine supplements and antacids are the other treatment modalities.

MOLAR PREGNANCY

Q1: Which of these would be the single most useful investigation to diagnose a molar pregnancy?
The correct answer is A. Abdominal ultrasound scan.

Clinical examination and investigations can lead to a suspected diagnosis of molar pregnancy. The diagnosis and the type of molar pregnancy can only be confirmed on histology.

A ✔ Abdominal ultrasound scan – Correct. Classically, scans will show excessive placental tissue, with cystic spaces in the placenta. The appearance may be described as 'a bunch or grapes' or 'a snowstorm'.

B Analysis of partner's semen – Incorrect. Molar pregnancies are caused by the presence of two copies of paternal DNA in the ovum. Semen analysis will not give any information as to whether this has occurred in this particular pregnancy. Semen analysis is usually only performed when assessing for a male cause of subfertility.

C Serum β hCG – **Incorrect.** A very high β hCG level can be suggestive of an underlying molar pregnancy. However, a twin pregnancy, or a pregnancy at a higher gestation than expected could lead to a higher than expected β hCG level.

D Serum human placental lactogen – **Incorrect.** This is a hormone produced by the placenta. It is not routinely tested for in pregnancy and knowing the level would have no bearing on the diagnosis of a molar pregnancy.

E Urine β hCG – **Incorrect.** This test is the most commonly used test to confirm or exclude the presence of an early pregnancy. It cannot differentiate between the types of pregnancy.

> ### Key Point
> β hCG is useful to confirm that a pregnancy exists, and a high level increases the suspicion of a molar pregnancy. However, pelvic ultrasound is the most commonly used investigation to diagnose molar pregnancy. The diagnosis is then confirmed on histology.

Q2: Which one of these statements is correct regarding a partial molar pregnancy?
The correct answer is A. Fetal tissue may be seen on an ultrasound scan.

A ✔ **Fetal tissue may be seen on ultrasound scan – Correct.** Some fetal tissue may develop in a partial molar pregnancy. There would be no fetal tissue in a complete molar pregnancy.

B Most commonly diagnosed after the birth of an otherwise healthy baby – **Incorrect.** Molar pregnancies occur in 1:700 pregnancies. They are almost exclusively diagnosed in early pregnancy, presenting with vaginal bleeding or hyperemesis. In rare asymptomatic cases, a dating scan, arranged at 12 weeks gestation in the UK, would identify the molar pregnancy.

C It contains 46 chromosomes – **Incorrect.** Partial molar pregnancies are created by two sperm with 23 chromosomes each entering an ovum containing maternal DNA (23 chromosomes). These all combine to create a developing embryo, in which each cell contains 69 chromosomes.

D It is caused by two sperm entering an empty ovum – **Incorrect.** A partial mole is created by two sperm entering an egg containing maternal DNA. A complete mole is caused by two sperm (or one sperm which self-replicates) entering an empty egg. Complete molar pregnancies have 46 chromosomes, but these are all paternal in origin.

E Chemotherapy treatment is likely to be offered after a partial molar pregnancy – **Incorrect.** Surgical evacuation of molar pregnancies is a curative procedure in the majority of cases. Only 15% of complete molar pregnancies and 0.5% of partial molar pregnancies require chemotherapy.

> ### Key Point
> Molar pregnancies are mostly identified in early pregnancy. They are caused by 46 chromosomes of paternal origin being present in the ovum.

Q3: What is the approximate 5-year survival after treatment of a molar pregnancy?
The correct answer is E. Over 99%.

The overall cure rate for molar pregnancies is over 99%. In patients who have severe high-stage disease or gestational choriocarcinoma, the 5-year survival rate is still over 90%. The reason the cure rate from these conditions is so high is that usually these pregnancies are symptomatic early in their development and are surgically removed. Even in cases where tissue remains after surgery, due to the rapid growth of the tissues, they are extremely susceptible to chemotherapy.

> ### Key Point
> Molar pregnancy responds well to chemotherapy if it is required. It has an overall cure rate approaching 100%.

> ### Important Learning Points
> - Molar pregnancies are an uncommon complication of pregnancy (1:700 pregnancies).
> - They usually present in early pregnancy with bleeding or hyperemesis.
> - Diagnosis is made by ultrasound scan.
> - Surgical evacuation of the uterus is the first-line management, after which products of conception are sent to histology to confirm the diagnosis.
> - Follow-up is required in all cases.
> - Chemotherapy is required in 5% of cases, with an overall cure rate of 99%.

ECTOPIC PREGNANCY

Q1: Given this presentation, what would be the most suitable investigation?
The correct answer is E. Transvaginal ultrasound.

This patient has symptoms suggestive of an ectopic pregnancy. The most common symptoms of an ectopic pregnancy are lower abdominal pain, vaginal bleeding and a missed period. It is important to remember that some ectopic pregnancies will present before a period has been missed. The positive urine β hCG test supports this diagnosis, as a negative urine β hCG test would exclude any type of pregnancy. β hCG is a hormone produced by the trophoblast cells of a fertilised egg. Its initial function is to stop the breakdown of the corpus luteum so that progesterone continues to be produced to maintain the lining of the uterus.

A transvaginal ultrasound (TVUS) would be the most useful investigation to carry out when an ectopic pregnancy is suspected. The TVUS looks for any evidence of an intrauterine pregnancy such as:

- Gestational sac.
- Yolk sac.
- Fetal pole and heartbeat.

A Abdominal CT scan – **Incorrect.** An abdominal CT scan would not be a suitable first-line investigation in a woman with a positive pregnancy test due to the levels of radiation the pregnancy would be exposed to.

B Abdominal ultrasound – **Incorrect.** Abdominal ultrasound would not be as accurate in the identification of an ectopic pregnancy as a transvaginal scan would, as it is more difficult to fully evaluate the adnexae, particularly in obese patients. It may sometimes be appropriate for women who find transvaginal ultrasound unacceptable after the limitations of abdominal ultrasound are discussed with them.

C Abdominal x-ray – **Incorrect.** An abdominal x-ray would not be a suitable first-line investigation in a pregnant woman and would offer little value for the diagnosis of ectopic pregnancy.

D Progesterone level – **Incorrect.** Low progesterone levels can indicate non-viable pregnancies but would not give any indication of the location of the pregnancy.

E ✔ **Transvaginal ultrasound – Correct.** The TVUS will look for the presence of any of the above signs of pregnancy outside of the uterus – for example, in the adnexae (the fallopian tubes and the ovaries) – which would point towards the diagnosis of an ectopic pregnancy. The ultrasound scan will also look for any free fluid, which may suggest intra-abdominal bleeding caused by a ruptured ectopic pregnancy.

💬 **Key Point**

A TVUS combined with serum β hCG measurement will allow you to make a confident diagnosis of ectopic pregnancy in most women, without having to resort to laparoscopy.

Q2: Which of these is not a risk factor for ectopic pregnancy?

The correct answer is A. Combined oral contraceptive pill (COCP).

Most of the risk factors can be recalled simply by remembering that they cause damage to the fallopian tubes, preventing the successful transfer of the fertilised blastocyst from the fertilisation site within the tube to the correct implantation site within the uterus.

A ✔ **Combined oral contraceptive pill – Correct.** Patients on the COCP, like any contraception, will be at a decreased risk of falling pregnant anyway, but unlike other contraceptive methods (such as the intrauterine devices), there is no evidence of an increased risk of an ectopic pregnancy if someone does become pregnant while on the COCP.

B Intrauterine contraceptive device (IUCD) – **Incorrect.** The use of an IUCD is a risk factor. Both the copper coil and the levonorgestrel-releasing intrauterine system (IUS) reduce the overall risk of falling pregnant, but if pregnancy occurs, there is a significant chance of it being an ectopic pregnancy (5% vs. 1% background risk). The exact reason for this increase is unknown.

C Pelvic inflammatory disease – **Incorrect.** PID causes damage to the fallopian tubes and can either delay the passage of the embryo or prevent it from exiting the tube. This results in a higher chance of the embryo implanting within the tube.

D Previous ectopic pregnancy – **Incorrect.** Women who have suffered a previous ectopic pregnancy are at an increased risk of having another one. This may be because whatever caused the first ectopic pregnancy increases the likelihood of another one. Also, the fallopian tubes may be damaged or blocked by having an ectopic pregnancy, thereby increasing the risk of a subsequent one.

E Smoking – **Incorrect.** Smoking has been shown to increase the number of ectopic pregnancies. Smoking reduces the efficiency of fallopian tube cilia in the transportation of the embryo along the tube.

 Key Point

The IUCD and Mirena IUS both have around a 99% success at preventing a pregnancy. However, within the 1% failure rate, these pregnancies have a higher chance of being ectopic. The risk is roughly 5% in this group, compared to a 1% overall population risk. This is due to the mode of action of these contraceptives, as they prevent intrauterine implantation of a pregnancy, but they do not prevent a pregnancy implanting in the tubes.

Q3: Which of these drugs is used first line in the medical management of ectopic pregnancy?

The correct answer is B. Methotrexate.

Around 75% of ectopic pregnancies can be managed without the need for surgery. Laparoscopy should be reserved for the patients who present as clinically unstable with a ruptured ectopic, or where medical management has either failed or been declined by the patient.

A Actinomycin D – **Incorrect.** Actinomycin D is a chemotherapy agent which is sometimes used in combination with other agents in the management of high-risk patients with gestational trophoblastic disease. It would not be used for the management of ectopic pregnancy.

B ✔ **Methotrexate – Correct.** Methotrexate is used as a first-line drug in the medical management of ectopic pregnancy. It has been shown to be as effective as surgery when used in stable patients, and fewer than 10% of women treated in this way will require subsequent surgical management. Methotrexate has anti-folate activity, as it is a folic acid analogue, and it is this interference with the functions of folic acid that will cause the termination of the ectopic pregnancy.

C Mifepristone – **Incorrect.** Mifepristone is a progesterone receptor antagonist and is used for induced medical abortion of an early pregnancy, usually combined with a prostaglandin. However, it is not recommended in the management of ectopic pregnancy.

D Oestrogen – **Incorrect.** Oestrogen would be ineffective in the management of ectopic pregnancy.

E Progesterone – **Incorrect.** Progesterone would be ineffective in the management of ectopic pregnancy.

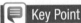 **Key Point**

Medical management with methotrexate is the preferred treatment for ectopic pregnancy. Around 15% of women will require more than one dose of methotrexate. Side effects include abdominal pain, conjunctivitis, stomatitis and gastrointestinal upset. For these reasons, women should be given clear information about the medical therapy if it is offered to them.

Q4: For the patient above, an ultrasound scan is inconclusive. Which investigation above would best indicate a diagnosis of miscarriage?

The correct answer is G. A serum β hCG drop of more than 50%.

When a pregnant patient has an ultrasound scan which cannot confirm the site of pregnancy, the pregnancy is termed a PUL. The next investigation to perform in the clinically stable patient is a serum β hCG, which is then repeated 48 hours later. The change in β hCG concentration can help to diagnose the location of the pregnancy. In a miscarriage, the pregnancy is failing, so the placental tissue stops producing β hCG; consequently, the levels fall over time. This patient would be advised to have a urine pregnancy test in 2 weeks' time, which would be negative to confirm a complete miscarriage.

Q5: For the patient above, an ultrasound scan is inconclusive. Further tests are performed, and the patient is then given methotrexate. Which test is most likely to have resulted in this management?

The correct answer is H. Serum β hCG concentration static.

In this PUL, the diagnosis has been presumed ectopic. Serial serum β hCG measurements taken 48 hours apart, with a rise of less than 63% or a fall of less than 50%, are suggestive of ectopic pregnancy. In a well patient, medical management of an ectopic pregnancy using methotrexate can be offered.

Q6: For the patient above, an ultrasound scan is inconclusive. Blood tests are then performed and following the tests, the doctor suggests that this is

likely to be an intrauterine pregnancy. Which test is required to confirm this?

The correct answer is E. Repeat ultrasound scan.

After the scan, the working diagnosis in this case is PUL. Serum β hCG measurements taken 48 hours apart would have been taken. For the doctor to suggest the pregnancy is intrauterine, the interval change between the two samples must have been more than 63%. NICE guidelines recommend a repeat ultrasound scan 1 week later to confirm the diagnosis.

Q7: For the patient above, an ultrasound scan is inconclusive. While talking to the patient, she complains of increased pain and briefly loses consciousness. Which option would represent the next step in her management?

The correct answer is A. Laparoscopy.

Following the scan, this patient has a PUL. At this stage, the pregnancy could be an ectopic, a viable pregnancy or a miscarriage. It should be presumed until proven otherwise, that all PULs are ectopic. This patient, therefore, has a presumed ectopic, and is now showing signs that she is clinically unstable. Definitive treatment is therefore required. The patient should be resuscitated using an ABC approach and then taken to theatre for laparoscopic treatment of an ectopic pregnancy.

Q8: For the patient above, an ultrasound scan shows a heterotopic pregnancy. Which option would represent the next step in her management?

The correct answer is A. Laparoscopy.

A heterotopic pregnancy is one viable intrauterine pregnancy plus a separate ectopic pregnancy occurring at the same time. These are rare, but important to be aware of for two reasons:

• A clinician who is not vigilant may see an intrauterine pregnancy but miss a small ectopic pregnancy, falsely reassuring the patient and clinician.

• In a PUL with a heterotopic pregnancy, if serum β hCG measurements are checked, the levels will rise by more than 63% in 48 hours because the intrauterine pregnancy will be growing normally. This may again falsely reassure the clinician, but the patient is at risk of ruptured ectopic and collapse.

This patient needs the ectopic pregnancy managed. Medical management cannot be used because this will also kill or damage the viable pregnancy, so surgical management is required. Laparoscopy is preferred to laparotomy, as it has a faster patient recovery period.

 Key Point

A PUL must be assumed to be an ectopic pregnancy until further testing proves otherwise. Beware that all diagnostic tests have their limitations, with no test having a 100% sensitivity or specificity. Clinical judgment is always required to manage patients most appropriately.

- An ectopic pregnancy is a pregnancy that occurs any-where outside of the uterus. In most cases, it is in the fallopian tubes.
- Symptoms may include lower abdominal pain, pelvic pain and suprapubic tenderness, shoulder tip pain, vaginal bleeding, presyncope, syncope, hypotension and shock.
- Key investigations to consider are a urine β hCG to con-firm the pregnancy and a TVUS to determine the location of the pregnancy and to check for free fluid.
- Signs of hypovolaemic shock are a bad prognostic indicator, and the patient must be treated as a medical emergency, following the ABC approach.
- Expectant management is first line in clinically stable women, but medical and surgical management remains an option under certain conditions.

MISCARRIAGE

Q1: A patient with a confirmed 8 week intrauterine pregnancy presents with vaginal bleeding; the cervical os is closed.
The correct answer is K. Threatened miscarriage.

A threatened miscarriage is the presence of symptoms of mis-carriage, but where the pregnancy may be able to continue. It can only be diagnosed when it is known that the pregnancy is intrauterine; symptoms without this knowledge should be classified as pregnancy of unknown location (PUL).

Q2: A patient with a confirmed 8 week intrauterine pregnancy presents with vaginal bleeding; the cervical os is open.
The correct answer is F. Inevitable miscarriage.

Inevitable miscarriage is diagnosed when the cervix is open in a patient with a known intrauterine pregnancy, where the products have not yet passed. This case presented in the exact same way as the example for threatened miscarriage, but on investigation in this case, it was noted that the cervical os is open, which means that the pregnancy will go on to miscarry.

An incomplete (or complete) miscarriage could present the same way, but some (or all) products would have passed through the os.

Q3: A patient who believes she is 8 weeks pregnant presents with light vaginal bleeding. An ultrasound scan reveals no pregnancy. A pregnancy test was positive 2 days ago.
The correct answer is J. Pregnancy of unknown location.

All pregnancies should be regarded as a PUL until their loca-tion has been identified, usually by ultrasound scan. When someone is pregnant, it is assumed that the pregnancy is intra-uterine if it is not causing any symptoms. If pain or bleeding occur, the diagnosis could be any type of miscarriage or an ectopic pregnancy, which would need further investigation to make the diagnosis. If a patient presents with bleeding, but on an ultrasound scan there is an empty uterus, it is possible that

there has been a complete miscarriage. Equally, it could be a very early intrauterine pregnancy which is too small to see on a scan or an ectopic pregnancy. For this reason, many com-plete miscarriages are initially investigated as a PUL, until the diagnosis can be supported by test results.

Q4: A patient who believes she is 8 weeks pregnant presents with light vaginal bleeding but had a heavy bleed the day before when she thinks she passed some products of conception; the cervical os is closed. An ultrasound scan reveals disorganised products of conception.
The correct answer is D. Incomplete miscarriage.

An incomplete miscarriage occurs when some products of conception have been passed, but some remain within the uterus. These may go on to pass naturally and become a complete miscarriage, or they may require medical or surgi-cal management to complete.

Q5: A patient attends for a dating scan at 12 weeks' gestation. A 12 week size fetus is seen within the uterus but no fetal heartbeat is detected.
The correct answer is G. Missed miscarriage.

A missed miscarriage is fetal demise which has occurred without symptoms of miscarriage, which has then been identified, classically, at a planned dating scan. The cervix may go on to open and pass the products and become a com-plete miscarriage. However, a missed miscarriage is the least likely of miscarriages to complete spontaneously, so it may need medical or surgical management.

In addition, an indelible miscarriage (option E) is not a real term.

 Key Point

Most patients presenting with a problem in early pregnancy will present with pain or bleeding. An understanding of the dif-ferential diagnoses and how to differentiate between them is needed to guide patients towards the correct management.

Q6: Which of the following statements regarding miscarriage are true or false?
A good understanding of the diagnostic terms used to describe miscarriages, and knowledge of the potential treatment options, are essential for a clinician to be able to discuss ongoing manage-ment with a patient. These patients are likely to present to doc-tors in primary care, emergency departments (EDs) or O&G.

A ✔ **Prostaglandin E₁ can be used to manage a mis-carriage – True.** The trade name for prostaglandin E₁ is misoprostol and it is commonly given vaginally to start the medical management of a miscarriage. It acts on the uterus, causing cervical dilatation and uterine contractions. Misoprostol can also be given (usually rectally) to control heavy bleeding follow-ing a miscarriage or following birth.

B Surgical management of miscarriage is the best treatment option for miscarriage – **False.** The three treatment options for miscarriage are expectant management, medical management and surgical management. Each option has its advantages and disadvantages, the importance of which often differs for each patient. It is important to explain fully to the patient about the different methods, with reference to their personal circumstances, so the patient can make an informed decision about the most suitable management option for her.

C Miscarriage is complete when there is no longer a fetal heartbeat seen on ultrasound – **False.** If a fetal heart was seen and then subsequently it is not seen, this implies the fetus is no longer viable. However, the miscarriage is not complete until the products of conception have been expelled or removed from the uterus.

D An incomplete miscarriage on ultrasound excludes the diagnosis of ectopic pregnancy – **False.** An incomplete miscarriage on ultrasound confirms that there has been an intrauterine pregnancy which has failed, but the miscarriage has not completed. It is likely that there is no ectopic in this case, but it does not 100% exclude ectopic pregnancy. In 1:10,000 cases, there can be an intrauterine pregnancy and an ectopic pregnancy. An ectopic with an intrauterine pregnancy can be difficult to diagnose but should be considered in a patient with ongoing symptoms or suddenly worsening abdominal pain in early pregnancy.

E ✔ **A threatened miscarriage may occur in a pregnancy which goes on to full term – True.** A threatened miscarriage increases the risk of a pregnancy going on to miscarry, but many women who have some bleeding in early pregnancy go on to have a full-term pregnancy.

> 💬 **Key Point**
>
> Complications and miscarriage often make early pregnancy a very stressful time for the patient. Awareness of the likely pregnancy outcome and treatments to complete a miscarriage are important so that the patient can be guided as smoothly as possible through this difficult time. Knowing when you can offer some reassurance about a positive outcome is also helpful.

Q7: In an emergency admission to the emergency department (ED), a patient who is miscarrying has profound hypotension and a heart rate of 50 bpm. Which is the most likely cause of these signs?

The correct answer is B. Cervical shock.

Managing the acutely unwell gynaecology patient is no different than managing any other patient. Follow the ABCDE approach. It is essential to look at the vaginal blood loss. A quick assessment of the patient's clothes, sanitary pads, the bed sheets and an external look at the vaginal bleeding will give a *good approximation of the recent loss. A speculum examination should then be performed to assess for blood collecting in the vagina and any blood clots or products of conception passing through the cervix which may need to be removed.*

A Beta blockade – **Incorrect.** Beta blockers can prevent a tachycardia even when a tachycardic response would be appropriate to the situation. This is not uncommonly seen in a beta blocked elderly patient who presents with classic signs and symptoms of a pulmonary embolus but no tachycardia. Similarly, a hypovolaemic beta blocked patient may present with signs of dehydration and hypotension, but no tachycardia. Occasionally, young patients are taking beta blockers (used for congenital heart problems, migraines, anxiety and blood pressure control in pregnancy), so it is possible that if the patient, in this case, were taking beta blockers, this could be the cause of or contributing to her symptoms. However, cervical shock is much more likely.

B ✔ **Cervical shock – Correct.** This classically presents with profound hypotension and bradycardia. Stimulation of the cervix, which commonly occurs as blood clots and products pass through the cervix, causes stimulation of the parasympathetic nervous system from within the brainstem, resulting in stimulation of the vagus nerve, which causes a bradycardia and resulting hypotension. A withdrawal of sympathetic stimulation of the vascular system is also thought to occur, which causes vasodilatation and further hypotension. The patient in this example has hypotension and a bradycardia, and a history which supports this diagnosis. This is why it is critically important to examine these patients vaginally when they present acutely unwell like this, as the hypotension can be easily resolved by removing the triggering item from the cervical os. However, it is important to remember that all causes of shock may contribute to a patient's collapse, so follow an ABCDE approach.

C Electrolyte disturbance – **Incorrect.** This is not a common cause of collapse. However, electrolyte disturbances can be difficult to diagnose clinically. By following the ABCDE approach, the common causes of collapse are assessed and treated. If, following initial management and investigations, the patient has not improved and diagnosis remains unclear, senior assistance should be requested and rarer causes considered. A venous blood gas will suggest any profound sodium, potassium or glucose abnormalities, although a formal lab sample will be more accurate. An Addisonian crisis can present with hypovolaemia, hypotension, hyperkalaemia and hyponatraemia. Hyper- and hypoglycaemia and hyper- and hypothyroid, and other electrolyte and endocrine disorders, can all present as emergencies. Remember to look for medical alert jewellery or alert cards in wallets.

D Hypovolaemic shock – **Incorrect.** This is characterised by hypotension, tachycardia, cool peripheries and a prolonged capillary refill time. The bradycardia in these cases does not support hypovolaemia as the main cause for hypotension. However, this patient will have had some bleeding, so there is likely to be an element of hypovolaemia contributing to the shock.

E Septic shock – **Incorrect.** Characterised by hypotension with tachycardia and warm peripheries with a fast capillary refill time. The pathophysiology of septic shock is due to systemic inflammation (systemic inflammatory response syndrome) in response to an infection, which causes generalised vasodilatation and resultant hypotension.

 Key Point

Managing an acutely unwell patient can be daunting. However, if an ABCDE approach is followed, even without confirmation of a diagnosis, the patient can be stabilised, thereby allowing time for the diagnosis to be found and for senior colleagues to review the patient.

Important Learning Points

- Pain and bleeding are common in early pregnancy.
- A miscarriage can be in various stages of completion: threatened, inevitable, incomplete or complete.
- A miscarriage may resolve spontaneously with complete expulsion, or it may require medical or surgical management to empty the uterus.
- Emergency admissions with haemorrhage and/or sepsis caused by a miscarriage need to be managed with an ABCDE approach in a timely manner to stabilise the patient.

RECURRENT MISCARRIAGE

Q1: Which statement is correct regarding miscarriage?
The correct answer is D. Miscarriage is defined as pregnancy loss up to 24 weeks' gestation.

Miscarriage itself is a distressing experience. Understandably, recurrent miscarriage can be devastating psychologically for a patient desperate to have a child. Sensitive management is needed, and where appropriate positive reassurance that in the majority of cases of recurrent miscarriage no cause is found, and the chance of a successful pregnancy are high.

A First trimester pregnancies end in miscarriage in 50% of cases – **Incorrect.** While first-trimester miscarriage is common, 20% is the correct number. In the second trimester, miscarriage is much less common, occurring in 1% to 2% of pregnancies. As a second-trimester miscarriage is uncommon, investigations to identify a cause are advised after a single second-trimester miscarriage.

B Miscarriage is defined as a pregnancy loss up to 12 weeks' gestation – **Incorrect.** Miscarriage is defined

as pregnancy loss before 24 weeks' gestation. A pregnancy loss up to 12 weeks' gestation has occurred in the first trimester. First-trimester miscarriages are common, affecting up to 20% of pregnancies.

C Miscarriage is defined as pregnancy loss up to 16 weeks' gestation – **Incorrect.** A second-trimester miscarriage occurs between 12 and 24 weeks. Bacterial vaginosis (BV) is associated with second-trimester miscarriages, so screening with vaginal swabs is advised in the first and second trimesters of subsequent pregnancies so BV can be identified and treated. However, outside of pregnancy unless symptomatic BV does not require treatment.

D ✔ **Miscarriage is defined as pregnancy loss up to 24 weeks' gestation – True.** Beyond 24 weeks' gestation, birth of a fetus without signs of life is defined as a stillbirth.

E Recurrent miscarriage investigations are advised if a patient has two or more consecutive first-trimester miscarriages – **Incorrect.** Investigations are advised after three or more miscarriages. The most common cause of a single miscarriage is a one-off genetic abnormality, which is unlikely to recur. After three miscarriages, the most common cause is still likely to be unfortunate sporadic genetic abnormalities. However, the chance of there being an underlying condition also increases, so this is the threshold at which investigations for causes are undertaken in most patients.

Key Point

Investigations into the cause of miscarriage should be undertaken after three first-trimester miscarriages or after a single second-trimester miscarriage.

Q2: Answer true or false: Which of these factors is associated with recurrent miscarriage?
The single most important risk factor for recurrent miscarriage is maternal age. It is important that women are aware of this so they can aim to complete their families at an age when successful pregnancy outcomes are likely.

A ✔ **Cocaine use – True.** Cocaine is associated with generalised vasoconstriction, which can occur in the placental bed, reducing blood supply to the developing fetus and resulting in miscarriage.

B Haemophilia – **False.** Thrombophilias are associated with blood clots causing reduced placental blood flow. Haemophilias, conversely, are not associated with miscarriage. If a patient with haemophilia has a miscarriage, she should be managed very carefully as she is likely to bleed heavily.

C ✔ **Hyperthyroidism – True.** Uncontrolled hypothyroidism and hyperthyroidism are associated with recurrent miscarriage. Adequately treating the condition reduces the miscarriage risk to that of the background population.

D ✔ **Maternal age more than 40 – True.** The average risk of a first-trimester miscarriage for all age groups is 20%. Over the age of 40, the risk is 50%, and over the age of 45, around 90% of pregnancies end in miscarriage. This is due to an increased rate of sporadic genetic abnormalities, often caused by meiotic nondisjunction.

E Vigorous exercise – **False.** Extreme exercise is associated with temporary hypothalamic failure, which can cause amenorrhoea and infertility but not miscarriage. Excessive trauma may increase the risk of miscarriage, so sports such as rugby, horse riding or motorsports should be avoided while pregnant.

> **Key Point**
>
> Most of the treatable causes of recurrent miscarriage are easy to identify and treat, to improve the chances of a future pregnancy.

Q3: No cause for recurrent miscarriages is found in Mrs Thompson. Which of the following medications would you advise her to take, either before or during a subsequent pregnancy?
The correct answer is C. Folic acid.

Any patient considering conception should be advised on how to optimise their chances of conceiving, and subsequently delivering, a healthy child. Stabilising chronic conditions, discontinuing teratogenic medications and commencing pre-pregnancy vitamin supplementation are some of the key ways to achieve this.

A Aspirin – **Incorrect.** Aspirin is used in pregnancy from 12 weeks' gestation for patients with antiphospholipid syndrome. Aspirin is also used in pregnancies at risk of developing pre-eclampsia. Some clinicians in the past have offered aspirin to patients with unexplained recurrent miscarriage; however, there is no evidence of benefit and aspirin may even increase miscarriage rates in this subgroup of patients.

B Carbimazole – **Incorrect.** This is a medical treatment for hyperthyroidism. It would be negligent to give Mrs Thompson this treatment, as it would cause hypothyroidism.

C ✔ **Folic acid – Correct.** All patients trying to conceive should be advised to take folic acid preconception and up until at least the 12th week of gestation. Folic acid does not reduce miscarriage rates, but it does reduce the risk of spina bifida in the fetus.

D Low molecular weight heparin (LMWH) – **Incorrect.** LMWH is offered to patients with recurrent miscarriage with known prothrombotic conditions, such as the thrombophilias and antiphospholipid syndrome. There is little evidence of benefit for use in patients with unexplained miscarriage.

E None of the above – **Incorrect.** Folic acid should be offered prenatally and antenatally. Along with folic acid, most pregnancy supplements in the UK also contain vitamin D, as a large number of the population are vitamin D deficient. There is little evidence of benefit in preventing miscarriage, but adequate levels of vitamin D will optimise conditions for a healthy pregnancy and neonate.

> **Key Point**
>
> Folic acid and vitamin D should be advised prenatally for all patients considering conceiving. Other medications should only be offered to treat specific causes of recurrent miscarriage. Progesterone pessaries may be commenced in a subsequent pregnancy if bleeding (threatened miscarriage) occurs in the first trimester.

> **Important Learning Points**
>
> - First-trimester miscarriage is common.
> - Investigations for causes of miscarriage should occur after three first-trimester miscarriages or after a single second-trimester miscarriage.
> - Many of the causes of recurrent miscarriage can be easily treated to optimise conditions for a future pregnancy.
> - The most common diagnosis after investigation is an unexplained cause of miscarriage. However, this may be a reassuring diagnosis, as 75% of patients under 40 with unexplained recurrent miscarriage will subsequently go on to have a successful pregnancy.

TERMINATION OF PREGNANCY

Q1: What is the maximum gestation at which most terminations can be legally performed in the UK?
The correct answer is D. 24 weeks.

Most terminations are sanctioned on the grounds that continuance of the pregnancy would involve risk, greater than if the pregnancy was terminated, of injury to the physical or mental health of the pregnant women. For this indication, the pregnancy must not have exceeded 24 weeks' gestation.

> **Key Point**
>
> One of the reasons UK law set 24 weeks as the limit for social terminations was, at that time or writing, the survival rate for babies born before this gestation was very low. This particular argument is now less clear, as medical advances are allowing increasing numbers of extremely preterm babies born under 24 weeks to survive.
>
> Regardless of a clinician's personal beliefs, it is important to ensure women are aware of the services available to them. If they are not comfortable providing an abortion when it is legally an option, they are duty bound to direct to another provider who can offer the service.

Q2: Answer true or false: The following statements could be valid reasons for a doctor to support the above patient's request for a termination of pregnancy.

All of the answers are true. Two doctors will need to review the case and assess the indication for termination. If both feel that the indication given suggests that continuing the pregnancy would involve a risk of physical or mental injury greater than if the pregnancy were terminated, then a termination can be certified, as long as it is before 24 weeks' gestation.

Key Point

Termination is a controversial topic, with many strong opinions on both sides of the argument. The wording of the Abortion Act allows doctors to certify for terminations of pregnancies less than 24 weeks gestation for a myriad of reasons, as almost anything may affect the mental health of the patient.

Q3: After careful consideration, Elizabeth decides to continue the pregnancy. The 20 week anomaly scan shows significant fetal abnormalities. An amniocentesis confirms the fetus has Down syndrome. Elizabeth is now 28 weeks pregnant. Which of the following statements is correct?

The correct answer is C. If Elizabeth decides to terminate the pregnancy, performing a feticide could be considered.

The decision to terminate a pregnancy with a known fetal abnormality is complex. When considering the options, the patient will need to think about the likely quality of life for the child if it were to be born, and the potential physical and mental distress caused to the patient and their relatives following either termination, adoption or keeping the child.

A If Elizabeth decides to terminate this pregnancy, she must do so by 34 weeks' gestation – **Incorrect.** When the indication for termination is that if the child were born it would be severely handicapped, then there is no limit to the gestation at which a termination can be legally performed. Allowing extra time for Elizabeth to think through the options and come to the correct decision for her may be very appropriate. However, the higher the gestation, the larger the fetus is likely to be, which may impact mode of birth and the risk of complications.

B Surgical termination would be the most appropriate method of termination at this gestation – **Incorrect.** It would be impossible to remove a fetus of this gestation using a vacuum curette because it is far too large. The technique to deliver surgically without performing major abdominal surgery would be to break the fetus up inside the womb and remove it gradually in pieces. This would be difficult for the surgeon and the patient and is highly likely to result in retained products and infection. Medical termination with feticide prior to termination would be the most appropriate termination strategy at this gestation.

C ✔ **If Elizabeth decides to terminate the pregnancy, performing a feticide could be considered – Correct.** Injecting potassium chloride into the fetal heart under ultrasound guidance would kill the fetus *in utero*. Following medical management (misoprostol), the fetus will be born stillborn.

D Three doctors are required to certify a termination at this gestation – **Incorrect.** At all gestations, two doctors are required to certify for a termination.

E The child could not be offered for adoption after birth – **Incorrect.** Termination is not the only option if a patient does not wish to keep the baby.

Key Point

Termination at advanced gestations is best achieved with feticide, followed by medical management. Emotional and psychological support is paramount during these difficult times in a patient's life.

Important Learning Points

• Most terminations in the UK are performed before 12 weeks' gestation.
• Unless there is severe maternal risk or a severe handicap is likely in the child, terminations cannot legally be performed in the UK beyond 24 weeks.
• The UK abortion laws allow significant scope for indications for abortion at gestations less than 24 weeks.
• Termination can be managed medically and surgically. At gestations beyond 15 weeks, surgical terminations become increasingly difficult, so medical management should be strongly considered as the termination method of choice beyond this gestation.

4 BENIGN GYNAECOLOGY

CONTRACEPTION

Q1: What advice should you give if a patient misses one COCP?
The correct answer is C. To take the missed pill and that day's pill at the same time, no additional contraception is required.

If one pill is missed, then the patient should take both the missed pill and the current pill and continue to take the rest of the pack as usual, with no need to double up on contraception. If two or more pills are missed, then the patient should take the last pill missed, leave any earlier pills and continue to take the rest of the pack as usual. She will, however, have to use an additional method of contraception for the next 7 days or consider emergency contraception if sexual intercourse has occurred in the previous 7 days. In addition, if there are 7 or more pills left in the pack, the patient should finish the pack and have the usual 7-day break. If there are fewer than seven pills left, the patient should finish the pack and begin a new one the next day.

Key Point

These recommendations apply to all COCPs except Qlaira®. Qlaira® has very specific advice for missing pills, depending on how long the pill has been missed and where in the menstrual cycle the individual is. It is unnecessary at an undergraduate level to know these guidelines, but it is important to appreciate that you would consult an experienced family planning clinician.

Q2: Answer true or false: For which of the following does the COCP have a protective effect?

The COCP contains an oestrogen and a progestogen. It acts by preventing ovulation. It also affects the lining of the womb and thickens the cervical mucus plug, preventing the entry of sperm into the uterus. Long-term benefits of taking the COCP are that it has been found to reduce the risk of ovarian and endometrial cancer, ovarian cysts and benign breast disease.

A Breast cancer – **False.** The COCP actually causes a slight increase in the risk of breast cancer. However, this risk is likely to be very small and will vary with age. This risk becomes the same as the background risk 10 years after stopping the COCP. Women with a strong family history of breast cancer may not be suitable candidates for taking the COCP or should take it with caution.

B Cervical cancer – **False.** Women on the COCP have a small increase in the risk of cervical cancer with a twofold increase in risk from the background level after 10 years of being on the pill.

C ✔ **Colorectal cancer – True.** The COCP also slightly reduces the risk of colorectal cancer.

D ✔ **Endometrial cancer – True.** The risk of endometrial cancer when on the COCP is halved.

E ✔ **Ovarian cancer – True.** The COCP has been found to halve the risk of ovarian cancer.

 Key Point

Another benefit of the COCP in many women is that it reduces menstrual discomfort and the quantity of each bleed. The COCP may be trialled for the treatment of endometriosis, dysmenorrhoea and menstrual problems in some women. Instead of taking one pill a day for 21 days and then having a 7-day break, women can tricycle the packets, taking 63 days' worth of pills before having 7 days off, enabling them to avoid a menstrual period for longer.

Q3: Answer true or false: Which of the following are contraindications for the COCP?

The COCP has multiple contraindications in addition to those mentioned in this question. It is also contraindicated for women with venous thrombosis or arterial disease, pro-thrombotic disorders and hypertension due to the increased risk of VTE when on the pill. It should also not be taken by women with hepatic impairment or if they are taking liver enzyme-inducing drugs because the COCP is metabolised by the hepatic CYP450 enzymes.

A ✔ **Age more than 50 years – True.** The COCP should not be taken by women over the age of 50 and should be taken with caution by women over 35 years of age.

B ✔ **BMI more than 35 kg/m² – True.** The COCP is contraindicated in women with a BMI over 35 kg/m² and should be taken with caution in women with a BMI above 30 kg/m².

C Migraine sufferer without aura – **False.** The COCP should not be taken by women who suffer from migraines with auras because of the cerebrovascular risks but can be taken with caution in women who suffer from migraines who have never suffered from an aura.

D Renal impairment – **False.** The COCP is metabolised by the liver, therefore renal impairment is not an issue.

E Smoker – **False.** Smokers can take the COCP, but with caution, as smoking reduces the bioavailability, and therefore the effectiveness, of the drug.

Key Point

Contraceptive choice can be difficult when patients have medical conditions which may contraindicate certain options. To help clinicians give appropriate information to their patient, the faculty of reproductive and sexual health have assessed the evidence and produced the UK Medical Eligibility Criteria (UKMEC) (Table 8.1). Each contraceptive option is given a criterion as to how safe the choice is likely to be, for patients with a range of medical conditions.

Q4: Which of the following is an advantage of the 52 mg IUS?

The correct answer is D. Reduces dysmenorrhoea.

An IUS is a very popular method of contraception amongst women of all ages, as it is relatively long-lasting and is not user dependent. A commonly used IUS is the 52 mg Mirena device; this is licensed for 5 years' use as contraception or as a treatment for menorrhagia. It is a small plastic device impregnated with the progestogen levonorgestrel and provides a continuous release of approximately 20 micrograms of hormone per day.

A Ensures regular menstrual cycles – **Incorrect.** One of the major disadvantages of the IUS is that for the first 3 months, and sometimes longer, the IUS can cause irregular bleeding which can be so significant to a patient's quality of life that they ask for the IUS to be removed.

B Lasts 10 years after insertion – **Incorrect.** The IUS does not last 10 years. The 52 mg IUS, is licensed for 5 years as a contraceptive. The 13.5 mg IUS (releases 6 micrograms of hormone a day) is licenced for 3 years. It is the copper coil that is licensed for up to 10 years after insertion.

C Protects against STIs – **Incorrect.** As with all non-barrier methods of contraception, patients need to be informed that although the IUS is a highly effective contraceptive, it does not protect against the transmission of STIs. Therefore, barrier protection should be used with sexual partners of unknown health status.

D ✔ **Reduces dysmenorrhoea – Correct.** An IUS may be fitted for contraceptive reasons, but it is also used as therapy for women with very heavy or painful periods. The reason for this is that the pro-gesterone released from the plastic frame thins the lining of the uterus, which may make a woman's period lighter. Approximately 90% of women have significantly reduced menstrual loss by 12 months of use, and in approximately one-fifth of women treated for menorrhagia, it causes amenorrhoea.

E Reduces PID – **Incorrect.** There is no firm evidence that the IUS decreases PID. It is contraindicated to put anything in the uterus when there is active PID, as this could worsen or prolong the PID. However, the IUS does not increase the risk of PID, and once PID has been treated, then an IUS is not contraindicated.

> 📑 **Key Point**
>
> A 52 mg IUS can also be used for hormone replacement therapy of progesterone. This may be used if a woman is taking oestrogen replacement treatment for symptoms of menopause. The role of the IUS is to protect the endometrium from the proliferative effect of oestrogen. Unopposed oestrogen therapy increases the risk of endometrial cancer.

Q5: Answer true or false: Which of the following are a contraindication for an IUS?

All forms of contraception have contraindications and cautions. This information needs to be balanced against the advantages and disadvantages for a patient to determine the best contraceptive device for them. With contraceptive use or prescribing, there is no "one size fits all" approach.

A Endometriosis – **False.** Endometriosis is a disease in which an IUS can be used. However, pain caused by endometriosis may be improved or worsened by the IUS.

B Heavy periods – **False.** In fact, heavy periods may be the very reason that an individual has an IUS fitted, as it is the first-line medical management for heavy periods. If a woman is having an extremely heavy period, then it may not be suitable to fit an IUS until the current period has completed due to the risk of expulsion.

C Nulliparity – **False.** The IUS requires special training for insertion and removal, and due to the smaller external os of a nulliparous woman, this can be more difficult. However, it is not a contraindication.

D ✔ **Pregnancy – True.** In the event that an IUS is fitted when there is an intrauterine pregnancy *in situ*, the risk of miscarriage and preterm labour is increased.

E ✔ **Uterine distortion – True.** In the case of a uterine cavity that is severely distorted, an IUS in contraindicated as the presence of this abnormality increases the risk of uterine perforation. If this does occur and the threads are not visible, then a TVUS can be used to find the location of the IUS. If ultrasound is not available, an abdominal x-ray can also identify an IUS as it is radio-opaque. An IUS which has perforated the uterus is likely to be within the abdominal cavity. A laparoscopy may be required to retrieve it.

> 📑 **Key Point**
>
> If pregnancy does occur after an IUS has been fitted, there is an increased risk of ectopic pregnancy.

Q6: What is the rate of spontaneous expulsion of an IUS?
The correct answer is B. 1 in 20.

Expulsion is an important factor to discuss with patients. Expulsion could be devastating for a patient who, if unaware that she has lost her contraceptive cover, could be at risk of an unplanned pregnancy. The patient needs to be educated on checking for threads from the cervix to check that the IUS is still in place. This should be done at the end of each period or once every month if she has an irregular cycle. If the woman cannot feel the threads, then she is advised to seek medical help as the IUS may have been expelled or incorrectly sited within the uterus. At that time, the IUS should not be relied on for contraceptive efficacy.

> **Key Point**
>
> Expulsion is most likely in the first 6–8 weeks after fitting, hence the timing of the 6-week appointment to check the threads.

Q7: Which is the only long-acting reversible contraception available that does not involve hormones?
The correct answer is B. Copper coil.

The copper coil, although a relatively older form of contraception, is still available for women wanting long-term contraception but for medical or personal reasons do not want hormones. The copper coil is an IUD which sits in the same location as an IUS, and it works because copper ions are toxic to sperm. The copper coil can also be used as an emergency contraception where it acts by its toxicity to sperm and a developing embryo, preventing implantation.

Q8: Which form of contraception is likely to need altering following pregnancy?
The correct answer is D. Diaphragm.

Diaphragms and caps need to be replaced annually to ensure efficacy. Women should also be advised to check their diaphragms regularly for holes, tears or any other damage. As well as annual assessment, they should also have their diaphragms reviewed if they have had any problems with the method, or if they have lost or gained more than 3 kg in weight, as these factors could all affect the fit of the device. Another important factor addressed in this question is if a woman has been pregnant, the shape and size of the cervix may have changed, so it is important to assess the fit of a previously used diaphragm.

Q9: Which form of contraception is usually inserted into the upper limb?
The correct answer is G. Implant.

The implant is a small, flexible rod that is placed in the upper arm. It is effective for 3 years, and the failure rate is the best

Table 8.1 UK Medical Eligibility Criteria Categories

UK MEDICAL ELIGIBILITY CRITERIA (UKMEC) CATEGORY	DEFINITION
UKMEC 1	A condition where there is no restriction for which kind of contraception can be used.
UKMEC 2	A condition for which the advantages of the proposed method should outweigh the risks.
UKMEC 3	A condition where the risks of a particular kind of contraception outweigh the benefits.
UKMEC 4	A condition where the risk is unacceptable if a certain method of contraception is used.

of all the reversible contraceptive options. It requires a small procedure to insert it and remove the implant involving a small incision. Some women do not like the implant as it can be felt through the skin, although being on the inside of the upper arm it is usually only felt when actually trying to feel for it.

Q10: Which female form of contraception has the lowest percentage efficacy?

The correct answer is E. Female condom.

According to the World Health Organisation data, female condoms are the least effective with the highest number of pregnancies per year when using contraception. This is a user-dependent form of contraception, so it has a higher percentage of pregnancies due to user errors. Overall, 20% of women experience an unintended pregnancy within the first year of typical use. The forms of contraception less effective than this are coitus interruptus (22%) (note: this is not technically a female form of contraception), fertility awareness-based methods (24%) (timing sexual intercourse around the menstrual cycle) and using spermicide alone (28%).

Q11: After use, which form of reversible contraception has the longest time period until optimum fertility is returned?

The correct answer is F. IM injection.

The IM injection lasts for approximately 8 to 12 weeks. However, after cessation of this contraceptive method, the mean time for return to normal fertility is 12 months. It is usually injected into the buttocks or thigh and is fat-soluble. This means that once it has been injected, it cannot be removed. For other forms, such as an IUS or COCP, return to normal fertility levels is relatively rapid. This may be a disadvantage of the injection if a woman's situation changes and she wants to become pregnant relatively rapidly. However, many women like it as a form of contraception because it is relatively painless. It is also almost impossible for a partner or anyone else to know they are using it and there is no user-dependent aspect.

Key Point

Quantifying contraceptive failure is expressed using 'per 100 woman years'. For example, if a particular method had a failure rate of 5 per 100 woman years, this means that if 100 women used that form of contraception for 1 year, then 5 of them would be become pregnant in that time when using the contraception correctly. This is for method failure; however, it is important to remember that for certain types of contraception, user failure is also possible, for example, pills or condoms.

Important Learning Points

- There are multiple methods of contraception, with no gold standard in the field. For this reason, the decision of what contraception to use needs to be made on a case-by-case basis to determine individualised needs.
- For each form of contraception, it is important to gain an overview of the method, advantages and disadvantages to help determine for whom the method might be most useful, the practicalities to ensure minimal user failure and the cautions and contraindications to establish who cannot use that form of contraception.
- Contraception is not only prescribed to ensure that a woman does not get pregnant. The hormonal component of many methods means they may also be given for a range of other gynaecological or medical reasons.
- The provision of appropriate contraception is crucial for family planning and in barrier forms, for the prevention of STIs. Globally, it also plays a large role in minimising the risk of dying during pregnancy or labour by enabling women to space out their pregnancies.

EMERGENCY CONTRACEPTION

Q1: As this patient is 15 years old, decide whether the following statements are true or false regarding prescribing her contraception.

Emergency contraception for girls under the age of 16 has been the source of much ethical debate. Maturity can vary greatly within young people of the same age; therefore, each decision needs to be made on an individual basis. The UK has the highest rates of teenage pregnancy in Western Europe and teenage pregnancy is a serious social problem. Having children at a young age can, in some circumstances, affect a young woman's health and wellbeing and severely limit their education and career prospects.

A ✔ **Emergency contraception can be provided to a competent young person aged under 16 years without parental consent or knowledge using the Fraser criteria – True.** The Fraser guidelines should be followed when making a decision regarding prescribing emergency contraception to an under 16-year-old. These state:

- That the young person understands the advice and has sufficient maturity to understand what is involved.
- That the doctor could not persuade the young person to inform her parents, nor to allow the doctor to inform them that the young person would be

very likely to begin or continue having sexual intercourse with or without contraceptive treatment.

- That without contraceptive advice or treatment, the young person's physical or mental health would suffer.
- That it would be in the young person's best interest to give such advice or treatment without parental consent.

B Emergency contraception can be provided to a competent young person aged under 16 years without parental consent or knowledge using the Gillick criteria – **False.** The term 'Gillick competence' comes from a case in 1985, when Victoria Gillick took her local health service to court because her daughter had been prescribed contraception under the age of 16 without her knowing. A child under the age of 16 is now assessed by Fraser guidelines to determine if they are Gillick competent, as there are no Gillick guidelines as such.

C Emergency contraception can be provided without parental consent; however, a termination requires a parent or carer to be informed – **False.** If an individual under 16 has been assessed by the Fraser guidelines and are deemed to understand the decision that they is making, then they are still entitled to the same healthcare that someone over 16 can have, including terminations. Young people are encouraged to tell an adult (this may not necessarily be their parents) to ensure that they get the appropriate support.

D ✔ **Emergency contraception may only be prescribed by a doctor or nurse for patients under 16 – True.** Individuals over 16 can buy oral emergency contraception (levonorgestrel) at a pharmacy without a consultation. If the individual has a consultation with a pharmacist, doctor or nurse, this service is free. However, for under 16-year-olds in the UK, emergency contraception is not available unless they attend a consultation.

E Copper intrauterine devices cannot be fitted in patients under the age of 16 – **False.** Copper IUDs are harder to fit in nulliparous women of any age, but some believe them to be an underutilised form of contraception in adolescents, an age when complying with the pill can often be difficult.

Key Point

Often teenagers' greatest fear is a lack of confidentiality, which may be a barrier to them accessing services. It is important to state that their confidentiality will be maintained at all times unless there is a circumstance where a health professional believes abuse may be occurring. In this circumstance, the child's safety comes before any right to confidentiality but this most likely will be discussed with the individual first.

Q2: How many days after unprotected sex can emergency contraception be prescribed?

The correct answer is D. Five days.

The progesterone modulator ulipristal acetate and the copper IUD are licensed for up to 5 days or 120 hours after unprotected sexual intercourse or failure of contraception. Levonorgestrel is licensed for up to 72 hours after unprotected sexual intercourse.

Key Point

The main effect of levonorgestrel and ulipristal acetate is to delay ovulation, allowing sperm to die before the oocyte is released. If the unprotected intercourse occurred after ovulation, these medications may be unsuitable.

Q3: Which of the following statements regarding emergency contraception are true?

Emergency contraception is an area of gynaecology where communication is vital. Many misconceptions exist surrounding emergency contraception and it is important that these are dispelled and that the patient is correctly counselled on the different forms of contraception, how to take these, future contraception and STI prevention and testing.

A Emergency contraception causes abortion of the embryo – **False.** In 2002, it was ruled that pregnancy begins at implantation; therefore, by preventing fertilisation, emergency contraception does not cause an abortion or termination by the legal definition in the UK (although this may not be the case with individual beliefs). This may be a common worry for some women, so it is very important to discuss clearly the mechanisms of action of different methods, as some may not be acceptable dependent on an individual's belief. Also, some forms of emergency contraception are thought to alter implantation; therefore, it is important that this is discussed relative to the time in the individual's menstrual cycle that emergency contraception is being sought.

B ✔ **Ulipristal acetate inhibits ovulation by blocking progesterone receptors – True.** The exact mechanism of ulipristal acetate is dependent on the timing of drug administration during the hormone cycle. If ulipristal acetate is taken before the LH peak, follicular rupture and ovum release will be delayed. Levonorgestrel also prevents ovulation by preventing the LH surge as a direct result of exogenous progesterone by negative feedback. During the luteal phase of the cycle, ulipristal acetate may also prevent pregnancy by decreasing endometrial thickness.

C ✔ **Women who take rifampicin should be advised that the copper IUD is the only method of emergency contraception that can reliably prevent pregnancy – True.** Rifampicin is a liver enzyme-inducing drug; therefore, caution should be taken when prescribing women emergency contraception and the following guidelines need to be considered:

- Women taking liver enzyme-inducing drugs, or who have stopped within the last 28 days, should be advised that a copper IUD is the only method of emergency contraception not affected by these drugs.
- Women taking liver enzyme-inducing drugs and who decline (or are not eligible) for a copper IUD should be advised to take 3 mg of levonorgestrel as soon as possible within 120 hours. This doubling of the usual dose is outside the product license, aiming to compensate for the increased metabolic rate of the liver.

D All three forms of emergency contraception give ongoing contraceptive efficacy for future acts of unprotected sexual intercourse in the next 72 hours – **False.** Only the copper IUD has ongoing contraceptive function.

E If the reason for taking levonorgestrel was two missed COCPs and the patient continues to take her COCP, then no extra precautions are required after taking this form of emergency contraception – **False.** Additional contraception, such as condoms, are required for 7 days with a patient on the COCP. If ulipristal was used, additional measures should be used for 2 weeks.

> **💬 Key Point**
>
> In order to give a patient the best care, the clinician must fully understand the patient's history, including when the unprotected intercourse occurred and medical history, in order to determine the suitable treatments available. The clinician then needs to be able to explain the options to the patient so she can make a decision based on her personal views as to the most appropriate treatment for her.

Q4: What is an absolute contraindication for hormonal forms of emergency contraception?
The correct answer is G. Pregnancy.

Pregnancy is the only contraindication listed above that applies to all forms of hormonal emergency contraception. If a woman is known to be pregnant, then emergency contraception is not appropriate.

Q5: What necessitates the dose of levonorgestrel to be doubled?
The correct answer is A. Carbamazepine.

Carbamazepine is an enzyme-inducing drug; therefore, any patient currently taking carbamazepine will need to double the dose of levonorgestrel used. However, treatment with levonorgestrel may not be as effective, so where possible the IUD should be used as treatment for emergency contraception in patients taking enzyme-inducing medications. People with epilepsy and other patients taking enzyme-inducing medications should avoid both forms of the contraceptive pill for long-term contraception as they are likely to be less

effective. The IUD, IUS and the depot injection are the advised methods to offer these women.

Q6: Which form of contraception is most likely to disrupt the next menstruation from its expected day the most?
The correct answer is D. Levonorgestrel.

Due to the high levels of progestogen, levonorgestrel is the form of emergency contraception most likely to disrupt the next menstruation by the most days.

Q7: Which oral form of emergency contraception can be offered if unprotected sexual intercourse has occurred and levonorgestrel was taken as emergency contraception 4 days ago?
The correct answer is D. Levonorgestrel.

Levonorgestrel is effective at preventing pregnancy following unprotected sexual intercourse up to 72 hours following the event. Therefore, further emergency contraception is required. It is safe to take repeated doses of levonorgestrel or ulipristal acetate within the same cycle. However, If a woman has already taken levonorgestrel, ulipristal could theoretically be less effective if taken in the following 7 days.

Q8: Which form of emergency contraception is contraindicated in Wilson's disease?
The correct answer is C. Copper IUD.

Wilson disease is a rare autosomal recessive inherited disorder of copper metabolism. The condition is characterised by excessive deposition of copper in the liver, brain and other tissues; therefore, the copper IUD is not suitable for women with this condition. However, Wilson disease can also cause hepatic impairment, reducing the efficacy of oral emergency contraception. Therefore, in cases of Wilson disease, specialist advice will need to be sought.

> **💬 Key Point**
>
> All emergency contraception should be prescribed on an individualised basis because, as demonstrated in these questions, there are a lot of factors to consider.

> **🔍 Important Learning Points**
>
> - Emergency contraception is effective at preventing unwanted pregnancy.
> - Pregnancy must be excluded before offering treatment.
> - Patients are at risk of STIs, so testing should be offered.
> - Levonorgestrel can be used up to 3 days after unprotected intercourse.
> - Ulipristal acetate can be used up to 5 days after unprotected intercourse.
> - A copper IUD can be used up to 5 days after unprotected intercourse. It is the only option that does not use hormones, and it offers long-term contraception.

MENORRHAGIA AND OTHER MENSTRUAL BLEEDING DISORDERS

Q1: What is the single most important investigation when managing menorrhagia in this patient?
The correct answer is D. Serum haemoglobin concentration.

Menorrhagia in young women is a very common presentation to the healthcare system via general practice, family planning services, ED and gynaecology services. The cause in most cases is usually physiological and treatment can be started quickly after presentation, with only simple investigations required prior to commencement.

A   Menstrual calendar – **Incorrect.** Patients are asked to record the length of their cycles, their days menstruating, amount of bleeding and any episodes of bleeding in between periods for two to three menstrual cycles. There is little evidence for their use in menorrhagia, but they may be of use to objectify a patient's symptoms and reassure a patient if they have normal menstrual cycles.

B   Pad weights to estimate menstrual loss – **Incorrect.** There is no evidence for estimating or calculating blood loss in menorrhagia outside of a research setting. The important factors are the subjective effect on a patients' life and the objective evidence of anaemia.

C   Pipelle endometrial biopsy – **Incorrect.** This can be taken in an outpatient clinic by passing a small biopsy tube through the cervix and gently scraping to remove a small sample of endometrium. Due to 'blind sampling' with pipelle biopsies, NICE now recommends hysteroscopy for the investigation of post-menopausal bleeding or in the premenopausal patient when there is an increased risk of endometrial dysplasia, for example, recurrent IMB, HMB in a patient aged 45 and over, or significant family history of endometrial or other associated cancers.

D   ✔ Serum haemoglobin concentration – **Correct.** A full blood count is the only necessary investigation in the majority of patients presenting with menorrhagia. The full blood count will show if the menorrhagia is clinically affecting the patient by causing anaemia (low serum haemoglobin concentration). Anaemia caused by menorrhagia is usually a microcytic anaemia as a result of iron deficiency, which is supported on an FBC by a low mean cell volume (MCV). Rarely, abnormally low platelets may be identified on an FBC, which may suggest a clotting abnormality and warrants further investigation.

E   Ultrasound scan – **Incorrect.** An ultrasound scan is of use when there are symptoms or signs suggestive of structural abnormality such as polyps or fibroids. Ultrasound scanning is also used in gynaecology as part of the initial investigations in post-menopausal bleeding (PMB).

> 💬 **Key Point**
>
> In patients with menorrhagia and no other associated symptoms, a full blood count is usually the only necessary investigation required prior to initial treatment.

Select the most appropriate investigation from the list above, for a patient presenting with menorrhagia and each of the following symptoms.

Q2: Constipation.
The correct answer is J. Thyroid stimulating hormone.

Persistent constipation can be a symptom of hypothyroidism. Both hyperthyroidism and hypothyroidism can cause menorrhagia. General screening symptoms that may be useful to discuss are excessive fatigue, weight gain, dry skin and depression in the case of hypothyroidism. Anxiety, weight loss, palpitations and diarrhoea should be asked about in the history in suspected hyperthyroidism.

Q3: Recurrent postcoital bleeding.
The correct answer is B. Colposcopy.

This involves a speculum examination to visualise the cervix and then, if needed, acetic acid and iodine are applied to the cervix to look for areas of dysplasia. The most common cause of postcoital bleeding in the young patient is an ectropion, however cervical cancer is an important differential. The ectocervix is usually made of stratified squamous epithelium, but in response to high oestrogen levels, for example, in young women, the delicate columnar epithelium of the cervical canal protrudes onto the ectocervix. This area can bleed on contact. It can be cauterised to prevent recurrent postcoital bleeding. Over time, the columnar epithelium will undergo metaplasia into squamous epithelium. It is this process which can lead to dysplasia in the presence of human papilloma virus (HPV).

[See 'Cervical Screening' page 150.]

Q4: History of heavy menstrual bleeding since menarche.
The correct answer is A. Clotting screen.

Menorrhagia from menarche suggests the possibility of a clotting abnormality. Clotting abnormalities can be de novo, but usually, there is a genetic abnormality within families. The most common bleeding disorder among patients presenting with menorrhagia is von Willebrand disease which, in clotting studies, will show a prolonged activated partial thromboplastin time (APTT), with a normal prothrombin time (PT) and bleeding time. Platelet numbers on full blood count are usually normal.

Q5: Uterus palpable abdominally.
The correct answer is K. Ultrasound scan.

A normal-sized uterus is not palpable abdominally. The most likely cause of a palpable uterus in a young patient is uterine fibroids (leiomyoma). These are benign growths of the uterine myometrium. They cause menorrhagia by bulging into the endometrial cavity. This increases the surface area of the endometrium, meaning there is more endometrium to menstruate. Fibroid growth is usually hormone-dependent, so fibroids tend to regress in size after menopause.

Q6: Vaginal discharge.
The correct answer is L. Vaginal swab for chlamydia.

Infection is an often-forgotten cause of uterine bleeding and menorrhagia. Any infection can cause inflammation and bleeding, but classically these are due to one of the sexually transmitted infections, usually chlamydia or gonorrhoea. Culturing or conducting a polymerase chain reaction (PCR) on a vaginal swab will detect the presence of an active infection. Testing for serum antibodies will demonstrate whether a patient has ever had a chlamydial infection, but not necessarily whether it is a current active infection.

 Key Point

Treatment of menorrhagia is only treating a symptom. If there are additional symptoms of an underlying cause, then this should be investigated and treated, as treatment of the cause may also treat the menorrhagia.

Q7: Answer true or false regarding the following statements about menorrhagia.
The initial treatment options for menorrhagia are mostly contraceptives which can be prescribed in general practice. Knowledge of the contraceptives' relative strengths in the management of menorrhagia is important, but so is knowledge of the cautions and contraindications for the use of each of the contraceptives.

[See 'Contraception' page 71.]

A The history of endometrial cancer in the family is likely to affect the clinical management of this patient – **False.** A single elderly relative diagnosed with a cancer is unlikely to represent an increased risk of cancer for a younger relative. However, if there is a significant family history (particularly if diagnosis was under the age of 50) or personal history of endometrial, breast, ovarian and/or bowel cancer, then there could well be a genetic predisposition to cancer and a change in menstruation may warrant further investigation. Lynch syndrome, formally called hereditary non-polyposis colorectal carcinoma (HNPCC), is the best-researched genetic cause of endometrial and bowel cancer in the younger age group. It is inherited in an autosomal dominant pattern. Recent advances in genetics have also found links to genes formerly just associated with breast cancer.

B ✔ **The levonorgestrel-releasing IUS is the first-line treatment for menorrhagia – True.** It is the most effective hormonal contraceptive option for menorrhagia. Like all progestogen hormonal contraceptives, its mechanism of action in treating menorrhagia is to prevent proliferation of the endometrium, using a combination of inhibition of the HPO axis, and direct action upon the endometrium.

C The progestogen-containing implant is an alternative to other progestogen-containing contraceptive treatments and has the added benefit of decreased serum concentrations of a progestogen compared to the other treatments – **False.** Progestogens act on the endometrium to prevent endometrial growth, which therefore reduces the amount of endometrial shedding at menstruation. The levonorgestrel-releasing IUS releases a progestogen into the endometrial cavity which acts locally on the endometrium, while little of the progestogen is systemically absorbed. Another method of giving progestogen is the implant, which is usually inserted in the upper arm. It requires the progestogen to be absorbed into the systemic circulation and then transported to the endometrium to have its effect. For this reason, the systemic concentration of progestogen is much higher in an implant than the IUS.

D **Mefenamic acid is a suitable treatment for a patient with menorrhagia and severe asthma – False.** Mefenamic acid is a non-steroidal anti-inflammatory drug. It can therefore induce bronchospasm or asthma exacerbation in some asthmatics. The name mefenamic acid can be confusing, in terms of its similarity to tranexamic acid. Tranexamic acid is a naturally occurring chemical in the body and forms part of the anti-fibrinolytic pathway, preventing clot breakdown. It should be used with caution in patients with a propensity to form abnormal clots, such as a deep vein thrombosis. There is no contraindication or cautions for its use in patients with asthma.

E A hysterectomy is not offered as first-line treatment for menorrhagia because other treatments are more effective and are cheaper – **False.** A hysterectomy results in the complete removal of the uterus, and with it, the endometrium. It almost always results in complete cessation of menstruation, and therefore menorrhagia, so could be considered the most effective option. It is not a sensible procedure for any patient wishing to maintain fertility. It is not a first-line treatment, because a hysterectomy is a major operation with significant risk of complications, and menorrhagia can be successfully managed in most cases with safe and effective alternatives.

 Key Point

Menorrhagia can be successfully managed in primary care in most cases, with a large variety of different pharmaceutical treatments available. As many of the treatments have an effect on fertility, either temporarily in the form of contraception or permanently in the case of surgery, it is imperative that the patient's fertility plans are discussed and considered when choosing the appropriate treatment for the individual patient.

Important Learning Points

- Menorrhagia is a clinical diagnosis.
- There is usually no sinister underlying cause, and a full blood count is usually the only initial investigation required.
- If an underlying cause is suspected, this should be investigated and treated together with the symptom of heavy menstrual bleeding.
- The levonorgestrel IUS is the most effective pharmaceutical treatment available.
- Treatment should be tailored to the individual patient; for a patient currently trying to conceive, the only treatment option available is tranexamic acid.
- Endometrial ablation and hysterectomy should not be considered for patients who have not completed their families.

FIBROIDS

Q1: Which is the most common type of uterine fibroid?
The correct answer is C. Intramural

Uterine fibroids are also known as uterine leiomyomas or leiomyomata. They are benign tumours of the uterine myometrium. They can grow towards or project away from the uterine cavity and are named based on their anatomical location. An individual woman may have multiple fibroids of different types.

A Cervical – **Incorrect.** Cervical fibroids arise from the cervix. Cervical fibroids are rare, but when they occur, they can be associated with dyspareunia. In childbirth, they can cause obstruction to a vaginal birth, and cause heavy bleeding if a caesarean is performed.

B Intraligamentous – **Incorrect.** Intraligamentous fibroids arise from the uterine myometrium and protrude outwards, extending to within the peritoneal folds of the broad ligament. Therefore, what was a subserous fibroid can develop into an intraligamentous fibroid as they extend. Intraligamentous fibroids are rare.

C ✔ **Intramural – Correct.** Intramural fibroids are fibroids that are within the muscle layer (myometrium). Therefore, as they grow, they distort the myometrium. Intramural fibroids are the most common type of uterine fibroid. Intramural fibroids account for approximately 70% of all fibroids.

D Submucosal – **Incorrect.** Submucosal fibroids arise from the myometrium but extend inwards towards the endometrial cavity. They remain covered by the endometrium. Submucosal fibroids distort the size and shape of the uterine cavity. Submucosal fibroids make up approximately 5% of all fibroids.

E Subserosal – **Incorrect.** Subserosal fibroids arise from the myometrium but protrude outwards towards the serosal layer of the uterus. Subserosal fibroids distort the size and shape of the external uterine wall. Subserosal fibroids make up approximately 20% of all fibroids.

Key Point

The common uterine fibroid types include intramural, subserosal and submucosal; rarer fibroids include cervical and intraligamentous.

Q2: Which of these presenting complaints is not an indication for surgery?
The correct answer is D. Red degeneration.

The symptoms and signs depend on the number of fibroids, their size and position. However, fibroids are usually asymptomatic. The common presenting symptoms include menstrual irregularities, dysmenorrhoea and dyspareunia. Torsion or red degeneration of fibroids can present in the emergency setting as acute pain and an acute abdomen.

A Failure of conservative medical management – **Incorrect.** If, despite all conservative measures, the patient is still having significant signs and symptoms, surgical treatments will be considered.

B Fibroid torsion – **Incorrect.** A pedunculated fibroid can undergo torsion on its pedicle, obstructing its blood supply and causing ischaemia, so the patient presents with acute pain. A torted fibroid is an indication for surgery to remove the fibroid.

C Heavy menstrual bleeding – **Incorrect.** Menorrhagia is an indication for surgery as the blood loss can be so severe that it leads to iron deficiency anaemia, as well as having a detrimental effect on the patient's quality of life. When a patient presents with fibroid symptoms, it is important to ask about blood loss, as well as the symptoms of anaemia, and if indicated, perform a full blood count.

D ✔ **Red degeneration – Correct.** Red degeneration is a complication of fibroids that most commonly occurs during pregnancy. In pregnancy, there are high levels of the sex hormones, oestrogen and progesterone, which promote rapid fibroid growth. This growth can exceed that supported by the blood supply, resulting in avascular necrosis of the fibroid. This presents with vomiting, pain and fever. Red degeneration usually settles with conservative measures of rest and analgesia. Surgery is avoided where possible in pregnancy, as the risks of the surgery in the expectant mother are higher than if she were not pregnant. There is also a risk of miscarriage or preterm birth.

E Very large fibroids causing pressure symptoms – **Incorrect.** Very large fibroids can cause the uterus to become excessively enlarged, resulting in pressure on the surrounding structures. This pressure can cause symptoms which include constipation and urinary retention, which can lead to further complications and is therefore an indication for surgery.

Key Point

Red degeneration can be treated conservatively with analgesia, anti-emetics and IV hydration. In rare cases where conservative measures fail to control the symptoms while the fibroid naturally degenerates, surgery may need to be considered. This means accepting the increased risks of operating if the patient is pregnant.

Q3: The patient above states these symptoms are having a significant impact on her quality of life, and she wishes to discuss a long-term solution. Which of the treatments below would you recommend to this patient?
The correct answer is D. Myomectomy.

The management of fibroids ranges from no treatment for small asymptomatic fibroids to the definitive treatment of hysterectomy. The management of fibroids depends on the symptoms, fibroid size, number and location. It is also determined by the patient's wishes, including her desire for fertility and uterine preservation. It also relies on co-morbidities, which determine the patient's fitness for surgical procedures, and her age relative to the menopause.

A Combined oral contraceptive pill – **Incorrect.** Although this medication is sometimes used for fibroid symptom control, it is also a contraceptive and this patient presented to the primary care physician as she was unable to conceive.

B Goserelin – **Incorrect.** Goserelin is a GnRH agonist, which is a drug class that temporarily prevents the menstrual cycle. It reduces oestrogen and progesterone levels, which reduces fibroid size. However, within 3 months of discontinuation of the medication, the fibroid could regrow. This is only a temporary solution, but it is often used pre-operatively to reduce fibroid bulk and blood loss. This medication may be used prior to surgery to improve surgical outcomes, but in itself is not a long-term treatment.

C Hysterectomy – **Incorrect.** Hysterectomy is a surgical procedure that removes both the fibroids and uterus. Although this procedure provides a definitive therapy for the fibroids, there is no ability for future childbearing, which is desired in this case.

D ✔ **Myomectomy – Correct.** Myomectomy is a surgical procedure that involves the "shelling" of a fibroid, leaving the rest of the uterus intact. As only the fibroid is removed, it allows future pregnancy, although it is not a procedure without its risks for a woman who wishes to conceive. These risks include haemorrhage which, if uncontrolled, can necessitate converting the operation into a life-saving hysterectomy. However, as this patient is developing fibroid complications, anaemia and pressure symptoms, as well as adverse impacts on her quality of life, it is important to discuss the risks and benefits of this treatment with this individual.

E Naproxen – **Incorrect.** Naproxen is a non-steroidal anti-inflammatory drug which is used for symptom control of fibroid-associated pain. This patient is not complaining of pain, but is presenting with menorrhagia, anaemia and pressure symptoms; therefore, this treatment is not appropriate.

Key Point

As many of the fibroid treatments are either a contraceptive or negatively affect fertility, it is important to take a full history and explore the patient's ideas, concerns and expectations prior to initiating a management plan.

Important Learning Points

- Uterine fibroids are very common and are benign tumours of the uterine myometrium.
- Uterine fibroids can produce a range of symptoms, from asymptomatic to acute pain (with fibroid torsion and red degeneration).
- Ultrasound is the first-line investigation.
- As fibroids are so prevalent, an asymptomatic fibroid can coexist with a more serious pathology. It is therefore always essential to perform a full history and examination to exclude alternative pathologies.

PREMENSTRUAL DISORDER

A good understanding of the HPO axis is essential to understand the cause and treatment of many gynaecological conditions. Premenstrual disorder is most likely caused by an increase in hormones in the luteal phase of the menstrual cycle, with some of the treatments being aimed at inhibiting different levels of the HPO axis to prevent ovulation.

[See 'The Menstrual Cycle and Physiology of the HPO Axis' page 8.]

Q1: Steroid hormone, which causes negative feedback on the hypothalamus and pituitary during the follicular phase of the menstrual cycle.
The correct answer is H. Oestradiol.

During the follicular phase, GnRH is released from the hypothalamus, which stimulates FSH release from the anterior pituitary. FSH stimulates ovarian follicle growth. Many follicles begin growing and produce oestradiol (an oestrogen). Oestradiol negatively feeds back on the hypothalamus and pituitary, resulting in less FSH being produced. Over the days in the follicular stage, FSH concentration falls in response to the ever-increasing oestradiol levels. Consequently, only the follicle with the most sensitivity to FSH is able to continue growing into the dominant follicle, which will go on to ovulate.

Q2: Hormone likely to be responsible for the symptoms of premenstrual disorder.
The correct answer is L. Progesterone.

Progesterone is produced in the luteal phase of the menstrual cycle by the corpus luteum of the ovary, in response to LH stimulation. The symptoms of premenstrual disorder coincide with the luteal phase when progesterone levels are highest, and symptoms resolve after menstruation when progesterone levels fall (the corpus luteum atrophies if implantation of a fertilised ovum does not occur because the corpus luteum needs stimulation from β hCG to prevent atrophy). Progesterone is believed to cause the symptoms of premenstrual disorder by interacting with neurotransmitters in the CNS.

Q3: The hormone responsible for inhibiting ovulation in the combined oral contraceptive.
The correct answer is H. Oestradiol.

Oestradiol (or very similar variations) is used in the combined oral contraceptive, together with a progestogen. A continuous heightened level of oestrogen causes negative feedback on the hypothalamus and pituitary, inhibiting FSH and LH release from the pituitary. This prevents follicular development, which in turn then prevents ovulation and formation of the corpus luteum, thereby preventing a rise in progesterone levels during the luteal phase. The combined oral contraceptives are an appropriate treatment for premenstrual disorder.

Q4: The hormone released in a pulsatile manner from the hypothalamus.
The correct answer is E. Gonadotropin-releasing hormone.

GnRH acts on the anterior pituitary, stimulating production and release of FSH and LH. GnRH analogues are used to inhibit the HPO axis. GnRH analogues are agonists which are given in a modified release preparation so that the levels in the blood are constant (rather than pulsatile). This causes a downregulation of receptors on the pituitary, resulting in a shutdown of the HPO axis. The inhibition of the HPO axis is so complete that the patient often gets menopausal symptoms.

Q5: The hormone which is in peak concentration just before ovulation.
The correct answer is G. Luteinising hormone.

Ovulation of the oocyte from the dominant follicle is caused by a sharp increase in the concentration of LH, called the 'LH surge'. The exact trigger for the pituitary to release the large concentration of LH is not clear, but it is believed to be a paradoxical response to the persistent negative feedback of oestrogen.

 Key Point

Progesterone is believed to be the likely factor causing the symptoms of premenstrual disorder. High levels of progesterone during the luteal phase tend to coincide with the highest level of premenstrual syndrome symptoms.

Q6: Which patient is most likely to suffer from premenstrual disorder?
The correct answer is C. A 27-year-old woman who is fit and well.

Premenstrual disorder is characterised by psychological, behavioural or physical symptoms severe enough to affect a woman's quality of life, associated with the luteal phase of the menstrual cycle. The answer is therefore the only person likely to be having menstrual cycles.

A A 60-year-old woman with angina – **Incorrect.** This patient is likely to be postmenopausal, since she is above the average age of menopause.
B A 29-year-old woman who is 4 months pregnant – **Incorrect.** This woman will not have menstrual cycles, since they cease during pregnancy.
C ✔ **A 27-year-old woman who is fit and well – Correct.** This patient is likely to have menstrual cycles so may suffer from premenstrual disorder.
D A 24-year-old man with gynaecomastia – **Incorrect.** Gynaecomastia is often driven by oestrogens. This patient may have an endocrinological disorder, but he will not be getting symptoms of premenstrual disorder and he will not be having menstrual cycles.
E A 16-year-old girl who has not had any pubertal changes – **Incorrect.** This girl has delayed puberty and may require investigation to identify any cause, but she will not be ovulating and so will not be suffering from premenstrual disorder (PMD).

 Key Point

You cannot get premenstrual disorder if you are not having menstrual cycles.

Q7: Answer true or false: These treatments may be of use in the treatment of premenstrual disorder.

Treatment of premenstrual syndrome is multifactorial. Simple lifestyle alterations, such as exercise, healthy diet, maintaining a healthy BMI, not smoking, and avoiding excess alcohol, will all improve symptoms. If they do not suitably improve symptoms, then other treatments are available.

A ✔ **Selective serotonin reuptake inhibitors – True.** Progesterone is believed to alter the effect of neurotransmitters such as serotonin. SSRIs have been shown to improve premenstrual symptoms, probably due to their effects on increasing the availability of serotonin in the CNS.
B Electroconvulsive therapy – **False.** ECT is used in very specific cases of severe psychiatric disease and is not used in the treatment of premenstrual disorder. However, cognitive behaviour therapy (CBT) is a recognised first-line treatment for premenstrual disorder, which is at least as effective as SSRIs at improving symptoms.
C Progestogen-only pill – **False.** Progesterone is believed to be the main cause of premenstrual disorder, so the POP and other progestogen-based contraceptives may exacerbate symptoms. Even when high doses of progestogen are used to inhibit

ovulation, patients can still get symptoms. These may be cyclical in nature, or because there is a constant raised level of progestogen, the symptoms may be more continual.

D ✔ **Third generation combined oral contraceptive – True.** The oestrogen component of the combined oral contraceptive causes negative feedback on the HPO axis, preventing follicle stimulation and ovulation, which prevents progression to the luteal phase where progesterone is in high concentration. The progestogen component of the third-generation combined pills does not cause premenstrual symptoms, but the older combined pills contain progestogens which do cause symptoms. The exact reason why these different progestogens act differently on premenstrual disorder symptoms is not well understood.

E ✔ **Nicotine patch – True.** Nicotine does not improve premenstrual disorder, but using a nicotine replacement to achieve smoking cessation can improve symptoms. Nicotine patches, gum and e-cigarettes are some of the over-the-counter treatments available to help people who wish to quit smoking.

 Key Point

Treating premenstrual syndrome involves lifestyle modification, pain management and other medications. These may include SSRIs and combined oral contraceptive pills. In more extreme cases, GnRH analogues or bilateral oophorectomy may be considered.

Important Learning Points

- Premenstrual disorder is characterised by physical, behavioural, or psychological symptoms which are severe enough to affect a woman's quality of life that occur regularly during the luteal phase of a woman's menstrual cycle, which then resolve after menstruation.
- Important differential diagnoses include psychiatric conditions (e.g. depression), and medical conditions (e.g. hypothyroidism).
- It is important to emphasise that premenstrual disorder will resolve around menstruation, with at least 1 week symptom-free (follicular phase) each menstrual cycle. Other differential diagnoses may still have exacerbations during the luteal phase like premenstrual disorder, but they will not fully resolve at menstruation.
- Overall, 5% of women have severe premenstrual symptoms; however, the majority of cases resolve or can be managed with simple treatment.

MENOPAUSE

Menopause is a physiological process resulting in significant changes in hormone levels. It occurs when the ovarian reserve of oocytes is depleted, so oestrogen is no longer produced in response to FSH.

Q1: The hormone raised at the perimenopause.
The correct answer is E. Follicle-stimulating hormone.

In the perimenopausal state, few oocytes are available for stimulation, and they require a higher level of serum FSH for them to undergo maturation and begin producing oestrogen.

Q2: The hormone replaced to reduce menopausal symptoms.
The correct answer is J. Oestrogen.

Once all the oocytes are depleted, the ovaries are then unable to produce oestradiol, which is the oestrogen present in high concentrations in the reproductive age group. The lack of this hormone is the cause of the menopausal symptoms.

Q3: The hormone given as part of hormone replacement therapy to reduce the risk of endometrial cancer.
The correct answer is L. Progesterone.

Unopposed oestrogen causes endometrial proliferation and hyperplasia, which can lead to neoplasia. Progesterone given with oestrogen significantly reduces the risk of endometrial cancer from HRT by preventing endometrial growth. In patients who have had a hysterectomy, oestrogen alone can be given to control menopausal symptoms.

Q4: The hormone released by the anterior pituitary.
The correct answer is E. Follicle stimulating hormone.

Other hormones released from the anterior pituitary are growth hormone, luteinising hormone, thyroid stimulating hormone, prolactin and adrenocorticotropic hormone. Antidiuretic hormone and oxytocin are released by the posterior pituitary.

Q5: The hormone which, if pathologically raised, is commonly associated with amenorrhoea and weight gain.
The correct answer is D. Cortisol.

Cushing disease is caused by an ACTH secreting tumour in the pituitary, whereas Cushing syndrome is chronically high cortisol levels for any other reason (including iatrogenic). Other symptoms include low mood, sleep disturbances and muscle weakness. Patients can also present as a result of osteoporosis, diabetes, hypertension and immune suppression. Clinicians should be aware that, in rare cases, menopausal symptoms may be attributable to an underlying systemic disease.

 Key Point

Knowledge of the HPO axis is very helpful in understanding the menopause. FSH rises in attempt to stimulate non-functioning ovarian tissue. Oestrogens are no longer produced by the ovaries, and this causes the symptoms.

Q6: What is the average age women go through the menopause in the UK?
The correct answer is D. 51 years old.

Overall, 80% of women will have gone through the menopause by age 54; 1% of women will be diagnosed with premature menopause, which is ovarian insufficiency diagnosed before the age of 40.

 Key Point

Menopausal symptoms from 45 years of age are likely to be caused by the physiological state of menopause. Symptoms occurring prior to the age of 40 will need to be investigated to exclude an underlying cause.

Q7: Answer true or false to the following statements regarding menopause and HRT.

The above woman is clearly demonstrating menopausal symptoms in the form of hot flushes. Other symptoms include night sweats, loss of sexual desire, low mood and vaginal dryness. Symptoms indicate a patient is going through the menopause, but it is a history of amenorrhoea for 1 year which is diagnostic of menopause.

A The above woman is now postmenopausal because she has now stopped having periods for 10 months – **False.** Menopause has occurred once a patient has not had a menstrual period for 12 months. However, menopausal symptoms can occur prior to the patient becoming postmenopausal.

B The progestogen part of combined HRT treatment reduces the menopausal symptoms – **False.** The role of the progestogen component in combined HRT is to oppose the stimulatory effect of the oestrogen component on the endometrium which, if left unopposed, could cause endometrial cancer. In patients who have had a hysterectomy, oestrogen can be used without a progestogen to control menopausal symptoms.

C ✔ **A recent deep vein thrombosis is a contraindication for oral HRT use – True.** Both the oestrogen and progestogen components of the replacement therapy appear to be prothrombotic. In a patient with a high risk of VTE, either a transdermal preparation or a non-hormonal treatment for symptoms is recommended.

D ✔ **It is reasonable to make the diagnosis of the menopause on history alone – True.** Usually, the diagnosis of menopause or the perimenopausal state can be diagnosed simply on a history of absent or erratic menstrual cycles, with symptoms of hot flushes, night sweats and vaginal dryness or pruritus. Only if there is doubt about the cause of the symptoms should other investigations be performed. A serum FSH is the most common investigation performed to assist in the diagnosis.

E ✔ **Woman with premature menopause but no symptoms may benefit from HRT – True.** Usually, hormone replacement therapy is only offered to patients with symptoms of menopause to improve their quality of life. However, in patients with early menopause, even if they have no symptoms, the benefit of treatment outweighs the risks, as HRT prevents early osteoporosis. The risks in this group are negligible because the treatment is simply replacing hormones which, if the women had not gone into menopause early, they would have produced anyway.

 Key Point

A woman can only be diagnosed as postmenopausal once she has had cessation of periods for 1 year. However, the ovaries will not suddenly stop; their function declines over time. This means that menopausal symptoms can occur for many years prior to the formal diagnosis of menopause.

🔍 **Important Learning Points**

- The diagnosis of menopause and perimenopause can be made clinically with a history of amenorrhoea, with or without symptoms (hot flushes, night sweats, dry skin, mood changes).
- A raised serum FSH supports the diagnosis of ovarian failure, as menopause is physiological ovarian failure.
- In rare cases where there is clinical suspicion, an underlying cause for symptoms may need investigation.
- Treatment of menopause is usually only required if a patient is having symptoms which impact on her quality of life.

VULVAL DISORDERS

Q1: The first-line medication for unprovoked vulvodynia.
The correct answer is A. Amitriptyline.

Amitriptyline is a tricyclic antidepressant which has analgesic properties and works well in the treatment of neuropathic pain. If a trial of amitriptyline is successful, then the dose can be titrated to optimise the effect of the drug. Patients often research the medication you have prescribed and can become distressed if they think you are secretly treating them for depression, so it is important to explain that although amitriptyline is used for depression in high doses, the low-dose preparation prescribed is for neuropathic pain.

Q2: A treatment for Bartholin cysts which may be performed by a 'window operation'.
The correct answer is J. Marsupialisation.

Marsupialisation of a Bartholin cyst involves creating an artificial mucocutaneous junction. In a window operation, this is done by removing an elliptical area of tissue to open the gland, and then the opening is sutured around to hold it open, allowing it to drain freely through a permanent connection to the vulva.

Q3: This may cause vulval dryness and is reserved for recurrent Bartholin cysts.
The correct answer is G. Excision of Bartholin gland.

The fluid produced in the Bartholin glands is useful for lubrication during sexual intercourse. The removal of the gland, and therefore the lack of lubrication around the vagina can cause pain and discomfort. Artificial lubricants may help after the operation, which is usually only performed as a last resort.

Q4: The initial treatment of choice for uncomplicated lichen sclerosus.

The correct answer is D. Clobetasol propionate ointment.

This is a potent corticosteroid ointment which helps to reduce the inflammation within the vulva. By sticking to the recommended regimen, patients can usually avoid the systemic side effects of the steroid.

 Key Point

Topical corticosteroids can cause exacerbations of local infections due to the immunosuppressive qualities of these drugs. Therefore, infections should be eliminated prior to using the ointment. If this is not possible, then preparations that contain an antibiotic or antifungal agent alongside a steroid may be used.

Q5: Beneficial in the context of vulvodynia if used prior to sexual intercourse

The correct answer is L. Topical local anaesthetic agent.

Topical local anaesthetic gel applied to the area 20 minutes prior to intercourse can be beneficial at managing the symptoms of provoked vulvodynia. There is also a role for lubricants and vaginal dilators.

Q6: Answer true or false: Which of the following associated features would support a diagnosis of lichen sclerosus in Janet?

The initial diagnosis of lichen sclerosus is based on the history and clinical findings. It is therefore important to be able to obtain a focused history, so that the diagnosis can be made without delay, and treatment begun.

A ✔ **Type 1 diabetes mellitus – True.** Type 1 diabetes mellitus is an autoimmune condition that tends to present in childhood. Although autoimmune thyroid diseases are most commonly associated with lichen sclerosus, other autoimmune conditions, including type 1 diabetes mellitus and vitiligo, are also associated.

B ✔ **Purpura – True.** Ecchymoses are large purpura which are associated with lichen sclerosus. They occur because the skin is atrophic. Atrophic skin is very fragile and can split very easily as a result of scratching, causing the patient to feel pain.

C Premenopause – **False.** Although young women can develop lichen sclerosus, it would be much lower down your list of differential diagnoses than in women who are postmenopausal.

D ✔ **Postmenopause – True.** Lichen sclerosus is most commonly seen in women who have undergone menopause. However, this is not as a result of hormonal changes or hormone replacement therapy.

E Recurrent vaginal fungal infections – **False.** Recurrent fungal infections, such as candida, are associated with vulvodynia but not associated with lichen sclerosus.

 Key Point

Treatment of lichen sclerosus is primarily by the use of topical corticosteroids. However, surgery may be necessary to remove any adhesions that have occurred as a result of the disease.

Q7: Which symptom would most suggest a diagnosis of provoked vulvodynia?

The correct answer is C. Pain upon touching the entrance to the vagina.

The key to diagnosing provoked vulvodynia is to remember that the pain will be localised and provoked.

A Constant widespread pain in the vulva – **Incorrect.** This sort of pain is suggestive of unprovoked vulvodynia. Provoked vulvodynia, previously called vestibulodynia, is localised to the vestibular area (the entrance to the vagina), rather than being widespread throughout the vulva. Additionally, as it is a provoked pain, it is not constant; rather, it occurs after an external stimulus.

B Deep pelvic pain during intercourse – **Incorrect.** Pain associated with vulvodynia is superficial and usually confined to the entrance of the vagina. Deep pelvic pain is often associated with causes such as pelvic inflammatory disease and endometriosis.

C ✔ **Pain upon touching the entrance to the vagina – Correct.** This correctly fits the diagnosis of localised (at the introitus) and provoked (upon touching) pain. The symptom can be reproduced on examination by touching the area with a cotton bud and asking the patient when and where they feel pain.

D Vulval itching – **Incorrect.** Itching is a common symptom of many vulval disorders. However, vulvodynia is a disorder of chronic pain, so itching does not feature as a direct result of the disease. However, vulvodynia may be precipitated by recurrent candidiasis, which frequently causes itching. Therefore, if candida is untreated at the time of presentation, the patient may complain of itching.

E A feeling of fullness in the vagina – **Incorrect.** A feeling of fullness is not associated with vulvodynia, but with an anatomical abnormality, most commonly a urogenital prolapse.

 Key Point

The previous names used for provoked vulvodynia were vestibulodynia and vestibulitis, suggesting that there is an underlying inflammatory process. Chronic inflammatory changes are not commonly seen on tissue samples; therefore, the name of the disease was modified, and biopsies do not form a part of the diagnostic process.

- Vulval disorders are common and can affect women of any age.
- Lichen sclerosus is an autoimmune skin condition which may lead to squamous cell carcinoma.
- Bartholin cysts occur at the entrance to the vagina and often require surgical intervention to prevent recurrence.
- Vulvodynia is vulvar discomfort, often described as burning pain, occurring in the absence of relevant visible findings or a specific, clinically identifiable, neurological disorder.
- Vulvodynia can be classified by whether or not it is provoked, and the site of the pain.
- The discomfort caused by vulval disorders may lead to psychological sequelae, including sexual dysfunction.

5 UROGYNAECOLOGY

PELVIC ORGAN PROLAPSE

Q1: Which of the following is not a risk factor for pelvic organ prolapse?

The correct answer is C. Congestive cardiac failure.

Prolapse is caused by damage to the structures supporting the vagina, such as the ligaments, fascia and levator ani muscles. However, factors that increase the intra-abdominal pressure, such as a chronic cough or obesity, can exacerbate symptoms.

A   Childbirth – **Incorrect.** Vaginal births stretch the muscles of the pelvic floor and can cause pelvic nerve damage. Large birth weights, multiple vaginal births and particularly difficult labours and births increase the risk of prolapse; for example, a prolonged second stage of labour or assisted vaginal birth.

B   Chronic obstructive pulmonary disease (COPD) – **Incorrect.** Anything that increases the intra-abdominal pressure increases the risk of pelvic organ prolapse, such as the chronic coughing experienced in COPD. The increased intra-abdominal pressure is transmitted to the pelvic floor musculature.

C   ✔ **Congestive cardiac failure – Correct.** Heart failure is not a risk factor for pelvic organ prolapse.

D   Menopause – **Incorrect.** Oestrogen deficiency which occurs after the menopause can cause atrophy of the vaginal fascia.

E   Obesity – **Incorrect.** Obesity places increased pressure upon the vagina, increasing the risk of failure of the supporting structures and leading to a prolapse.

Key Point

The risk of prolapse can be reduced by patients regularly performing pelvic floor exercises following childbirth to maintain perineal muscle tone. Maintaining a healthy lifestyle and normal BMI, and treating chronic conditions such as constipation and coughing, will reduce Valsalva manoeuvres.

Q2: What is the correct description of a cystocoele?

The correct answer is B. Prolapse of the bladder.

It is difficult to diagnose the type of prolapse just from the history. Diagnosis is made by clinical examination using a C-shaped speculum. However, the history is very important in helping to decide the management option.

A   Prolapse of the urethra – **Incorrect.** Prolapse of the urethra is known as a urethrocoele. The defect lies in the lower anterior vaginal wall.

B   ✔ **Prolapse of the bladder – Correct.** Prolapse of the bladder is known as a cystocoele with the defect in the upper anterior vaginal wall.

C   Prolapse of the rectum – **Incorrect.** Prolapse of the rectum is known as a rectocoele with a defect in the posterior vaginal wall.

D   Prolapse of the pouch of Douglas – **Incorrect.** Prolapse of the pouch of Douglas often contains small bowel or omentum and is known as an enterocoele.

E   Prolapse of the vaginal vault – **Incorrect.** The vault is the apex of the vagina. It most commonly prolapses after hysterectomy.

Key Point

In vaginal prolapse, when we discuss prolapse of an organ such as the bladder, we do not mean that the bladder is visible inside the vagina. Damage to the vaginal fascia weakens the vagina, so pressure from other pelvic organs pushes on the vaginal wall. This causes the vagina to bulge into itself, with the associated pelvic organ pushing into the space, but this organ remains on the other side of the vaginal wall.

Q3: Answer true or false: The following are treatment options for pelvic organ prolapse.

A prolapse is not a life-threatening condition. If the patient's quality of life is not affected, a prolapse does not need treating. Treatment options include conservative management, vaginal pessaries, and vaginal surgery.

A   ✔ **Weight loss – True.** Any degree of prolapse is exacerbated if the patient is overweight. Excess weight increases the intra-abdominal pressure and this increase in pressure is transmitted to the pelvic floor muscles. Therefore, losing weight will reduce the stress on the pelvic floor anatomy.

B   ✔ **Pelvic floor muscle exercises – True.** Pelvic floor muscle exercises aim to increase the strength and duration of the muscle contractions. If the walls of the vagina are weak, the pelvic organs can protrude into the vagina more easily. A strict programme of pelvic floor exercises needs to be followed in order to see a benefit. A minimum of 3 months of eight contractions at least three times daily is advised. A referral to a physiotherapist can be very helpful to teach these exercises. These exercises are very important in the prevention of prolapse and should be strongly encouraged for all women postpartum.

C Mid-urethral sling – **False.** Sling operations such as tension-free vaginal tape (TVT) are used in the treatment of stress incontinence. This procedure aims to stabilise the urethra and is not a procedure used to treat pelvic organ prolapse.

D ✔ **Vaginal ring pessary – True.** A pessary is a plastic or silicone device that fits into the vagina to support the vaginal wall and pelvic organs. It is a good option if surgery is not wanted; for example, in women who are considering having children in the future. Pessaries need to be sized correctly, cleaned and re-inserted regularly.

E ✔ **Laxatives – True.** Avoiding constipation and straining to defecate can help prevent pelvic organ prolapse. They also reduce the exacerbation of symptoms and may reduce the sensation of a bulge.

> 💬 **Key Point**
>
> Treatment of prolapse is based upon many factors, such as age, possible future pregnancies and sexual activity. Therefore, a thorough history is important.

Q4: Which surgical procedure would be a treatment option for a cystocoele?

The correct answer is A. Anterior repair.

Surgery offers a more definitive treatment for prolapse. The type of surgery offered depends on the patient and the prolapse that exists. Recurrence of a prolapse following surgical correction is common, with up to 30% requiring a further procedure. The high recurrence rate may be due to the fact that the tissues are already weak prior to the repair.

A ✔ **Anterior repair – Correct.** An anterior repair is indicated for repair of a cystocoele (a prolapse of the bladder through the anterior vaginal wall fascia). This procedure uses stitches to repair or strengthen the tissue, similarly in a posterior repair.

B Hysterectomy – **Incorrect.** Hysterectomy can be used to treat a uterine prolapse. This can be done through a vaginal or an abdominal approach.

C Manchester repair – **Incorrect.** This procedure is indicated to treat a uterine prolapse. This is a uterus-sparing procedure, but it is very rarely carried out due to the high complication rate. The procedure involves removing some of the cervix and tightly suturing together the ligaments which support the uterus on its lower aspect (uterosacral and cardinal ligaments). This lifts the uterus and increases the strength of the support.

D Posterior repair – **Incorrect.** A posterior repair, also known as a posterior colporrhaphy, is indicated for a repair of a rectocoele (a prolapse of the posterior vaginal wall). Stitches are used to repair or strengthen the tissues.

E Sacrocolpopexy – **Incorrect.** Sacrocolpopexy is a procedure to fix the vaginal vault (following a hysterectomy) to the sacrum using a mesh. A similar procedure can be performed attaching the uterus to the sacrum in patients with a uterus; this is called a hysterosacropexy.

> 💬 **Key Point**
>
> The use of mesh as part of anterior and posterior repair surgery decreases the recurrence rate of prolapse, but mesh use for this has stopped in the UK due to a high number of complications associated from mesh erosion. However, mesh is used for sacrocolpopexy, but the erosion appears to be less frequent. Mesh is commonly used in other surgical procedures, most commonly for hernia repair in general surgery where it more rarely causes mesh erosion.

> 🔍 **Important Learning Points**
>
> - Vaginal prolapse is common in women, with around 50% of parous women showing signs of prolapse. However, less than 10% of affected women will actually require an operation.
> - Common symptoms are a dragging sensation or the feeling of a bulge in the vagina. Urinary and bowel symptoms can also occur with a large prolapse.
> - Pelvic floor exercises and maintaining a healthy BMI are key ways to prevent a symptomatic prolapse.
> - A variety of pessaries and surgical interventions are available, depending on the type of prolapse and the patient's preference.

URINARY INCONTINENCE

Q1: Answer true or false: When initially assessing the urinary incontinence in this lady, which of the following would you carry out as a primary investigation?

When assessing a patient complaining of urinary incontinence, it is important to take a detailed history. This will help to categorise the type of urinary incontinence the patient is experiencing and help decide on a management plan.

A ✔ **Bladder diary – True.** Bladder diaries help to measure the frequency and severity of a patient's symptoms. Quantifying symptoms help to support a diagnosis and counsel patients on lifestyle changes.

B ✔ **Post-void residual volume – True.** PVR is the amount of urine remaining in the bladder after voiding. It can be measured using a handheld bladder scanner or catheterisation following voiding.

C Renal ultrasound – **False.** Imaging is not required for routine assessment for urinary incontinence. However, a pelvic ultrasound would be warranted if a pelvic mass is identified on examination.

D ✔ **Urinalysis – True.** Urinary tract infections (UTIs) can cause or exacerbate urinary incontinence. A urine dip is a quick and simple way to assess for a UTI, with a urine dip positive for both nitrites and leucocytes being the most convincing.

E Urodynamics – **False.** Urodynamics includes multichannel cystometry, ambulatory monitoring and video dynamics. These tests assess the intravesical and intra-abdominal pressures and how they relate to the patient's voiding, filling and storing. This type of testing is not required prior to starting first-line treatments in most patients.

> **Key Point**
>
> It is also important to exclude other causes or exacerbating conditions of urinary incontinence, such as UTIs, diabetes, chronic cough, pelvic organ prolapse or a pelvic mass. Therefore, a full examination includes an abdominal examination, as well as an evaluation for prolapse.

Q2: Which of the following is not a risk factor for stress incontinence in this lady?

The correct answer is A. Alcohol.

Risk factors for stress incontinence can be categorised into factors that increase the intra-abdominal pressure and factors that reduce the strength of the pelvic floor muscles, ligaments and fascia. An obstetric history is vital, as this identifies a risk for injury to the pelvic floor.

A ✔ **Alcohol – Correct.** Drinks containing alcohol or caffeine cause diuresis and detrusor muscle contractions and overactivity. A reduction in caffeinated drinks and alcohol, as well as limiting fluid intake, can improve symptoms of urgency and frequency. This is advised as a first-line treatment for overactive bladder. However, there is no evidence that this lifestyle choice is a risk factor for stress incontinence.

B Chronic cough – **Incorrect.** Coughing increases the abdominal pressure which in turn can increase the intravesical pressure and cause stress incontinence. It is therefore important to ensure that COPD and asthma patients have their respiratory disease well managed and that all patients are advised to stop smoking.

C Lack of oestrogen – **Incorrect.** Post-menopause, there is a lack of oestrogen, and this can decrease the strength of the urethra. Therefore, oestrogen given vaginally can improve symptoms of urinary incontinence if associated with vaginal atrophy.

D Obesity – **Incorrect.** Anything that increases the intra-abdominal pressure increases the risk of stress urinary incontinence. When the intravesical pressure overcomes the threshold of the bladder sphincters, urine is voided. Therefore, increased weight can cause increased intravesical pressure and stress urinary incontinence. Patients with stress urinary incontinence or overactive bladder with a BMI greater than 30 kg/m² should be advised to lose weight.

E Vaginal birth – **Incorrect.** Vaginal birth stretches the muscles of the pelvic floor as the baby descends down the vaginal tract. Multiple vaginal births and large birth weights increase the risk of damage to the pelvic floor muscles. Women should be encouraged to do pelvic floor exercises following vaginal birth. Supervised pelvic floor muscle training of at least 3 months' duration is a first-line treatment for women with stress incontinence.

> **Key Point**
>
> Stress incontinence often coexists with uterovaginal prolapse, as many of the risk factors are the same. These include increasing age, obesity, smoking, pregnancy, vaginal births, pelvic surgery and a chronic cough.

Q3: Some presentations of urinary incontinence require referral immediately to secondary care without first trying conservative management. Which of the following situations could be managed initially in primary care?

The correct answer is B. Mixed incontinence picture.

If a patient presents with red flag symptoms, they will need to be referred straight to secondary care in order to exclude a malignancy. In patients who have had previous pelvic surgery or have a pelvic organ prolapse, their management may be more complex and their symptoms will often not improve with conservative measures. Therefore, these patients warrant a secondary care referral.

A Haematuria – **Incorrect.** Haematuria without the presence of infection can indicate a malignancy of the urinary tract, so this needs urgent further investigations with cystoscopy and an ultrasound scan.

B ✔ **Mixed incontinence picture – Correct.** If a patient presents with symptoms of both stress and urge incontinence, management can be challenging. A bladder diary can be helpful to decipher exactly what the patient is experiencing. Treating the most bothersome symptom using conservative measures can be done in primary care. If this fails, referral can be made to secondary care, where further investigation with urodynamic studies may be considered.

C Previous surgery for urinary incontinence – **Incorrect.** When a patient has had previous surgery, referral is indicated to assess the anatomy and condition of the previous repair. The patient will have already tried conservative management previously, prior to surgery, so repeating this is unlikely to be successful.

D Recurrent UTIs – **Incorrect.** Recurrent UTIs are traditionally defined as two or more laboratory-confirmed urinary infections within 6 months. Recurrent UTIs are common, especially in sexually active women and postmenopausal women. Recurrent UTIs need further workup in a primary care setting to exclude diagnoses such as diabetes or STIs. However, if these diagnoses have been excluded and symptoms have not settled with antibiotics, then patients require an ultrasound and referral to secondary care for cystoscopy to exclude bladder cancer.

E Symptomatic pelvic organ prolapse – **Incorrect.** Women with urinary incontinence who have symptomatic prolapse that is visible at or below the vaginal introitus should be referred to a specialist. Conservative management for incontinence will have little effect in these women, and surgical management is often necessary.

> ### Key Point
>
> Red flag symptoms which could suggest a malignancy include:
> - Suspected mass arising from the urinary tract.
> - Macroscopic (visible) haematuria in an adult.
> - Microscopic (not visible) haematuria if the patient is 50 years or older or has recurrent episodes.
> - Persistent or recurring UTIs associated with haematuria if the patient is older than 40 years.

If a patient is noted to have any of these symptoms, an urgent referral to secondary care is required.

Q4: Answer true or false: Which of the following are treatment options for stress incontinence?

The treatment for urinary incontinence differs depending on the type of incontinence the patient is experiencing. Lifestyle measures are important in all patients and should be advised; for example, fluid intake reduction and achieving a healthy BMI. However, more invasive treatments are recommended if conservative measures do not improve symptoms.

A Botulinum toxin – **False.** Botulinum toxin blocks the release of acetylcholine and temporarily paralyses muscles where it is injected. It can be used in the treatment of idiopathic detrusor overactivity when conservative management has been unsuccessful in the management of urge incontinence.

B ✔ **Duloxetine – True.** Duloxetine is a serotonin and noradrenaline reuptake inhibitor. It can be used as a second-line treatment for stress incontinence if surgery is contraindicated. It acts by increasing internal urethral sphincter contractility. Side effects of duloxetine include nausea, dry mouth, constipation and insomnia.

C Oxybutynin – **False.** Oxybutynin is an antimuscarinic medication. It is a treatment used for overactive bladder and urge incontinence if bladder training has been ineffective. The side effects include dry mouth, constipation, blurred vision, fatigue and cognitive dysfunction.

D ✔ **Pelvic floor muscle training – True.** Pelvic floor muscle training aims to increase the strength and length of contraction of the pelvic floor muscles, helping to stabilise the urethra. Supervised pelvic floor muscle training is advised for a minimum of 3 months as first-line treatment for stress and mixed urinary incontinence.

E ✔ **Colposuspension – True.** Surgery is considered in stress incontinence after the failure of conservative management.

> ### Key Point
>
> There are many treatment options to consider when treating urinary incontinence. Non-invasive treatments can be considered with only minimal investigation. Urodynamics should be performed if symptoms have not been controlled with simple measures and surgical treatment is being considered.

> ### Important Learning Points
>
> - A thorough history will identify the type of incontinence in the majority of cases.
> - Urinalysis and bladder diaries are essential first-line investigations.
> - Simple lifestyle measures, including treating constipation, optimising fluid intake and treating comorbidities, can help incontinence. Maintaining a healthy BMI is helpful in stress incontinence and cutting out caffeine and alcohol improves urge incontinence.
> - Pelvic floor exercises form part of the primary management of stress incontinence. Further treatments may include urethral bulking agents, sling surgery or duloxetine.
> - Bladder retraining is the primary management for urge incontinence. Further treatments are antimuscarinic and selective beta agonist medications.
> - Urodynamic studies should be undertaken prior to operative treatment options if primary treatments have failed.

6 PELVIC PAIN

ENDOMETRIOSIS

Q1: What is the best investigation for diagnosing endometriosis?

The correct answer is C. Laparoscopy.

The common symptoms associated with endometriosis are chronic pelvic pain, dysmenorrhoea and deep dyspareunia. Unfortunately, this collection of symptoms is not specific to endometriosis, and examination also does not give a definitive diagnosis. Investigations are required to confirm the presence of endometriosis, although even the presence of the disease does not necessarily mean it is responsible for the symptoms.

A CA-125 – **Incorrect.** CA-125 is a serum biomarker of ovarian cancer and as such should be requested as part of a workup if an atypical cyst or mass is identified on an ovary. CA-125 is also elevated in anything which causes peritoneal inflammation, including PID, endometriosis and even menstruation during a normal cycle. While elevated CA-125 levels may support the diagnosis of endometriosis, it is obviously not diagnostic.

B History and examination alone – **Incorrect.** A thorough history may raise the suspicion of endometriosis, and in some cases, simple pain relief or hormonal treatments may be successful in treating the symptoms without recourse to laparoscopy. However, the history and examination alone is not sufficient for an accurate and reliable diagnosis of endometriosis.

C ✔ **Laparoscopy – Correct.** Direct visualisation of lesions via laparoscopy and biopsy remains the gold standard diagnostic test. In addition to this, it is also possible to 'see and treat' these lesions during laparoscopy, either by resecting the endometriosis out of the tissues or by destroying the endometriosis in situ using laser ablation or diathermy. However, medical treatments may be started before a diagnostic laparoscopy is performed. If this treatment is successful, surgery may be avoided, which would be preferable in patients at high risk of surgical complications.

D MRI – **Incorrect.** MRI can be useful to assess the extent of endometriosis, particularly when it infiltrates deep into tissues. However, for the majority of superficial peritoneal endometriosis, the evidence supports laparoscopy as the more sensitive diagnostic modality.

E Transvaginal ultrasound – **Incorrect.** Transvaginal ultrasound is routinely used in the workup of these patients. It is good at demonstrating large endometriotic lesions, most commonly endometrioma cysts on the ovaries, and rarely for identifying lesions in the rectum or bladder. It is also good at identifying pelvic masses and collections not caused by endometriosis that may be responsible for a patient's symptoms. However, the commonest location for endometriosis is peritoneal, and ultrasound is poor at detecting these, as they are often very small lesions which cannot be differentiated from normal tissue.

> 💬 **Key Point**
>
> Patients are often exposed to multiple investigations; however, direct visualisation by laparoscopy remains the gold standard. Patients who are not suitable for laparoscopy, or who choose not to have one, can be offered medical treatments without confirmation by laparoscopy.

Q2: Answer true or false: Which of these non-surgical treatment options are recommended for endometriosis?

Many women opt for medical treatment before a diagnosis is confirmed with laparoscopy. After a diagnosis is made at laparoscopy, medical management may subsequently be commenced if symptoms are not relieved after the surgery. The management choice should be based on the severity of the disease, the patient's health beliefs and the side effect profiles of the various treatment options. Symptoms often reoccur following the cessation of non-surgical management options.

A ✔ **Combined oral contraceptives – True.** The combined oral contraceptives are effective at reducing pain in patients with endometriosis. They negatively

feedback on the HPO axis, preventing ovulation and halting the rise in oestrogen levels during the normal menstrual cycle. Like the normal endometrium, endometriosis growth is driven by oestrogen, so these treatments can cause the resolution of endometriosis. The systemic progestogen-only contraceptives have equally been shown to improve endometriosis symptoms. Similarly, progestogens inhibit the proliferative effect of oestrogens on endometriosis (and normal endometrium). Some of the preparations also inhibit follicular development and ovulation, thereby decreasing oestrogen production by the ovaries in the follicular phase.

B ✔ **Levonorgestrel intrauterine system – True.** IUSs have been shown to significantly lower the amount of pain experienced by endometriosis sufferers for between 3 to 5 years. The progestogen released by the IUS inhibits the effect of oestrogen on the endometrium (and also endometriosis), preventing tissue proliferation. The IUS can also downregulate the HPO axis in some patients, reducing oestrogen production.

C Non-steroidal anti-inflammatory drugs (NSAIDs) – **False.** NSAIDs are commonly prescribed for patients with pelvic pain, as there is good evidence for their use in menorrhagia and dysmenorrhoea. There is no good evidence for their beneficial use in endometriosis but given that symptoms may be multifactorial and confirming the correct diagnosis can be difficult, clinicians often still prescribe them. The likely benefit is weighed up against the potential risks of prolonged NSAID use, in particular gastrointestinal ulceration.

D ✔ **Patient support groups – True.** Patient self-help groups play an invaluable role in supporting patients with counselling and advice.

E Statins – **False.** Some preliminary studies suggest statins may prevent the onset and progression of endometriosis, but this is currently an area requiring further research before statins can be used for this indication.

> 💬 **Key Point**
>
> Hormonal therapies make up the mainstay of treatment options, reducing hormonal stimulation of endometrial tissue. Which treatment is offered depends heavily on the side effect profiles of the drugs used.

[See 'Contraception' page 71.]

Q3: Answer true or false: If the patient would like to become pregnant, which of the following are appropriate options to offer?

There is debate as to the effect of endometriosis on fertility. There is evidence that treating endometriosis surgically improves fertility, but the mechanism is poorly understood.

A Hormonal therapies – **False.** Continuous hormonal therapy treatments, including danazol, gestrinone, medroxyprogesterone acetate and GnRH analogues, all act to downregulate the HPO axis. So while they may treat endometriosis, they also prevent ovulation and possible pregnancy. One theory (and limited research) suggests that giving a hormone to cause ovarian suppression and anovulation for a few months prior to either attempting spontaneous conception or IVF may improve pregnancy outcomes in patients with endometriosis. However, further research is required before this can be considered as routine practice.

B ✔ **Intrauterine insemination (IUI) – True.** In patients who have had surgically treated mild to moderate disease and who have patent fallopian tubes, IUI, particularly with ovarian stimulation, has been shown to increase fertility in patients with endometriosis.

C ✔ ***In vitro* fertilisation (IVF) – True.** IVF is considered an appropriate option in patients with endometriosis who are struggling to conceive and have no other identifiable, treatable causes of infertility or whose tubal function is compromised.

D ✔ **Laparoscopic ablation and adhesiolysis – True.** Surgical treatment of endometriosis has been shown to be effective at increasing fertility in some patients with endometriosis.

E ✔ **Tubal flushing – True.** Tubal flushing has long been used to assess fallopian tube patency. However, tubal flushing with oil-soluble media has also been shown to improve fertility in small studies, although the mechanisms behind this are unknown.

> ### 🗩 Key Point
>
> Many patients end up undergoing IVF; however, in suitable patients, IUI may be attempted before this.

> ### 🔍 Important Learning Points
>
> - Endometriosis is the presence of endometrial tissue outside the uterus.
> - Important symptoms include pain, dysmenorrhea and dyspareunia.
> - Examination findings and results from investigations correlate poorly with symptoms.
> - There is an association with infertility.
> - Management is often trialled before definitive diagnosis.
> - Direct visualisation by laparoscopy and biopsy is the gold standard investigation.
> - Management is usually hormone based to reduce endometrial tissue stimulation, although in severe cases surgical options are available.

SEXUALLY TRANSMITTED INFECTIONS

Q1: A 22-year-old female presents with a known history of recurrent chlamydia. She has now developed pelvic pain ongoing for the last two months and has a temperature of 39.5°C.

The correct answer is I. PID.

It is most likely that this patient has developed PID after recurrent episodes of chlamydia infection that may not have been adequately treated. The young age is important in this question, as chlamydia is most common under the age of 25. Chlamydia and gonorrhoea are the commonest causes of PID, which can cause significant loss in quality of life due to chronic pelvic pain. It is also associated with infertility, hence the importance of treating chlamydial infections promptly. Patients should also be educated regarding safe sex practices and retested after treatment. This is to ensure the initial infection has resolved and there has been no reinfection of the patient.

Q2: A 35-year-old female who is a commercial sex worker develops a painless ulcer on her vulva. She has no other symptoms.

The correct answer is J. Syphilis.

This is highlighting the importance of knowledge regarding a chancre; a painless ulcer that develops as part of primary syphilis. It is important that any individual with a painless ulcer is investigated for syphilis because the chancre often resolves, and due to its painless nature, it may not trouble a patient. If left undiagnosed and untreated at this early stage, syphilis can develop to the later stages with significant associated health morbidities. A particular risk factor highlighted in this question is the detail that this patient is paid for sex. Many sex workers will be open about this with clinicians; however, you should never make assumptions and when taking a sexual history, it is routine to ask everybody this question.

Q3: A 25-year-old female has had a change in her discharge over the past 3 weeks; it has an offensive smell and on microscopy, mobile organisms are seen.

The correct answer is K. *Trichomonas vaginalis (TV).*

A change in vaginal discharge can occur for many reasons, including physiological changes, BV, TV, candidiasis, and many other STIs. Many genitourinary medicine (GUM) clinics will have access to microscopy on site, allowing vaginal swab smears to be viewed instantly. Identifying flagellated, mobile organisms in the specimen confirms the diagnosis of TV, allowing timely treatment.

Q4: A 27-year-old female returns after having cryotherapy treatment 2 months ago; her STI has reoccurred.

The correct answer is A. Anogenital warts.

This patient previously had cryotherapy – liquid nitrogen at very cold temperatures touched onto localised areas – often used to cause necrosis of warts. However, the treatment for warts is often unsuccessful and this patient has returned, most likely to discuss future treatment options. Depending on how she found the treatment previously and how florid her warts are, cryotherapy could be offered again or another treatment option could be explored. There is currently no gold standard, as all options have disadvantages.

Q5: A 12-year-old female has a vaccine called Gardasil® administered. Which STI is she protected against?

The correct answer is A. Anogenital warts.

Gardasil® is the name for a quadrivalent HPV vaccine, effective against types 6 and 11 that cause warts, as well as 16 and 18 that cause cervical cancer. Vaccines are offered in the UK to girls aged 11 to 14, with a second dose given 6 months to 2 years later. Another vaccine, Cervarix®, protects against types 16 and 18 but not against anogenital warts.

 Key Point

Although in real life it may be very difficult to distinguish the differences between STIs by the clinical history and examination, exams often have stereotypes to help determine which answer is most likely. It is important, as a student preparing for exams, to start to determine the 'buzz words' often used by examiners, and describing STIs are a good example of this.

Q6: Answer true or false to the following statements regarding contact tracing.

Contact tracing is a very important aspect of genitourinary medicine. While taking a sexual history, think beyond the patient in front of you and include all who may be infected. It is also important to consider that just because an individual is in a relationship, this does not always mean that they are only having sexual intercourse with that person. A thorough sexual history is required, obtained in a non-judgemental manner.

A ✔ **Patients should be encouraged to contact people possibly at risk of having an STI themselves – True.** Although other services can be offered it is important to first discuss with the patient whether they would feel able to communicate with any possible contacts. Ensure they are counselled correctly regarding what information to give this person or people, and it might be beneficial to provide resources or written information for the contacts to read and use.

B As long as both partners are undergoing treatment, they can engage in sexual intercourse – **False.** This is a common misconception. Patients should ideally refrain from any sexual intercourse until both partners have completed their treatment and have reached the prescribed time after treatment has passed. This is to prevent partners from reinfecting one another.

C ✔ **Many GUM clinics offer a service to contact people who could be at risk of having an STI – True.** Many people will feel unable to communicate with contacts that may potentially have contracted an STI. In some cases, this may also mean contacting individuals who have not been in touch with the patient for a significant amount of time. Most GUM clinics will offer services where they can anonymously make contact with other at-risk individuals, often using text messages that simply tell the contacts that they should get tested, without commenting on the potential source.

D With all STIs, individuals should only consider contacting those with whom they have had sexual intercourse within the last 6 months – **False.** The time period over which contacts will need to be traced depends on the STI, the likely time of infection and the incubation period of the infection.

E Only those who have engaged in vaginal and anal sexual intercourse need to be contacted – **False.** Oral sex is also a possible method of transmitting STIs, although it is rare to transmit chlamydia, gonorrhoea and TV by this route.

 Key Point

Ultimately, the determination of what contact tracing is required depends on taking a thorough, comprehensive sexual history from the patient.

Q7: Which of the following is the triad of symptoms in reactive arthritis?

The correct answer is C. Arthritis, urethritis and uveitis.

Reactive arthritis is a triad of urethritis, uveitis and arthritis. Urethritis may also occur as cervicitis in women. This is commonly remembered as 'cannot see, cannot pee, cannot climb a tree.' Reactive arthritis, is an autoimmune condition that develops following an infection elsewhere in the body. It commonly occurs in individuals between the age of 20 and 40 and is more common in men.

 Key Point

The commonest causes of reactive arthritis are intestinal infections, such as Salmonella or Campylobacter or STIs such as chlamydia or gonorrhoea.

Q8: Which of the following statements describes Fitz-Hugh Curtis syndrome?

The correct answer is D. Liver capsule inflammation and adhesions following PID.

PID is the inflammatory process caused by an STI, most commonly chlamydia, but gonorrhoea and other bacteria have also been implicated. The most common specific symptom is right upper quadrant pain, which may be pleuritic in nature.

A Areas of endometrial tissue outside of the uterus in the pelvic cavity – **Incorrect.** This describes the finding of endometriosis. This condition is also associated with chronic pain, inflammation, adhesions and infertility. The mechanism behind endometriosis formation is unclear, but no infective process is involved.

[See 'Endometriosis' page 202.]

B Atony of the bladder resulting from autonomic neuropathy following pelvic inflammatory disease – **Incorrect.** This is not a recognised complication of PID.

C Infertility developing due to tubal scarring following PID – **Incorrect.** Infertility is a common long-term complication of PID. The inflammation caused by infection results in fibrous scar tissue formation within the pelvis. The clinical picture can be subtle, with only the loss of cilia within the fallopian tubes, but this reduces oocyte transfer. Conversely, PID can cause significant fibrosis and obliteration of the canal of the tubes. Fibrous adhesions can also surround the ovary, preventing oocyte release to the tubes, or cause ovarian damage and anovulation.

D ✔ **Liver capsule inflammation and adhesions following PID – Correct.** Liver function tests and ultrasound scans are usually normal as the inflammation only affects the capsule, not the underlying parenchyma. Treatment is usually antibiotics to treat the underlying infection. Adhesions develop shortly after the infection has occurred, and can remain lifelong after the infection has resolved; they are often seen at diagnostic laparoscopy.

E Renal failure developing due to ascending infection following PID – **Incorrect.** PID can cause severe sepsis, which can cause renal failure due to end-organ hypoperfusion caused by vasodilatation and hypotension. Severe pelvic abscesses and adhesions can rarely cause ureteric obstruction causing renal failure.

> 💬 **Key Point**
>
> Fitz-Hugh Curtis syndrome presents as right upper quadrant pain, which is often worse on breathing or movement; it is caused by adhesions and inflammation of the liver capsule. It is a rare complication of PID, most commonly caused by chlamydia.

> 🔍 **Important Learning Points**
>
> - The severity of STIs can vary significantly. However, often the dangers of these infections are in their complications rather than the acute phase of the disease.
> - Contact tracing is a crucial part of the management of STIs.
> - If one STI is diagnosed in an individual, a thorough sexual health screen should be performed to rule out the existence of any other STIs.
> - Management is often with antimicrobials; however, always check the dose, route, frequency and any contra-indications with local guidelines.
> - It is important not to forget the psychosexual impact that STIs can have and to be sensitive to this during consultations.

BENIGN OVARIAN CYSTS

Q1: Answer true or false to the following statements with regards to benign ovarian cysts.

A large number of ovarian cysts identified on ultrasound are simple in nature and often require little or no follow-up. Having a good understanding of the diagnostic criteria will reduce unnecessary investigations and referrals and reduce both patient and clinician anxieties over normal findings.

A A benign ovarian cyst is a fluid-filled sac with a diameter of more than 5 cm, arising on, or within, an ovary – **False.** The definition of a benign ovarian cyst is a fluid-filled sac with a diameter of greater than 30 mm (3 cm), arising on, or within an ovary.

B ✔ **The gold standard investigation is a transvaginal ultrasound of the ovaries – True.** The most appropriate investigation of a benign ovarian cyst is an ultrasound. Ideally, this is a transvaginal scan due to the increased sensitivity when compared to a transabdominal one. An ultrasound can help identify the size, location and contents of an ovarian cyst and therefore guide the necessary treatment options.

C ✔ **A unilocular cyst with no blood flow is indicative of a benign cyst – True.** According to the IOTA group criteria for a benign ovarian cyst, the positive indicators include a unilocular cyst and the lack of blood flow. Other indications for a benign cyst include an acoustic shadow, a smooth multilocular cyst of less than 10 cm diameter, and the largest solid component (if present) being less than 7 mm.

D CA-125, lactate dehydrogenase, alpha-fetoprotein and hCG should be measured in all patients with an ovarian cyst seen on ultrasound – **False.** Lactate dehydrogenase, alpha-fetoprotein and hCG determinations are only necessary in patients younger than 40 years old with a complex cyst seen on ultrasound, due to the increased risk of a germ cell tumour. Although CA-125 is commonly measured, it has a low specificity and its results should be interpreted with caution in premenopausal women. It is important to remember that other conditions, such as endometriosis, can cause CA-125 to increase. If CA-125 is significantly raised, further investigation may be required to rule out cancer.

E Transvaginal aspiration of a benign ovarian cyst is a common treatment of choice – **False.** Due to the high recurrence rate following aspiration, this treatment is not commonly used.

> **Key Point**
>
> Differentiating between a benign and malignant cyst is of prime importance for deciding on the urgency of treatment.

Q2: Simple cyst less than 5 cm.
The correct answer is H. No treatment.

Most of these cysts are physiological and will remit sponta-
neously within a few months. Due to their small size, they
are at low risk for cyst accidents.

Q3: Simple cyst 5 to 7 cm.
The correct answer is L. Watchful waiting.

An ultrasound should be repeated in 1 year to identify any
growth or change in the cyst. They are at low risk of ovarian
torsion, and many will spontaneously resolve and therefore
do not require immediate treatment.

Q4: Simple cyst more than 7 cm.
The correct answer is E. Laparoscopic cystectomy.

Large cysts are at risk of ovarian torsion and causing chronic
pain, so they should be removed. A cystectomy approach is
preferable but must be based on each individual patient's cir-
cumstances.

Q5: Dermoid cyst.
The correct answer is E. Laparoscopic cystectomy.

These cysts tend to grow with time and are unlikely to
resolve, so surgery should be offered. Again, laparoscopic
surgery is preferred; however, this depends on the individual
patient.

Q6: Haemorrhagic cyst 3 cm diameter.
The correct answer is L. Watchful waiting.

Ultrasound should be repeated in 8 weeks, as haemorrhagic
cysts should have resolved in this time period. If the cyst has
not resolved, it should be treated as a complex ovarian cyst
and investigated with tumour markers and possible surgical
management.

> **Key Point**
>
> Simple cysts less than 5 cm in diameter do not require any
> follow-up as they are likely to resolve spontaneously. Large
> simple cysts (larger than 7 cm) and dermoid cysts are unlikely
> to resolve, so surgical management is offered to prevent
> complications from occurring.

Q7: Answer true or false: Which of the following are
complications of benign ovarian cysts?
Small benign ovarian cysts regularly grow and resolve
asymptomatically during the menstrual cycle without ever
being identified. A small minority of cysts can cause pain,
which is usually transient and requires no medical atten-
tion. However, occasionally, a cyst can cause severe pain,
which requires hospital admission and may require interven-
tion to prevent complications of ovarian damage.

A ✔ **Cyst rupture – True.** This may present with pain
and occasionally with an acute abdomen. This
can be treated easily with analgesia but requires
prompt investigations to rule out sinister causes for
the symptoms.
B PCOS – **False.** Polycystic ovaries is one of the diagnostic criteria for polycystic ovarian syndrome
(PCOS), but the multiple small cysts seen are a
complicaton of the syndrome not a cause of it.
C Cervical cancer – **False.** The process of PCOS can
lead to endometrial cancer due to the lack of withdrawal bleeds and the consequent endometrial
hyperplasia. Cervical cancer has no known link to
ovarian cysts.
D ✔ **Ovarian torsion – True.** A large cyst is at
increased risk of causing the ovary to twist. A high
index of suspicion is required, as ovarian torsion
can present with non-specific abdominal pain or an
acute abdomen. Urgent diagnosis and laparoscopy
is required to prevent necrosis of the ovary.
E ✔ **Cyst haemorrhage – True.** This may present with
acute pain. It can be treated easily with analgesia,
but urgent investigation is required to rule out
other causes of pain, such as appendicitis or ovarian torsion, which would require urgent surgery.

> **Key Point**
>
> Cyst accidents may present with acute pain and should be in-
> vestigated and treated urgently. Early recognition and treatment
> of ovarian torsion can prevent necrosis and loss of the ovary.

> **Important Learning Points**
>
> - Ovarian cysts are common in premenopausal women,
>   and most of these cysts are benign.
> - Ovarian cysts may present with symptoms or may be an
>   incidental finding on an ultrasound being performed for
>   an alternate reason.
> - The first-line investigation is ultrasound, preferably trans-
>   vaginal. Ultrasound is useful to assess the size, location
>   and consistency of a cyst.
> - Simple cysts often do not require any treatment.
> - The COCP may be used for long-term prevention of
>   cysts.
> - Cyst accidents may present with an acute abdomen.
>   Ovarian torsion, cyst haemorrhage and cyst rupture are
>   examples of cyst accidents. Early treatment of ovarian
>   torsion is required to prevent loss of the ovary.

7 ONCO-GYNAECOLOGY

OVARIAN CANCER

Q1: Answer true or false: Which of the following are risk
factors for ovarian cancer?
There is no reliable screening test for ovarian cancer and the
symptoms are often vague, leading to a delayed diagnosis. A
good understanding of the risk factors may improve identifi-
cation of symptomatic patients at an earlier stage.

A Early menopause – **False.** Early menopause reduces the number of times a woman is likely to ovulate and decreases the amount of time a woman has high oestrogen levels. The risk of ovarian cancer is increased by the number of times a patient has ovulated in her life. It is believed that ovulation causes damage to the epithelial lining, which is then repaired by new epithelial growth. The more times regrowth is required, the higher the chance there is of abnormal growth occurring, leading to cancer.

B ✔ **Infertility – True.** Not having children increases the risk of ovarian cancer. During pregnancy, the HPO axis stops, meaning a reduction in ovulation and ovarian epithelial damage. Treatments for infertility, such as clomiphene, may also increase ovarian cancer risk.

C Irritable bowel syndrome (IBS) – **False.** New onset of IBS symptoms (change in bowel habits, abdominal bloating and pain) in a postmenopausal woman should prompt investigation to exclude ovarian cancer as the cause of these symptoms, as ovarian cancer can present with these vague symptoms. IBS itself, however, does not increase a patient's risk for ovarian cancer.

D Multiparity – **False.** During pregnancy and breast-feeding, a woman will not be ovulating, thereby reducing ovarian damage, which actually decreases her risk of ovarian malignancy.

E ✔ **Use of hormone replacement therapy (HRT) – True.** Additional oestrogen increases ovarian cancer risk. However, the increased risk is small, with only one extra ovarian cancer per thousand patients taking HRT. Also, after 5 years following discontinuation of HRT, a patient's risk drops back to the background risk.

> 📧 **Key Point**
>
> The key risk factors for ovarian cancer are:
> - Prolonged oestrogen exposure.
> - Increased lifetime number of ovulations.
> - Family history – a genetic cause is implicated in 10% of ovarian cancers.

Q2: Using the history above, which of the following would be the most appropriate course of action?
The correct answer is **B.** Organise a CA-125 test.

Symptoms of ovarian cancer are vague, and can easily be attributed to other conditions, with IBS being the most common misdiagnosis. Clinical vigilance is therefore essential. Symptoms such as abdominal discomfort, abdominal bloating, change in bowel habits, nausea, lethargy or decreased appetite all warrant investigation.

A Dismiss the symptoms, they are too vague – **Incorrect.** Ovarian cancer presents with vague symptoms, so clinicians must have a low threshold for considering the diagnosis of ovarian cancer in any postmenopausal woman with vague symptoms. This woman, however, has unexplained weight loss, which is a symptom suggestive of underlying pathology.

B ✔ **Organise a CA-125 test – Correct.** This is the recommended first-line blood test. If the test is positive, an ultrasound of the pelvis should be organised to look for pelvic masses. If the blood test is normal and there is low clinical suspicion of malignancy, identification and treatment for other causes of the patient's symptoms should be undertaken.

C Organise an urgent CT scan – **Incorrect.** This is not a recognised first-line investigation. CT scans are used to stage ovarian cancer once a cyst or mass is identified on an ultrasound scan.

D Review the patient in 2 weeks to assess if the symptoms improve – **Incorrect.** Persistent symptoms in postmenopausal women should be investigated. The patient has been having unintentional weight loss now for 3 months, so it is very unlikely that waiting 2 weeks will improve her symptoms. Investigation should be started promptly.

E Send the patient to the emergency department (ED) – **Incorrect.** ED is an acute service not set up to arrange investigations for cancer or provide psychological support. Care should be coordinated by the primary care physician.

> 📧 **Key Point**
>
> A clinician needs to know when to investigate and how to do so. Incorrect investigation could lead to delayed diagnosis and a worse prognosis for the patient. Every general practitioner should be aware of national guidelines detailing symptoms and signs which warrant urgent referral for suspected cancers.

Q3: What is the most common type of ovarian cancer?
The correct answer is **C.** Epithelial tumour.

Histological diagnosis is usually only made after surgery. The type of cancer (along with grading and staging) is required to correctly plan ongoing management and advise on likely prognosis.

A Choriocarcinoma – **Incorrect.** This is a rare germ cell tumour of the ovary. Choriocarcinoma is the presence of malignant placental cell types which produces β hCG. They most commonly occur following malignant change of a molar pregnancy, rather than a primary ovarian cancer.

B Embryonal carcinoma – **Incorrect.** This is a very rare germ cell tumour of the ovary. The tumour contains early embryonic tissue, often containing a yolk sac. β hCG is commonly produced by this type of tumour.

C ✔ **Epithelial tumour – Correct.** Epithelial tumours account for 90% of ovarian cancers. They are most common in postmenopausal women and are rare in women below the age of 40. There are many different types, but the most common is the papillary serous cystadenocarcinoma.

D Immature malignant teratoma – **Incorrect.** This is a germ cell tumour which has the ability to form any cell type. They are the malignant form of dermoid cysts. They account for less than 1% of ovarian tumours.

E Stromal tumour – **Incorrect.** Stromal tumours arise from the fibrous ovarian tissue and the ovarian tissues responsible for hormone production. They account for approximately 8% of ovarian cancer.

> **Key Point**
>
> Epithelial tumours account for over 90% of ovarian cancer and predominantly occur in postmenopausal women. They are the most likely to cause an elevated CA-125 level, although CA-125 is normal in over 50% of early-stage epithelial ovarian cancers.

Q4: What is the optimal first-line treatment option for stage 1 ovarian cancer?

The correct answer is D. Total abdominal hysterectomy and bilateral salpingo-oophorectomy (BSO).

Most cancers are managed in a similar way. A multidisciplinary team allows expertise from many medical fields to combine to create the optimal treatment plan. Treatment may involve surgery, chemotherapy and radiotherapy either to cure or to improve and prolong quality of life. It is important to remember the psychological impact of cancer on patients and their families and to provide adequate support. The palliative care specialists are also a very important part of the team, offering treatment to improve symptoms either as side effects of the disease or from treatment.

A Chemotherapy and radiotherapy – **Incorrect.** Chemotherapy may occasionally be used as a primary treatment, but radiotherapy is rarely used to treat ovarian cancer.

B Platinum-based chemotherapy – **Incorrect.** Surgery is usually the primary treatment, followed by adjuvant chemotherapy if required. Where surgery is not possible – for example, where a patient has significant medical co-morbidities – stand-alone chemotherapy may be used. There is research ongoing into the possible benefits of neoadjuvant chemotherapy prior to surgery.

C Radiotherapy – **Incorrect.** Radiotherapy is rarely used for ovarian cancer because high doses of radiation are required to be effective. Due to the proximity of radiotherapy-sensitive organs like the bowel, the potentially severe side effects outweigh the potential benefits.

D ✔ **Total abdominal hysterectomy and bilateral salpingo-oophorectomy – Correct.** The aims of surgery are:
- To obtain a tissue sample to confirm the diagnosis and identify the cell type.
- To attempt to remove all of the tumour, as a curative procedure.
- To remove as much tumour as possible (debulking) where complete resection is not possible, to improve the duration and quality of life.

A course of adjuvant platinum-based chemotherapy often follows surgery to reduce recurrence rates.

E Unilateral salpingo-oophorectomy – **Incorrect.** There is a risk of cancer being present in the contralateral ovary at the time of surgery, and there is also a higher risk of recurrence leaving an ovary *in situ*. Very occasionally, this is considered when a woman has a low-grade and low-stage cancer and wishes to preserve fertility.

> **Key Point**
>
> The best chance of achieving complete disease resection is by removing both ovaries, both fallopian tubes and the uterus. Lymph nodes and the omentum may also be excised as part of a curative procedure, depending on the tumour stage.

> **Important Learning Points**
>
> - Symptoms of ovarian cancer are vague; therefore, high clinical suspicion is required.
> - Initial investigation is CA-125. If this is elevated, a pelvic ultrasound is arranged, and the patient is referred to gynaecology if a mass is identified.
> - Epithelial cell tumours are the most common form of ovarian cancer and occur primarily in the postmenopausal patient.
> - Key risk factors for ovarian cancer are an increased number of ovulations, age and oestrogen exposure.
> - Ovarian cancer often presents as advanced-stage disease, meaning surgery and chemotherapy usually have a palliative intent, as survival rates in high stage disease are low.

ENDOMETRIAL CANCER

Q1: Answer true or false: Which of the following are risk factors for endometrial cancer?

Endometrial cancer is extremely rare in women under 40 years of age, with over 90% occurring in postmenopausal women. However, in premenopausal women with symptoms and other risk factors, the differential diagnosis of endometrial cancer should be considered.

A Early menopause – **False.** Early menopause reduces the number of times a woman is likely to ovulate and decreases the amount of exposure to oestrogen.

B Multiparity – **False.** During pregnancy, the menstrual cycle and ovulation both stop. There are raised levels of oestrogen (mainly oestriol) while pregnant, but also very high levels of progesterone, so the endometrium is not stimulated to proliferate during pregnancy.

C   ✔ **Nulliparity – True.** This risk of endometrial cancer is inversely related to parity. Pregnancy, breastfeeding and use of the combined oral contraceptive are all protective against endometrial cancer because they stop ovulation, which reduces the physiological oestrogen exposure during the menstrual cycle.

D   ✔ **Raised BMI – True.** Adipose tissue makes oestrone, which is a form of oestrogen. This is outside the control of the HPO axis, and there is no equivalent production of progesterone to protect the endometrium from stimulation by oestrogen. Obese women, therefore, have increased levels of oestrogen in their bodies, which stimulates the endometrium, increasing the risk of endometrial cancer.

E   Smoking – **False.** Smoking has a protective effect; however, the exact mechanism is unclear.

 Key Point

Oestrogen exposure is a major risk factor for endometrial cancer. This may be from physiological causes such as the menstrual cycle, iatrogenic causes such as hormone replacement therapy and pathological causes such as obesity. The other key risk factor for endometrial cancer is increasing age.

Q2: Which one of the following options would not be of use to the clinician assessing this patient?

The correct answer is B. Cervical smear.

A thorough history identifying risk factors for endometrial cancer should be sought. A careful examination, including a vaginal examination, is required to rule out vulval, vaginal and cervical causes of bleeding. Transvaginal ultrasound is then usually requested to assess the endometrium. A pipelle biopsy should then be obtained if there is evidence of endometrial thickening. If it is not possible to obtain a biopsy, then a hysteroscopy is undertaken to visualise and biopsy the endometrium.

A   Cervical examination – **Incorrect.** History and examination are the essential first steps in diagnosing the cause of PMB. Abdominal examination should assess for masses and pelvic lymphadenopathy. Speculum examination and digital vaginal examination are required to assess the vulva, vagina and cervix for any abnormality that may be responsible for the bleeding.

B   ✔ **Cervical smear – Correct.** The history states that the patient had a normal cervical smear 4 years ago, so a repeat is not due as part of routine screening. It is important to visualise the cervix as part of an examination for any patient with PMB, as bleeding from a cervical cancer is a differential diagnosis. If on examination this was considered, then the next

step in the management plan should be to refer a patient for a colposcopy. A smear should not be performed.

C   Hysteroscopy – **Incorrect.** This is commonly performed for patients presenting with PMB, where it is either not possible to obtain an adequate endometrial biopsy during a routine examination or where ultrasound indicates a possible focal lesion, such as a polyp. In these cases, hysteroscopy can view the entire uterine cavity, take a biopsy of the endometrium and facilitate removal of the polyps.

D   Pipelle biopsy – **Incorrect.** If a transvaginal ultrasound scan demonstrates an endometrial thickness of at least 4 mm in a patient presenting with PMB, a biopsy of endometrium should be taken to assess for endometrial hyperplasia or cancer. Using a Cuscoe speculum, the cervix can be visualised during a routine clinical appointment and a biopsy probe passed in through the cervical os. Gentle scraping of the endometrial lining allows a biopsy to be obtained within the probe.

E   Transvaginal ultrasound – **Incorrect.** This is usually the first-line investigation to view the endometrium in a patient with PMB. If the endometrial thickness is 4 mm or greater on the ultrasound, then a biopsy is required for further assessment of the endometrium. If the endometrium is less than 4 mm thick, the cause of the PMB is unlikely to be from the endometrium and another differential diagnosis should be considered.

 Key Point

Colposcopy of the cervix is indicated only if there is evidence of cervical abnormality. There is no rationale for obtaining a cervical smear in PMB patients unless the patient is not up to date with smears within the cervical screening programme.

Q3: Answer true or false, considering each of the following statements regarding postmenopausal bleeding.

Any woman reporting PMB should be urgently investigated with a pelvic ultrasound scan, which may then be followed by an endometrial biopsy. Diagnosis in early-stage disease is possible with prompt investigation, which can significantly improve a patient's chance of having curative surgery.

A   Endometrial thickness on TVUS of less than 10 mm is considered benign – **False.** An endometrial thickness of less than 4 mm is unlikely to be due to endometrial pathology and so further investigation is not required. If the endometrium is at least 4 mm thick, then an endometrial biopsy is warranted.

B   Approximately 30% of patients presenting with PMB have endometrial cancer – **False.** Of the patients presenting with the symptom of PMB, 10% will be found to have endometrial cancer. When investigating a patient for PMB, it is important to explain that cancer is what is being 'looked for', but in the vast majority of cases, a non-sinister cause of bleeding is identified.

C ✔ **Reinvestigation of recurrent PMB should be considered after 6 months – True.** If investigations for endometrial cancer were normal, but PMB recurs, the patient should be reinvestigated, with most clinicians obtaining an endometrial biopsy. Although small, all investigations have a false negative rate, so recurrent symptoms should not be ignored because of previous normal investigations.

D PMB is defined as an episode of bleeding 6 months or more after the last period – **False.** The definition of PMB is vaginal bleeding following 12 months of amenorrhoea in women of an age where the menopause can be expected.

E The 5-year survival rate for a patient diagnosed with endometrial cancer after presenting with PMB is 20% – **False.** Survival depends on a number of factors. Endometrial cancer usually presents early with PMB when the cancer is still confined to the uterus with stage I disease. The overall 5-year survival rate for endometrial cancer is around 80%.

Key Point

Patients presenting with PMB have a 10% chance of being diagnosed with endometrial cancer on subsequent investigations. Fortunately, the vast majority of these patients will have early-stage disease, where a hysterectomy (with or without radiotherapy) is likely to be curative in most cases. If a patient ignores PMB and does not present, the cancer is more likely to have spread at the time of eventual diagnosis, and the 5-year survival rate is much lower.

Important Learning Points

- Uterine cancer is the most common gynaecological cancer in high income countries.
- Overall prognosis is good, largely due to early presentation with PMB.
- Unopposed oestrogen is a key risk factor for the development of endometrial cancer.
- There is no screening test for endometrial cancer; TVUS and endometrial biopsy are first-line investigations for PMB.
- Stage I disease is treated surgically with hysterectomy and BSO, with radiotherapy often not being necessary.

CERVICAL SCREENING

Q1: Ideally when should cervical screenings take place during a typical menstrual cycle?
The correct answer is B. Day 14.

Ideally, a cervical smear should be taken mid-cycle, on day 14. This is because the mucus plug is thinnest at this time in the menstrual cycle, so the sample is least likely to have contamination that could mask any subtle differences in the cells.

Also, the epithelium of the cervix is at its thickest, so samples taken will contain a full range of cells. Ideally, a cervical smear should not be taken during menstruation, because if endometrial cells are seen on a cervical smear report, the patient may need to be investigated to rule out endometrial cancer, as it is presumed that the patient is shedding endometrial tissue outside of menstruation. Many women will have a smear taken at times other than day 14 with no issues; however, the question asked for the ideal time for the screening test.

Key Point

Like all screening tests, the cervical smear is not a diagnostic test for cervical cancer. It is very important that you communicate this to women, ensuring that they know that you are looking for the HPV virus and "changes in the cells". This is relatively common, as 1:20 tests show dyskaryosis, which may be for a variety of reasons. It is thought that cervical screening allows early detection, which prevents 75% of cervical cancer.

Q2: Answer true or false: In the following situations is cervical screening not required?
Cervical screening may not be appropriate for all women. When determining if it is necessary for a woman to have smear tests, it is important to consider what causes cervical cancer: HPV. Therefore, with the introduction of a vaccination for cervical cancer, it is hoped that in the future screening using smear tests will become unnecessary.

A Over the age of 55 – **False.** This is too young; it is women aged 65 and over who have had three normal test results in a row who are not invited for further cervical screening tests. This is due to the low risk for women in this group to go on and develop cervical cancer. Women aged over 64 who have had abnormal test results in the past will continue to be invited for screening until no further abnormal cells are detected. And finally, women aged 65 and over who have never had screening and have previously been sexually active are entitled to a test, no matter what age they are.

B Previous cervical ablation – **False.** Similar to partial hysterectomy, cervical ablations do not remove the risk of dyskaryosis or cervical cancer in the remaining cervix. Women who have undergone ablation for previous abnormal histology should in fact have an increased regimen of smear tests, as they are at increased risk for future abnormal results.

C ✔ **Sexually inactive lifelong – True.** Most cervical cancer is caused by HPV, which is a sexually transmitted virus. Therefore, women who have never had sex may choose to ignore their invitation to screening, as the risk of cancer is very low. However, women that are not currently in a sexual relationship but have been in the past should have regular cervical screening, as they are at risk of HPV exposure.

D Three previous negative results – False. Unless the woman is over the age of 64, then three previous negative results alone is not a reason for women not to attend future screening appointments.

E ✔ Total hysterectomy – True. Women who have had a total hysterectomy do not need to attend screening. Women who have had a hysterectomy due to cervical cancer may need to have a vault smear to assess for evidence of recurrence as part of the follow-up management. If, however, the hysterectomy is partial and the woman has either all or part of her cervix remaining, then smear test appointments should still be made.

 Key Point

Cases where cervical screening is usually not appropriate:
- Before the age of 25 (in England).
- Over the age of 65.
- Lifelong sexually inactive women.
- Pregnant women.
- Women who have had a total hysterectomy.

Q3: If this patient had received only negative results from their previous cervical smears, how often should they be screened?
The correct answer is C. Once every 3 years.

Screening for cervical cancer is offered for free to women between the ages of 25 and 64 in the UK. Screening before the age of 25 is offered in some parts of the UK, but there is controversy as to the risks and benefits of this, as a significant number of patients have false-positive screening results in this age group.

Unless there have been previous abnormalities or a woman has never had a smear, women over the age of 65 are not usually offered screening. This is because the aetiology and progression of cervical cancer suggests that it is highly unlikely that women of this age will go on to develop the disease.

 Key Point

- Women aged 25 to 49 are invited for screening every 3 years.
- Women aged 50 to 64 are invited for screening every 5 years.
- Women aged 65 or over are only screened if they have not been screened since they were 50 or if they have had recent abnormal test results.

Q4: Which of the following HPV vaccine and virus pairings are correct?

The correct answer is D. Gardasil® HPV subtypes 6, 11, 16 and 18.

The vaccination offered to a patient depends on the cost of that vaccination and also the range of diseases that the patient is at risk of.

 Key Point

The two HPV subtypes responsible for causing the majority of cervical cancer cases are 16 and 18. The Cervarix® vaccine protects against HPV subtypes 16 and 18. The Gardasil® vaccine also protects against subtypes 16 and 18 but also protects the patient against HPV subtypes 6 and 11, which are responsible for many cases of genital warts. HPV subtypes 2 and 7 are also linked to common warts and are not carcinogenic and therefore not vaccinated against.

Important Learning Points

- HPV is the biggest risk factor for the development of cervical cancer in the UK.
- Cervical screening is offered to women from 25 to 65 years of age in England, and from 20 to 65 in the rest of the UK.
- Screening is not looking for cancer; it is looking for HPV infection and then cell changes (dyskaryosis) which, if left untreated, may develop into cancer.
- A cervical smear takes cells from the cervix. The subsequent result from a smear is a cytology report, which describes any dyskaryosis seen in the smear.
- Patients with abnormal smear results are referred to colposcopy where the cervix is examined. If needed, they undergo treatment for the abnormality, most commonly with a large loop excision of transformation zone (LLETZ) procedure.
- CIN is a grading system for histological samples of the cervix. Histology cannot be obtained from a smear. It is usually obtained from a biopsy or after an LLETZ procedure.

CERVICAL CANCER

Q1: Answer true or false: Which of the following women are at an increased risk of developing cervical cancer?
All women are offered cervical screening in the UK, but unfortunately, some patients will go on to develop cervical cancer in spite of this. It is important to be able to identify women who are at increased risk of cervical cancer so that they can adapt their lifestyle to minimise these risks, if possible.

A ✔ A woman who is HIV positive – True. Patients with HIV may be immunocompromised. Immunocompromised patients are at increased risk of contracting HPV and also of developing subsequent precancerous and cancerous lesions. HIV increases a patient's risk of cervical cancer sixfold. Other forms of immunosuppression, such as treatments for inflammatory bowel disease and following organ transplantation, also increase the risk of cervical cancer, but to a lesser degree.

B ✔ A woman in her 60s who tells you her mother took treatment to increase her oestrogen levels to prevent a miscarriage – True. This patient's mother probably took diethylstilbestrol whilst she was pregnant. This was taken during the 1940s and 1950s in order to increase a woman's oestrogen levels and therefore, theoretically, to prevent miscarriage. It has since been shown that women who were exposed to this *in utero* are two to three times more likely to develop invasive cervical cancer than those who were not.

C A woman whose two older sisters have been diagnosed with cervical cancer – **False.** Unlike many cancers, cervical cancer does not appear to have a genetic link. If the patients have a very similar lifestyle, then this may indeed lead to them having similar risk factors, but simply having siblings or other close female relatives with cervical cancer does not affect one's risk of cervical cancer.

D ✔ **A woman in her early thirties who has had several sexual partners, she has been using a COCP for 7 years and does not use barrier contraception – True.** This woman has had several sexual partners and does not use condoms, meaning that the chances of her having HPV are high. Additionally, she has been taking oral contraception for over 5 years, which increases the risk of HPV infections.

E ✔ **A woman who has previously tested positive for Chlamydia trachomatis antibodies – True.** Women who have had chlamydia through unprotected sexual intercourse will also be at risk for HPV. Women with HPV who also test positive for *Chlamydia trachomatis* or herpes simplex antibodies are more likely to develop cervical cancer.

Key Point

A detailed history should be performed in order to elicit possible risk factors. such as sexually transmitted diseases and smoking status. The age at which a woman becomes sexually active affects her risk of having HPV, as around 50% of women are infected with HPV within 4 years of initially having intercourse (coitarche).

Q2: Which of the following characteristics does not increase the risk of psychosocial problems in women diagnosed with cervical cancer?

The correct answer is E. Older patient.

The diagnosis of cancer is extremely distressing for any patient. However, some patients may go on to experience a more severe psychological response. It is important for medical staff to be able to identify them so that they are offered appropriate help as soon as possible.

A Having a child who is under 21 years of age – **Incorrect.** Women with children under the age of 21 are more likely to experience psychosocial complications. This may be because younger children are more dependent on their parents and so they may develop more anxiety related to their disease and its effect on the children.

B History of psychiatric illness – **Incorrect.** Patients with a history of psychiatric illness are more likely

to develop a psychiatric illness in the future than those with no psychiatric history. A cancer diagnosis can often trigger a depressive episode in these patients.

C Living alone – **Incorrect.** Poor social support, either perceived or real, is an indicator that patients may experience more extreme psychological distress.

D Lymphoedema – **Incorrect.** Lymphoedema may be present in up to 50% of cervical cancer patients. It is often distressing, as it can limit the patient's mobility and may alter their body image. These issues increase the likelihood of a patient experiencing high levels of psychological distress.

E ✔ **Older patient – Correct.** Younger patients are more at risk of extreme psychological distress relating to their cervical cancer.

Key Point

A multidisciplinary team should be involved in the management of all cervical cancer patients. They should regularly screen the patients for psychological problems. If the patient is experiencing psychological distress, then they should be offered support accordingly. This may include counselling, support groups, and in more severe cases, the involvement of liaison psychiatrists.

Q3: Which of the following surgical treatment options for cervical cancer is the most appropriate for a young woman who wishes to retain her fertility?

The correct answer is E. Radical trachelectomy.

Surgical treatment is often the first-line treatment for women with cervical cancer. Whether or not the patient wishes to have children after treatment, it is important to understand the components of each procedure and which anatomical structures are going to be affected. This allows you to discuss competently the procedure with the patient and choose the most appropriate treatment option together.

A Bilateral salpingo-oophorectomy – **Incorrect.** This involves the removal of both ovaries. Even if the uterus remains *in situ*, the patient will no longer produce eggs for fertilisation. Additionally, this procedure alone is not a treatment for cervical cancer, although it is often performed along with a radical hysterectomy.

B Mastectomy – **Incorrect.** This is an operation in which the breast is removed, usually after a diagnosis of breast cancer. Although this treatment does not alter a patient's fertility, it is not an appropriate treatment for cervical cancer.

C Pelvic exenteration – **Incorrect.** This is drastic surgery involving the removal of the uterus and ovaries (along with other pelvic organs), so the patient would not be able to become pregnant.

D Radical hysterectomy – **Incorrect.** This procedure involves the removal of the uterus, so the patient will not be capable of carrying a pregnancy even if her ovaries remain and continue to release eggs.

E ✔ **Radical trachelectomy – Correct.** This procedure is specifically designed for women with cervical cancer who wish to retain their fertility. The cervix is removed, but the uterus is still able to accommodate a pregnancy. The patient would then usually require a specialist to monitor her throughout her pregnancy and a caesarean birth. Only early-stage cervical cancer would be suitable for this operation.

 Key Point

Women who wish to retain their fertility after treatment should be counselled carefully prior to surgery. They should be aware of all the options of having children and the risks and benefits of the treatment that they are offered. In this way, the patient is able to make an informed decision.

 Important Learning Points

- Squamous cell carcinoma is the most common form of cervical cancer, accounting for two-thirds of cases.
- A woman's risk of developing cervical cancer during her lifetime is around 1 in 130.
- HPV and inadequate cervical screening are the biggest risk factors for cervical cancer.
- The symptoms of cervical cancer are often very non-specific so there should be a high level of suspicion for this disease.
- Surgery is often the initial treatment offered to cervical cancer patients.
- It is possible for fertility to be retained following the treatment of early cervical cancer, but recurrence is more likely than with a radical hysterectomy.
- The 5-year survival rate for cervical cancer is around 65%.

VULVAL AND VAGINAL CANCERS

Q1: What is the most likely cause for this patient's symptoms?

The correct answer is A. Atrophic vaginitis.

The patient has had a postmenopausal bleed. This is commonly the presenting symptom of endometrial cancer and this pathology needs to be ruled out. The patient also has a history of lichen sclerosus, which increases her risk of developing vulval intraepithelial neoplasia (VIN), so this should also be considered in the differential diagnosis for this patient. However, the question asks for the most likely diagnosis.

A ✔ **Atrophic vaginitis – Correct.** This is by far the most likely diagnosis and accounts for the majority of cases of postmenopausal bleeding. The epithelium of the vagina is weaker and drier after the menopause, due to a reduction in oestrogen levels. Abrasions, bleeding and vaginal discomfort during intercourse are common symptoms. It can be treated with local oestrogen creams and, if needed, lubricants during intercourse.

B Endometrial cancer – **Incorrect.** Overall, 10% of patients presenting with postmenopausal bleeding will have endometrial cancer, so it is essential to investigate to rule this pathology out. However, 90% of patients with postmenopausal bleeding do not have endometrial cancer, so it is not the most likely diagnosis.

C Vaginal cancer – **Incorrect.** While vaginal cancer could present with postmenopausal bleeding and should be looked for during an examination of this patient, it is a very rare diagnosis, with an incidence of less than 1 per 100,000.

D Vaginal intraepithelial neoplasia (VAIN) – **Incorrect.** This is a pre-cancerous condition within the vaginal epithelium, which may present with vaginal bleeding. Like vaginal cancer, it too is rare.

E VIN – **Incorrect.** This is a pre-cancerous change of the vulval epithelial cells, which is associated with both the human papillomavirus and lichen sclerosus. This diagnosis is more likely than either VAIN or vaginal cancer, but VIN is seen in less than 5% of cases of lichen sclerosus, so it is less likely than either endometrial cancer or atrophic vaginitis.

 Key Point

Although sinister pathologies are important to rule out, they are not always the most likely diagnosis. In any patient presenting with postmenopausal bleeding, a history should be taken, followed by a careful examination. In this case, the vulva should be inspected with great care, given the increased risk of VIN or vulval cancer developing within lichen sclerosus. The vagina and cervix should also be examined and an ultrasound arranged to assess the endometrium. Once sinister pathology has been excluded, the patient can be reassured and treated for atrophic vaginitis.

Q2: A biopsy subsequently taken from a suspicious area of lichen sclerosus on the patient's vulva has been reported as containing VIN. Answer true or false, regarding VIN and the management of this patient.

Vulval intraepithelial neoplasia is a pre-cancerous condition that, if left untreated, can progress to vulval cancer. It is a rare condition, but the diagnosis is being made more frequently, which is thought to be due to the increased exposure to HPV in the population.

A ✔ **VIN may have been caused by lichen sclerosus – True.** VIN most commonly develops due to HPV infection, but can also form from skin conditions such as lichen sclerosus. Yearly examination is advised to monitor for VIN or vulval cancer development in lichen sclerosus.

B VIN may have been caused by the human herpes virus (HHV) – **False.** VIN can be caused by HPV, types 16, 18 and 31 most commonly. HSV types 1 and 2 are associated with oral and genital herpes ulcers, but no herpes viruses have been associated with VIN.

C ✔ **VIN may progress to vulval cancer in around 20% of cases – True.** Treatment may be offered to excise VIN or to medically treat it to reduce the chance of progression to squamous cell vulval cancer.

D ✔ **This patient should be offered a colposcopy – True.** VIN may be caused by HPV, which can also cause pre-cancerous cervical intraepithelial neoplasia (CIN) changes in the cervix. At colposcopy, the vagina can also be examined for the much rarer VAIN, which is also associated with HPV infection.

E ✔ **Surgery could be avoided as the patient is sexually active – True.** Where possible, surgical excision should be considered as it is the treatment most likely to prevent progression of VIN to cancer, particularly where the disease is localised to a single lesion. However, extensive surgery is likely to have a profound effect on sexual function. There is the option of treating the patient conservatively or medically with regular follow-up, but the patient should be counselled fully about benefits and risks of each management option so she can choose the best treatment for her personal circumstances.

> 💬 **Key Point**
>
> VIN is a pre-cancerous condition commonly associated with HPV infection and lichen sclerosus. Surgical excision is the preferred treatment of VIN, but where this is declined or not technically possible, medical therapies can be used to reduce the risk of progression to vulval cancer.

Q3: With a diagnosis of VIN, which of the conditions is the patient not at an increased risk of developing?

The correct answer is C. Endometrial cancer.

VIN can be caused by lichen sclerosus or HPV. HPV can also cause the pre-cancerous conditions VAIN and CIN, which can then progress to cancer of the vagina or cervix. For this reason, when VIN is diagnosed the patient should be advised to have regular colposcopy follow-up to assess the cervix and vagina for these changes. There is no association between VIN and endometrial cancer.

> **Key Point**
>
> When either VIN or VAIN has been diagnosed, colposcopy should be performed to assess the cervix, as there is likely to be cervical dysplasia associated with HPV infection.

> 🔍 **Important Learning Points**
>
> - Vulval and vaginal cancers are rare conditions, but failure to consider them in a differential diagnosis may delay appropriate treatment.
> - Vigilant follow-up in 'at risk' groups will help to identify pre-cancerous change and allow treatment to prevent cancer development.
> - HPV is associated with CIN, VIN and VAIN, so if any are diagnosed, it is important to examine the patient for any signs of the others.
> - Biopsy confirms the diagnosis of these skin lesions and can usually be performed under local anaesthetic as an outpatient.
> - Surgery is the primary treatment of vulval and vaginal cancer, with adjuvant radiotherapy and/or chemotherapy for advanced disease.

9

Antenatal Care

Outline

ORGANISATION AND PRINCIPLES OF ANTENATAL CARE

The World Health Organisation (WHO) advises that all pregnant women should be offered antenatal care (Fig. 9.1). In the UK, this is primarily provided by midwives, with the support of primary care physicians, within the community setting.

SCHEDULE OF APPOINTMENTS

Routine antenatal appointments are planned throughout a woman's pregnancy with a midwife to provide continuity of care. All pregnant women should plan to schedule seven antenatal appointments. Nulliparous women are offered 10 antenatal appointments. Additional or longer antenatal appointments are offered depending on the woman's medical, social and emotional needs. Appointments are then held with doctors as required for the woman's biopsychosocial needs.

FIRST CONTACT WITH A HEALTHCARE PROFESSIONAL

The first contact is almost always with the woman's primary care physician. Primary care physicians are crucial in antenatal and postnatal care throughout a woman's pregnancy.

Upon initial contact, information regarding the following should be given to women:
- Folic acid and vitamin supplements.
- Smoking, recreational drug use and alcohol intake.
- Antenatal screening.
- Diet and exercise.
- Maternity benefits.
- Antenatal classes.
- The pregnancy care pathway.

BOOKING APPOINTMENT

Early in antenatal care is the 'booking appointment', and ideally, this should take place within 10 weeks. It is usually carried out by a midwife who will be assigned to the patient throughout the pregnancy. At this appointment, the woman should receive information regarding the pregnancy, particularly the screening tests available. Early appointments facilitate rapid identification of the woman's needs and for any extra support to be put in place early. If a woman books late in pregnancy, it is important to find out why, as this may highlight unmet social, psychological and medical needs. If risk factors that require obstetric input are identified, then the obstetrics team may see the patient throughout the pregnancy in addition to her routine appointments.

The primary outcomes are to:
- Identify women who may need additional care or obstetric input according to:
  - Past medical history, for example, epilepsy and hypertension.
  - Previous or current mental health conditions, for example, depression, anxiety and bipolar disorder.
  - Past obstetric history, for example, previous caesarean and pre-eclampsia.
  - Current and recent medicine, including over-the-counter medicines, health supplements and herbal remedies.
  - Allergies.
  - Family history, for example, puerperal psychosis and diabetes.
  - Social history, for example, occupation, family and home situation, physical activity, smoking, alcohol consumption and recreational drug use.
- Assess risk factors for:
  - Gestational diabetes – if at risk, offer referral for an oral glucose tolerance test.
  - Pre-eclampsia – if at risk, advise to take aspirin.
  - Fetal growth restriction – if at risk, offer additional ultrasound scans.
  - Venous thromboembolism – where significant risk is identified, low molecular weight heparin prophylaxis may be offered antenatally.
  - Female genital mutilation (FGM).

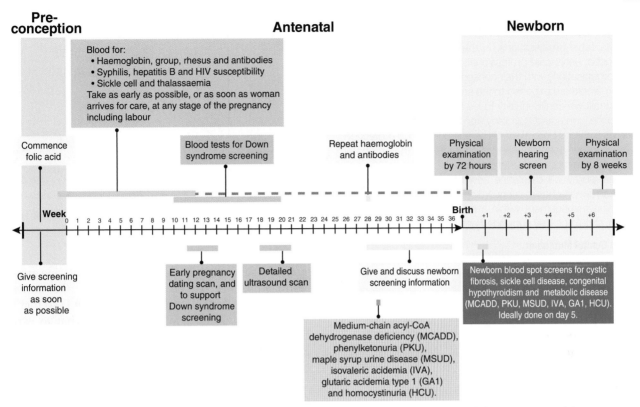

Fig. 9.1 Timeline of Antenatal Care From Conception to Birth. This includes pre-conception, during pregnancy and the postpartum period (Adapted from www.nhs.screening.uk).

- Domestic abuse – asking at the earliest opportunity when alone.
- Measure height and weight to calculate body mass index (BMI).
- Measure blood pressure to identify pre-existing hypertension.
- Dip the urine for protein, nitrites and glucose to identify underlying renal disease, urinary tract infection or diabetes, respectively.
- Offer booking blood tests:
  - Full blood count (FBC) – assess for anaemia, platelet count and haemoglobinopathies (sickle cell and thalassaemia).
  - Group and save (G&S) – blood group, rhesus D status, red cell alloantibodies.
  - Microbiology – hepatitis B virus (HBV), human immunodeficiency virus (HIV), syphilis.
- Offer urinalysis and mid-stream urine microscopy, culture and sensitivity (MC&S) to screen for asymptomatic bacteriuria.
- Offer screening for Down, Edward and Patau syndromes – either blood tests or combined ultrasound and blood tests.
- Offer an early ultrasound scan (between 11^{+2} weeks and 14^{+1} weeks gestation) to obtain an accurate estimation of gestational age, identify large structural abnormalities, determine the number of fetuses, and, if the patient wishes, undertake the ultrasound part of the Down, Edward and Patau syndromes screening.

- The anomaly scan (between 18 weeks and 20^{+6} weeks gestation) enables further assessment of congenital abnormalities that may be more readily detected at this later gestation and to determine the location of the placenta.

[See 'Antenatal Screening and Diagnostic Tests' page 223.]

 Sensitivity in Antenatal Consultations

Domestic Violence and Abuse

Domestic abuse is any incident of controlling, coercive, or threatening behaviour, violence or abuse between adults who are, or have been, partners or family members. Abuse can be psychological, physical, sexual, financial or emotional. Abuse is poorly reported, but it is estimated that at least 30% of women and 15% of men have at some point been victims of domestic abuse.

Risk factors for being the victim of domestic abuse include being female, suffering from a physical disability or mental health problem, social isolation and financial dependence. Significant life changes can also increase the risk, with pregnancy being a pertinent example.

Antenatal screening is a critical time to identify domestic abuse. Healthcare professionals should directly ask all women presenting for care about it, and be aware that it might affect their partners as well. Many centres in the UK have advertising campaigns promoting the reporting of domestic abuse, with many methods for private disclosure away from partners who may also be attending hospital. When a woman identifies herself or staff suspect abuse, they must find a way to meet with the woman alone, in an environment created to allow disclosure.

Where abuse is taking place, there are multiple agencies who can offer support, including social services, the police and charitable organisations. In the UK, if someone is being abused, healthcare professionals can usually only refer to other organisations with their consent. However, if children in the household are exposed to the same abuse, child protection law allows confidentiality to be broken and other agencies to be contacted. Similarly, for a pregnant woman, as soon as a child is born, they will be subject to child protection laws, so other agencies can be contacted in the antenatal period to plan for the postnatal period.

Local policy will determine how each case is managed, and each hospital has a safeguarding lead. The level of risk will determine management within a multidisciplinary team. The woman should be fully supported and informed throughout.

Female Genital Mutilation

Female genital mutilation (FGM), also known as female genital cutting, is any procedure that involves partial or complete removal, or other injuries, of the external female genitalia for non-medical reasons. The WHO has classified FGM into four types:

- Type I involves the clitoris.
- Type II is partial or total removal of the clitoris and labia minora, with or without excision of the labia majora.
- Type III involves narrowing of the vaginal orifice (infibulation), often to the point where there is an opening just large enough to allow urination and menstruation.
- Type IV is all other harmful procedures to the female genitalia.

It is estimated that 125 million women have undergone FGM. As a cultural practice, it is sometimes performed in early childhood in some East African countries (including Kenya, Tanzania, Egypt and Ethiopia) and others (e.g., Yemen, Indonesia and Malaysia).

FGM is illegal in the UK, and there is a campaign by the WHO to eradicate FGM worldwide. There are many complications of FGM, including infection, dyspareunia, menstrual difficulties, infertility, obstetric complications, including perineal trauma and psychological sequelae.

It is routine practice to ask about FGM antenatally, regardless of cultural background as this is often the first time a woman is identified as having undergone FGM. For obstetric management, it is essential to identify the type of FGM so that surgery (de-infibulation) can be offered to open up the closed vagina of FGM type III to allow for a vaginal birth. This can be offered at any point in the pregnancy or labour but is often offered at approximately 20 weeks' gestation.

A risk assessment also needs to take place for the unborn child and any existing children to identify their risk of being subjected to FGM. Depending on the level of risk identified, other agencies, including the safeguarding team, social services and the police may need to be informed. Many hospitals have a lead midwife for FGM.

AT EVERY APPOINTMENT

At each appointment, the midwife should enquire about the patient's general health and regular fetal movements. The patient's blood pressure should be checked, and the urine should be dipped to check for protein. After 25 weeks' gestation, a symphysis fundal height (SFH) should be measured to assess fetal growth. This should be plotted on a growth chart (Fig. 9.2) to highlight the

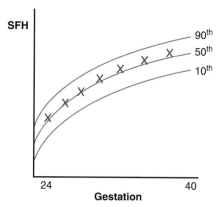

Fig. 9.2 A Normal Growth Chart Plotting the Symphysis Fundal Height Measurements.

potential small for gestational age or intrauterine growth restricted babies. At each appointment, the midwife can provide essential information (Table 9.1) so that the woman is educated and prepared for what to expect based on the stage of pregnancy. Educating the woman and/or partner on getting ready for labour, birth, the postnatal period and breastfeeding is beneficial.

[See 'Small-for-Gestational-Age Babies and Intrauterine Growth Restriction' page 316.]

Fetal movements should be felt with a regular pattern by 24 weeks' gestation, although many feel movements prior to this. The patient should be encouraged to monitor fetal movements throughout the pregnancy and contact her midwife or local hospital if she has concerns about the frequency of movements.

 Testosterone and Pregnancy

Transgender men may be on testosterone supplementation, which is currently not recommended during pregnancy, so it is often stopped when conceiving. Overall, this can be challenging and lead to menstrual cycles returning and changes in body shape. Together with the pregnancy, it may trigger feelings of gender dysphoria, which need to be sensitively managed.

28 WEEK APPOINTMENT

The 28 week appointment is for all pregnant women. Along with routine blood pressure, urinalysis and SFH measurements, women should be offered another opportunity to screen for anaemia and atypical red cell allo-antibodies. Any anaemia detected at this stage (less than 10.5 g/dL) should be investigated and treated. Identifying the blood group, rhesus (D) status and red cell antibodies in pregnant women is important to prevent haemolytic disease of the newborn and to identify possible issues with any future transfusion.

In many countries, including the UK, women who are rhesus negative are offered anti-D prophylaxis at the 28 week appointment, and a plan is put in place for a further course of prophylaxis after birth.

Table 9.1	Advice to Women During Their Antenatal Care
ISSUE	**ADVICE**
Work	It is generally safe to continue working, and women should be educated on their maternity rights and benefits.
Medicines	As few medicines as possible should be prescribed where the benefit outweighs the risk.
Nutritional supplements	400 mcg of folic acid before conception until 12 weeks gestation is advised, and women should be informed to increase their vitamin D intake during pregnancy and when breastfeeding. In comparison, vitamin A is known to be harmful as it is teratogenic. Iron supplementation is not routinely recommended but is offered as supplementation if a blood test identifies anaemia.
Food	The risk of listeriosis and salmonella should be minimised by ensuring food is thoroughly cooked before eating and not eating some types of cheeses, meats, paté and unpasteurised milk.
Exercise	Moderate exercise is not harmful. However, sports that risk abdominal trauma or falls should be avoided.
Sexual intercourse	Sex is thought to be safe during pregnancy.
Alcohol	Alcohol should be avoided for 3 months prior to a planned pregnancy and during pregnancy. If women choose to drink, advise no more than one to two UK units twice a week and avoid binge drinking. It is important to highlight that evidence suggests no safe level of alcohol during pregnancy.
Smoking	Smoking should be avoided, and women should be helped to quit if they smoke; nicotine replacement can be used.
Cannabis	Cannabis and all illicit medications should be avoided during pregnancy.
Car travel	Seatbelts should be worn above and below the bump, not over it.
Travelling abroad	The additional risk of venous thrombo-embolism with long haul travel can be reduced with compression stockings, mobilising where possible and keeping hydrated. Women should be advised to discuss flying and vaccinations with their midwife or doctor.

More recently, in countries like the UK, women are also offered the pertussis vaccination due to a public health outbreak of whooping cough in neonates. This should be given ideally between 28 weeks and 32 weeks' gestation for optimum transplacental delivery of antibodies to the fetus.

28 Week Summary

- Measure blood pressure and dip the urine for protein.
- Measure and plot SFH.
- Offer a second round of screening blood tests:
  - FBC to assess for anaemia and platelet count.
  - G&S to assess for atypical red cell alloantibodies.
- Offer anti-D prophylaxis to rhesus-D negative women.
- Offer oral glucose tolerance test to diagnose gestational diabetes if clinically indicated.

APPOINTMENTS BETWEEN 28 AND 40 WEEKS

After 28 weeks, appointments will involve discussions on antenatal preparation for labour, including information about labour, pain relief, creating a birth plan and discussing the benefits and risks of all options. Women receive advice on perineal massage and pelvic floor exercises to minimise the chance of perineal tears during labour. In addition, women are given information on recognising active labour and the postnatal period, including care of a newborn, breastfeeding and newborn screening.

28–40 Weeks Summary

- Discuss birth plan and preparation for labour.
- Discuss the postnatal period.
- Measure blood pressure and dip the urine for protein.
- Measure and plot SFH.

APPOINTMENTS AFTER 41 WEEKS

The risk of intrauterine death and stillbirth increases significantly 14 days beyond the due date. As well as routine monitoring of the pregnancy, appointments after 41 weeks focus on initiating birth. Initially, women are offered a membrane sweep; this involves introducing the examining fingers into the cervical os (opening) during a vaginal examination. This should separate the membranes from their attachment to the cervix, resulting in the release of local mediators, such as prostaglandins, increasing the probability of the onset of labour. This increases the likelihood of labour commencing within 48 hours to 1 week.

If women do not wish to have a membrane sweep, or if it does not stimulate labour, then women should be offered a labour induction. It should be offered routinely at term plus 10–12 days. Women are assessed using the Bishop score to help decide the method of induction. Induction is often initiated by introducing prostaglandins vaginally. The cervix is then re-examined after 6 hours (if gel or tablets were administered) or after 24 hours (if a pessary was given). These iatrogenic prostaglandins are given with the aim of ripening the cervix so that it is favourable (soft, dilated and effaced for the delivery of the fetus) and to stimulate uterine contractions. In some cases, this is sufficient to bring about the onset of active labour. However, in the majority, further steps, such as amniotomy and intravenous oxytocin infusion, are required to initiate labour. Women can also choose to have a caesarean if this is their preference after appropriate counselling.

[See 'Induction and Augmentation' page 270.]

Beyond Week 41 Summary

- Offer a membrane sweep.
- Offer induction of labour.
- Measure blood pressure and dip the urine for protein.
- Measure and plot SFH.

AFTER 42 WEEKS

If induction of labour is declined from 42 weeks' gestation, women should be offered increased monitoring with cardiotocography (CTG) and ultrasound examination at least twice weekly. However, it should be emphasised to the patient that no monitoring can prevent a stillbirth.

Information in Pregnancy

During the pregnancy, information should be given on:
- The development of the baby during pregnancy.
- Nutrition and diet.
- Exercise, including pelvic floor exercises.
- Maternity benefits.
- The pregnancy care pathway.
- Antenatal screening.
- Fetal movements.
- Antenatal classes.
- Planning place of birth.
- Breastfeeding.
- Vitamin K.
- Options for prolonged pregnancy.
- 'Baby blues'.
- Contraception.

QUESTIONS

Heidi is a 22-year-old nulliparous woman who thinks she is approximately 8 weeks pregnant after taking a home pregnancy test. She is unsure about the organisation of antenatal care in her area. Heidi approaches her primary care physician for some advice.

Q1   Which of the following are suitable for midwife-led care?

A A nulliparous woman with a family history of diabetes mellitus.

B A multiparous woman with sickle cell disease.

C A multiparous woman with a previous history of pre-eclampsia.

D A primiparous woman with a consistent blood pressure of above 130/90.

E A multiparous woman with well controlled epilepsy.

Q2   Answer true or false: What advice should be given to the woman during antenatal care?

A She should carry her own case notes.

B If drinking milk, it should be pasteurised.

C She should be advised that flying is contraindicated during the later stages of pregnancy.

D Folic acid should be taken up to 20 weeks' gestation.

E Regularly wearing compression stockings will prevent the occurrence of varicose veins.

Q3   If this pregnancy continues to be uncomplicated, how many antenatal appointments should she attend?

A 7.

B 9.

C 10.

D 12.

E 13.

[Answers on page 369.]

OBSTETRIC ABDOMINAL PALPATION

Obstetric palpation can be used to detect a vast amount of information about an ongoing pregnancy. It is most useful in the third trimester, as fetal growth is sufficient to enable accurate palpation findings. This examination assesses aspects of both maternal and fetal conditions.

Before the examination, an obstetric history should be taken. This will include questions regarding the woman's gravidity and parity, including asking about stillbirths and fetal losses. The current pregnancy should also be explored, asking about any difficulties they are experiencing, such as nausea, vomiting, bleeding or pain and about fetal movements.

AN OVERVIEW OF ABDOMINAL PALPATION

INTRODUCTION

- Introduce yourself and confirm the patient's name and age.
- Explain what you are going to do and obtain consent.
- Check the estimated date of delivery with the woman and determine gestation.
- Wash your hands.
- Place the woman in a comfortable position, ideally lying flat. Usually, the patient's head will need to be elevated due to the physiological breathlessness of pregnancy. In addition, in late pregnancy, lying completely flat may cause aortocaval compression resulting in pre-syncope, so lying on her left side may be more appropriate.
- Expose the abdomen appropriately from the xiphisternum to the pubic symphysis.

INSPECTION

- Determine if the distension of the abdomen is symmetrical and appropriate for gestation.
- Look for any signs of pregnancy, such as linea nigra and striae gravidarum.
- Look for fetal movements.
- Observe any scars from previous surgery and previous caesareans, as this may be important in determining the mode of birth.

PALPATION

- Ask the patient if she has any abdominal pain before beginning to palpate. Feel for the fundus of the uterus with the ulnar border of your hand. This is called the Leopold manoeuvre.
- Measure the SFH. Using a tape measure, measure this from the top of the fundus to the top of the symphysis pubis. To avoid measurement bias, the tape measure should be used upside down until it is time to read the measurement. This is often referred to as 'blind measurement' (Fig. 9.3).
- Lie – start from the fundus and palpate in a circle around the abdomen (Fig. 9.4). Anchor the fetus in position with one hand on one side of the abdomen and palpate the abdomen from the other side to determine the lie. If the baby is in a longitudinal lie, one side should feel firm (fetal back), and the other should feel emptier (fetal limbs).
- Presentation – turn to face the woman's feet and palpate for the two fetal poles (head and bottom) (Fig. 9.5). The head should be firmer and more ballotable. The part of the fetus that can be felt suprapubically is the presenting part.
- Engagement – feel, with both hands, either side of the presenting part (usually the head) and assess how much of the presenting part is palpable above the pelvic brim. Warn the patient that this might be slightly uncomfortable. Engagement is measured in fifths palpable.
- Liquor volume – gain an impression of the liquor volume by how easy the fetal limbs are to palpate. If they are very easy to feel, there may be reduced liquor (oligohydramnios); conversely, if the abdomen is very tense and fetal extremities are difficult to palpate, this may indicate excess liquor (polyhydramnios).

> 💡 **Symphysis Fundal Height**
>
> After 24 weeks gestation, the SFH should correlate with the gestation of the pregnancy ±2 cm. For example, a patient with a gestational age of 36 weeks would be expected to measure from 34 to 38 cm to be within the normal range.

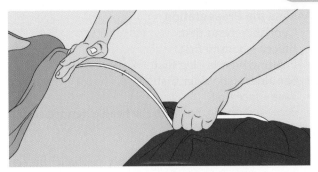

Fig. 9.3 Taking a Blind Measurement of the Symphysis Fundal Height.

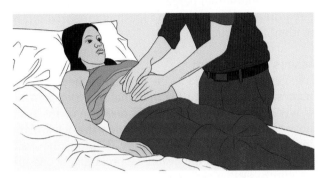

Fig. 9.4 Assessing the Lie by Palpating Around the Abdomen in a Circle With Both Hands.

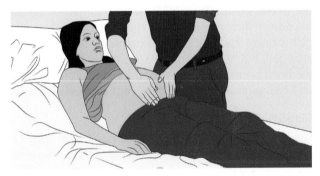

Fig. 9.5 Assessing the Fetal Presentation.

Assess the Lie (Fig. 9.6)

- Longitudinal – the head and bottom are palpable at the top and bottom of the uterus.
- Transverse – the fetus is lying across the uterus.
- Oblique – the lie is between longitudinal and transverse.

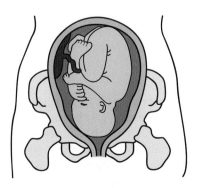
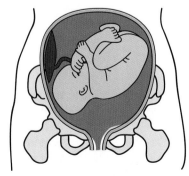
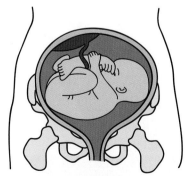

| Longitudinal | Oblique | Transverse |

Fig. 9.6 Fetal lie.

Assess the Presentation
- Cephalic – head first.
- Breech – bottom first.
- Footling breech – leg first.
- Shoulder – shoulder first.
- Face – face first.
- Brow – cephalic, but with the head extended so that the brow presents first.

It is important to note that only cephalic, breech, and in some cases, shoulder presentation can be diagnosed by abdominal palpation. A vaginal examination is required for face, brow and footling presentations to be identified clinically.

Assess Engagement
Engagement is defined as the descent of the fetal head or presenting part into the maternal true pelvis. After 37 weeks, the fundal height will decrease as the head moves further into the pelvis and below the pelvic brim. Engagement can be quantified by dividing the head into fifths. A fifth of the head is approximately one finger width, so this can be used as a proxy marker; 5/5 palpable means that no part of the head is below the pelvic brim. When 0/5 palpable, the head is fully below the pelvic brim. The fetal head is engaged when the maximum diameter of the fetal head has passed into the pelvic brim. Therefore, at 3/5 palpable, the head is not engaged, but at 2/5 palpable (3/5 engaged), it is. Once the head is engaged, it is very unlikely that the fetal lie will change from a longitudinal cephalic presentation.

AUSCULTATION
Using a handheld Doppler probe or Pinard, listen to the fetal heart. The instrument is placed over the anterior shoulder to hear the fetal heart, using the firm fetal back and head as markers to locate the shoulder. The maternal pulse should also be felt to ensure you are hearing the fetal heart separately from the maternal heart. Note that a Pinard should be held onto the abdomen with an ear, leaving both hands free (Fig. 9.7). A normal fetal heart rate should be 100–160 bpm.

At the end of the examination, ensure that the woman is comfortable and cover her up. Check if she has any questions and thank her.

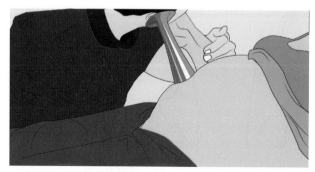

Fig. 9.7 Auscultating the Fetal Heart With a Pinard and Palpating the Maternal Pulse Simultaneously.

Table 9.2	Abnormal Findings and the Underlying Cause
FINDING	**CAUSE**
Excoriation or scratch marks on the abdomen	Associated pruritus, which could be due to obstetric cholestasis.
Fetal limbs easy to palpate	Oligohydramnios, because less liquor is surrounding the fetus, therefore the fetal parts are easy to feel.
SFH not as big as expected	Poor fetal growth, for example, intrauterine growth restriction.
Abnormal mass felt on abdominal palpation	All the causes of an abdominal mass in a non-pregnant woman can also occur in a pregnant woman. However, due to the gravid uterus, they may not be in the expected position.
Pain on palpation	Although the examination may be uncomfortable, it should not be painful; therefore, think of potential causes, such as a concealed placental abruption or appendicitis.

Further assessment or investigation may include blood pressure measurement, urinalysis, speculum examination, CTG or ultrasound scanning.

 An Example Summary

I examined Imogen Percy, a 25-year-old female, currently 38 weeks gestation, gravidity one, parity zero. On examination, she was comfortable at rest. The symphysis fundal height was 38 cm, which is in keeping with her current gestation. The lie was longitudinal and the presentation cephalic. The fetal head was not engaged, with 5/5 palpable. On auscultation, a regular heart rate of 120 bpm was noted, with no added sounds.

POTENTIAL ABNORMAL FINDINGS

This list (Table 9.2) is not exhaustive; however, it includes some abnormalities that indicate maternal or fetal disease:

❓ QUESTIONS

Amrita is a 32-year-old woman who presents to triage. She reports that usually she feels the baby move at least five times in the morning when it is most active, but this has not been the case for 3 days. She is gravidity three, parity two, and is 37^{+5} weeks gestation. She is known to have gestational diabetes, but otherwise her pregnancy is going well.

Q1   What is the most important reason for examining the woman in the left lateral position later in pregnancy?
   A It makes it easier to palpate the uterus.
   B It is more comfortable for the woman.
   C It reduces compression of the vena cava.
   D It means that assessment of the SFH is more accurate.
   E It makes it easier to auscultate the fetal heart.

Q2 Which of the following could cause SFH to be larger than expected?

A Oligohydramnios.
B Polyhydramnios.
C Gestational diabetes.
D Raised blood pressure.
E Raised BMI.

Q3 What is the name of the scar indicated in the diagram?

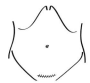

A Midline.
B Pfannenstiel.
C Kocher.
D Paramedian.
E Lanz.

[Answers on page 371.]

ANTENATAL SCREENING AND DIAGNOSTIC TESTS

Antenatal screening is the process of testing for conditions, diseases or abnormalities in the mother or fetus. After screening tests, women can be offered information, additional tests and appropriate treatment, if necessary, to reduce their risk and/or any complications arising from the disease or condition.

All antenatal screening tests are optional, and this must be communicated. In addition, not all screening tests are diagnostic, and this needs to be made very clear to couples. It must also be explained that all screening tests carry a risk of false positives and false negatives.

Screening is the process of identifying apparently healthy or asymptomatic individuals within a population who may be at an increased risk of a disease or condition. Several key concepts need to be grasped to understand screening. These apply not only in obstetrics but across medicine. These are outlined in Table 9.3.

Traditionally, screening tests are inexpensive, non-invasive tests, but they are not as sensitive or specific as more expensive or invasive diagnostic 'gold standard' tests. If a traditional screening test is positive, the patient is then offered further assessment and investigation with the gold standard test to confirm the diagnosis. Examples of screening tests include cervical smear tests, which would determine the need for a further, more-invasive colposcopy or biopsy.

As screening has developed, inexpensive non-invasive diagnostic tests have been introduced and now form part of screening for the population. In these cases, positive test results do not require further investigation, as the diagnosis is made from the 'screening' test alone. An example of a diagnostic screening test, outside of obstetrics and gynaecology, is ultrasound scans for an abdominal aortic aneurysm. The result

Table 9.3	Important Definitions for Understanding Screening Tests
TERM	**DEFINITION**
False positive	An individual who is referred for further assessment after a positive screening test but does not have the target condition when the gold standard diagnostic test is performed.
False negative	An individual who is not referred for further assessment after a negative screening test but does have the condition.
Sensitivity	The number of people identified with a positive screening test who actually have the disease.
Specificity	The number of people with a negative screening test who do not have the disease when tested with the gold standard diagnostic test.
Positive predictive value	A ratio of people with the disease receiving a positive screening test to all people with a positive screening test.
Negative predictive value	The ratio of people without the disease receiving a negative screening test to all people with a negative screening test.

Table 9.4	Basic Antenatal Investigation Tools
SCREENING TOOL	**POTENTIAL DISEASES DETECTED**
Blood pressure	Hypertension and pre-eclampsia.
Urine dipstick	Urinary tract infections (UTIs), pre-gestational and gestational diabetes, renal disease and pre-eclampsia.
Glucose tolerance test (GTT)	Gestational diabetes.
Infectious blood screen	HIV, syphilis and hepatitis B are tested in routine antenatal screening. Other infectious diseases, including hepatitis C, parvovirus and toxoplasmosis, may be tested for specific antenatal conditions.
Maternal haemoglobin	Maternal anaemia and haemo-globinopathies (higher risk in Afro-Caribbean populations).
Group and save	Red cell antibodies for Rhesus D status (Rhesus disease)

diagnoses the condition and guides whether surgical intervention is offered.

INVESTIGATIONS OFFERED IN PREGNANCY

Multiple investigations are offered during pregnancy to asymptomatic women, which are used for the pre-emptive detection of diseases or complications in the mother or baby (Table 9.4). While many of these tests are often considered screening tools for obstetric diseases, they may double up as the final diagnostic tests themselves. However, further investigations may be needed. For example, elevated blood pressure is diagnostic for hypertension but does not determine the underlying cause or whether the hypertension is part of a larger disease process, such as pre-eclampsia.

Multiple other screening tools are also used to detect medical complications, social issues and psychological issues that may affect a woman during pregnancy. For example, questions are asked regarding diet and alcohol intake, psychiatric disorders, domestic violence and family medical history. These questions should be asked at or before the first antenatal appointment.

If the results of any tests during pregnancy are positive, further investigation may be offered to that woman to determine any further diagnoses and guide future management. Nonetheless, any woman can refuse to have any of these tests and has no obligation to act in any particular way on the results.

SCREENING WITH ULTRASOUND

In a pregnancy with no complications, two screening ultrasound scans are offered. The dating scan, which in most hospitals includes the nuchal translucency scan, and the fetal anomaly scan (Table 9.5). Additional ultrasound scans may be required if there are any complications during the pregnancy.

Ultrasound is a good screening tool, as it is relatively quick and poses virtually no risk to the mother or baby. Multiple images and measurements are taken

and stored during the anomaly scan. Ultrasound scans are screening tests and, as such, carry a degree of risk that some conditions may be missed (a false negative result). Similarly, for a number of conditions, further investigation is required to confirm the diagnosis suggested by the ultrasound, as some of the ultrasound scans will produce a false positive result. The major limitation of any ultrasound scan is that the accuracy of the test is operator dependent. Early gestational age, certain positions of the fetus, raised maternal BMI, presence of fibroids, polyhydramnios, oligohydramnios and multiple pregnancies may all decrease the accuracy of the scan.

Key conditions identified on the fetal anomaly ultrasound scan have a predicted detection rate (the percentage of cases detected by ultrasound) of more than 50%, ordered by the percentage detection rate from high to low, see Table 9.6:

Table 9.5 The Dates and Purpose of Antenatal Ultrasound Scans Offered to all Women

DATE (APPROXIMATELY)	PURPOSE
8–14 weeks	Dating scan – the primary aims of this scan are to determine an accurate gestational age, ensure the viability of the pregnancy, identify the number of fetuses and detect any gross fetal abnormalities.
	Nuchal translucency scan – ultrasound measurement of the thickness of the fluid beneath the skin overlying the back of the fetal neck, used along with blood tests in the screening for Down syndrome.
18–21 weeks	Fetal anomaly scan – a more detailed assessment to examine fetal anatomy and screen for fetal anomalies. Not all anomalies can be detected accurately on ultrasound at approximately 20 weeks, and the sensitivity and specificity of detecting each anomaly vary.

Table 9.6 Key Conditions Identified on the Fetal Anomaly Ultrasound Scan

Anencephaly	A severe type of neural tube anomaly where the neural tube fails to close at the base of the skull, resulting in the absence of significant areas of the brain and skull.
Gastroschisis	A type of abdominal wall anomaly where the intestine protrudes through the abdominal wall.
Edward syndrome	Trisomy 18, a genetic disorder where babies are often born with a small head and severe intellectual disabilities.
Open spina bifida	A severe type of neural tube anomaly, also known as myelomeningocele, where the spinal canal is open, forming a sac exposing tissues and nerves.
Bilateral renal agenesis	A genetic disorder of the absence of both kidneys at birth.
Exomphalos	A type of abdominal wall anomaly where there is an anomaly at the umbilical cord insertion into the fetus, allowing the bowel to herniate into the umbilical cord.
Cleft lip	A birth anomaly with an opening or split in the upper lip.
Diaphragmatic hernia	A birth anomaly where abdominal organs can move into the chest due to a hole in the diaphragm.
Lethal skeletal dysplasia	A genetic condition of abnormal bone growth where the chest and lungs do not develop fully.
Severe cardiac abnormalities	A severe congenital anomaly affecting the heart.
Patau syndrome	Trisomy 13, a genetic disorder which affects facial features, microcephaly (small head) and other abnormalities.

DOWN SYNDROME SCREENING

Two different blood tests can be offered to screen for Down syndrome, depending on fetal gestation.

Combined test (blood tests and ultrasound): 10^{+0} weeks to 14^{+1} weeks:

- Free beta human chorionic gonadotrophin (β hCG).
- Pregnancy associated plasma protein A (PAPP-A).
- Nuchal translucency on ultrasound (see Fig. 9.8).

Quadruple test (blood tests alone): 14^{+2} weeks to 20 weeks:

- Free β hCG.
- Unconjugated oestriol.
- Alpha fetoprotein (AFP).
- Inhibin-A.

The combined test is more accurate than the quadruple test and can be carried out at an earlier gestation. The results will indicate a woman's chance of having a baby with Down syndrome. The chance is calculated using the results of the screening tests and other factors in the medical history, most notably maternal age. A risk of one in 150 is used as the cut off level for defining a high chance. A chance of less than one in 150 is a lower chance result, meaning that the patient will not be offered diagnostic testing. However, this does not mean that the baby has no chance of being born with Down syndrome. Diagnostic testing may be offered if the screen shows a chance greater than 1 in 150.

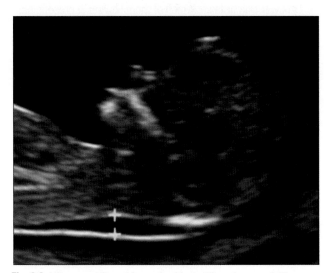

Fig. 9.8 Ultrasound Scan Measuring Nuchal Translucency (NT).

CHORIONIC VILLOUS SAMPLING AND AMNIOCENTESIS

Further diagnostic tests are required to diagnose Down syndrome and other chromosomal abnormalities, as outlined in Table 9.7.

In the near future, screening blood tests and chorionic villous sampling (CVS) will likely become much less common. Free fetal deoxyribonucleic acid (DNA)

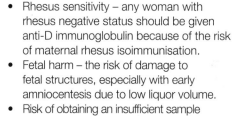

Table 9.7	Key Concepts of Amniocentesis and Chorionic Villous Sampling	
	CHORIONIC VILLOUS SAMPLING (CVS)	**AMNIOCENTESIS**
Definition	Chorionic villus (a sample of the placental tissue) is used to enable the prenatal diagnosis of conditions such as chromosomal abnormalities (see Fig. 9.9).	Amniotic fluid is used to enable the prenatal diagnosis of conditions such as chromosomal abnormalities or intrauterine infections (see Fig. 9.10).
Timing	11^{+0}–13^{+6} weeks gestation.	15 weeks gestation onwards.
Benefits	It can be performed at earlier gestations than amniocentesis.	Lower risk of miscarriage (1% risk as opposed to 2% in CVS).
Risks	The risks for amniocentesis and CVS are similar in principle, but the degree of risk differs between the two procedures. • Miscarriage – this is the most significant risk: approximately 1% in amniocentesis and 2% in CVS. • Infection – infection can be introduced at the time of the procedure as a needle is inserted through the abdomen to obtain the samples. • Rhesus sensitivity – any woman with rhesus negative status should be given anti-D immunoglobulin because of the risk of maternal rhesus isoimmunisation. • Fetal harm – the risk of damage to fetal structures, especially with early amniocentesis due to low liquor volume. • Risk of obtaining an insufficient sample to analyse – in this case, the risk to the pregnancy has therefore occurred for no substantial benefit, and the couple will have to decide whether to undergo a repeat attempt.	

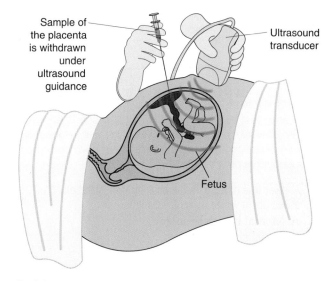

Sample of the placenta is withdrawn under ultrasound guidance

Ultrasound transducer

Fetus

Fig. 9.9 Chorionic Villous Sampling.

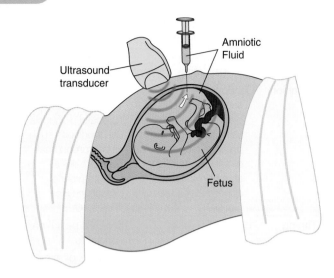

Fig. 9.10 Amniocentesis.

can be identified and processed from maternal blood, which can easily be taken without the invasive sampling risks to the fetus. The results from free fetal DNA analysis are at least as sensitive and specific as those from CVS. The cost of free fetal DNA analysis is currently too great to use on a large scale, but the cost is falling dramatically each year.

Placental Mosaicism

In around 1% of pregnancies, there is an error in DNA replication during the placental development, leading to some or all of the placenta having a different genotype from that of the fetus. The most common mosaicism is triploidy; however, it is rare for abnormal placental genetics to have a detrimental effect on the development of a normal fetus.

Awareness of placental mosaicism is important when interpreting the results of CVS and free fetal DNA testing (free fetal DNA in maternal blood is actually of placental origin). Where testing demonstrates a genetic abnormality, there is a 1% chance that the placenta is abnormal but not the fetus. Amniocentesis may then be offered in these cases, particularly if termination is considered, as the DNA collected from the amniotic fluid is primarily from fetal skin cells, so it is more likely to identify the correct fetal genotype.

 QUESTIONS

Julia is a 35-year-old primiparous woman attending her booking visit with the midwife. She had a positive home pregnancy test last week. She thinks that she is approximately 10 weeks pregnant. At this booking visit, information is given regarding the screening tests that she will be offered throughout her pregnancy.

Q1 Answer true or false: At the booking visit, questions are asked about which of the following?
A Mental health problems.
B Social support.
C Diet and nutrition.
D Pregnancy intentions.
E Medical comorbidities.

Q2 Tests for Down syndrome screening are offered between which weeks of gestation?
A Weeks 6 and 10.
B Weeks 8 and 14.
C Weeks 10 and 14.
D Weeks 16 and 24.
E Weeks 14 and 20.

Q3 Which of the following disorders is a greater risk in Afro-Caribbean women than in white Northern European women?
A Hepatitis B.
B Syphilis.
C HIV.
D Haemoglobinopathies.
E Rubella.

Q4 Answer true or false: In a pregnancy progressing normally with no complications, a woman will be offered her first ultrasound scan in the first trimester. What are the primary purposes of this scan?
A To detect twins.
B To date the pregnancy.
C To detect miscarriages.
D To detect fetal abnormalities.
E Down syndrome screening.

Q5 At what week of gestation is a woman ideally offered a fetal anomaly scan?
A 16 weeks.
B 18 weeks.
C 20 weeks.
D 22 weeks.
E 24 weeks.

Q6 Answer true or false: Which of the following, if present, has a greater than 50% chance of being detected by the fetal anomaly scan?
A Anencephaly.
B Cerebral palsy.
C Spina bifida.
D Gastroschisis.
E Autism.

Julia is now 18 weeks pregnant. She had the combined test screening for Down syndrome and was found to have increased nuchal translucency on ultrasound scan and low levels of PAPP-A in comparison to β hCG. She is therefore considering going on to have further diagnostic tests to try to diagnose whether Down syndrome affects her pregnancy.

Q7 At 18^{+4} weeks' gestation, which diagnostic test is most suitable for this patient?
A Amniocentesis.
B Chorionic villous sampling.
C Anomaly ultrasound scan.
D Quadruple test.
E Maternal chromosome analysis.

Q8   Julia is told about the risk of miscarriage. Which are the correct percentages quoted for amniocentesis and CVS?

A Amniocentesis 3% and CVS 2%.

B Amniocentesis 1% and CVS 2%.

C Amniocentesis 2% and CVS 1%.

D Amniocentesis 5% and CVS 4%.

E There is no risk of miscarriage at this gestation.

Q9   She also undergoes a test for Edward syndrome. Which chromosome is a trisomy in this syndrome?

A 13.

B 21.

C 15.

D 18.

E 12.

[Answers on page 372.]

KEY REFERENCES

ORGANISATION AND PRINCIPLES OF ANTENATAL CARE

National Institute for Health and Clinical Excellence, 2014. Domestic Violence and Abuse: Multi-Agency Working. Public Health Guideline (PH50).

National Institute for Health and Clinical Excellence, 2021. Antenatal Care. NICE Clinical Guidance (NG201).

National Institute for Health and Clinical Excellence, 2021. Inducing Labour. NICE Clinical Guidance (NH207).

Public Health England, 2021. Pertussis (Whooping Cough) Vaccination Programme for Pregnant Women [Internet]. https://www.gov.uk/government/publications/vaccination-against-pertussis-whooping-cough-for-pregnant-women/pertussis-whooping-cough-vaccination-programme-for-pregnant-women

Royal College of Obstetrics and Gynaecologists, 2015. Female Genital Mutilation and its Management. RCOG Green Top Guideline (GTG 53).

OBSTETRIC ABDOMINAL PALPATION

National Institute for Health and Clinical Excellence, 2021. Antenatal Care. NICE Clinical Guideline (NG201).

ANTENATAL SCREENING AND DIAGNOSTIC TESTS

National Institute for Health and Clinical Excellence, 2021. Antenatal Care. NICE Clinical Guideline (NG201).

Royal College of Obstetricians and Gynaecologists, 2010. Amniocentesis and Chorionic Villous Sampling. RCOG Green Top Guideline (GTG 8).

Screening Programmes (Online). http://www.fetalanomaly.screening.nhs.uk

UK Screening Portal (Online). http://www.screening.nhs.uk

10 Medical Disorders in Pregnancy

Outline

DIABETES

GESTATIONAL DIABETES

Gestational diabetes mellitus (GDM) refers to glucose intolerance, with the first onset and diagnosis in pregnancy. GDM resolves shortly after birth; it accounts for 90% of diabetes mellitus (DM) in pregnancy and affects 4 to 5 in 100 women during pregnancy. Pre-existing DM (type 1 and type 2) refers to glucose intolerance with first onset and diagnosis before pregnancy. It affects 0.3% to 1% of pregnant women.

RISK FACTORS

Screening for GDM is determined by elucidating any pre-existing risk factors. If any of these risk factors exist, then in the UK, testing for gestational diabetes is recommended:
- Body mass index (BMI) more than 30 kg/m^2.
- Previous macrosomic baby (more than 4.5 kg).
- Previous GDM.
- Family history of DM (first-degree relative).
- Ethnic background associated with higher incidence of DM.
  - South Asian.
  - Afro-Caribbean.
  - Middle Eastern.
- Personal history of polycystic ovarian syndrome (PCOS).

Testing is also considered if persistent glycosuria is identified on antenatal urinalysis screening.

 Diabetes Aetiology

Diabetes arises through a complex relationship of genetic and environmental factors. 400+ genomic variants have been associated with Type 2 diabetes. In the context of ethnicity, associated environmental factors are probably more important. 7% of Pima Indians have diabetes in Mexico. In the USA, where the Pima Indian population were found to be less active and more obese, the figure is 38%.

AETIOLOGY

To understand why GDM occurs, it is first important to understand the physiology of normal pregnancy with regards to glucose metabolism. Extra energy is required not only for the growing fetus but also to support the changes in maternal physiology. Therefore, an increased sensitivity to insulin initially occurs, which leads to glycogen synthesis and fat deposition. However, a degree of insulin resistance develops midway through pregnancy. In addition, cortisol, progesterone, oestrogen and human placental lactogen (hPL) are all antagonists of insulin. Therefore, in the second half of pregnancy, serum glucose levels may rise. The exact pathophysiology is not clearly defined; however, the processes involved are thought to be the same as those in type 2 diabetes mellitus (T2DM), propagated by the diabetogenic effects of hormones involved in pregnancy.

- GDM occurs in 2% to 5% of pregnant women and is the commonest metabolic complication associated with pregnancy.
- The increase in the incidence of GDM within the last decade is largely attributable to increased screening and improved diagnosis, along with an increase in obesity that is coupled with the sedentary lifestyles within the general population.
- All pregnancies are associated with an increased insulin resistance, and up to a two- to three-fold increase in pancreatic beta cell insulin secretion. GDM results when insulin secretion cannot overcome peripheral insulin resistance, which is primarily driven by the placenta as an adaptive response to ensure availability of glucose for the developing fetus.
- When the glucose levels are excessive, fetal complications may develop. This occurs because maternal hyperglycaemia will result in fetal hyperglycaemia, resulting in fetal hyperinsulinaemia that leads to multiple negative implications.

INVESTIGATIONS

If any of the risk factors (as discussed) are identified, testing for GDM should be carried out with a 2-hour oral glucose tolerance test (OGTT) at 24 to 28 weeks' gestation (women with GDM in a previous pregnancy are also offered an initial OGTT at booking). The fasting blood glucose is measured, then a 75 g load of glucose is given (usually as a drink), followed by a further blood glucose measurement 2 hours after the glucose dose.

GDM can be diagnosed if either of the following is observed:

1 A fasting plasma glucose level of 5.6 mmol/L or above **or**
2 A 2-hour plasma glucose level of 7.8 mmol/L or above.

If at any point during pregnancy glycosuria is detected on routine antenatal urine dipsticks (more than or equal to 2+ glucose on one occasion or 1+ on two or more occasions), then this may also be an indicator of GDM. If glycosuria is found, even in women without risk factors, then testing for GDM with an OGTT should be considered.

COMPLICATIONS

Maternal

Skin and urinary tract infections are more common due to hyperglycaemia. Pre-eclampsia and pregnancy-induced hypertension are also associated with GDM, although these are not true complications.

[See 'Pre-Eclampsia and Pregnancy-Induced Hypertension' page 301.]

Fetal

- Polyhydramnios, caused by fetal polyuria (which has the same pathology as seen in adults with diabetic polyuria).
- Macrosomia (increased growth) secondary to the fetal hyperinsulinaemia that results from maternal hyperglycaemia.
- Small for gestational age and intrauterine growth restriction, secondary to placental vascular dysfunction.
- Intrauterine death.

Neonatal

- Respiratory distress syndrome can develop because of delayed pulmonary surfactant production.
- Hypoglycaemia secondary to persistent hyperinsulinaemia
- Polycythaemia can result from intrauterine hypoxia causing elevated erythropoietin levels.
- Jaundice as a complication of liver immaturity and excessive breakdown of red blood cells.
- Death.

Obstetric

- Increased risk of induction of labour, often offered to reduce the risk of stillbirth.

- Macrosomia significantly increases the risk of assisted vaginal birth and shoulder dystocia, which can cause both fetal and maternal trauma.
- Caesarean birth is more likely due to fetal distress, failed induction of labour or suspected cephalopelvic disproportion.

MANAGEMENT

General

The woman should be managed with a multidisciplinary approach, under consultant-led care at a joint obstetric and endocrinology clinic. Educating and motivating the woman to optimise her blood sugar control and diet is essential, and emphasising the benefits of these lifestyle changes should be a priority.

Pregnancy

- GDM is initially managed with conservative measures such as diet and exercise, and all women should be referred to a dietician. If adequate targets are not met, then women are managed with metformin which can be added to or replaced by insulin to obtain optimum glucose control.
- Blood glucose levels should be checked regularly, as doses of insulin may gradually need to be increased throughout the pregnancy.
- The aim for antenatal glucose management should be for monitoring of preprandial and nightly glucose.
  - For monitoring purposes, fasting blood glucose should be between 4 and 5.9 mmol/L, and 1-hour postprandial blood glucose should be less than 7.8 mmol/L.
- Monitor blood pressure, as patients with hypertension and DM have an increased risk of intrauterine growth restriction, pre-eclampsia, placental abruption and maternal stroke.
- Women should be more closely monitored for pre-eclampsia as it is more frequent in women with DM.
- Serial ultrasound examinations are needed to monitor fetal growth and liquor volume.

Birth

- Birth should be in a hospital with a neonatal intensive care unit.
- Induction of labour is usually offered to women with GDM from 38 weeks' gestation. Some clinicians advocate allowing women with GDM not requiring metformin or insulin to continue the pregnancy up to 40+6 weeks. Induction is offered to reduce the risk of stillbirth at later gestations.
- GDM alone is not an indication for a caesarean. However, a caesarean is offered where there is evidence of a macrosomic or large for gestational age (>4.5 kg) baby, as this is linked with in increased risk of cephalopelvic disproportion and shoulder dystocia.
- GDM with good glucose control can be managed normally in labour. It is generally accepted that if the mother has a blood glucose level greater than

7 mmol/L, she requires an insulin sliding scale, regardless of previous therapy. Good control is important as it reduces the chance of uncontrolled neonatal blood sugars and neonatal hypoglycaemia.
- During labour, continuous monitoring with cardiotocography (CTG) is advised.

Postpartum
- Stop insulin after birth, as the maternal insulin requirement falls immediately.
- The neonate should be kept with the mother unless clinical complications develop, with regular blood glucose testing to identify hypoglycaemia early. Neonatal feeding should be initiated at the earliest opportunity.
- Monitor the baby for respiratory distress, encephalopathy and jaundice.
- Reassess maternal fasting blood glucose levels after 6 weeks to ensure that the woman does not have ongoing T2DM that was labelled as GDM because it was diagnosed for the first time in pregnancy.

PROGNOSIS

Mothers who have had gestational diabetes have an increased risk of T2DM postpartum: 50% will develop DM within the next 5 to 10 years. There is also an increased rate of GDM recurrence (1:3 women) in future pregnancies. Therefore, women should be advised on lifestyle factors such as diet, exercise and maintaining a healthy BMI to reduce the risk. They should have a fasting glucose test with their primary care physician 6 weeks after the birth (and if normal, a blood test for HbA1c taken yearly thereafter). The mother also has an increased risk in the long term of cardiovascular disease, stroke, renal disease and retinopathy. The neonate has an increased risk of childhood obesity and developing T2DM in adulthood.

PRE-EXISTING DIABETES AND PREGNANCY

PRENATAL ADVICE

Women with diabetes should be advised to plan for their pregnancies. Should they be hoping to conceive, it is crucial that they maintain good blood glucose control prior to conception and throughout pregnancy to minimise the risk of miscarriage, congenital malformation, stillbirth and neonatal death. The recommended HBA1c level is less than 48 mmol/L prior to conception; those whose level is greater than 86 mmol/L are strongly advised not to conceive until this is lower due to the increased risk of congenital malformation. This can be managed in part by diet, exercise and lifestyle factors. In addition, women should take 5 mg of folic acid daily until 12 weeks' gestation to minimise the risk of neural tube defects. Their medication may need to be reviewed and optimised; metformin and insulin are safe during pregnancy. However, other oral blood glucose lowering agents should be discontinued prior to conception and insulin used instead. In addition, other medications that women might be taking for comorbidities (particularly angiotensin-converting enzyme (ACE) inhibitors and statins) should also be stopped.

EARLY PREGNANCY
- Women should be seen within the first trimester at a joint diabetic and obstetric clinic for joint care throughout the pregnancy.
- Women with diabetes should be evaluated for diabetic nephropathy, neuropathy, retinopathy, hypertension and thyroid disease.
- Aspirin 150 mg daily will often be given after 12 weeks' gestation to reduce the risk of developing pre-eclampsia.

COMPLICATIONS

All the risks discussed in GDM above apply to pre-existing DM, as well as the following additional complications.

Additional Maternal Complications
- Increased insulin requirements – due to the insulin resistant state of pregnancy.
- Hypoglycaemia – this may be asymptomatic; therefore, women should be advised to check their blood glucose levels regularly. Regular hypoglycaemic episodes and a decreasing requirement for insulin is worrisome, as this may suggest placental insufficiency and impending fetal demise.
- Progression of any pre-existing nephropathy, neuropathy and retinopathy – pregnancy can accelerate the microvascular complications of diabetes; therefore, careful surveillance is crucial. Retinal screening should be offered following their first antenatal clinic appointment (unless already performed in the last 3 months) and then again at 28 weeks. If any diabetic retinopathy is present at booking, an additional assessment is offered between 16 and 20 weeks.
- Progression of any pre-existing nephropathy – if renal function (U&Es, urine protein) has not been assessed in 3 months preceding pregnancy, then it should be offered at the first contact. A nephrologist should be involved if creatinine is more than 120 μmol/L or protein excretion is more than 2 g/24 hours, except in the context of pre-eclampsia.
- Increased risk of pre-eclampsia – increased monitoring of maternal blood pressure and proteinuria, in addition to aspirin administration.

Additional Fetal Complications
- Increased risk of congenital abnormalities given the influence of insulin resistance during organogenesis; the majority of these are related to the cardiovascular and central nervous systems. Therefore, a detailed cardiac scan is also performed at the time of the anomaly scan.
- Either macrosomia or intrauterine growth restriction are more likely in women with pre-existing diabetes. Regular growth scans are arranged to monitor this and are individualised to the clinical situation.

BIRTH

Women with pre-existing diabetes should be seen regularly by the joint obstetrics and diabetic team to review fetal growth scans and to oversee glucose monitoring. Medication doses should be altered to optimise diabetic management throughout pregnancy, particularly in the lead up to birth, to ensure that blood sugar levels are optimum. Women who have diabetes and no other complications are advised to have an elective birth by induction of labour, or by caesarean if clinically indicated, between 37^{+0} weeks and 38^{+6} weeks of pregnancy. This is because of the increasing risk of stillbirth and other complications.

Immediately after birth, women should return to their pre-pregnancy regime with regular blood sugar monitoring as the metabolic requirements of pregnancy resolve quickly. If breastfeeding the risk of hypoglycaemic episodes for the woman is high due to increased metabolic demand.

PROGNOSIS

Despite the increased risks of complications in the antenatal and intrapartum periods, most women with pre-existing diabetes do well, as do their newborns. However, the risk of the child developing T1DM is increased if its mother also has T1DM.

❓ QUESTIONS

Emma, a 34-year-old, gravida two, para one, is seen in clinic at 28 weeks' gestation. Her BMI is 35 kg/m² and 3+ glucose was detected in her urinalysis. She has had an otherwise normal pregnancy so far; her last pregnancy was uncomplicated. She has no other past medical history and her mother has type 2 diabetes.

Q1 Answer true or false: which of the following risk factors put Emma at increased risk of gestational diabetes?
  A Age >30 years.
  B BMI ≥35 kg/m².
  C Multiparity.
  D Family history of diabetes.
  E Glycosuria 3+ on urine dipstick.

Q2 Which of the following statements are correct regarding factors driving increased insulin resistance in pregnancy?
  A Decreased production of thyroid hormones.
  B Decreased placental lactogen.
  C Increased placental progesterone.
  D Decreased cortisol and growth hormone.
  E Increased weight gain.

Q3 Answer true or false: What antenatal management options could be applied to this woman?
  A Consistently high blood glucose levels merit the use of metformin or insulin.
  B Measurement of glycosylated haemoglobin every 4 to 6 weeks.
  C Ultrasound examinations every 2 weeks in the first trimester.

  D Involvement of a dietician in the multidisciplinary team.
  E Regular maternal fundoscopy.

Q4 Answer true or false: Which management options could be applied to this woman regarding birth?
  A The aim for the mode of birth should always be a caesarean.
  B The estimated timing of birth in women requiring insulin is 38 to 39 weeks following the absence of obstetric complications.
  C GDM women with blood glucose greater than 7 mmol/L during labour require an insulin sliding scale.
  D Women with GDM have decreased rates of assisted vaginal birth.
  E There should be a continuation of pregnancy doses of insulin and diabetic medication for a minimum of 6 weeks postpartum.

A Autonomic neuropathy.	**H** Random plasma glucose measurement.
B Macrosomia.	
C 7 mmol/L.	**I** Gastroenteritis.
D 7.8 mmol/L.	**J** Fasting plasma glucose measurement.
E 11.1 mmol/L.	
F Diabetic nephropathy.	**K** Polycythaemia.
G Hyperbilirubinaemia.	**L** Oral glucose tolerance test.

Select the most appropriate option from the above list that corresponds to the following statements. Each answer can be used once, more than once or not at all.

Q5 The minimum glucose concentration needed for the diagnosis of GDM with the 2-hour OGTT.

Q6 Phototherapy is the first-line treatment for this neonatal complication of diabetes.

Q7 This complication of diabetes causes reduced gastric motility leading to protracted vomiting.

Q8 A fetal complication associated with prolonged labour and shoulder dystocia.

Q9 Women diagnosed with GDM are offered this test at 6 weeks postpartum to assess for T2DM.

[Answers on page 376.]

EPILEPSY

Epilepsy is usually defined as a clinical diagnosis of two or more seizures more than 24 hours apart, or a single seizure with characteristic features of an epilepsy syndrome. Approximately 1% to 2% of the UK population suffers from epilepsy. Seizures are the result of the hyperexcitability of cortical neurons, with subsequent symptoms depending on the area of cortex affected. Seizures can be diagnosed as a primary condition, often congenital, or they may result from reversible causes of a lowered seizure threshold, such as drug use, hypoglycaemia, infection and pregnancy. A seizure in pregnancy may represent an epileptic seizure in a known epileptic or a first episode of epilepsy. If occurring after 24 weeks' gestation, it is also necessary to consider eclamptic seizures.

In pregnancy, seizure frequency generally improves in 10% of women and worsens in 30%. Seizures may become more frequent during pregnancy because of factors relating to both a decreased seizure threshold and alterations in anti-epileptic drug (AED) regimens or levels.

Mechanisms include:
- Lack of sleep.
- Vomiting, causing altered AED levels.
- Lowered concentrations of AEDs in pregnancy due to increased plasma volume.
- Adjustment of AED doses due to adverse effects during pregnancy.
- Steroid hormone changes associated with pregnancy causing alteration of AED levels.

In general, if seizures are well controlled in the 12 months leading up to pregnancy they are likely to remain so during pregnancy.

Epilepsy and other neurological causes are the second most common cause of maternal mortality in the UK. Women with epilepsy are 10 times more likely to die in pregnancy and childbirth than those without; most of these cases are due to SUDEP (sudden unexplained death in epilepsy). The biggest risk factor for SUDEP is poorly controlled generalised epilepsy and therefore it is important to carefully counsel women about the importance of continuing their AEDs in pregnancy.

MANAGEMENT

PRENATAL MANAGEMENT

- Women considering pregnancy should aim to be seizure free, ideally for at least 2 months prior to conception. Their pregnancy should be monitored in an obstetrician-led clinic, with input from an epilepsy specialist.
- Drug treatment should be optimised with a balance between reducing the risks of seizures and minimising the increased risk of malformations attributed to many AEDs. Monotherapy is safer than polytherapy, and different AEDs vary in how safe they are in pregnancy. Lamotrigine and carbamazepine are generally regarded as two of the safer AEDs for use during pregnancy.
- A higher prophylactic dose of 5 mg folic acid should be given prior to conception and continued for at least the first 12 weeks of pregnancy, as epilepsy is associated with increased rates of spina bifida and other neural tube defects.
- Lifestyle advice should be provided that minimises the risk to health if a seizure were to occur. This includes advice on avoiding swimming as a form of exercise, on taking showers instead of baths, on

getting adequate sleep and regarding vomiting and AEDs.

ANTENATAL MANAGEMENT

Key fetal malformations include neural tube defects, cleft lips/palates and heart defects. A detailed fetal cardiac ultrasound may be offered from 16 weeks' gestation or included as part of the anomaly ultrasound. Some units offer this scan earlier than offered for routine pregnancies, at around 18 weeks.

Women with epilepsy are reviewed at regular joint obstetric and neurology antenatal clinics, where seizure frequency is discussed and medications altered to reduce seizure frequency. Growth scans are also advised in the third trimester to detect fetal growth restriction.

INTRAPARTUM MANAGEMENT

- The risk of seizure in labour is 1% to 2% due to pain, stress and often fatigue. Hence, women should be managed in a consultant-led obstetric unit, unless they have been seizure free and off medication for more than 10 years.
- Consider avoidance of pethidine during labour, as this may lower seizure threshold. Diamorphine may be used as an alternative.
- Continuous CTG monitoring should be provided during labour.
- Good hydration and adequate pain relief in labour are mandatory to help avoid seizures. An early epidural may be recommended.

POSTPARTUM MANAGEMENT

- The risk of seizures is cited as highest in the early postpartum period, in comparison to the antenatal period. This is often due to ongoing stresses such as sleep deprivation and pain.
- Breastfeeding is safe while on AEDs.
- Women should be advised regarding postnatal management of AEDs, to ensure optimal management with respect to their ongoing epilepsy.
- Postpartum contraceptive requirements – Mirena©, contraceptive injections and implants are all compatible for use with AEDs. Note that the combined oral contraceptive pill and progesterone only pill are affected by cytochrome P450 (CYP450) enzyme inducing AEDs. Therefore if these AEDs are used, the doses of both the contraceptive pill and AEDs may need adjustment.

SEIZURES IN PREGNANCY

INITIAL MANAGEMENT

Initial management of any seizure in pregnancy will always involve an ABCDE approach. Specific treatment for the seizure will depend on the clinical picture and whether the seizure is deemed primary epilepsy or eclampsia. A case of suspected epilepsy should be treated with a benzodiazepine given rectally (such as diazepam) or intravenously (such as lorazepam) in repeated doses. This should be followed by a phenytoin infusion if the benzodiazepine alone is unsuccessful at terminating the seizure. Suspected eclampsia is managed by an intravenous infusion of magnesium sulphate. In cases of status epilepticus that is unresponsive to treatment, intubation is usually required and birth is likely to be necessary.

> ### 💡 Status Epilepticus
>
> Status epilepticus is defined as a generalised tonic-clonic convulsion lasting 30 minutes or more, or repeated convulsions occurring over a period of at least 30 minutes without recovery of consciousness in this time. However, NICE guidelines now state that an individual who has been having a tonic-clonic convulsion for 5 minutes or more should be treated the same as if they fulfil the definition for established status epilepticus, i.e. with prompt escalation of treatment.

INVESTIGATIONS

If epilepsy has already been diagnosed, limited investigations are required, particularly if seizures are infrequent and brief. If seizure frequency is increasing, it is important to review anti-epileptic medications and potentially check drug levels to ensure that they are within the therapeutic window. If the diagnosis of epilepsy is in doubt, an electroencephalogram (EEG) may show characteristic changes, particularly if recorded during a seizure; however, do not exclude the diagnosis if the EEG is normal.

If no pre-existing epilepsy is diagnosed, further tests should be carried out to determine the cause of any seizure in pregnancy. These should only be carried out once the initial seizure episode has been managed appropriately. These further investigations may include:

- Bloods (including an FBC, U&Es, LFTs), glucose, a group and save, and a urine dipstick to help rule out important differentials, such as intracranial infection, electrolyte abnormalities (such as hyponatraemia), pre-eclampsia and hypoglycaemia.
- Consider a head CT or MRI if less common differentials are considered, such as an acute intracranial haemorrhage, venous sinus thrombosis or emboli, or a space occupying lesion.
- EEG may be useful; however, this may remain normal between seizure episodes.
- CTG to check on the fetal wellbeing. This is likely to show abnormalities during an acute seizure, but once the mother stabilises, the fetus should also stabilise. If not stable after the mother has stabilised, then birth should be considered.

In a patient with recurrent atypical seizures and negative investigation results, a diagnosis of pseudoseizures may be considered, but this is a diagnosis of exclusion. Vigilance is important in this patient group, as pseudoseizures are often associated with significant mental health issues, social problems or domestic violence.

COMPLICATIONS

Although the vast majority of women with epilepsy will have healthy pregnancies, epilepsy does confer some additional risks for the pregnancy and the fetus, as detailed below.

FETAL COMPLICATIONS

- Miscarriage and threatened miscarriage.
- Congenital malformations associated with AED use, including the following:
  - Neural tube defects.
  - Microcephaly.
  - Cardiac defects.
- Low intelligence quotient (IQ).
- Low birthweight and intrauterine growth restriction.
- Neonatal death.
- Developmental delay.
- Childhood epilepsy (4% vs. background risk of 0.5%).

MATERNAL COMPLICATIONS

- Increased seizure frequency.
- SUDEP.
- Pre-eclampsia.
- Placental abruption.

PROGNOSIS

More than 90% of women with epilepsy have a successful and healthy pregnancy with no fetal abnormalities.

❓ QUESTIONS

Azra, a 25-year-old primigravida woman, has attended her primary care physician for pre-conception advice. She suffered from several idiopathic focal seizures as a child and was subsequently diagnosed with epilepsy. Her current medication regimen includes lamotrigine and sodium valproate. Her last seizure was 2 months ago, at which time the dose of sodium valproate was increased from 600 to 1000 mg/day. Her only past medical history of note is asthma, which is currently well controlled with salmeterol inhalers. She also takes the combined oral contraceptive pill.

Q1 Regarding the AED sodium valproate, which of the following are correct?

   A Valproate should, if possible, be stopped completely prior to conception.

   B If on valproate the woman should have a discussion with an epilepsy specialist regarding an alternative AED prior to conception.

   C Valproate levels must be monitored at least once per trimester in those taking it during pregnancy.

D Adverse effects of valproate may be avoided if the dose is reduced.

E Breastfeeding is not recommended for women taking valproate.

Q2 Answer true or false: Which of these statements would constitute appropriate pre-conception advice for this mother?

A Stopping the oral contraceptive may significantly alter lamotrigine levels.

B Monotherapy should be adopted, as it is always the most appropriate option.

C Optimising seizure control prior to conception is important, because uncontrolled generalised seizures during pregnancy can increase the risk of SUDEP.

D Pregnancy itself may lower the seizure threshold, causing increased seizure frequency if not treated adequately.

E The patient should be made aware that women with epilepsy are predisposed to a higher risk of complications during pregnancy and labour.

Q3 Which aspects of management during the pregnancy would be recommended in this case?

A High-resolution ultrasound scan at 12 weeks.

B All AED levels should be routinely monitored.

C Folate supplementation should not be commenced until a positive pregnancy test.

D Lamotrigine and carbamazepine are largely considered safe to use during pregnancy.

E The neonate should not be given 1 mg vitamin K parenterally at birth.

[Answers on page 379.]

CARDIAC DISORDERS

Cardiac disorders fall into three main categories: electrical (arrhythmias), structural (damage to the heart muscles or valves) or circulatory. Cardiac disorders during pregnancy can be pre-existing or acquired. Congenital heart defects are the most common pre-existing condition in pregnancy, and hypertension is the most common acquired condition.

Due to advances in neonatal and paediatric cardiac surgery over the last 30 years, an increasing number of babies born with severe congenital heart defects, such as tetralogy of Fallot, transposition of the great arteries, pulmonary atresia and hypoplastic left heart syndrome, are surviving into adulthood. As a result, an increasing number of women with severe congenital cardiac problems are reaching adulthood and going on to become pregnant.

In addition, the average age at which women have children is increasing, as are obesity rates. The result is an increased incidence of hypertension, ischaemic heart disease and heart failure in pregnancy. Cardiac disease is one of the leading causes of maternal mortality and therefore it is very important to appropriately risk assess and identify these patients in pregnancy.

NORMAL CARDIAC CHANGES

The physiological and haemodynamic changes that occur during pregnancy hugely affect the cardiovascular system. These changes begin in the first 8 weeks of gestation.

Increased cardiac output (by approximately 40%) occurs to allow an increased blood flow of up to 500 mL/min to the uterus. This is achieved by:

1 An increase in stroke volume (30%) in the first and second trimester (this increases again in the third trimester).

2 An increase in heart rate (10 to 15 bpm).

3 An increased plasma volume, increasing from approximately 70 mL/kg when not pregnant up to 100 mL/kg in the pregnant woman.

4 A decrease in systemic vascular resistance (SVR). There is systemic vessel dilatation and the placenta acts as a low resistance shunt, lowering total peripheral resistance.

These changes cause a decrease in blood pressure until approximately 22 to 24 weeks' gestation, when the blood pressure again increases until term. Relative anaemia also occurs, for although the red cell number increases, this increase is less than that of the plasma volume. This aggravates the hyperdynamic circulation.

Normal findings in a healthy pregnant woman include:

- Increased heart rate.
- Peripheral oedema.
- Slight increase of venous pressure.
- Widened pulse pressure.
- Fixed splitting of the second heart sound (S2) during later stages of pregnancy.
- Systolic 'flow' murmurs due to an increased pressure and flow through the aortic valve in particular.

Investigations also need to be interpreted cautiously due to normal physiological changes. For example, left axis deviation is observed on an ECG due to the elevation of the diaphragm caused by the increasing size of the uterus. A chest x-ray may also show cardiac enlargement. Echocardiography will show an increased left ventricular end diastolic volume and a small increase in the left ventricular wall thickness.

IDENTIFYING CARDIAC DISEASE

Most women with cardiac disease in pregnancy will have it as a pre-existing condition. However, it is important to monitor the disease for deterioration, and to be aware of possible new onset disease. Symptoms in pregnancy are similar to those in the non-pregnant population, including fatigue, orthopnoea, decreased exercise tolerance, chest pain and palpitations. Clinical signs, such as a raised jugular venous pressure (JVP) and oedema, may be seen. Cyanosis is a particularly worrying sign and should always be investigated.

Investigation of cardiac disease in pregnancy is usually the same as in the non-pregnant population. Investigations may include blood tests (FBC, U&Es, troponin, BNP), ECG, echocardiography, chest x-ray, MRI and cardiac catheterisation. The most likely complications to arise during pregnancy are arrhythmias and heart failure. In addition, women who have congenital heart problems themselves should be offered a detailed fetal cardiac scan during pregnancy because of an increased risk of congenital heart disease in the fetus.

Red flag cardiac symptoms in pregnancy:
- Chest pain requiring opioids or radiating to arm, shoulder or jaw/associated with haemoptysis or abnormal observations.
- Sudden onset, tearing or exertional chest pain.
- Persistent sinus tachycardia.
- Paroxysmal nocturnal dyspnoea.
- Orthopnoea.
- New wheeze or no improvement with asthma medication.

If any of these are present they should be investigated urgently and be managed with an MDT approach.

 Peripartum Cardiomyopathy

Peripartum cardiomyopathy is a rare form of dilated cardiomyopathy where the heart dilates and weakens during pregnancy, inducing the symptoms of heart failure. Peripartum cardiomyopathy usually occurs in the last month of pregnancy until approximately 5 months postpartum. It may occur in patients with no previous cardiac disease, possibly resulting in a diagnostic delay and patient death. The main symptoms include fatigue, shortness of breath and fluid retention, as in heart failure. Investigation involves history, examination, bloods (including B-type natriuretic peptide (BNP) and troponin), ECG, chest x-ray and further imaging such as an echocardiogram, CT and cardiac catheterisation. Medical management may involve vasodilators, diuretics, beta blockers, anticoagulants and antiarrhythmics; however, some medications are contraindicated in pregnancy. Some women may present in acute heart failure and will require aggressive management. In these cases, if medical management fails, mechanical support may be required. In severe cases, cardiac transplantation may be needed.

Hypertrophic Obstructive Cardiomyopathy

Hypertrophic cardiomyopathy is increasingly being diagnosed in pregnant women. Women with hypertrophic cardiomyopathy tend to tolerate pregnancy well; however, a multidisciplinary team should manage them, as there is a risk of sudden cardiac arrest and death. A family history is strongly associated with this condition, although even if the abnormal gene is passed on, it will have no effect on the heart of the fetus or newborn since the disease is adult onset. Genetic testing may be offered to close relatives of a patient diagnosed with hypertrophic cardiomyopathy.

MANAGEMENT

The management of cardiac disease can be complex and dependent on the specific cardiac abnormality. A condition like paroxysmal atrial fibrillation may require no specific additional care, whereas pulmonary stenosis will require close monitoring in a dedicated cardiac-obstetric clinic.

Ideally, patients with a pre-existing heart condition will be seen by a cardiologist prior to conception to discuss the risks pregnancy may pose and to optimise treatments to limit any risk. In some cases, such as in those with severe heart failure or severe congenital heart disease, patients may be informed of significant maternal risks and advised to avoid pregnancy. The highest-risk cases are those with pulmonary hypertension and right to left shunting, where pregnancy carries at least a 50% risk of maternal mortality.

Antenatally, patients should be reviewed regularly in joint obstetric and cardiac antenatal clinics. The key aims of the clinics are:
- Regular review of cardiac symptoms during pregnancy.
- Follow up with echocardiograms or other investigations to monitor disease progression; the frequency will depend on the severity of the disease.
- To discuss timing and mode of birth. Birth should be closely monitored in a consultant-led unit. Labour, and in particular pushing in the second stage, is a significant stressor on the cardiovascular system.
- Vaginal birth may be a viable option for some women. To limit the cardiac stress, early use of epidural anaesthesia may be suggested, reduced time pushing in the second stage of labour, or early recourse to an assisted vaginal birth.
- Caesarean may be considered the safer option in some cases.

Postnatal follow up is crucial, as changes in the cardiovascular system and fluid shifts in the postnatal period can increase the risk of deterioration of cardiac disease.

TREATMENT OPTIONS FOR DETERIORATING HEART DISEASE

The methods of treating most conditions are broadly the same for pregnant and non-pregnant women. Conservative measures, such as rest or salt and fluid restriction, may be considered in heart failure. Medications can be used to treat heart failure, ischaemic heart disease or arrhythmias. However, some drugs are contraindicated in pregnancy due to potential fetal effects. For example, ACE inhibitors are contraindicated as they can cause fetal anuria, pulmonary hypoplasia and skull deformities. Where possible, alternative safer medications should be used.

Rarely, in severe cases, surgical interventions like balloon angioplasty, stenting, pacemakers, balloon pumps or transplantation may be required. In these severe life-threatening cases, serious consideration should be given to early birth to reduce cardiac demand.

PROGNOSIS

Outcome depends on the cardiac disorder underlying the symptoms, and it varies. Cardiac disorders during pregnancy are one of the leading causes of maternal deaths in the UK.

❓ QUESTIONS

Rebecca, a 29-year-old who is 28 weeks pregnant, comes to see the primary care physician as she is concerned because there is a family history of heart disease. Her aunt died as a result of developing heart failure during pregnancy. She is currently well and has had a normal pregnancy up to date.

Q1 Answer true or false: Which of the following could be considered normal when investigating a pregnant woman?
   A Enlarged cardiac borders on chest x-ray.
   B Changing cardiac axis on ECG.
   C ST wave elevation on ECG.
   D Palmar erythema.
   E Flow murmurs.

Q2 Answer true or false: Which of these factors is a risk factor for developing a cardiac disorder in pregnancy?
   A Increased maternal age (more than 35).
   B Smoking.
   C Pre-existing cardiac disorder.
   D Pre-existing diagnosis of asthma.
   E Busy lifestyle.

Q3 Which of these blood tests, when there are increased levels, indicate possible myocardial damage?
   A Thyroid hormones.
   B Troponin I.
   C Iron levels.
   D Carbon dioxide.
   E Potassium.

[Answers on page 381.]

MATERNAL WEIGHT

BMI is calculated using the patient's weight in kilograms divided by the square of their height in metres. Obesity during pregnancy is defined as a BMI of 30 kg/m² or higher at the patient's first antenatal consultation. Patients with a BMI of 25.0 to 29.9 kg/m² are classed as overweight. A high maternal BMI at the time of conception increases risks for both mother and baby.

As seen in the general population, obesity during pregnancy can be further divided into:
- Obesity class 1 – BMI 30.0 to 34.9 kg/m².
- Obesity class 2 – BMI 35.0 to 39.9 kg/m².
- Obesity class 3 – BMI ≥ 40 kg/m² (morbidly obese).

AETIOLOGY

The proportion of pregnant women who are obese has risen significantly over recent years, mirroring the increase in rates amongst the general population. In the early 1990s 8% of pregnant women were obese, rising to 16% in the 2000's, and currently around 23% in the early 2020's. This increase can partially be attributed to higher-calorie, fat-laden diets, coupled with reduced exercise levels. With such a high proportion of pregnant women affected, obesity is one of the most commonly seen conditions that leads to a high-risk pregnancy. It is important to also consider that while obese women may eat additional calories, they also have a higher risk of malnourishment due to the types of food typically eaten.

CLINICAL FEATURES

Excess adipose tissue within the body is generally detected on inspection during a clinical examination. Some women with obesity will be asymptomatic. However, patients may have symptoms such as:
- Breathlessness.
- Pain in load bearing joints.
- Increased sweating.
- Skin breakdown and ulcers.
- Fatigue.
- Gastroesophageal reflux.
- Psychological distress.

If the patient has any complications as a result of obesity, such as gallstones, they may describe additional symptoms associated with these pathological states.

INVESTIGATIONS

All women should have their weight and height measured starting at their booking appointment, meaning that screening for obesity will be routine early in pregnancy. If the patient has a raised BMI, taking a medical history is important to ascertain any underlying aetiology, as this will guide treatment advice.

DIFFERENTIAL DIAGNOSIS

In a few cases, a BMI increase is not due to excess adipose tissue. Other reasons include:
- Mesomorphic state – highly muscular state (body builders).
- Anasarca – highly oedematous state.
- Acromegaly.

Rarely, associated symptoms may warrant further investigation into the cause for obesity, such as:
- Hypothyroidism.
- Cushing syndrome.

However, obesity due to these factors is much less common than obesity due to excess calories.

COMPLICATIONS

The risks of obesity in the general population include gallstones, osteoarthritis, cardiovascular disease, stroke and increased cancer risk. Pregnant women who are obese carry those risks as well as the risks of other problems related to their pregnancies. These conditions, highlighted below, are significant and can affect both the mother and baby throughout pregnancy and labour and after birth.

MATERNAL COMPLICATIONS

- Venous thromboembolism (VTE).
- Hypertension.
- Pre-eclampsia.
- Gestational diabetes.
- Premature birth.
- Induced labour.
- Anaesthetic complications – decreased success rate of epidural and spinal anaesthesia, and increased general anaesthetic risks.
- Assisted vaginal birth or caesarean.
- Postpartum haemorrhage.
- Infection of wounds.
- Difficulties in breastfeeding.
- Admission to intensive care.
- Cardiovascular disease.
- Death.

FETAL COMPLICATIONS

- Shoulder dystocia.
- Stillbirth and miscarriage.
- Congenital abnormalities.
- Macrosomia.
- Intrauterine growth restriction.
- Neonatal death.
- Childhood obesity.

MANAGEMENT

PRE-CONCEPTION

Women of childbearing age should ideally be counselled regarding their BMI and be encouraged to reach an optimum BMI level before becoming pregnant. If they are overweight or obese prior to pregnancy, the loss of 5% to 10% of their weight would be significant enough to improve health during pregnancy. Nonetheless, the ideal BMI range for a woman looking to conceive would be 18.5% to 24.9 kg/m². Furthermore, a reduction in BMI in overweight or obese women can improve the chance of conceiving a baby.

DURING PREGNANCY

Weight Management

- If a woman is deemed to be obese during pregnancy, she should be advised of the risks of this condition.
- Regular weight measurement during pregnancy is only necessary if body weight will impact clinical management, for example, in the planning of equipment requirements for birth.

- There is no standardised expected weight gain in pregnancy. If a woman is deemed as obese, the emphasis should be on a healthy diet and lifestyle and minimising any weight gain in pregnancy.

Diet and Lifestyle

- Lifestyle advice about diet and exercise should be given to all women when booking in with their midwives.
- Dispel the 'eating for two' myth and explain that there is no requirement to increase calorific intake until 6 months' gestation, at which point approximately 200 extra calories per day is sufficient.
- Women who were physically active prior to the pregnancy should be able to continue as normal, providing they feel able to do so. If previously inactive, women should aim to start with 15 minutes of continuous exercise three times per week and gradually increase this to 30 minutes of moderate intensity activity per day.
- All obese women should be commenced on 10 µg of vitamin D daily and encouraged to continue taking high-dose folic acid supplementation until 12 weeks' gestation.

Implications for Antenatal Care

- All women with a BMI over 30 kg/m² should have a VTE assessment at their booking appointment. If they have three or more additional risk factors for VTE, they should be prescribed low molecular weight heparin (LMWH) as soon as possible and continue this treatment for 6 weeks following birth.
- A patient who is deemed at high risk of pre-eclampsia should receive a daily dose of 150 mg aspirin throughout pregnancy. Women with a BMI more than 35 kg/m² should be informed of the symptoms of pre-eclampsia. Increased blood pressure and urinalysis measurements may be considered, in addition to routine antenatal care appointments.
- Due to the increased risk of gestational diabetes, all obese women should have an OGTT between 24 and 28 weeks' gestation.
- Antenatal ultrasound screening is not as accurate in obese women as it is in non-obese women. This can lead to missed abnormalities on the 20 week anomaly scan and is coupled with an increased risk of congenital abnormalities, such as neural tube defects.
- Measurement of the symphysis fundal height is not accurate in obese women, so fetal growth is monitored by serial ultrasound scans performed beginning at 28 weeks.

[See 'Venous Thromboembolism' page 355.]
[See 'Pre-Eclampsia and Pregnancy-Induced Hypertension' page 301.]

DURING LABOUR

Obese women can often have a vaginal birth without medical intervention, but they are at increased risk of complications during labour and postpartum.

- If the patient's BMI is more than 35 kg/m², the current recommendation is that she should deliver in an obstetrician-led birth unit rather than a midwife-led suite.
- Senior anaesthetists and obstetricians should be made aware of morbidly obese patients (BMI over 40 kg/m²) who are in labour so that they can be prepared to undertake urgent interventions if necessary. Early venous access should also be considered in these patients as they are more difficult to cannulate in emergency situations.
- Fetal monitoring in labour can be more challenging in the obese women. Maintaining a good fetal heart rate trace can be difficult using normal abdominal CTG transducers, so a fetal scalp electrode (FSE) is often attached to improve fetal monitoring.

AFTER BIRTH

Obesity still poses risks to the woman's health in the postpartum period and beyond, so encouraging a healthy lifestyle is important. Obese women are also at increased risk of VTE, so they may require 7 days to 6 weeks of thromboprophylaxis (usually with LMWH) after birth. After pregnancy, the 6-week postpartum check provides a good opportunity to discuss weight management with the mother, including conservative and medical options for treatment.

PROGNOSIS

Obesity in pregnancy has many associated risks, as outlined above. Lifestyle modifications after birth can dramatically reduce the risk of complications in subsequent pregnancies. Prognosis for the mother is good, provided she makes appropriate lifestyle changes. The child should be monitored for signs of obesity and other metabolic problems throughout childhood.

LOW BMI IN PREGNANCY

Mothers who are underweight (BMI <18.5 kg/m²) also face risks before and during pregnancy. Prior to pregnancy, underweight women are at risk of amenorrhoea. This means that their chances of conception are likely lower than those of women with a normal BMI. This underscores the importance of advising women to adopt healthy diets and optimise their BMI prior to conception.

MANAGEMENT

Active attempts to alter the woman's BMI towards the normal range during pregnancy are often advised, typically with the help of a dietician and nutritional supplements. The women should also have regular monitoring by their midwives. Birth in a consultant-led unit should be considered for underweight women, but it may not always be necessary if fetal growth is deemed to be within normal ranges. In contrast to obese women, those with a low BMI appear to have a lower risk of pre-eclampsia, gestational diabetes and assisted vaginal birth or caesarean when compared to women who have a normal weight. Regardless, the serious risks of pregnancy with a low BMI support the recommendation that women should have a normal BMI for their pregnancy.

COMPLICATIONS

Maternal
- Anaemia.
- Malnutrition.

Fetal
- Preterm birth.
- Low birth weight.
- Hypoxic ischemic encephalopathy.
- Stillbirth.

The most significant risks associated with a low BMI are preterm birth and low birth weight. Preterm birth is the most frequent cause of neonatal death, so low maternal BMI presents a significant risk of mortality for the baby.

PROGNOSIS

Low BMI is sometimes associated with an underlying, often severe, psychiatric illness. If this is the case, careful liaison with psychiatry services is vital in order to protect the mother and baby throughout the pregnancy.

❓ QUESTIONS

Rachel is a 29-year-old who has recently discovered she is unexpectedly pregnant with her first child. She is 160 cm tall and weighs 92.5 kg at her booking appointment but is otherwise fit and well. She is concerned about the effect her weight may have on her and the baby during the pregnancy.

Q1 Which of these BMI calculations and classification pairings is correct for Rachel (160 cm tall and 92.5 kg)?
    A 36.1 kg/m²; morbidly obese.
    B 36.1 kg/m²; obese class 2.
    C 57.8 kg/m²; morbidly obese.
    D 57.8 kg/m²; obese class 2.
    E 32.6 kg/m²; obese class 1.

Q2 Using the correct BMI for Rachel, select which additional monitoring or treatments should be offered throughout her pregnancy.
    A OGTT between 24 and 28 weeks.
    B Seven days thromboprophylaxis following birth.
    C Birth in a consultant-led unit.
    D Routine measurement of maternal weight at every midwife and medical consultation.
    E Monitoring for pre-eclampsia every 3 weeks from 24 to 32 weeks and every 2 weeks thereafter.

[Answers on page 382.]

Q3 Answer true or false: Obese women are likely to be at risk of which of the following obstetric complications?

   A Seizures.
   B A large baby.
   C Pulmonary embolism.
   D A baby with a flat philtrum.
   E Requirement of ventouse for birth.

THYROID DISEASE

HYPERTHYROIDISM

Hyperthyroidism is defined as functional overactivity of the thyroid gland. It affects approximately 1 in 500 pregnancies. Note that pregnancy is associated with hypertrophy and increased vascularity of the thyroid gland and that these changes reverse postnatally. True clinical hyperthyroidism should be differentiated from transient gestational hyperthyroidism, which is usually milder and rarely requires treatment.

RISK FACTORS

- Family history of thyroid disease, particularly Graves disease.
- Previously treated thyroid disease, even if well controlled.
- Subclinical thyroid disease prior to pregnancy.

AETIOLOGY

Hyperthyroidism in pregnancy has several possible causes:
- Graves disease (more than 90%) – autoimmune hyperthyroidism is caused by immunoglobulin G (IgG) autoantibodies, which stimulate thyroxine production by binding to thyroid stimulating hormone (TSH) receptors. Signs specific to Graves disease include exophthalmos, proptosis, thyroid acropachy and pretibial myxoedema. The IgG antibodies are able to cross the placenta and potentially cause fetal hyperthyroidism.
- Transient gestational hyperthyroidism – this is caused by high levels of hCG, which contains the same alpha subunit as TSH, causing some cross reactivity at the TSH receptors. Blood tests show a biochemical hyperthyroid state but patients are rarely symptomatic and this requires no treatment. It usually occurs in the first trimester when hCG levels are highest, and has normally resolved by 20 weeks' gestation as hCG levels fall. It is commonly identified in patients with hyperemesis, which is also associated with high hCG levels.
- Rare causes
  - Toxic adenoma or multinodular goitre – adenomas, which are benign tumours, are classified as 'toxic' if they produce excessive thyroid hormone.
  - Toxic adenocarcinomas.
  - De Quervain subacute thyroiditis – this is also known as 'painful subacute thyroiditis,' as the thyroid may be tender. It often occurs following viral infections, especially Coxsackie, mumps and adenoviruses. It is usually transient but may develop later into hypothyroidism.

COMPLICATIONS

- Thyroid storm.
- Maternal tachycardia or arrhythmia.
- Miscarriage and stillbirth.
- Premature birth.
- Pre-eclampsia.
- Fetal thyrotoxicosis.
- Low birth weight and growth restriction.
- Both neonatal hyperthyroidism and hypothyroidism.

INVESTIGATION

- Symptoms and signs lead to suspicion of thyroid disease, with thyroid function tests confirming the diagnosis.
- Total T4 and T3 will be artificially increased secondary to raised thyroid binding globulin (TBG), particularly in the first trimester, and therefore cannot be relied upon for diagnosis. As a result, free T4 is most useful in diagnosing hyperthyroidism.
- Rarely, where doubt exists about the diagnosis, serum levels of TSH receptor antibodies can be checked. Clinicians will often routinely check for these antibodies in pregnancy to guide the level of monitoring, as higher levels increase the risk of fetal and neonatal complications.

MANAGEMENT

- All pregnant women with thyroid disease, whether newly diagnosed or long standing, should be referred to an endocrinologist for:
  - Close monitoring of symptoms.
  - Repeated thyroid function tests (TFTs) throughout pregnancy to guide treatment adjustments.
- Medications are given to inhibit thyroid hormone synthesis to maintain a euthyroid status:
  - Propylthiouracil – commonly used in pregnancy as not known to be teratogenic, but it can in rare instances cause maternal liver failure, so it is not used outside of pregnancy.
  - Carbimazole – in rare instances it can cause a fetal bone disorder. It is usually a safer medication for the mother, so it is often commenced after initial bone development is completed (from the second trimester) and is commonly used in non-pregnant patients.
  - Outside of pregnancy, a 'block and replace' regimen is used where high doses of these medications are used to completely inhibit thyroid function, with thyroxine given back to maintain a euthyroid state. However, anti-thyroid medication crosses

the placenta in higher concentrations than thyroxine, so a block and replace regimen in pregnancy would cause fetal hypothyroidism. To reduce the chance of this, lower doses of anti-thyroid medications are used in pregnancy so that some function remains for both the maternal and fetal thyroid glands. In other words, the 'block' is not complete, so no replacement thyroxine is needed.

Other treatments:
- Beta blockers can be used to help in symptom control. In rare cases, they can cause fetal growth restriction.
- If thyroid surgery is needed due to poor medical control, this is possible in pregnancy.
- Radioactive iodine, which is commonly used outside of pregnancy, is absolutely contraindicated in pregnancy, as the radiation is teratogenic and the iodine will accumulate in both fetal and maternal thyroids, destroying fetal thyroid tissue.

Obstetricians should:
- Counsel the patient regarding the increased risk associated with hyperthyroidism.
- Consider organising regular growth scans, particularly where medical control is poor, as growth restriction is a risk.
- The fetal heart should be listened to every 4 to 6 weeks, as a tachycardia or arrhythmia may be the first sign of fetal thyrotoxicosis. This occurs in approximately 1% of pregnancies complicated by hyperthyroidism, and it is caused by antibodies crossing the placenta. If left untreated, it can lead to high output cardiac failure, hydrops and stillbirth.
- As long as no complications arise during the antenatal period, birth options remain the same as for a low-risk pregnancy.

Plans should be made antenatally for monitoring of thyroid function after birth. Both carbimazole and propylthiouracil are safe during breastfeeding.

PROGNOSIS

Gestational outcome depends on the severity of thyroid disease and the ability to adequately control thyroid hormone levels. Where patients have been stabilised preconception and monitored carefully throughout pregnancy, outcomes are good.

HYPOTHYROIDISM

Hypothyroidism is the second most common endocrinological disorder in pregnancy after diabetes. It occurs in 3% of pregnancies, with 0.5% being overtly symptomatic (Table 10.1) and a further 2.5% having biochemical evidence of hypothyroidism, but no symptoms, termed subclinical hypothyroidism. The physiological changes in pregnancy predispose to a hypothyroid state by creating an increased iodine demand due to active transport of iodine to the placenta and increased glomerular filtration rate.

AETIOLOGY

There are several possible causes of hypothyroidism in pregnancy:
- Hashimoto thyroiditis – this is the most common cause of hypothyroidism in the UK. It is an autoimmune hypothyroidism, with thyroid peroxidase (TPO) antibodies present in 95% of patients with Hashimoto's. However, they are also present in over 10% of the normal population. A goitre is commonly seen due to lymphocytic infiltration. The immune reaction destroys thyroid follicles causing hypothyroidism.
- Iodine deficiency – this is the most common cause of hypothyroidism in lower income countries. Classically, it presents with a goitre caused by excessive TSH causing hyperplasia, but as iodine is essential for thyroxine production, the hyperplasia does not increase output of hormones.
- Treated Graves disease – patients who have previously had radioiodine or thyroid surgery for hyperthyroidism later develop hypothyroidism. It is important to identify these patients, as they may

Table 10.1	Symptoms of Thyroid Disease				
HYPOTHYROIDISM			**HYPERTHYROIDISM**		
SYMPTOMS	**SIGNS**		**SYMPTOMS**	**SIGNS**	
• Depression	• Goitre		• Anxiety and psychosis	• Goitre (± bruit)	
• Cold intolerance	• Weight gain		• Heat intolerance	• Weight loss	
• Dry skin	• Hair thinning		• Diaphoresis	• Hair thinning	
• Mental slowing and tiredness	• Carpal tunnel		• Palpitations	• Lid lag	
	• Bradycardia		• Tremor	• Exophthalmos and proptosis	
• Constipation	• Mental slowing		• Less satiable	• Tachycardia or arrhythmias	
• Easy satiety	• Slow reflexes		• Weight loss	• Systolic flow murmur	
• Weight gain	• Myxoedema		• Hair thinning	• Resting tremor	
• Hair thinning	• Coma		• Menstrual irregularity	• Proximal myopathy	
• Menstrual irregularity			• Loss of libido	• Pretibial myxoedema	
• Loss of libido				• Brisk reflexes	

have TSH receptor IgG antibodies which can cross the placenta and cause fetal thyrotoxicosis.

- Rarer causes:
  - Drugs – including lithium and amiodarone.
  - Radiotherapy or surgery.
  - Atrophic hypothyroidism – sometimes caused by inhibitory TSH receptor antibodies.
  - Infiltrative diseases such as sarcoidosis.
  - Disease affecting the hypothalamic pituitary axis.

COMPLICATIONS

- Miscarriage and stillbirth.
- Postpartum haemorrhage.
- Preterm birth.
- Slightly reduced infant IQ if hypothyroidism is poorly treated. The risk is greatest if treatment is inadequate in the first 12 weeks' gestation, due to fetal neurological development during this time being dependent on maternal thyroxine.
- Severe thyroid deficiency can cause fetal cretinism:
  - Severe neurodevelopmental dysfunction.
  - Deafness.
  - Growth restriction.

INVESTIGATIONS

- Symptoms and signs lead to suspicion of thyroid disease, with thyroid function tests confirming the diagnosis (low T4, raised TSH).
- Rarely antibody testing may be considered:
  - TPO antibodies – multiple studies have shown that the presence of these antibodies can affect fetal outcomes as they can cross the placenta. Therefore, women with hypothyroidism are often checked for the presence of these.
  - TSH receptor antibodies – this may be checked in patients with hypothyroidism following treatment for Graves disease.

MANAGEMENT

- Women with known hypothyroidism should have stable thyroid function prior to conceiving.
- As soon as a woman with hypothyroidism learns she is pregnant, she should immediately increase the dose of her levothyroxine replacement by approximately 25%.
  - This is because the fetal thyroid does not begin to function until 12 weeks, but thyroxine is essential for early fetal brain development. In these early weeks, the fetus is completely dependent on maternal thyroxine, which can cross the placenta. Increasing the dose early ensures there is adequate thyroxine and dramatically reduces fetal complications.
- Thyroid function should be checked at booking and subsequently every 4 weeks, until the treatment dose remains stable. Following stabilisation, checking once per trimester is sufficient.

- Growth scans may occasionally be considered in patients with severe hypothyroidism or high antibody titres.
- If all remains well antenatally, patients with hypothyroidism can be treated similarly to low-risk pregnancies during labour.
- After birth, the levothyroxine dose should be returned to the pre-pregnancy dose. The primary care physician should recheck thyroid function 12 weeks after birth. Primary care physicians should also be aware that these patients are at an increased risk of developing postpartum thyroiditis.

Postpartum Thyroiditis

- This occurs after pregnancy in 5% of women, the majority of whom will not have an existing thyroid condition.
- It occurs approximately 3 to 6 months postpartum.
- It is more likely to occur in the presence of TPO antibodies.
- The exact aetiology is unknown, but some believe it is part of the process of the immune system 'correcting' after the downregulation required to support pregnancy; the result is a mild autoimmune condition.
- It is a transient process which causes a mild hyperthyroidism, sometimes followed by hypothyroidism before resolving to a euthyroid state.
- It usually lasts 3 to 6 months, rarely needing treatment.
  - It can present with mild hyperthyroid symptoms or hypothyroid symptoms.
  - The hypothyroid symptoms can often be misdiagnosed as postnatal depression.
  - It can present with painless thyroid enlargement, in contrast to other transient thyroiditis causes, which often cause a tender thyroid.
- A patient who develops postpartum thyroiditis has a significant chance of developing hypothyroidism in the future. Primary care physicians should undertake long-term monitoring for this.

PROGNOSIS

With appropriate treatment, prognosis remains excellent for women with hypothyroidism during pregnancy.

❓ QUESTIONS

Sophie, a 28-year-old in her first pregnancy, has come to see her primary care doctor at 12 weeks' gestation. She has had loose stools for 2 weeks and is very anxious. She is worried about the possibility of thyroid disease, given a family history of Graves disease. She has no significant past medical history and takes no regular medications.

Q1 Answer true or false regarding the following statements concerning hyperthyroidism in pregnancy.

  A Thyroid function is routinely screened for in the antenatal booking visit.

  B Free T4 is the active thyroid hormone exerting the main physiological effect.

C Free T4 is the most useful investigation in diagnosing hyperthyroidism in pregnancy.

D Carbimazole is the first-line treatment for hyperthyroidism in the first trimester.

E Graves disease is the most common cause of hyperthyroidism in pregnancy.

Q2 During pregnancy, levels of which of the following would be expected to increase?

A TSH.

B Free T4.

C Total T4.

D Maternal iodide.

E TBG.

Q3 Answer true or false: The risk of which of the following are increased with hyperthyroidism in pregnancy?

A Fetal growth restriction.

B Deep vein thrombosis (DVT).

C Neonatal hypothyroidism.

D Miscarriage.

E Congenital malformations.

[Answers on page 384.]

HEPATITIS B

Hepatitis is an inflammatory condition of the liver. Over half of all cases of acute hepatitis are attributable to viral infection; however, it can be secondary to autoimmune, vascular or metabolic conditions. Hepatitis B virus (HBV) is transmitted through contact with blood or other bodily fluids of an infected person. Risk factors include sexual contact, needle sharing and maternal hepatitis B at the time of birth. Needle stick injuries and other workplace-based exposures present a particularly high risk in the healthcare setting. The prevalence of hepatitis B among pregnant women in the UK is 0.4 to 1%.

BACKGROUND

Routine screening for HBV status is offered to all pregnant women in early pregnancy, ideally at their first contact with antenatal services. In some countries, all babies get routine hepatitis B vaccinations, but in the UK, only babies in high-risk situations are offered vaccination. In the UK, screening is done by testing maternal blood for the hepatitis B surface antigen (HBsAg). If this is positive, a specialist referral should be made. Further testing should then occur for hepatitis B envelope antigen (HBeAg), anti-hepatitis B envelope (anti-HBe), hepatitis B viral load, other hepatitis types (C and D) and HIV. A liver ultrasound is also advised, as well as checking liver function tests. The serological tests are summarised in Table 10.2.

In early acute infection, the presence of HBsAg will often precede any symptoms or detectable rise in serum transaminases. Hepatitis B infection is rarely symptomatic; however, if left untreated or if severe,

Table 10.2 Interpreting Hepatitis B Serology Results

SEROLOGICAL MARKER	DETECTION AND INFECTION STAGE	ACUTE INFECTION	CHRONIC INFECTION	RESOLVED INFECTION	VACCINATED	UNVACCINATED/ NO PREVIOUS DISEASE
HBsAg	Hepatitis B surface antigen – marker of infection. Persistent for more than 6 months in chronic infection.	+	+	–	–	–
Anti-HBc immunoglobulin M (IgM)	Antibody to hepatitis B core protein – seen in acute infection only.	+	–	–	–	–
Anti-HBc IgG	Antibody to hepatitis B core protein – follows IgM and persists as IgG in chronic infection.	–	+	+	–	–
HBeAg	Hepatitis B envelope antigen – presence associated with higher rates of viral replication and infectivity.	+/–	+/–	–	–	–
Anti-HBe	Antibody to envelope antigen – associated with significant decrease in likelihood of transmission.	–	–	+/–	–	–
Anti-HBs	Antibody to surface antigen – indicates immunity to infection. May be obtained after clearing the virus or through vaccination.	–	–	+	+	–
HBV DNA	Viral load can be quantified and used to detect level of current viral replication.	Variable	Variable but higher if HbeAg +	Undetectable	–	–

HBeAg, Hepatitis B envelope antigen; *HBV*, hepatitis B virus; *HBsAg*, hepatitis B surface antigen; *IgG*, immunoglobulin G.

it may lead to significant liver disease, both acutely and chronically, and the development of hepatocellular carcinoma. Co-infection with another virus can occur along with HBV (for example, with hepatitis D), increasing the risk of complications.

If a patient is HBsAg positive, then the patient has active hepatitis and is at risk of transmission to the fetus. If, however, they are HBsAg negative, then there is no risk of transmission. Screening alone cannot determine whether someone has been vaccinated, never been exposed to the virus, or been exposed to it and cleared it. The important point is that there is no additional risk to the pregnancy.

MOTHER TO CHILD TRANSMISSION

The risk of transmission from mother to infant depends on maternal infectivity. Women who have a high viral load, and are both HBsAg and HBeAg positive, have the highest risk of transmission. Anti-HBe is protective. HBV DNA is the most accurate measure of infectivity, and in cases of high infectivity, antiviral agents may be considered in the third trimester to decrease maternal viral load. One antiviral that could be considered is the reverse transcriptase inhibitor tenofovir.

All infants born to HBsAg positive mothers should receive hepatitis B vaccination at birth and complete the schedule consisting of three further doses at 1, 2 and 12 months. In those that are at higher risk – for example, if the mother has a high viral load or is HBeAg positive – immunoglobulin therapy should be administered shortly after birth to further reduce the risk of hepatitis B transmission. Infants born to a mother with hepatitis B should be tested for the disease at 12 months of age, after completing the vaccination schedule. Breastfeeding is not associated with increased risk of infection in infants receiving HBV vaccination.

MANAGEMENT IN LABOUR

Women should be encouraged to birth vaginally unless there are other obstetric indications for a caesarean, as the transmission risk is not affected by a caesarean. In labour, clinicians should avoid, where possible, the use of a fetal scalp electrode or fetal blood sampling, as well as midcavity or rotational assisted vaginal births. These increase the chance of fetal trauma, which could increase the risk of transmission. This risk of transmission is greater if the woman is HBeAg positive.

PROGNOSIS

If a woman with hepatitis B (HBsAg positive) does not receive optimum health care and treatment, her neonate has an approximately 10% risk of developing chronic hepatitis B, which rises to over 90% if HBeAg is also present. Treatment of both mother and neonate reduces transmission by over 90%.

? QUESTIONS

Rose is a 29-year-old, gravidity one, parity zero, who presents to the clinic at 18 weeks' gestation. She has been feeling tired and run down for a while, and has recently been experiencing frequent nausea and headaches, following a period of feeling particularly unwell for the past week or two. She does not drink alcohol and denies any drug use. She was born in Indonesia and previously worked as a nurse before moving to the UK 7 years ago. On examination, she shows poorly localised abdominal tenderness with guarding, and mild scleral icterus. Her blood results from her booking appointment reveal that she is HBsAg positive.

Q1 Which option is the most appropriate immediate step in Rose's management?

   A Lamivudine, zidovudine and lopinavir.
   B Commence tenofovir disoproxil at 28 weeks.
   C Ribavirin and PEG-IFNα-2a.
   D Refer to a hepatologist or relevant specialist and arrange further tests.
   E Sofosbuvir oral medication and referral to specialist.

On further testing, the following results are obtained.

AST	765 IU/
ALT	880 IU/L
ALP	190 IU/L
HIV-ab	–
Anti-HAV IgM	–
Anti-HAV IgG	+
HBsAg	+
Anti-HBs	–
Anti-HBc IgM	–
Anti-HBc IgG	+
HBeAg	+
Anti-HCV IgM	–
Anti-HCV IgG	–

Q2 Answer true or false to the following statements regarding this woman's results.

   A She was vaccinated against HBV when training as a nurse.
   B She may need to commence antiviral treatment in the third trimester to prevent transmission.
   C She was probably infected with hepatitis B early in life.
   D Her baby requires the hepatitis B vaccine at birth.
   E She is likely to be a chronic carrier of HBV.

Select the most appropriate option from the list below that corresponds to the following statements. Each answer can be used once, more than once or not at all.

A	HDV-RNA.	G	Anti-HBe.
B	HBeAg.	H	Anti-HBc IgM.
C	Anti-HDV IgM.	I	ALP.
D	HBsAg.	J	ALT.
E	ANA.	K	HBV-DNA.
F	AST.	L	Albumin.

Q3 The presence of this indicates a markedly lower likelihood of vertical transmission of HBV.

Q4 Chronic infection is identified by its persistence past 6 months.

Q5 The most reliable predictor of infectivity and viral replication in HBV.

Q6 A significant elevation of this enzyme is commonly associated with viral hepatitis.

[Answers on page 385.]

HIV

The most concerning issue with human immunodeficiency virus (HIV) in pregnancy is transmission to the fetus (Table 10.3), although other pregnancy complications may arise due to HIV, such as maternal susceptibility to infection. The risk of HIV transmission is highest during labour, although intrauterine and breastfeeding transmission may also occur, particularly when a high maternal viral load exists.

RISK FACTORS

Table 10.3	Factors Affecting Risk of Vertical HIV Transmission	
DECREASE RISK OF TRANSMISSION		**INCREASE RISK OF TRANSMISSION**
• Combination antiretroviral therapy. • Neonatal zidovudine treatment. • Caesarean– where viral load is high. • Avoidance of breastfeeding.		• Decreased CD4 count or increased viral load. • Membrane rupture more than 4 hours. • Preterm labour. • Low birth weight.

INVESTIGATIONS

- All pregnant women in the UK should be offered screening for HIV at their antenatal booking visit, usually at around 8 to 10 weeks.
- If the patient is confirmed as HIV positive, her CD4 count and viral load must also be established. Viral load is the most important indicator for transmission. It should be monitored at least once every trimester, at 36 weeks and around the time of birth. All HIV positive mothers should also be screened for hepatitis B, hepatitis C, varicella, syphilis, rubella, measles and toxoplasmosis.
- Once the mother is commenced on medication, regular antenatal monitoring of drug toxicity is required, including FBC, U&Es and LFTs.
- Other STIs and opportunistic infections or comorbidities should also be investigated.
- Contact tracing is crucial in women with a new diagnosis of HIV in pregnancy.

COMPLICATIONS

Pregnancies affected by HIV are associated with an increased risk of:
- Intrauterine growth restriction.
- Prematurity.
- Stillbirth.
- Neonatal infections.
- Congenital malformations.

MANAGEMENT

- Prenatal planning is required if the women is known to be HIV positive. This may include optimising the patient's antiretroviral therapy (ART). ART is a combination of at least three antiretroviral drugs, usually comprising two nucleoside reverse transcriptase inhibitors (NRTIs) and one protease inhibitor.
- If previously undiagnosed with a detectable HIV viral load, appropriate ART should be started during pregnancy.
- Care of all pregnant women with HIV is shared between HIV specialists and obstetricians, with more regular antenatal reviews than in HIV negative women.
- A decision regarding the mode of birth (Fig. 10.1) should be made by 36 weeks, following a discussion with the patient, particularly regarding the most recent blood results.
- After birth, the neonate is likely to be commenced on ART. Treatment should be commenced as soon as practicable after birth (preferably within 4 hours), and it is usually continued for 2 or 4 weeks or longer dependent on risk of transmission at birth. Even where the maternal viral load is less than 50 copies/mL, zidovudine monotherapy is often considered and commenced in the neonate because a small risk of HIV vertical transmission still exists. Where the risk of transmission is high, multiple drug ART is prescribed.
- Women are recommended not to breastfeed in the UK because of the risk of transmission through breast milk.
- It is also important to stress the ongoing importance of barrier contraception.

PROGNOSIS

The overall prognosis of HIV infection for the mother is not affected by pregnancy. Outcomes for the fetus depend strongly on whether the infection is transmitted. In the UK, with correct management, transmission occurs in less than 1.4% of cases. HIV infection is sometimes fatal in children, particularly in developing countries, where transmission rates are up to 30%.

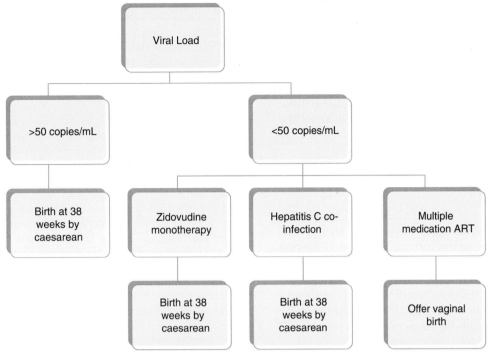

Fig. 10.1 Flow chart regarding birth planning in HIV positive women. In certain cases, caesarean birth is required to reduce transmission risk. Note that in vaginal birth, ventouse, fetal blood sampling and fetal scalp electrode monitoring must be carefully considered prior to use. Emerging data shows there is little or no increased risk of HIV transmission using these methods. *ART,* Antiretroviral therapy.

❓ QUESTIONS

Louise, a 32-year-old primigravida, is attending their 16 week antenatal check-up. Louise is currently well, but is known to be HIV positive, taking ART and co-trimoxazole prophylaxis for *Pneumocystis jirovecii*. There is no other past medical history of note. Louise has some concerns and would like your advice regarding the effects of their medications on the fetus and the risk of transmission of HIV to the baby.

Q1 Answer true or false: Which of the following would represent correct advice to the woman?

A Screening for hepatitis B and C should be performed.

B Smoking should be discontinued, as it may increase risk of vertical HIV transmission.

C ART should be continued pre- and postpartum.

D Birth by planned caesarean is advisable depending on viral load.

E Pneumocystis pneumonia (PCP) prophylaxis should be discontinued due to its teratogenicity.

Q2 This woman decides to continue taking antiretroviral medications and undergoes a planned caesarean. They also choose not to breastfeed. What is the approximate risk of vertical HIV transmission in this case?

A 1%.

B 8%.

C 15%.

D 25%.

E 40%.

Q3 Answer true or false: Which of the following are risks to the fetus posed by maternal HIV infection?

A Intrauterine growth restriction.

B Prematurity.

C Neonatal bradycardia.

D Neonatal acute respiratory distress syndrome (ARDS).

E Acquired immunodeficiency syndrome (AIDS) dysmorphic syndrome.

[Answers on page 387.]

SICKLE CELL DISEASE

Haemoglobinopathies are inherited diseases characterised by an abnormality in haemoglobin production. The most common of these conditions are sickle cell disease (SCD) and thalassaemia. SCD refers to the group of haemoglobinopathies in which abnormal haemoglobin S (HbS) molecules are formed. In the UK, the average lifespan of someone with SCD lies in the mid-50s, so most people with SCD will reach reproductive age. Over 300 infants with SCD are born in the UK each year. Individuals with sickle cell disease are symptomatic, whereas those with sickle cell trait inherit one sickle cell gene but the other is unaffected. They are therefore asymptomatic but can have children born with SCD.

RISK FACTORS

SCD is the most commonly inherited disease world-wide. The mutated gene is inherited in an autosomal recessive pattern. It is more prevalent in individuals with ancestry from high malaria prone areas, which predominantly affects Black individuals, but also those with ancestry from non-Black populations in areas like Greece and Italy.

PATHOPHYSIOLOGY

HbS takes the place of normal HbA in red blood cells (RBCs). The HbS molecules polymerise in hypoxic conditions, leading to the formation of sickle-shaped RBCs. These sickle cells are rigid and unable to deform as they pass through narrow capillaries. This can cause vaso-occlusions, resulting in ischaemia and painful acute 'sickle cell crises'. Sickle cells typically survive only 10 to 20 days (normal RBCs survive 90 to 120 days). The spleen destroys the sickle cells faster than bone marrow can synthesise new RBCs, causing haemolytic anaemia. Most patients are considered asplenic, either because of rupture of the spleen (as a result of a sickle cell crisis), or hyposplenism (atrophy of the spleen due to chronic damage). Asplenia puts patients at increased risk of infections, particularly from encapsulated microorganisms such as *Streptococcus pneumoniae* and *Haemophilus influenzae*.

INVESTIGATIONS

All pregnant women are offered screening for SCD and thalassaemia in early pregnancy (ideally, <10 weeks).

- In high-prevalence areas – a blood test for SCD, thalassaemia and other haemoglobinopathies.
- In low-prevalence areas – a blood test for thalassaemia and a questionnaire to determine likelihood of other haemoglobinopathies (and then a blood test if there is significant risk).
- The baby's father is offered testing if the mother is affected or a carrier to determine the likelihood of the baby being affected.

Following genetic counselling, if there is a high risk of thalassaemia major, the mother could choose to undergo CVS or amniocentesis to determine the haemoglobinopathy status of the fetus, particularly if they would consider termination for the condition. In the near future, it may also be possible to assess this using free fetal DNA found in maternal serum. Postnatally, a blood spot (heel prick) test is offered for all newborns, which screens for SCD. Screening for other haemoglobinopathies is only carried out if indicated.

 Thalassaemias

Thalassaemias are the other common autosomal recessive haemoglobinopathies. These inherited disorders cause reduced globin chain synthesis, resulting in reduced haemoglobin in RBCs. Mutations of the α globin genes give rise to α thalassaemia, whereas mutations of the β globin gene give rise to β thalassaemia. The terms thalassaemia major, intermedia and minor refer to disease severity. Patients with severe thalassaemia require greater numbers of regular blood transfusions when compared to those with minor disease. Patients have microcytic, hypochromic anaemia, as is also seen with iron deficiency anaemia. However, thalassaemia will not respond to iron supplementation and giving iron will only aggravate the condition. Antenatal care involves monitoring iron levels in those who receive blood transfusions. Overloading of iron can cause maternal cardiomyopathy and new endocrinopathies, particularly DM, hypothyroidism and hypoparathyroidism, while intrauterine growth restriction can be seen in the developing child. All iron chelation therapy is potentially teratogenic in the first trimester. Deferoxamine is the only chelation agent advised for use in the second and third trimester. Ideally, aggressive chelation therapy should occur before conception.

COMPLICATIONS

- Increased risk of sickle cell crises – nausea and vomiting in pregnancy can result in dehydration. This, as well as overexertion, stress and the hypercoagulable status of pregnant women can cause an increased frequency in sickle cell crises.
- Risk of worsening anaemia – in an uncomplicated pregnancy, there is an increase in the red cell count as well as an even greater increase in the amount of plasma. This disproportionate increase results in haemodilution and can cause anaemia. The growing fetus also puts increased demand for iron and folate on the mother, both of which are already in high demand in haemolytic anaemia.
- Increased risk of infection – the immune system is compromised in normal pregnancy, and SCD patients are asplenic.
- Increased risk of having a growth restricted baby, and consequently, increased likelihood of fetal distress, labour induction and caesarean birth.
- Reduced options for birth positions if hips have been replaced – femoral head necrosis can result from SCD-related ischaemia.
- Increased chance of the baby having SCD.

MANAGEMENT

- Outside of pregnancy, patients with SCD are reviewed at least annually by specialists. At each visit, the intentions of women regarding pregnancy and contraception should be discussed. Women should be well informed of the maternal and fetal complications.

- Assessments for chronic disease are carried out regularly. It should include:
  - Nephropathy and retinopathy screening.
  - Screening for iron overload – aggressive iron chelation is advised before conception.
  - Screening for red cell antibodies due to increased risk of haemolytic disease of the newborn.

These test results should be up to date if a woman is thinking of becoming pregnant. Patients with SCD usually take penicillin prophylactically and have up to date immunisations due to asplenia. If not, these should be prescribed prior to conception.

- Most patients also take folic acid outside pregnancy (for haemolytic anaemia), but this should be increased to 5 mg daily prior to conception and throughout pregnancy. This reduces the risk of neural defects and compensates for the increased demand for folate during pregnancy.
- Other medications should be reviewed. Hydroxycarbamide, used to reduce the complications of SCD, is possibly teratogenic, and so its use should be stopped 3 months before conception. ACE inhibitors and angiotensin receptor blockers (used to reduce progression of nephropathy) may also be stopped before conception if the mother's clinical condition is stable, as they have been shown to cause fetal abnormalities.
- Individuals with SCD are also encouraged to know the haemoglobinopathy status of their partner before becoming pregnant, and they should be offered counselling and advice about reproductive options.
- SCD can increase the risk of pre-eclampsia; all women should therefore be commenced on aspirin from 12 weeks.

- Careful consideration of VTE prophylaxis as SCD can increase the risk in pregnancy, especially during a crisis.
- Many women will become pregnant without preconception care, and so these measures should take place as early as possible during antenatal care (Table 10.4).
- Care should involve an obstetrician, haematologist and midwives experienced in high-risk care.

ANTENATAL CARE

Iron supplements are only given if there is evidence of iron deficiency to minimise the risk of iron overload. Blood transfusions are only indicated for women with acute anaemia.

- Women are advised to avoid sickle cell crises by staying hydrated, warm, avoiding stress and not overexerting themselves. Painful crises are the most frequent cause of hospital admission. Analgesia is given according to the severity of pain.
- Acute chest syndrome (ACS) is the second most common complication, presenting with tachypnoea, chest pain, cough, shortness of breath and new infiltrate seen on chest x-ray, and there is an increased risk of hypoxia. The presentation is similar to pneumonia, so both are treated simultaneously.

INTRAPARTUM CARE

- Women should be encouraged to give birth in hospital in a consultant-led unit.
- If the fetus is growing normally, induction of labour (or planned caesarean, if there are other obstetric indications) is advised from 38+0 weeks gestation to avoid late pregnancy complications.
- Women need to be kept warm and well hydrated throughout labour.
- Avoid pethidine.

Table 10.4 Routine Antenatal Care Given, in Addition to the Following Measures

WHAT?	WHEN?	WHY?
Blood pressure and urinalysis	At each consultation and more frequently if patient had pre-existing proteinuria	Monitor for pregnancy-induced hypertension
Mid-stream urine for cultures	Monthly	Monitor for urinary tract infections – more common in SCD.
Viability scan	Seven to 9 weeks gestation	In view of increased risk of miscarriage
Aspirin prophylaxis	From 12 weeks gestation (adverse effects on fetal development before this period)	May reduce risk of developing pre-eclampsia
Growth scan	Every 3–4 weeks from 24 weeks gestation	Monitor risk of fetal growth restriction
Discuss pain management	Third trimester	Pethidine should not be given due to risk of pethidine-associated seizures in patients with SCD
Low molecular weight heparin (LMWH)	Any antenatal hospital admissions or throughout pregnancy if other risk factors coexist	Thromboprophylaxis
Crossmatch blood	Before birth	If atypical antibodies are present from previous recurrent transfusions, blood crossmatching is likely to take time

SCD, Sickle cell disease.

POSTPARTUM CARE

Thromboprophylaxis should be given with LMWH, compression stockings, non-steroidal anti-inflammatory drugs (NSAIDs) to encourage early mobilisation.

PROGNOSIS

Most pregnancies complicated by maternal SCD are likely to result in a live birth; however, these pregnancies are at increased risk of obstetric and fetal complications. Specialist multidisciplinary care is imperative to minimise the risks.

❓ QUESTIONS

Ifemelu is a 37-year-old who moved to England 2 years ago from Nigeria. Ifemelu was diagnosed with sickle cell anaemia as an infant and has needed numerous hospital stays due to sickling crises throughout their life. Ifemelu has been married for 5 years, and has previously not wanted children. Their husband has never had symptoms of sickle cell anaemia. Ifemelu has recently become unintentionally pregnant so is anxious as to how this will affect their health. The couple are worried about whether the baby will have SCD, and are thinking about terminating the pregnancy.

Q1   At what stage in a pregnancy could this woman first know whether their baby has inherited SCD?
A After conception, following haemoglobinopathy screening of the father.
B During the first trimester, following blood testing of the mother.
C At the end of the first trimester, following CVS.
D During labour, following fetal blood sample (FBS) from the baby.
E After the birth of the baby, following the heel prick test.

Q2   At the antenatal clinic, Ifemelu has a medication review. Which of the following changes does not need to be implemented?
A An increase in folic acid dosage.
B Commencement of iron tablets.
C Commencement of low-dose aspirin.
D Stopping of hydroxycarbamide.
E Stopping of ramipril.

Q3   Ifemelu attends the emergency department at 28 weeks, presenting with worsening shortness of breath, a cough and feeling generally unwell over the past 48 hours.

On examination her respiratory rate is 24, SaO$_2$ 93% on air, heart rate 92 bpm, temperature 37.6°C, BP – 115/60. You notice bibasal crackles and arrange a chest x-ray. The chest x-ray shows new infiltrates and you suspect acute coronary syndrome.

Which of the following treatments would you commence first?
A IV antibiotics, analgesia and nebulisers
B IV antibiotics, oxygen, blood transfusion and involvement of haematology.
C Oxygen, treatment dose LMWH and involvement of haematology.

D Oxygen, IV antibiotics, treatment dose LMWH and analgesia.
E Involvement of ITU, oxygen and IV antibiotics.

Q4   The results of a heel prick test show that a newborn boy does not have SCD, nor is he a carrier. His parents had been concerned because the condition exists in both sides of the family. After testing the parents antenatally, the obstetrician had told the parents that there had been a 50% chance of the baby having a normal haemoglobinopathy status. What are the most likely statuses of the baby's parents?
A Both parents occasionally suffer from sickle cell crises.
B Both parents have SCD and a spontaneous mutation has occurred.
C One parent has SCD, and one parent is a carrier.
D Both parents have sickle cell trait.
E One parent is a carrier, and one parent has normal haemoglobin.

[Answers on page 388.]

INTRAHEPATIC CHOLESTASIS

Intrahepatic cholestasis of pregnancy (ICP) (previously referred to as obstetric cholestasis) is a multifactorial condition which is characterised by pruritus in the absence of a skin rash or primary skin condition and raised bile acids. LFTs may be abnormal but are not part of the diagnostic criteria.

Pruritis is common in pregnancy with 25% of women reporting it but the incidence of ICP in the UK is around 0.7% in multi-ethnic populations. Alternative causes for pruritus, therefore, must be excluded. In ICP, the pruritis and raised bile acids should return to normal postnatally.

RISK FACTORS

- Personal or family history of ICP.
- Multiple pregnancy.
- Hepatitis C.
- GDM.

PATHOPHYSIOLOGY

ICP most commonly presents in the third trimester. It may be linked to a genetic predisposition to the cholestatic effect of oestrogen. However, the exact aetiology remains unknown.

In ICP, the movement of bile through the bile ducts is decreased. This results in a build-up of bile acids in the body and reduced uptake of fat-soluble vitamins, such as vitamin K, which require bile to aid their absorption. This is rarely clinically significant for the mother, but severe vitamin K deficiency may cause fetal bleeding complications, as vitamin K is required for production of coagulation factors II, VII, IX and X.

ICP has been found to have an increased risk of stillbirth in singleton pregnancies when the bile acid concentration reaches above 100 µmol/L (or > 40 µmol/L after 38 weeks) in singleton pregnancies. It is not entirely clear what the pathophysiology of this is, but it is thought that the accumulation of bile acids causes an acute anoxic event due to possible fetal arrythmia or placental vessel spasm. It is therefore important to monitor bile acid concentrations in pregnancy.

SYMPTOMS

Primary pruritus often presents widespread, particularly affecting the palms of the hands and soles of the feet. Itching is typically worse at night. The bile acids or LFTs may take weeks to change after the pruritis, therefore any pregnant woman with persistent pruritis should have their LFTs and bile acids rechecked if symptoms persist.

SIGNS

- Dermatographia artefacta – skin trauma from intense scratching.
- Pale stool and dark urine.
- Jaundice.

These symptoms and signs resolve after birth.

INVESTIGATIONS

- LFTs and bile acids – pregnancy-specific ranges should be used.
  - Increased serum bile acid concentration – usually increases soon after the onset and serves as the optimum marker of the disease. Diagnostic level is a random bile acid level ≥ 19 µmol/L. A level greater than 40 µmol/L signifies moderate disease, and greater than 100 µmol/L severe.
  - Abnormal transaminase (ALT) and gamma glutamyl transferase (gamma GT). Alkaline phosphatase (ALP) is not used, as it increases physiologically due to production by the placenta. Clinical jaundice does not commonly occur in women with obstetric cholestasis; if it does, it tends to be mild, with bilirubin levels rarely exceeding 100 µmol/L.
- Tests to be considered if an atypical presentation of ICP or clinical suspicion:
  - Clotting screen.
  - Viral screen for hepatitis A, B and C and Epstein-Barr virus (EBV).
- Liver autoimmune panel for:
  - Chronic active autoimmune hepatitis.
    - Anti-nuclear antibodies.
    - Anti-liver or kidney microsomal antibodies.
    - Anti-smooth muscle antibodies.
  - Primary biliary cirrhosis.
    - Anti-mitochondrial antibodies.
  - Liver ultrasound – for gallstones as the cause.

DIFFERENTIAL DIAGNOSES

RASH AND PRURITUS

- Eczema.
- Atopic eruption of pregnancy.
- Polymorphic eruption of pregnancy – pruritic, papular rash, usually occurring in and around the striae gravidarum with umbilical sparing on the abdomen in the third trimester, which settles shortly after birth.
- Pemphigoid gestationis – rare autoimmune condition where blistering of the skin occurs in pregnancy, typically there is no umbilical sparing.
- Shingles.

DERANGED LIVER FUNCTION

- Pre-eclampsia.
- Acute fatty liver of pregnancy – check glucose levels as hypoglycaemia occurs with this condition.
- Gallstones or cholecystitis.
- Intrinsic liver problem – viral or autoimmune.

COMPLICATIONS

The clinical importance of ICP primarily lies in the potential dangers to the fetus.

FETAL RISKS

- Spontaneous preterm birth.
- Iatrogenic preterm birth.
- Stillbirth.
- Fetal distress.
- Meconium-stained liquor at a lower gestation.

These risks can be caused by both the disease and suboptimal management. A poor outcome is more likely for woman whose bile acids are above 40 (moderate disease), or other comorbidities or those with multiple pregnancies. It is therefore important to tailor care to each individual for the best possible outcome.

No specific form of antenatal fetal monitoring is recommended, and neither ultrasound nor CTG improve the outcome when performed during pregnancy to monitor ICP.

MATERNAL RISKS

The maternal risks are relatively minimal, the main ones being sleep deprivation from severe pruritus and anxiety. More recent studies have shown that ICP has been associated with a higher incidence of pre-eclampsia and GDM. No extra testing is required for this however. There may also be a small link between ICP and developing certain autoimmune conditions such as diabetes, psoriasis and thyroid problems in later life.

ICP does remain a diagnosis of exclusion, which cannot be definitively made until after birth, when the symptoms and biochemical derangements resolve. The maternal risks of other conditions which cause a similar clinical picture can be much greater.

MANAGEMENT

Managing these women should be consultant-led care and birth should occur in a hospital setting. All management and monitoring should be done on an individual basis with attention to the impact on the patient and decision for birth.

- Monitoring –
  - Bile acids and LFTs – to be repeated after 1 week to confirm diagnosis. Thereafter when considering timing of birth those with mild disease (bile acids <39), consider weekly testing from 38 weeks and from 35 weeks for those with moderate disease.
  - CTG during labour should be offered. However, there is little evidence that monitoring the fetus antenatally is of any benefit, as stillbirth in ICP often occurs suddenly and with no precipitating warning.
- Medications – drugs can be prescribed, but they only offer symptomatic relief for pruritus with no effect on outcome. The options include:
  - Topical emollients.
  - Antihistamines.
  - Ursodeoxycholic acid – the mechanism of action for this drug is not clear in the context of ICP.
- Vitamin K – this should be given if there is evidence of deficiency (prolonged prothrombin time).
- Birth – should be individualised according to the severity of disease and other comorbidities. Mild disease (bile acids 19 to 39), consider planned birth by 40 weeks. Moderate disease (bile acids 40 to 99), consider planned birth at 38 to 39 weeks. Severe disease (bile acids >100), consider planned birth at 35 to 36 weeks.
- Postpartum – postnatal resolution of pruritus and return to normal levels of LFTs should be confirmed. LFTs should not be measured until at least 10 days after birth, as LFT levels may have naturally risen in the first 10 days of puerperium. LFTs may take up to 6 weeks to normalise. If there is not complete resolution, the patient should be referred to a hepatologist for further investigation.

PROGNOSIS

Pruritus affects 25% of pregnancies. However, only a small proportion (0.7%) of these women will have ICP. The major concern in ICP is the risk of stillbirth. The perinatal mortality is approximately 1:200 cases, which is similar to the general population. Following birth, the outlook for women is generally positive, with only a few patients suffering from long-term sequelae, however, the recurrence rate in future pregnancies is high, ranging from 45% to 90%.

❓ QUESTIONS

Malika, a 32-year-old primiparous woman at 32^{+5} weeks gestation, presents with severe pruritus affecting her arms and feet. On examination, no rash is visible. Following LFTs, it is found that her ALT, ALP and bile salt levels are elevated. She is aware that her mother, who attends the hospital with her, had obstetric cholestasis. She has a BMI of 35 kg/m^2 and smoked before pregnancy, but states that she had stopped when she found out that she was pregnant.

Q1   The main hepatic duct joins with which other duct to form the common bile duct?
  - **A** Ampulla of Vater.
  - **B** Cystic duct.
  - **C** Left main hepatic duct.
  - **D** Pancreatic duct.
  - **E** Right main hepatic duct.

Q2   Which of the following liver function test components are increased during pregnancy as part of a normal physiological response?
  - **A** ALT.
  - **B** ALP.
  - **C** Gamma GT.
  - **D** Bilirubin.
  - **E** Serum cholesterol.

Q3   Answer true or false: Which of the following aspects of this woman's case are risk factors for ICP?
  - **A** Primiparous.
  - **B** Family history.
  - **C** Maternal age more than 30.
  - **D** Male fetus.
  - **E** Previous history of smoking.

Q4   What is the primary reason for considering induction of labour before 36 weeks' gestation in a woman with known ICP?
  - **A** Fetal distress.
  - **B** Fetal growth restriction.
  - **C** Maternal sleep deprivation.
  - **D** Total bile acids >100 μmol/L.
  - **E** Meconium.

Q5   Answer true or false regarding the following management options.
  - **A** Emollient creams are both safe and highly effective.
  - **B** Dexamethasone is the first-line treatment option for ICP.
  - **C** Activated charcoal improves pruritus.
  - **D** Ursodeoxycholic acid improves pruritus but has no effect on liver function.
  - **E** No treatment options have been found to improve fetal or neonatal outcomes.

[Answers on page 390.]

KEY REFERENCES

DIABETES

Bottalico, J.N., 2007. Recurrent gestational diabetes: risk factors, diagnosis, management, and implications. Semin. Perinatol. 31 (3), 176–184.

National Institute for Health and Clinical Excellence, 2015. Diabetes in Pregnancy: Management of Diabetes and Its Complications From Preconception to the Postnatal Period. NICE Clinical Guidance (CG 63).

National Institute for Health and Clinical Excellence, 2021. Caesarean Section. NICE Clinical Guidance (NG192).

Royal College of Obstetrics and Gynaecology Green Top Guideline, 2012. Shoulder Dystocia Guideline (CTG 42).

EPILEPSY

Knight, M., Bunch, K., Tuffnell, D., Patel, R., Shakespeare, J., Kotnis, R., et al., 2020. Saving Loves, Improving Mother's care. MBRRACE, Oxford.

National Institute for Health and Clinical Excellence, 2012. The Epilepsies: The Diagnosis and Management of the Epilepsies in Adults and Children in Primary and Secondary Care. NICE Clinical Guideline (CG 20).

Royal College of Obstetricians and Gynaecologists, 2016. Epilepsy in Pregnancy. RCOG Green Top Guideline (GTG 68).

Walker, S.P., Permezel, M., Berkovic, S.F., 2009. The management of epilepsy in pregnancy. BJOG 116, 758–767.

CARDIAC DISORDERS

Abbas, A.E., Lester, S.J., Connolly, H., 2005. Pregnancy and the cardiovascular system. Int. J. Cardiol. 98 (2), 179–189.

Bowater, S.E., Thorne, S.A., 2010. Management of pregnancy in women with acquired and congenital heart disease. Postgrad. Med. J. 86, 100–105.

Givertz, M.M., 2013. Peripartum cardiomyopathy. Circulation 127, 622–626.

Knight, M., Bunch, K., Tuffnell, D., Patel, R., Shakespeare, J., Kotnis, R., et al., 2020. Saving Loves, Improving Mother's care. MBRRACE.

MATERNAL WEIGHT

Han, Z., Mulla, S., Beyene, J., Liao, G., McDonald, S.D., et al., 2011. Maternal underweight and the risk of preterm birth and low birth weight: a systematic review and meta-analyses. Int. J. Epidemiol. 40 (1), 65–101.

National Institute for Health and Clinical Excellence, 2010. Weight Management Before, During and After Pregnancy. NICE Public Health Guideline (PH 27).

National Institute for Health and Clinical Excellence, 2012. Obesity. NICE Clinical Guideline (CG 43).

Royal College of Obstetricians and Gynaecologists, 2018. Management of Women With Obesity in Pregnancy. Green Top Guideline (GTG 72).

Sebire, NJ, Jolly, M, Harris, J., Regan, L., Robinson, S., 2001. Is maternal underweight really a risk factor for adverse pregnancy outcome? A population-based study in London. BJOG 108 (1), 61–66.

THYROID DISEASE

Dhillon-Smith, R., Boelaert, K., Jeve, Y.B., Maheshwari, A., Coomarasamy, A., Royal College of Obstetricians and Gynaecologists, 2022. Subclinical hypothyroidism and antithyroid autoantibodies in women with subfertility or recurrent pregnancy loss. RCOG scientific impact paper. BJOG 129 (12), e75–e88.

Girling, J., 2008. Thyroid disease in pregnancy. Obstet. Gynaecol. 10, 237–243.

Jefferys, A., Vanderpump, M., Yasmin, E., 2015. Thyroid dysfunction and reproductive health. Obstet. Gynaecol. 17, 39–45.

HEPATITIS B

British Viral Hepatitis Group, Maternal and Paediatric subgroup, 2021. Guideline for the management of hepatitis B in pregnancy and the exposed infant. UK Guideline.

National Institute for Health and Care Excellence, 2013. Diagnosis and Management of Chronic Hepatitis B in Children, Young People and Adults. NICE Clinical Guideline (CG 165).

HIV

British HIV Association, 2018. Management of HIV infection in pregnant women. 2020.

Royal College of Obstetrics and Gynaecology, 2010. HIV in Pregnancy. RCOG Green Top Guideline (GTG 39).

SICKLE CELL DISEASE

Claster, S., Vichinsky, E.P., 2003. Managing sickle cell disease. BMJ 327 (7424), 1151–1155.

Royal College of Obstetricians and Gynaecologists, 2011. Management of Sickle Cell Disease in Pregnancy. RCOG Green Top Guideline (GTG 61).

Royal College of Obstetricians and Gynaecologists, 2014. Management of Beta Thalassaemia in Pregnancy. RCOG Green Top Guideline (GTG 66).

INTRAHEPATIC CHOLESTASIS

Girling, J., Knight, C., et al. (on behalf of the Royal College of Obstetrcians and Gynaecologists), June 2022. Intrahepatic Cholestasis of Pregnancy RCOG Green Top Guideline (GTG 43).

Walker, I., Chappell, L.C., Williamson, C., 2013. Abnormal liver function tests in pregnancy. BMJ 347, f6055.

TWIN PREGNANCY

Multiple pregnancy is defined as a pregnancy with more than one fetus. The focus of this chapter will be the development of twins (the most common multiple pregnancy, currently accounting for around 1.5% of livebirths). However, the principles covered can also be applied to higher order pregnancies, such as triplets and quadruplets.

Twins can be monozygotic ('identical'), where one fertilised zygote splits and forms two embryos or dizygotic ('non-identical'), whereby two embryos develop from two distinct zygotes, each fertilised by separate sperm cells.

Key definitions are:
- Zygosity – number of ova.
- Chorionicity – number of placentae (think chorionic plate of the placenta).
- Amnionicity – number of fetal membranes (think amniotic sac).

AETIOLOGY

The fetus is surrounded by two membranes, the chorion (which develops first) and the amnion (Fig. 11.1). The chorion is the outer membrane surrounding the fetuses (developed from trophoblastic tissue that becomes the placenta). The amnion is the inner membrane that encloses the fetus and amniotic fluid (characterised by the amniotic sac). At birth, these two membranes lie adjacent to each other, so they are impossible to tell apart on ultrasound scanning, but during the first trimester it is possible to differentiate them.

Dizygotic twins are always dichorionic diamniotic (DCDA), with separate placentas and amniotic sacs. Monozygotic twins can be DCDA (10%) or, more commonly, monochorionic diamniotic (MCDA) (90%). When MCDA, both fetuses share a placenta but have separate amniotic sacs. Rarely, monozygotic twins are monochorionic monoamniotic (MCMA) (0.01% of all pregnancies), when they share both a placenta and an amniotic sac.

Clinically, determining whether the fetuses share chorions or amniotic sacs is critical to providing increased surveillance for those at higher risk of pathology.

For monozygotic twinning, the incidence of amniotic or chorionic sharing is determined by the stage of embryonic development at which zygote splitting occurs (Table 11.1).

RISK FACTORS

Likelihood of having a pregnancy with twins is increased by:
- Increasing maternal age.
- Increasing parity.
- Family history.
- Fertility treatment – approximately 25% of twin pregnancies in the UK are following *in vitro* fertilisation (IVF).

 Incidence of Twin Pregnancy

The natural incidence of dizygotic ('non-identical') twinning is 12/1000 in the UK; 54/1000 in Nigeria and 4/1000 in Japan. By comparison, the rate of monozygotic ('identical') twins is 3/1000 almost universally.

The overall incidence of twin pregnancy is significantly affected by the availability of assisted conception in a country and their rules on how many embryos can be implanted per cycle. In the UK, where single embryo transfer is advised in most cases, the overall incidence of twin pregnancy is 16/1000.

INVESTIGATIONS

Overall, 50% of the twins born worldwide are only identified as twin pregnancies at birth. However, detection at an earlier gestation is possible in high income countries where ultrasound scanning is routinely used. In the UK, most twins are detected at the 12-week dating scan.

Table 11.1	Number of Days That Splitting Occurs, and Its Effect on Chorionicity and Amnionicity in Monozygotic Twinning		
NUMBER OF DAYS POST-FERTILISATION	**STAGE OF DEVELOPMENT**	**NUMBER OF CHORIONS**	**NUMBER OF AMNIONS**
Less than 4 days	Eight cell stage	Dichorionic	Diamniotic
4 to 8 days	Blastocyst stage	Monochorionic	Diamniotic
8 to 14 days	Inner cell mass has started to form	Monochorionic	Monoamniotic
More than 14 days (conjoined twins)	Amniotic cavity and yolk sac forms	Monochorionic	Monoamniotic

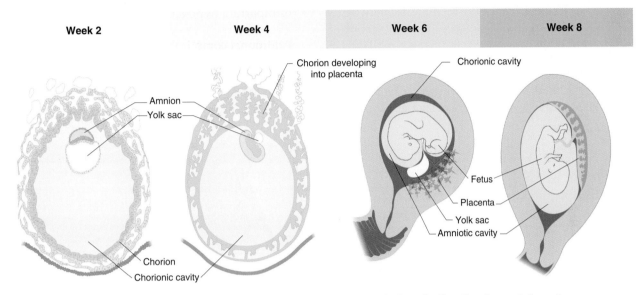

Fig. 11.1 **Early Embryological Development**. Initially chorion and chorionic cavity. Over time the amniotic cavity grows and obliterates the chorionic cavity.

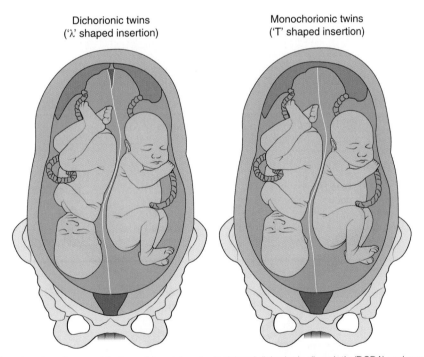

Fig. 11.2 First trimester ultrasound findings determining chorionicity of dichorionic diamniotic (DCDA) and monochorionic diamniotic (MCDA) twins.

At the dating ultrasound:
- Multiple fetuses can be seen, confirming multiple pregnancy.
- The amniotic membranes can usually be observed to assess diamnioticity or monoamnioticity.
- Assessing chorionicity (Fig. 11.2) can be difficult:

- In the first and early second trimester, the shape of the membrane insertion points can identify chorionicity:
  - Lambda (λ) shape insertions are dichorionic. The triangular appearance is formed by the two separate chorionic membranes meeting with their

separate amnions, forming a thick membrane. Note that DCDA twins may be monozygotic or dizygotic. Differentiating between them is only possible if fetuses are of different sexes, where observation of fetal genitalia will allow differentiation. Different sexes are indicative of dizygoticity, while identical sexes remain indeterminate.

- 'T' shape membrane insertions are monochorionic. This is because the membranes between the twins are thinner, as they are made up only of amnion.
- Beyond 20 weeks, two discrete placentas may be seen, diagnosing dichorionicity. However, if the placentas lie adjacent to each other, it can be difficult to distinguish them separately at later gestations.

COMPLICATIONS

Complications for both monozygotic and dizygotic twins:
- Preterm birth.
- Fetal growth restriction – can occur in one or both twins.
- Increased perinatal mortality – four times that for singleton births.
- Increased risk of chromosomal abnormalities.
- Intrapartum hypoxia.

Additional complications for monochorionic twins:
- Feto-fetal transfusion syndrome (FFTS) (Fig. 11.3).
- Twin anaemia polycythaemia sequence (TAPS) – a large haemoglobin difference between twins (donor has anaemia, recipient has polycythaemia).

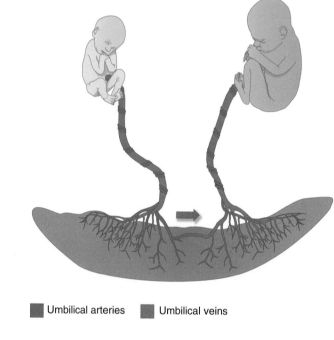

■ Umbilical arteries   ■ Umbilical veins

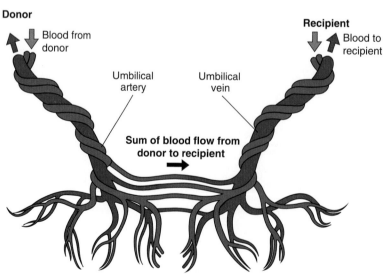

Fig. 11.3 Feto-Fetal Transfusion Syndrome Vessels and Fetuses. In reality, there are often multiple anastomotic vessels, with some blood flowing from twin A to twin B and some flowing the other way. Feto-fetal transfusion syndrome occurs when a mismatch arises in the amount being 'swapped' between the two twins.

- Twin reversed arterial perfusion (TRAP) – in this rare condition, one twin has either an absent or non-functioning heart and is usually maldeveloped. The other twin usually develops healthily but is at risk of cardiac failure as it supplies the blood for both twins.
- Further increased incidence of structural fetal abnormalities.

Additional complications for monoamniotic twins:
- Cord entanglement and associated *in utero* demise.

In addition, all maternal complications present with an increased incidence in multiple pregnancies in comparison to singleton pregnancies. Those of particular clinical importance include:
- Anaemia.
- Hyperemesis gravidarum.
- Hypertension in pregnancy.
- Pre-eclampsia.
- Placenta praevia.
- Antepartum and postpartum haemorrhage.
- Assisted vaginal birth.
- Increased maternal mortality; two and a half times that of singleton births.

 Feto-Fetal Transfusion Syndrome

Feto-fetal transfusion syndrome (FFTS), also known as twin-to-twin transfusion syndrome (TTTS), is caused by the anastomoses of the umbilical vessels between the two fetuses within the placenta. This develops in the first and second trimesters of monochorionic twin pregnancies. One fetus (the donor) loses blood to the other twin (recipient) (see Fig. 11.3). This causes both fetuses to be affected, with the donor appearing small, suffering growth restriction, anaemia and oligohydramnios (less liquor) and the recipient presenting with a hyperdynamic circulation causing polyhydramnios (increased liquor). In severe forms, the recipient develops fluid overload, resulting in hydrops (effusions in multiple body cavities such as the abdomen, chest, or skull) and heart failure. The donor twin can sometimes also develop hydrops from high-output cardiac failure caused by severe anaemia. Untreated FFTS has a high mortality rate (more than 90%) for both twins; and the recipient twin is the more likely to die. If intervention is required for FFTS, the problem vessels are transected using lasers *in utero* at specialist centres. However, even with early treatment there is a high risk of mortality for at least one twin.

MANAGEMENT

ANTENATAL CARE

- 10% of twin pregnancies diagnosed in the first trimester will continue only as singleton pregnancies; hence, this needs to be communicated sensitively to parents.
- All women diagnosed with a twin pregnancy should have an ultrasound scan between 10 and 13 weeks' gestation (the routine dating scan) to assess viability, chorionicity, major congenital malformations

and nuchal translucency. The timing of this examination is critical, as chorionicity is most accurately determined before 14 weeks. In addition, the timing of the screening is essential to determine subsequent monitoring protocols. In particular, women diagnosed with twin pregnancy will undergo more antenatal growth scans for the following reasons:
- Antenatal screening may be complex, as there are multiple fetuses to consider.
- The increased risk of complications, as outlined above.
- Growth assessment of both fetuses is much harder than in singleton pregnancies. Ultrasound scans should be used to monitor fetal growth, as symphysial fundal height (SFH) measurements are unreliable in multiple pregnancies.
- If growth discordance between twins or small for gestational age (SGA) on growth charts is identified, increased monitoring is required for growth restriction.

Monochorionic twins ultrasound regimen:
- Dating scan at approximately 12 weeks.
- Every 2 weeks from 16 weeks until birth to survey for FFTS. The first signs often identified are discordance in the amount of liquor each twin is making and the relative size of their bladders.
  - Alongside FFTS, simultaneous monitoring for fetal growth restriction and TAPS should be offered at every ultrasound assessment from 16 weeks to monitor for complications of monochorionicity.
- Structural survey including detailed cardiac scan at 18–22 weeks' gestation.
- Every 2 weeks from 24 weeks for fetal growth assessment.

Dichorionic twins' ultrasound regime:
- Dating scan at approximately 12 weeks.
- Detailed structural survey at 18 to 22 weeks gestation.
- Every 2 to 4 weeks from 24 weeks onwards for fetal growth assessment.

TIMING OF BIRTH

- In uncomplicated pregnancies, planned birth can be offered:
  - At 37 weeks in DCDA twins.
  - At 36 weeks in MCDA twins.
  - Between 32^{+0} and 33^{+6} weeks in MCMA twins.
- The timing of birth should be considered on an individual basis for complicated pregnancies.
- Parents should be counselled that multiple pregnancies should not go beyond 37 to 38 weeks' gestation, as the risk of perinatal mortality and morbidity increases with gestational age.

MODE OF BIRTH

- Parents of twin pregnancies should be advised that approximately 60% of cases result in spontaneous birth before 37 weeks.

- The mode of birth is usually finalised at approximately 32 weeks' gestation in uncomplicated twin pregnancies, when fetal presentations are unlikely to change.
- In uncomplicated DCDA or MCDA twin pregnancies after 32 weeks: both planned vaginal and caesarean birth are safe options, as long as the first baby is in a cephalic presentation and there is no significant intertwin size difference. Any obstetric contraindications to labour must also be considered. If the first twin is not cephalic at the time of planned birth, caesarean is recommended.
- In the rare case of MCMA pregnancies, there is a high risk of cord entanglement that can cause fetal hypoxia and intrauterine death. Due to this risk, a planned caesarean is offered from 32 weeks, even if no complications have occurred. This needs to be carefully balanced against fetal maturity. If a complication occurs prior to 32 weeks, necessitating earlier birth, a caesarean should also be offered.

INTRAPARTUM CARE

- It is important that a senior obstetrician and a senior anaesthetist are involved during intrapartum care. There should be two midwives and two paediatricians at the time of birth.
- An epidural can be beneficial in vaginal birth of multiple pregnancies: it increases the likelihood of success of assisted vaginal birth and enables a quicker transition to delivery by caesarean if required.
- Syntocinon should be ready if uterine activity decreases after birth of the first twin.
- During labour, cardiotocography (CTG) monitoring of both twins is crucial to monitor fetal well-being. This can be difficult, and it is not uncommon for the heartbeat of one twin to be monitored by both transducers. To minimise this possibility, a fetal scalp electrode can be applied to the head of the presenting twin (contraindicated if below 34 weeks), and an abdominal transducer can be used to monitor the second twin. Difficulty monitoring both twins may contribute to the increased risk of fetal hypoxia.
- If there is an abnormal CTG trace for the presenting twin, a fetal blood sample can be undertaken to further assess the fetal condition. However, if the second twin's CTG trace is abnormal, there is no way to further assess its condition, so fetal compromise should be assumed and birth expedited. Usually, caesarean section is the fastest mode of birth, unless delivery of the first twin is imminent, whereby vaginal birth may be facilitated.
- After birth of the first twin, the additional space created in the uterus allows the second twin to freely turn, ending up in any lie and position. Abdominal palpation and ultrasound can identify the lie of the second twin, and external cephalic version can be attempted to guide the second twin's head into the pelvis. Two hands can be kept on the pregnant abdomen to keep the twin in position while an amniotomy is performed. Once the lie is fixed, pushing can recommence and the second twin can be born.
- An alternative method to correct an abnormal lie is for the obstetrician to attempt internal podalic version: a manoeuvre where the obstetrician inserts a hand into the uterus to grasp one or both feet and draw them through the cervix to deliver the baby in the breech position. These manoeuvres are easier to both perform and undergo if an epidural has been given.
- There is an association with the second twin being more likely to suffer hypoxia if there is a long delay between the birth of the first and second twin. For this reason, syntocinon infusion can be used to increase uterine contractions after the first twin has been delivered. If birth is not imminent within about 40 minutes of delivery of the first twin, most obstetricians would offer intervention to expedite birth.
- If the lie cannot be stabilised to allow vaginal birth, or if there is cord prolapse or CTG abnormalities suggesting fetal distress, an emergency caesarean may be required to deliver the second twin. This occurs in approximately 2% of cases after the successful vaginal birth of the first twin.

Twin pregnancies are at an increased risk of postpartum haemorrhage because the uterus is larger than for a singleton pregnancy and is less able to quickly contract, resulting in bleeding secondary to atony of the uterus. To reduce the chance of this, active management of the third stage of labour with uterotonic medications, such as a syntocinon infusion, should be recommended.

Higher Order Pregnancies

Triplets or higher order pregnancies are rare and are usually managed in specialist centres due to high levels of complications, including mortality of all the fetuses and mother. To reduce the rate of complications, women with higher order pregnancies can be offered selective reduction, which is the intentional termination of one or more fetuses to improve the survival chances of the remaining fetuses. Delivery of higher order pregnancies is almost exclusively done by planned caesarean birth.

PROGNOSIS

Uncomplicated multiple pregnancies have a marginally worse prognosis than singleton pregnancies, as the risks of complications are increased. Timing of birth is also critical, as the increase in perinatal mortality and morbidity seen in twin pregnancies beyond 37 weeks of gestation parallels that seen in singleton pregnancies beyond 41 weeks.

? QUESTIONS

Dheepa is a 32-year-old woman who is currently pregnant with twins. She is 22^{+6} weeks gestation, and the pregnancy has had no complications to date. She is gravidity three, parity two, and her previous pregnancies were singletons with no complications.

Q1   If the two fetuses have separate membranes but share the same placenta, how is this pregnancy described?

   A Monochorionic monoamniotic.
   B Monochorionic diamniotic.
   C Dichorionic monoamniotic.
   D Dichorionic diamniotic.
   E Twin to twin transfusion.

Q2   Which structure gives rise to the placenta during embryological development?

   A Trophoblast.
   B Morula.
   C Blastocyst.
   D Inner cell mass.
   E Zona pellucida.

Q3   If Dheepa's pregnancy was diagnosed with FFTS, what is the best management at this gestation?

   A Conservative management.
   B Laser ablation.
   C Amnioreduction.
   D Septostomy.
   E Bipolar diathermy.

[Answers on page 392.]

KEY REFERENCES

Dodd, J.M., Crowther, C.A., Haslam, R.R., Robinson, J.S., Twins Timing of Birth Trial Group, 2012. Elective birth at 37 weeks of gestation versus standard care for women with an uncomplicated twin pregnancy at term: the twins timing of birth randomised trial. BJOG. 119 (8), 964–974.

Royal College of Obstetricians and Gynaecologists, 2016. Management of Monochorionic Twin Pregnancy. RCOG Green Top Guideline (GTG 51).

National Institute for Health and Clinical Excellence, 2019. Twin and Triplet Pregnancy. NICE Clinical Guideline (NG137).

Management of Labour

Outline

SPONTANEOUS VAGINAL BIRTH

A spontaneous vaginal birth refers to birth of the fetus in a vertex (head-first) position without assisted vaginal birth or caesarean. Spontaneous vaginal birth includes labours that are induced. In this chapter, we will be discussing term deliveries (37 to 42 weeks).

In antenatal care and labour, pregnancies are stratified as high or low risk depending on certain key factors. However, some low-risk women may go on to have complications, and conversely, many high-risk women will go on to have no difficulties.

Low-risk pregnancies will:
- Have no significant long-term medical, psychiatric or social concerns – for example, raised BMI, epilepsy, chronic kidney disease or hyperthyroidism.
- Have normal routine pregnancy screening tests.
- Have no significant complications with the current or previous pregnancies.

STAGES OF LABOUR

LATENT PHASE (EARLY LABOUR)

This stage of labour is when the cervix is effacing and dilating from a closed os to 4 cm in diameter. It can last hours to several days.

ESTABLISHED LABOUR

- First stage – 4 to 10 cm (10 cm is equivalent to full cervical dilatation).
- Second stage – from full cervical dilatation until complete birth of the fetus. This can be split into two stages:
  - Passive second stage is defined as the examination finding of a fully dilated cervix before or in the absence of involuntary expulsive contractions. This stage does not happen in all labours.
  - Active second stage occurs in all women, where the woman actively 'pushes' with expulsive contractions.

- Third stage – from birth of the baby until delivery of the placenta and membranes.

In a spontaneous, established labour, the rate of dilation should be no slower than 0.5 cm/h for primigravidous women and 1 cm/h for multiparous. From the onset of the second stage of labour (full dilatation), National Institute for Health and Clinical Excellence (NICE) guidelines state that the baby should be delivered within 4 hours. It is recommended that a primiparous woman be given 1 hour of passive second stage to allow for descent of the fetal head before commencing active pushing. A further hour of passive descent is advised for anyone with epidural analgesia.

It is expected that a primiparous woman should have delivered within 2 hours of active pushing, and a multiparous woman should deliver within 1 hour of active second stage. If birth is not imminent after this, then an obstetrician should review the woman with consideration of an operative birth (assisted vaginal birth or caesarean) checking for any signs of an obstructed labour or fetal distress.

MECHANISM OF LABOUR

Labour is characterised by regular, painful uterine contractions, which cause the cervix to efface (shorten) and dilate (open). The presenting part of the fetus is pushed against the cervix during a contraction, causing the cervical changes. Once the cervix is fully effaced and dilated (10 cm), the second stage of labour commences, and the fetus is delivered by maternal pushing with contractions.

In a vertex (head first) labour, the fetal position is determined relative to where the occiput (the back of the skull) is in relation to the maternal pelvis, particularly the pubic symphysis. For example, occipitoanterior (OA) means that the fetal occiput is closest to the anterior part of the maternal pelvis.

It is important to remember that the fetal head is not a sphere shape but instead a rugby ball shape.

Throughout labour, the largest diameter of the fetal skull needs to be presenting in the direction of the widest diameter of the maternal pelvis, which is not round either, and the widest plane changes throughout the J-shaped canal of the pelvis. The inlet of the female pelvis is widest in the transverse plane requiring the fetus to be in an occipitotransverse (OT) position, but the pelvic outlet is widest in the anterior to posterior direction requiring the fetal head to ideally be OA at this stage. Therefore, to achieve a successful vaginal birth, the fetal head may be required to move into different positions at the different stages of labour.

For a typical cephalic presentation (OA position), the fetus manoeuvres within the uterus in relation to the pelvis to allow the vaginal birth. This process, often called the 'mechanism of labour', can be broken down into nine steps (Fig. 12.1):

1 Pre-engagement of the fetal head with the pelvis – the fetal head is 'floating' in the uterus, away from the pelvis.
2 Engagement – the fetus descends into the pelvis in the OT position, as the pelvic inlet is widest in this plane.

The fetal head flexes, narrowing the diameter of the head that is traversing the birth canal. Fetal engagement is determined by the amount of fetal head palpable (measured in fifths) above the pelvic brim. Once two-fifths or less of the fetal head are palpable above the pelvic brim then the head is engaged. In the vast majority of women, the fetal head has engaged before the commencement of established labour.

3 Internal rotation – as the fetus descends further into the pelvis and towards the pelvic outlet, the shape of the pelvis changes, with the widest diameter in the anterior-posterior plane. The fetus rotates through 90 degrees to enter the OA position to accommodate the change in dimensions of the pelvis.
4 Extension – once the fetal head descends further, it is then visible as it begins to part the labia. As the head is pushed onto the maternal perineum, this causes extension of the fetal neck, which then allows for the head to deliver.
5 Birth of the fetal head by extension.
6 External rotation – the fetal shoulders, which have entered the pelvic inlet in the transverse position,

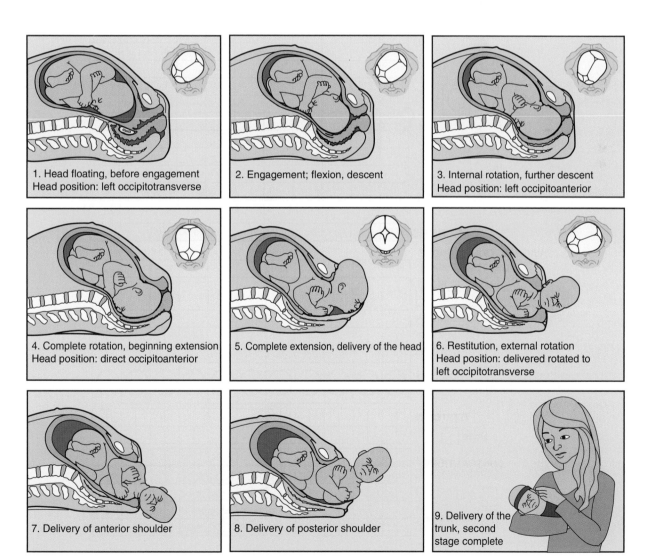

1. Head floating, before engagement
Head position: left occipitotransverse

2. Engagement; flexion, descent

3. Internal rotation, further descent
Head position: left occipitoanterior

4. Complete rotation, beginning extension
Head position: direct occipitoanterior

5. Complete extension, delivery of the head

6. Restitution, external rotation
Head position: delivered rotated to left occipitotransverse

7. Delivery of anterior shoulder

8. Delivery of posterior shoulder

9. Delivery of the trunk, second stage complete

Fig. 12.1 The Mechanism of Labour.

rotate to the anteroposterior position for passage through the pelvic outlet. As they do this, the head can be seen rotating to align with the shoulders; this is referred to as restitution.

7 Anterior shoulder delivery – with the next contraction, the anterior shoulder is delivered. A birth assistant can help guide the shoulder under the pubic symphysis by applying gentle axial traction to the fetal head.

8 Posterior shoulder delivery – the posterior shoulder should then deliver after the anterior shoulder but again may be assisted with gentle traction on the fetal head.

9 Trunk delivery – following birth of the shoulders, the rest of the body usually follows without difficulty (because of its narrower diameter).

ASSESSMENT

Clinical progression of labour is documented on a partogram (Fig. 12.2). This is an important graphical representation of how the labour is progressing, allowing early recognition of any delay in labour or any maternal or fetal complications, which can then be acted upon.

Monitoring throughout labour involves the following:
- Fetal heart rate (FHR) – in low-risk pregnancies, this is monitored with intermittent auscultation every 15 minutes in the first stage of labour and every 5 minutes after a contraction in the second stage.
- Uterine contractions – length, strength and frequency.
- Routine maternal observations – blood pressure, pulse and temperature.
- Assessment of the woman's pain.
- Vaginal loss – liquor (including colour and the presence of meconium) and blood.
- Bladder care – ensure the mother is passing urine regularly.
- Fluid balance.
- Cervical dilatation, station and position of the fetal head – usually examined every 4 hours. The fetal station is measured in centimetres in reference to the maternal ischial spines; for example, –2 is above the spines and +2 is below the spines.

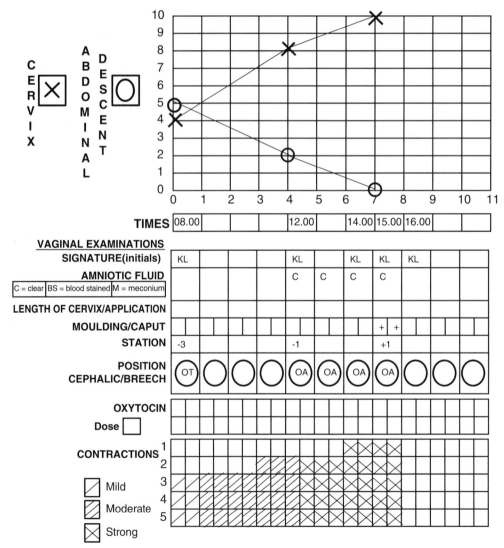

Fig. 12.2 A Partogram Demonstrating Spontaneous Labour.

If there are potential concerns, additional assessment may be needed by an obstetrician.

 Meconium

Meconium is the first faeces passed by the newborn. It is dark in colour. If it is passed *in utero*, it will change the appearance of the liquor, which is usually clear. Meconium is more likely at term and post-dates. Meconium can, however, be a sign of fetal distress, so women with thick meconium are recommended to have a cardiotocography (CTG). Meconium can be aspirated by the fetus *in utero*, which may lead to respiratory distress as it can be irritating to the fetal lungs.

DELIVERY OF THE PLACENTA

Management of the third stage of labour can be active or physiological. This decision is made after careful consideration of clinical factors and maternal choice.

Active management:
1 Routine use of uterotonic drugs such as oxytocin.
2 Controlled cord traction (gently pulling on the cord).

Physiological management:
1 No routine use of uterotonic drugs.
2 Delivery of the placenta by maternal effort.

The decision of whether to actively or physiologically manage the third stage of labour is a contentious subject; however, worldwide the biggest cause of maternal death is postpartum haemorrhage, and active management of labour may reduce this risk. Active management may also be indicated if there is failure to deliver the placenta passively. However, some women may be opposed to being actively managed, as they may feel that labour should be a natural process.

MANAGEMENT

The key aspects to managing a spontaneous vaginal birth are:
• Planning place of birth – women should be offered the choice of planning birth at home, in a midwife-led unit or in an obstetric unit. An obstetric unit will be recommended if the woman has any indication for high-risk care.
• Clinical intervention – this does not need to be offered or advised where labour is progressing normally.
• Communication – all women in labour should be in control of and involved in the decisions regarding their care.
• Support in labour – a woman in established labour should receive supportive one-to-one care.
• Pain relief – pain relief should be offered after women are informed of the implications that it may have on their labour.

DELAY DURING BIRTH

Delay during a vaginal birth can occur at any stage. At the first stage, the cervix may not be dilating at the expected rate of at least 0.5 cm/h. An obstetrician will be asked to review the woman. Delay can be treated in the first stage with an oxytocin infusion to increase the frequency and strength of contractions. If this is unsuccessful, birth by caesarean will be required.

In the second stage, delay is diagnosed if the fetal cephalic station (descent) is not progressing.
• Primiparous labour – 2 hours of active second stage of labour before delay of this stage can be diagnosed and an obstetrician called.
• Multiparous labour – 1 hour before obstetric review.

Management options for the obstetrician to consider at this point are oxytocin infusion, assisted vaginal birth or caesarean.

An additional sign of possible delayed labour or obstruction is caput and moulding of the fetal head. Caput (or caput succedaneum) is swelling of the fetal scalp caused by the pressure during labour. The presence of significant caput is a sign that labour may be delayed. Moulding is overlapping of the fetal skull bones; some degree of moulding during labour is normal but excessive amounts suggest obstruction.

The degree of moulding can be classified in four stages, in increasing severity of pathology:
1 The bones are separated normally.
2 The bones are touching each other.
3 The bones are overlapping but can be easily separated using the examiner's hands.
4 The bones are overlapping and cannot be separated by digital pressure.

❓ QUESTIONS

Alice is a 31-year-old multiparous lady; she is gravidity four, parity two. She is 38⁺⁴ weeks gestation, and she thinks that her labour started a few hours ago, so she presents to the obstetric ward at her local hospital. She is planning on having a vaginal birth and is relatively calm, as she had delivered her two previous children vaginally as well. There have been no complications during her current pregnancy.

Q1 Answer true or false: How is progress in the first stage of labour measured?
  A Descent of the fetal head.
  B Pain scales.
  C Cervical dilatation.
  D Fetal heart rate.
  E Rate of contractions.

Q2 What is the definition for established labour?
  A Regular contractions and cervical dilatation of 3 cm or more.
  B When the fetal head descends below the ischial spines.
  C When the mother feels the urge to push.

D Regular, painful contractions and cervical dilatation of 4 cm or more.

E Regular, painful contractions and cervical dilatation of 5 cm or more.

Q3 What can be given to 'actively manage' the third stage of labour?

A Oestrogen.

B Vitamin K.

C Progesterone.

D Nitric oxide.

E Oxytocics.

A Anterior rotation.	G Internal rotation.
B Effacement.	H Occipitoanterior.
C Engagement.	I Occipitoposterior.
D Extension.	J Occipitotransverse.
E External rotation.	K Posterior rotation.
F Flexion.	L Restitution.

Select the most appropriate option from the above list that corresponds to the following statements. Each answer can be used once, more than once or not at all.

Q4 What is the term for the fetal head descending into the maternal pelvis?

Q5 What action of the fetal head is caused by the contracting uterus above to ensure that the minimum head diameter is presented for delivery?

Q6 What movement of the fetal neck enables the fetal head to be delivered completely?

Q7 What is the name of the action describing the fetal head realigning with the shoulders?

Q8 What change in the cervix is required to enable birth of the fetus vaginally?

[Answers on page 394.]

MONITORING THE FETUS

The main modalities for monitoring the fetus in the antenatal and intrapartum periods are:
1 Fetal movements.
2 Pinard stethoscope.
3 Handheld Doppler fetal monitoring.
4 Ultrasound imaging.
5 Cardiotocography (CTG).
6 Fetal blood sampling (FBS).

MATERNAL PERCEPTION OF FETAL MOVEMENTS

For most of the time in pregnancy, women are not with a healthcare provider. Assessment of fetal well-being is carried out by women themselves monitoring their fetal movements. Fetal movements can be felt by the mother from approximately 20 weeks' gestation. The intensity of movements usually increases until about 32 weeks' gestation and then plateaus. The frequency of movements should remain the same throughout the pregnancy. Women are advised that if the movement frequency decreases, they should contact a healthcare provider so further assessments of fetal well-being can be established. Decreased movements can be a sign of growth restriction and acute fetal compromise which, if identified with further investigation, can be appropriately managed. Unfortunately, in some cases, decreased fetal movements can be the first sign of an intrauterine death.

PINARD STETHOSCOPE

A Pinard stethoscope is a horn-like instrument used to auscultate the FHR. It is a hollow object about 8 inches long and works by amplifying sound. The examiner listens through the narrow end of the instrument whilst the wide end is placed against the pregnant abdomen, at approximately the level of the fetal anterior shoulder. It is non-invasive and, therefore, a very safe device which can be used throughout the antenatal and intrapartum periods.

DOPPLER FETAL MONITORING

Doppler fetal monitors may be used to augment or replace the use of the Pinard stethoscope. These are simple handheld devices that use ultrasound technology to measure the FHR. Their use normally requires a lubricating jelly interface between the probe and the skin. Similarly, these devices are non-invasive and very safe to use. Either the Pinard or Doppler can be used for monitoring fetal well-being in the labour of low-risk women.

ULTRASOUND IMAGING

Ultrasound imaging requires training to perform, and the machines are expensive. Ultrasound assessments are recommended in every pregnancy in the UK to calculate the due date (dating scan), and at around 20 weeks, when an anomaly scan is performed. This scan also confirms placental location. In pregnancies at high risk of growth restriction, ultrasound is used in the third trimester to monitor fetal growth. Amniotic volume and umbilical artery Doppler images can also be assessed; abnormal images may indicate fetal compromise.

Ultrasound scanning can be performed to confirm fetal presentation, and when other modalities have failed to find a fetal heartbeat, ultrasound is the gold standard modality to assess for intrauterine death.

CARDIOTOCOGRAPHY

CTG records the FHR and its temporal relationship to the maternal uterine contractions. It is used in the antenatal period where there is an increased risk of adverse neonatal outcomes – for example, to assess fetal well-being in a woman presenting with decreased fetal movements.

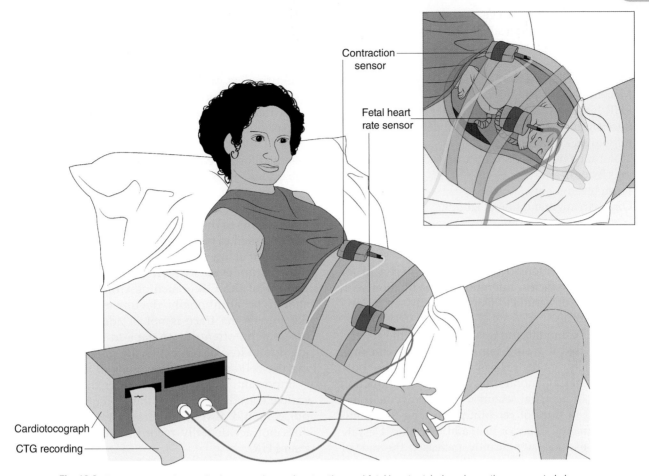

Contraction sensor

Fetal heart rate sensor

Cardiotocograph

CTG recording

Fig. 12.3 Cardiotocography monitoring transducers (contraction and fetal heart rate) placed over the pregnant abdomen.

In high-risk pregnancies, CTG is the fetal monitoring modality of choice during labour, as fetal condition can be monitored continuously.

The CTG trace is recorded using two transducers placed over the pregnant abdomen. A pressure transducer (tocometer) overlies the uterine fundus, where contractions are initiated. The other, a Doppler ultrasound transducer, is placed on the abdomen over the approximate site of the fetal anterior shoulder to ascertain the FHR (Fig. 12.3). This transducer works in exactly the same way as the handheld Doppler fetal monitoring device, but it can be left monitoring the FHR continuously.

Alternatively, if the cervix is favourable, a much smaller Doppler transducer, known as a fetal scalp electrode, may be placed on the fetal scalp. This is particularly useful if abdominal monitoring is difficult due to fetal positioning or maternal obesity. Uterine contractions and the FHR are then recorded on the same paper trace, known as a cardiotocograph, and these traces are reviewed regularly by the midwife or obstetrician.

INDICATIONS FOR CARDIOTOCOGRAPHY IN THE ANTENATAL PERIOD

CTG may be employed in the antenatal period to assess the fetal well-being in complicated and high-risk pregnancies. The frequency of CTG recording will depend on the clinician and local guidance, gestational age and the level of risk associated with the pregnancy. Computerised analysis of CTGs is now available and advised to support human analysis of the CTG. At present, no computer algorithm has been designed which can assist in CTG analysis in labour.

INDICATIONS FOR CONTINUOUS CARDIOTOCOGRAPHY MONITORING IN LABOUR

Fetal Antenatal Risks
- Breech presentation.
- Multiple pregnancy.
- Prematurity.
- Fetal intrauterine growth restriction.
- Ultrasound findings suggesting compromised placental function, such as oligohydramnios or abnormal umbilical artery Dopplers.

Maternal Antenatal Risk Factors
- Previous caesarean.
- Pre-eclampsia.
- Pregnancy more than 42 weeks' gestation.
- Premature rupture of membranes more than 24 hours.
- Induction of labour.
- Diabetes including GDM.

- Antepartum haemorrhage.
- Other maternal medical illness which may affect fetal well-being.

Intrapartum Risk Factors
- Meconium-stained liquor.
- FHR less than 100 bpm or more than 160 bpm, or decelerations after a contraction, detected by intermittent auscultation.
- Maternal pyrexia of 38°C once or 37.5°C twice, readings 2 hours apart.
- Fresh bleeding in labour.
- Oxytocin augmentation of labour.

DISADVANTAGES OF CARDIOTOCOGRAPHY MONITORING

In the UK, CTG monitoring in labour is reserved for high-risk pregnancies. Intermittent auscultation with either Pinard or handheld Doppler is advised in low-risk pregnancies.

When CTG monitoring was introduced, the general belief was that it would improve neonatal outcome. Unfortunately, evidence has shown that the only improvement CTG monitoring has made is a reduction in the rate of neonatal seizures. No improvement has been noted in rates of cerebral palsy, long-term neurodevelopmental delay or neonatal mortality. Despite this, CTG use has significantly increased the rate of obstetric interventions, including assisted vaginal birth and caesarean section.

A major functional limitation of CTG is the significant interindividual variation among healthcare professionals in the interpretation of abnormal traces. To improve this, some centres now attach electrodes to the fetal head during labour to monitor the ST segment of the fetal electrocardiogram (ECG) waveform. This is used as an adjunct to CTG and is aimed at better guiding birth decisions, but more research is needed before this is considered for use more widely.

CARDIOTOCOGRAPHY INTERPRETATION

For the fetus, labour is stressful. For example, the uterine contractions interrupt the placental blood flow. A healthy fetus will cope with these interruptions, while conversely, a fetus which is compromised will be less able to cope. The CTG shows changes in the FHR that indicate signs of the fetus becoming acidotic in labour. The purpose of monitoring is to identify when this occurs, and either alter the situation to improve the condition of the fetus, or where that is not possible, to deliver the fetus before it suffers long-term injury from hypoxia or dies.

Interpreting a CTG is complex. Only with experience can healthcare professionals become proficient at assessing fetal well-being in labour.

The mnemonic 'DR C BRaVADO' is a simple way to perform a systematic assessment of a CTG trace. This is described below (Table 12.1). Refer to Figs. 12.4 to 12.10 for example CTG traces.

OVERALL ASSESSMENT OF A CARDIOTOCOGRAPHY

The overall assessment of the CTG trace requires the classification of the FHR pattern as 'reassuring', 'non-reassuring' or 'abnormal' (also termed normal, suspicious and pathological). The four indices of baseline heart rate, variability, decelerations and accelerations are specifically considered in order to define the CTG trace (Table 12.2). The overall CTG classification is essential for the early recognition of fetal distress and subsequent emergency management.

Women who are undergoing continuous CTG monitoring must have hourly, systematic overall assessments of the trace. Any healthcare professional who is asked to provide an opinion on the trace must document it on the CTG and medical notes. Any intrapartum events which may affect or explain the pattern of the CTG, such as siting of an epidural, should be additionally documented on the trace. Sometimes the trace is not of adequate quality for assessment, often due to gaps in the FHR monitoring due to loss of contact of the transducers. Checking the contacts and connections of the transducers is important. In addition, consider the use of a fetal scalp electrode to improve the CTG quality. Maternal pulse should also be monitored to ensure the CTG does not accidentally record maternal pulse rather than FHR.

- Normal – a FHR trace in which all features are classified as reassuring.
- Suspicious – a FHR trace with one feature classified as non-reassuring and the remaining features classified as reassuring.
- Abnormal – a FHR trace with two or more features classified as non-reassuring or at least one classified as abnormal.

MANAGING THE CARDIOTOCOGRAPHY IN LABOUR

Normal – continue care.
- Suspicious – assess for and treat any cause of fetal distress.
- Maternal position – lying supine can cause aortocaval compression by the gravid uterus, reducing maternal cardiac output. Changing to left lateral position relieves this.
- Dehydration – give intravenous (IV) fluids to improve maternal cardiac output.
- Low blood pressure – common after an epidural is sited. Give IV fluids to improve maternal cardiac output.
- Hyperstimulation – if contraction frequency is greater than 5 in 10 minutes and synthetic oxytocin is being used, the infusion rate should be reduced or stopped. If required, medication such as the β-agonist terbutaline can be given to further reduce contraction frequency.
- Infection – investigate for the cause. Treat with IV antibiotics and IV fluids.

Table 12.1   Interpreting Cardiotocography Traces

DR: Define Risk	High or low risk – are there any risk factors present?
C: Contractions per 10 min	The number, length, strength and frequency should be monitored over 10-min periods. • Four to five contractions in 10 min are normal. • More than five contractions in 10 min indicate hyperstimulation of the uterus. The more contractions there are, the less time the fetus has to recover between contractions, so it is more likely to become compromised.
BRa: Baseline Rate	The average fetal heart rate (FHR) over a 10-min period. • Normal FHR is 110–160 bpm.
V: Variability	This is the variation of the FHR from one beat to another. This can be seen as small deviations in the baseline rate, which can be assessed looking at the width of the baseline rate over 30 seconds to 1 minute intervals. • Normal variability is more than 5 bpm.
A: Accelerations	These are transient episodes of increased FHR of at least 15 bpm for at least 15 seconds. • This cardiotocography (CTG) feature is reassuring and predictive of a fetus that is not suffering from hypoxia. • Accelerations must be present on an antenatal CTG to regard it as normal, but they can be absent on a normal CTG in labour.

D: Decelerations	These are transient episodes of decreased FHR of at least 15 bpm for at least 15 seconds. These may be classified into different patterns:
	• Early decelerations – short-lasting decelerations occurring with the contractions, recovering quickly. These are associated with fetal head compression and are a normal feature in labour. They have a similar appearance to typical variables, but always occur at the same time in relation to contractions.
	• Variable – intermittent periodic slowing of the FHR, with rapid onset and a variable recovery phase back to the baseline rate.
	  • These classically vary in length, depth and timing compared to the uterine contractions, occurring from the start, middle or after contractions.
	  • Most decelerations seen in labour are classified as variable.
	  • Variable decelerations are classified based on their duration and depth of drop in heart rate during the deceleration.
	  • Variable decelerations without concerning characteristics (previously called typical variables)
	    • They last for less than 60 seconds, and variability is maintained throughout the deceleration.
	    • Usually have 'shoulders' – these are seen as a brief rise in FHR prior to and after a deceleration.
	    • These types of decelerations are a normal physiological response to transient acute hypoxia from cord compression during a contraction reflecting a well-oxygenated fetus and are not a cause for concern in isolation.
	  • Variable decelerations with one or more concerning characteristics (previously called atypical variables)
	    • Concerning features include the following: lasts longer than 60 seconds, a loss of shoulders, slow return to baseline FHR following contraction, prolonged secondary rise in baseline rate, biphasic (W shaped) deceleration, loss of variability during deceleration and continuation of a baseline rate at a lower rate post contraction.
	    • If these decelerations occur for a prolonged period, they may indicate fetal hypoxia.
	• Late decelerations
	  • Uniform, repetitive and periodic slowing of the FHR. Begin during the middle or end of a contraction and recover after the contraction is completed.
	  • These are the most likely features of a CTG to be associated with fetal hypoxia.
	• Prolonged decelerations are decreases in FHR which last at least 90 seconds.
	  • They become pathological if they last more than 3 minutes.
	  • This is a worrying sign – if they persist despite attempts to improve the fetal condition, birth should be expedited.

O: Overall assessment	• Reassuring. • Non-reassuring. • Abnormal.

• Rapid progress – vaginal examination as sudden head descent or the head pressing on the perineum can cause temporary changes to CTG.

Abnormal (Table 12.3) – significant risk of fetal compromise.
• Assess and treat any cause as in non-reassuring.

• If cervix is fully dilated and the fetus is easily deliverable, then consider an assisted vaginal birth.
• If not immediately deliverable, consider on vaginal examination using a finger to rub the fetal head. This 'fetal scalp stimulation' causes an acceleration on the CTG and a normalising of the CTG in a non-compromised fetus. If the CTG does not improve on

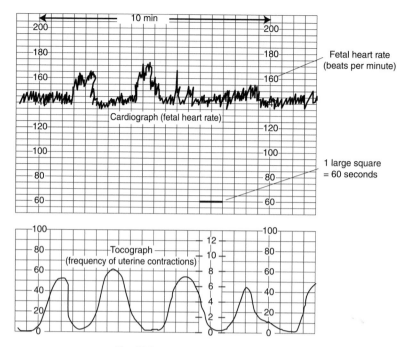

Fig. 12.4 Reassuring Cardiotocography.

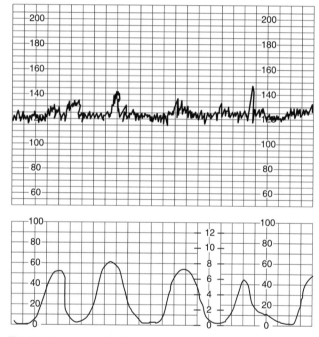

Fig. 12.5 Reassuring Cardiotocography – normal baseline rate (120 bpm), normal variability (5 bpm), accelerations present and no decelerations.

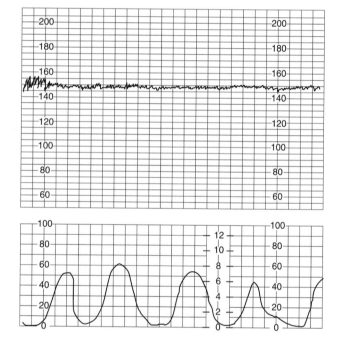

Fig. 12.6 Cardiotocography Showing Reduced Variability.

fetal scalp stimulation or after treating suspected underlying causes, then there are two courses of action depending on the local hospital policy. These are either:

- Deliver by the quickest available method (assisted vaginal birth or caesarean).
- Undertake FBS to assess fetal acidaemia. If the result is normal, continue with the labour. If the result is not obtainable or abnormal, then deliver by the quickest available method.

Uncommon Cardiotocography Abnormalities

Increased variability, also known as saltatory pattern, on CTG is thought to be a finding in rapidly evolving hypoxia. The pathophysiology is not fully understood but is thought to be due to sympathetic overdrive in the fetus in response to rapidly dropping oxygen levels where the variability is markedly increased greater than 25 bpm for more than 25 minutes.

Sinusoidal pattern resembles a sine wave (an oscillating pattern that is smooth and regular); it is rare but is associated with severe fetal anaemia or hypoxia.

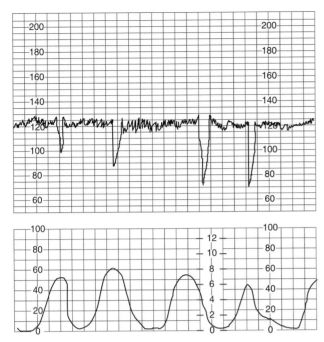

Fig. 12.7 Cardiotocography Showing Variable Decelerations Without Concerning Characteristics. Features seen here include decelerations lasting less than 60 seconds, and the presence of shouldering.

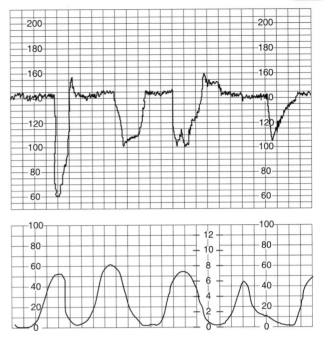

Fig. 12.9 Cardiotocography Showing Variable Decelerations with Concerning Characteristics. Features seen here include decelerations lasting longer than 60 seconds, loss of variability within decelerations, loss of shouldering, and biphasic 'W' shape.

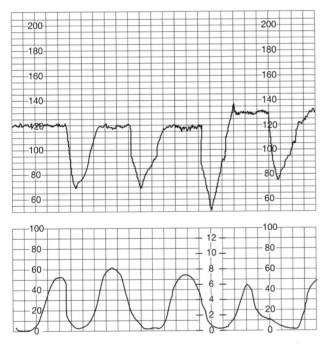

Fig. 12.8 Cardiotocography Showing Late Decelerations – trough of each deceleration is after the peak of each contraction, usually uniform in nature.

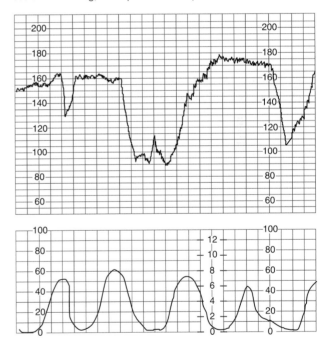

Fig. 12.10 Cardiotocography Showing Prolonged Deceleration.

FETAL BLOOD SAMPLING

The use of FBS in the UK has declined in recent years with advancement in the interpretation of CTGs, negating the need for additional testing to decide on timing of birth. There is also concern that performing an FBS will, in some cases, delay the birth of a compromised fetus to obtain the FBS, resulting in a worse neonatal outcome than if birth had been expedited instead.

In units where FBS is still used, the rationale is that in some cases an abnormal CTG pattern does not always represent a compromised fetus, so an FBS can help assess whether or not it is safe to continue the labour or proceed to urgent delivery.

Provided there is sufficient cervical dilatation (more than 3 to 4 cm), an obstetrician can view the fetal head using an amnioscope. Subsequently, a small scratch made on the fetal head can provide a sample of a few drops of blood. The blood is rapidly analysed for pH and base excess measurements. In some units, lactate is also being

Table 12.2 Reassuring, Non-Reassuring and Abnormal Features on a Cardiotocography

FEATURE	BASELINE RATE (bpm)	VARIABILITY (bpm)	DECELERATIONS	ACCELERATIONS
Reassuring	110–160	5–25	None or early Variable decelerations without concerning characteristics (last less than 1 minute, variability is maintained within the deceleration, heart rate returns to baseline, shouldering usually present) with over 50% of contractions occurring for less than 90 minutes.	Present
Non-reassuring	161–180 100–109	<5 for 30–50 minutes or >25 for 15–25 minutes	Variable decelerations without concerning characteristics with over 50% of contractions occurring for more than 90 minutes. Single prolonged deceleration for up to 3 minutes.	
Abnormal	<100 >180 Sinusoidal pattern for ≥10 minutes	<5 for over 50 minutes or >25 for more than 25 minutes	Variable decelerations with concerning characteristics (one or more of: last longer than 1 minute, loss of shouldering, loss of variability within the deceleration, failure to return to baseline, biphasic) with more than 50% of contractions for more than 30 minutes despite changing maternal position and treating any other immediate cause of cardiotocography deterioration. Late decelerations with more than 50% of contractions for more than 30 minutes. Single prolonged deceleration for more than 3 minutes.	Antenatally, the absence of accelerations is abnormal. Intrapartum lack of accelerations is of no significance.

Table 12.3 Common Cardiotocography Abnormalities and Their Interpretation

CARDIOTOCOGRAPHY ABNORMALITY	POTENTIAL CAUSES
Fetal tachycardia (more than 160 bpm)	Prematurity, fetal hypoxia, fetal anaemia, maternal anaemia, maternal fever, hyperthyroidism, drugs including tocolytic terbutaline and chorioamnionitis.
Bradycardia (less than 100 bpm)	Pregnancy more than 42 weeks, congenital heart abnormalities, cord prolapse and compression resulting in fetal hypoxia, fetal acidosis, epidural and spinal anaesthesia, maternal seizures and rapid descent of the fetus.
Reduced baseline variability (less than 5 bpm)	Variability may be less during periods of fetal sleep; normally last less than 45 minutes. Prolonged, reduced variability is concerning and may suggest fetal hypoxia, particularly if there are other abnormalities detected on the trace. Prematurity, drugs such as opiates, magnesium sulphate (used in pre-eclampsia) and benzodiazepines can also reduce the baseline variability.
Variable decelerations without concerning characteristics	Typical variable decelerations occur due to compression of the fetal head and umbilical cord during contractions, which increases vagal tone and thus causes a significant drop in fetal heart rate.
Variable decelerations with concerning characteristics	These may indicate fetal hypoxaemia and are associated with an increased risk of umbilical artery acidosis and low Apgar scores at 5 minutes.
Late decelerations	Persistent late decelerations indicate fetal hypoxia and acidosis, secondary to uteroplacental blood flow insufficiency. The presence of repeated late decelerations is associated with poor neonatal outcomes, increased risk of cerebral palsy and reduced Apgar scores following birth.
Uterine hypercontractility	Uterine hypercontractility compromises uteroplacental blood flow and thus fetal oxygenation. Hypercontractility in the presence of oxytocin augmentation can produce abnormal fetal heart rate patterns. Hence, if more than five contractions are taking place every 10 minutes, oxytocin infusion should be slowed or stopped. Uterine relaxation should allow the cardiotocography trace to return to normal in the absence of another cause. If oxytocin is not in use or altering the infusion rate has not been effective and uterine hypercontractility is causing fetal distress, the benefits of a tocolytic which causes uterine relaxation, such as the beta-2 adrenergic agonist terbutaline should be considered.

Table 12.4 Fetal Blood Sampling Results

CLASSIFICATION OF FBS RESULT	pH	LACTATE (mmol/L)	ACTION
Reassuring	≥7.25	≤4.1	Continue labour. Repeat FBS in 1 hour if CTG remains abnormal.
Borderline	7.21–7.24	4.2–4.8	Continue labour. Repeat FBS in 30 minutes if CTG remains abnormal.
Abnormal	≤7.20	≥4.9	Urgent birth of the fetus is indicated, as significant fetal acidosis present.

CTG, Cardiotocography; *FBS*, fetal blood sampling.

measured either along with or instead of pH (Table 12.4). The results are considered in the context of the clinical features of the woman and baby, the progress of labour and any previous scalp blood pH measurements.

Contraindications to FBS include:
- Maternal infection – for example, human immunodeficiency virus (HIV), hepatitis and herpes simplex virus.
- Fetal bleeding disorders – for example, haemophilia.
- Breech position.
- Prematurity – gestation less than 34 weeks.

FBS is additionally not advised in cases of suspected sepsis, as a normal FBS result in this situation cannot reliably confirm fetal well-being.

FETAL BRADYCARDIA

A sustained fetal bradycardia (over 3 minutes) is an emergency requiring immediate obstetric review to prevent significant fetal hypoxia.
- Abdominal and vaginal exam to assess for cause of bradycardia.
- Maternal position should be changed.
- Rapid IV fluid may be given to correct an acute hypotension.
- If the heart rate does not recover, birth should be achieved within 10 to 12 minutes.
- If the heart rate does recover, an FBS may be undertaken prior to considering continuing with labour.

You can consider a 'rule of three' for severe fetal bradycardia:
- Three minutes – call for help, including theatre team and anaesthetist.
- Six minutes – move to theatre.
- Nine minutes – prepare for birth (assisted vaginal birth or caesarean).
- Ten to 12 minutes – aim to deliver the baby.

❓ QUESTIONS

Jenny is a 34-year-old nulliparous lady, who is currently at 39 weeks' gestation. She and her partner arrived at the labour ward following a spontaneous onset of labour and rupture of membranes. She is now experiencing a delay in the first stage of labour. An oxytocin infusion is started and CTG monitoring is commenced. When reviewing the CTG an hour later, the midwife notes:
- Five to six contractions every 10 minutes for 30 minutes.
- Baseline heart rate: 114 bpm.
- Absent accelerations.
- Baseline variability: 10 bpm.
- Late decelerations with majority of contractions for 30 minutes.

Q1 You have been asked to review the CTG. What is the most appropriate management?
A Call for obstetrician review immediately and continue oxytocin.
B Call for obstetrician review immediately, and stop oxytocin.
C Administer terbutaline: a tocolytic drug to stop contractions.
D Continue current management with a 'watch and wait' approach with careful assessment of CTG.
E Call obstetrician with preparation for an urgent assisted vaginal birth or caesarean section.

Q2 What are late decelerations?
A Episodes of decreased FHR for 30 seconds, of at least 20 bpm from baseline heart rate, which occur in the middle of the contraction and return to baseline at the end of the contraction. If all other features are reassuring, they do not reflect fetal compromise.
B A baseline FHR of less than 100 bpm in the second stage of labour, which may be due to cord compression or prolapse.
C Episodes of decreased FHR for 15 seconds, of at least 15 bpm from baseline heart rate, which appear to have little relationship to the contraction pattern, reflecting umbilical cord compression.
D Episodes of decreased FHR for 15 seconds, of at least 15 bpm from baseline heart rate, which occur during the middle of the contraction's peak and end after the termination of the contraction. It is associated with poor neonatal outcome.
E Episodes of increased FHR for 15 seconds, of at least 15 bpm from baseline heart rate, which occur during the contraction's peak and end following the contraction. These are pathological and are associated with increased risk of cerebral palsy.

Q3 At what time point does a bradycardia become abnormal by NICE classification?
A 30 seconds.
B 1 minute.
C 2 minutes.
D 3 minutes.
E 5 minutes.

[Answers on page 396.]

INDUCTION AND AUGMENTATION

INDUCTION OF LABOUR

Induction of labour is the artificial initiation of labour. It is offered when the risk of continuing the pregnancy is higher than the risk of delivering for either the mother or the fetus (Table 12.5). Induction is most commonly performed for post-term women. However, many inductions occur at preterm gestations, where the risk of continuing the pregnancy is greater to the mother or baby than the risks of preterm labour for the baby. Examples of this include severe pre-eclampsia and intrauterine growth restriction.

Augmentation of labour is the speeding up of labour that is already established (either spontaneously or after induction). This is conventionally done using an infusion of synthetic oxytocin and may be carried out if the labour is not progressing.

Augmentation of Labour

The WHO advises that augmentation is indicated where there is a cervical dilatation of less than 0.5–1 cm/h during the active phase of the first stage of labour (where the cervix dilates from 4 to 10 cm).

Women should be counselled carefully before being induced, with treatment and care based on the woman's individual needs and preferences. The risks of continuing the pregnancy and the risks of induction should be discussed so the patient can make an informed decision. As an example, post-term gestation is one of the commonest reasons that induction is offered. The risks of continuing the pregnancy (beyond 42 weeks) include:

- Fetal compromise and potential admission to the neonatal intensive care unit.
- Placental insufficiency.
- Stillbirth and neonatal death.
- Increased likelihood of caesarean birth.

Table 12.5   Potential Indications for Inducing Labour

INDICATIONS	EXPLANATION
Post-term gestation	The risk of placental insufficiency and stillbirth doubles after 42 weeks' gestation. To avoid this risk, induction is offered to deliver the baby prior to this date.
Diabetes	If the mother has diabetes, the fetus is at increased risk of stillbirth and neonatal hypoglycaemia, with this risk increasing significantly as gestation extends beyond term. Induction may be indicated at around 38 weeks if the mother has poor glycaemic control or there is evidence of macrosomia.
Maternal age	Maternal age over 40 is associated with an increased risk of stillbirth after 40 weeks gestation. Induction may be offered by 40 weeks to reduce the risk of stillbirth.
Reduced fetal movements	This can be a sign of placental insufficiency, which if left unmanaged can lead to fetal compromise and intrauterine death. Induction is offered to prevent stillbirth.
Multiple gestations	Pregnancies carrying more than one fetus are usually induced by 38 weeks. This is due to the higher rate of stillbirth if gestation is allowed to continue.
Rupture of membranes	To prevent ascending infection causing fetal and/or maternal sepsis. The risks of infection need to be balanced against the risks of prematurity. In early preterm rupture (before 34 weeks gestation), the risk of prematurity is greater than the risk of infection, so pregnancy may be continued for several weeks prior to induction. In pregnancies with ruptured membranes beyond 37 weeks' gestation, the risk of prematurity complications is minimal. Therefore, if labour does not occur spontaneously within 24 hours, induction is offered to minimise the risk of ascending infection.
Hypertensive disorders	Induction would be considered in women after 37 weeks of pregnancy with uncontrolled hypertension. This is chiefly due to the risks associated with development of pre-eclampsia and subsequent eclampsia. Worsening pre-eclampsia may be an indication for induction prior to 37 weeks if there is a risk of maternal or fetal compromise.
Pre-existing medical conditions	Induction from 37 weeks gestation is offered in a number of other medical conditions which may increase the risk of stillbirth at term. These include systemic lupus erythematosus and antiphospholipid syndrome. Induction may be offered for medical conditions which have worsened as a result of pregnancy, where birth may improve the maternal condition. These include poorly controlled epilepsy, renal disease and heart failure.
Antepartum haemorrhage	Induction is usually offered for term pregnancies in the presence of a small antepartum haemorrhage due to the risk of developing a large haemorrhage if the pregnancy were continued, which could compromise mother and fetus. Induction at earlier gestations may be considered with a large haemorrhage. However, in a life-threatening situation, the quickest delivery would be a caesarean not induction.

However, induction also has risks, including:

- Uterine hyperstimulation and fetal distress.
- Increased analgesia requirements.
- Failed induction.
- Longer hospital stay.
- Choice of place of birth limited, usually to the obstetric-led delivery suite.

The risks of continuing the pregnancy will vary depending on the indication for induction. The risks of induction are broadly similar for all inductions. However, the earlier in gestation that the induction occurs, the higher the risk of failed induction and increased risk of requiring a caesarean section.

Earlier birth also increases the risk of neonatal complications associated with prematurity. Before 34 weeks, these risks are significant, so severe risks to mother or baby have to be present to consider birth prior to this gestation. Conversely, after 37 weeks' gestation, the risks of prematurity are very low, so the risk of continuing the pregnancy does not have to be as significant for an obstetrician to offer birth beyond this gestation.

PRE-INDUCTION

MEMBRANE SWEEPING

- This can be performed a few days before an induction of labour as a helpful adjunct, as it may trigger spontaneous labour, thereby negating the need for induction. It is most commonly performed around 40 and 41 weeks' gestation, prior to a woman being induced for post-dates or post-term. During vaginal examination, a finger is swept around the cervix, separating the membranes of the amniotic sac from the cervix.
- This stimulates the release of prostaglandins and increases the likelihood of labour commencing within the following 48 hours.

The following are not recommended, as there is no evidence that they have any more effect than placebo in starting labour: herbal supplements, acupuncture, homoeopathy, castor oil or warm baths.

ASSESSING THE CERVIX

Before a decision is made to induce labour, it is useful to calculate a Bishop's score (Table 12.6). This is a clinical score used to assess cervical ripeness, which can be used to predict the likelihood of spontaneous labour from that point and subsequent need for induction. It is calculated using five parameters assessed via a vaginal examination. Any score above eight increases the probability that the cervix is ripe or 'favourable' and a vaginal birth is therefore more likely to be successful.

Table 12.6 Calculating a Bishop's Score

SCORE	0	1	2	3
Cervical dilatation (cm)	<1	1–2	3–4	>4
Length of cervix (cm)	>4	2–4	1–2	<1
Station (relative to ischial spines) (cm)	−3	−2	−1 or 0	+1/+2
Consistency	Firm	Average	Soft	—
Position	Posterior	Mid/anterior	—	—

FEATURES OF A BISHOP'S SCORE

- Fetal station – the relationship between the presenting part of the baby and the maternal ischial spines. The ischial spines are the narrowest part of the pelvis. If the presenting parts are above the spines, they are graded negatively; and if below, they are graded positively.
- Consistency – the texture of the cervix.
- Position – the position of the cervix relative to the vaginal walls. Anterior positions are better aligned with the uterus and therefore are associated with an increased likelihood of spontaneous birth.

Once the decision to induce labour has been made, several methods can be considered as detailed below. Analgesia should be given if requested, as induced labour tends to be more painful than spontaneous labour.

METHODS OF INDUCING LABOUR

The aim of induction of labour is to ripen the cervix so that the membranes can be ruptured (amniotomy), followed by an IV oxytocin infusion which will then cause regular uterine contractions and establish labour.

PROSTAGLANDIN E$_2$ ADMINISTRATION

- These medications are conventionally administered into the vagina. They increase cervical ripeness.
- They are used when the clinician's assessment of the woman's cervix is that rupturing the membranes would not be possible or very difficult.
- Occasionally prostaglandins can be sufficient to induce labour alone, but normally amniotomy (artificial rupture of membranes (ARM)) and oxytocin infusion are required to complete the induction of labour.
- Prostaglandins can be administered in different regimes. The most common options are either vaginal tablets inserted at 6-hourly intervals or a pessary containing a slow-release prostaglandin, which is left in the vagina for 24 hours (Fig. 12.11).
- While the prostaglandin is *in situ*, it often causes uterine tightening. If the tightening becomes painful, analgesia should be given and a CTG applied to assess the fetal condition. The main risk associated with prostaglandin use is uterine hyperstimulation,

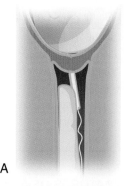
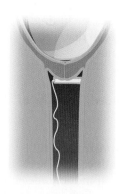

A

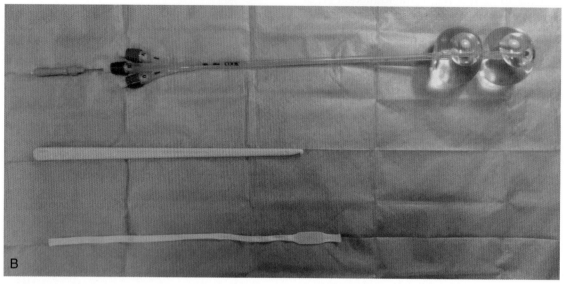

B

Fig. 12.11 A. The vaginal sustained-release prostaglandin pessary is placed behind the cervix to release prostaglandins adjacent to the cervix. B. Upper: The cervical ripening balloon is shown with both balloons filled; Middle: Amniotomy hook; Bottom: Sustained release PGE2 vaginal insert, with 25cm tail to aid removal. (Source: Layden, Elizabeth A., et al., eds. Clinical Obstetrics and Gynaecology. Elsevier Ltd, 2022.)

which refers to uterine contractions becoming excessively frequent and strong. This can cause fetal compromise (demonstrated in CTG changes), uterine rupture or placental abruption. It is treated by removing the prostaglandins and considering the use of beta agonists, most commonly terbutaline, as tocolytics to reduce the rate of contractions.

MECHANICAL INDUCTION METHODS

- Sometimes mechanical dilation with a catheter is offered.
- This involves passing a catheter through the cervix, then inflating the balloon with fluid. If the catheter falls out, the cervix has opened enough that an amniotomy can be performed.
- The catheter (often called a balloon) is licensed for a particular time period, for example, 12 hours, and when this has been reached, it is recommended to be removed.
- Where prostaglandins are contraindicated or used with caution (for example, in a patient with brittle asthma or previous caesarean birth), mechanical dilation may be used first-line for induction.

AMNIOTOMY

- Amniotomy is the ARM. It is done during a vaginal examination with a small, sharp hook on the end of a plastic stick (Fig. 12.11).
- Amniotomy can only be performed when the cervix is ripe enough (high enough Bishop's score) to allow the midwife or doctor to pass a finger and hook through the cervix to reach the membranes.
- If the Bishop's score is sufficient at first examination, then amniotomy may be performed as the initial method of induction. If the Bishop's score is low, prostaglandins or mechanical methods can be used to ripen the cervix before amniotomy is conducted.
- Amniotomy can be uncomfortable for the patient, so Entonox® or other analgesia should be available.

Once amniotomy has been performed, an IV infusion of oxytocin should be commenced. The infusion rate is gradually increased to a level where the uterus is regularly contracting around four times every 10 minutes. This should result in active labour. During the labour, continuous CTG monitoring should be performed, as there is increased risk of hyperstimulation and fetal compromise when using the oxytocin infusion.

FAILED INDUCTION

If the induction process fails, a number of options remain:

- Conservative management, watching and waiting after a stretch and sweep may be an option, but the woman and clinician would need to consider the urgency of the induction.
- If prostaglandins have been used, a repeat course of prostaglandins can be given to ripen the cervix. This is done if it is safe to do so and both the obstetrician and the woman are in agreement. However, most prostaglandins are not licensed for repeated courses, so this should be explained.
- The alternative would be to try mechanical methods. If mechanical method was the primary option used, then prostaglandins can be considered.
- Caesarean birth.

AUGMENTATION OF LABOUR

Augmentation of labour is the process of uterine stimulation to increase the duration, frequency and intensity of uterine contractions in a spontaneous labour. It is commonly used in slowly progressing labour, where contractions are assessed as insufficiently strong or where there is inappropriate coordination for cervical dilatation to occur.

If the membranes are still intact, an amniotomy should be performed. If slow progress is the only indication for augmentation, then a vaginal examination can be performed 2 hours later to assess progress. If progress remains slow, or the membranes had previously been ruptured, then labour can be augmented using an IV oxytocin infusion. The infusion rate is increased to cause four regular contractions every 10 minutes.

The aims of augmentation are to:

- Shorten the labour.
- Prevent complications associated with prolongation of labour.
- Avoid caesarean birth.

Augmentation increases the risk of fetal distress and hyperstimulation. Continuous CTG monitoring should be performed to monitor for these risks and managed quickly if they occur. Due to these risks, augmentation is associated with increased obstetric intervention, including assisted vaginal birth and caesarean.

Another complication of oxytocin is that prolonged use can cause decreased maternal urine output and fluid retention. This occurs because oxytocin is similar in structure to antidiuretic hormone (ADH), both of which are released from the posterior pituitary and act upon ADH receptors in the kidney.

Contraindications to augmentation:

- Hypertonic uterine activity – contractions more than five times in 10 minutes and/or no relaxation between contractions.
- Suspected obstructed labour – evidence includes significant caput or oedema and haematuria.
- Suspected fetal distress.
- Breech presentation.
- Intact membranes – increased risk of amniotic fluid embolus, therefore amniotomy should be performed prior to augmentation with oxytocin.

Cautions:

- Previous caesarean – increased risk of scar rupture, particularly if prostaglandins were used to induce the labour.
- Compound fetal presentation.
- Prematurity.

PROGNOSIS

Prognosis following induction or augmentation of labour is usually excellent, assuming there are no other complications associated with the pregnancy or birth. Labour can be more painful for the mother, as contractions may start more quickly and are often stronger than spontaneous contractions. The earlier the gestation induction is attempted, the less likely it is to be successful. This is because the uterus has fewer oxytocin and prostaglandin receptors at earlier gestations. Additionally, a woman who has never laboured is less likely than a multiparous woman to have a successful induction.

❓ QUESTIONS

Vanessa, a 38-year-old woman, 40 weeks pregnant, gravidity five, parity two, has arrived for a scheduled induction. Her baby is normally grown and is active. She gave birth vaginally to two sons in the last 5 years without any complications. She put on 12 kg after her second son was born and has since developed type 2 diabetes.

Q1   Which of the following are indications for induction?
   A Pre-eclampsia.
   B Breech presentation.
   C History of precipitate labour.
   D Maternal request.
   E History of previous caesarean section.

Q2   Answer true or false: Which of the following statements include accurate information that should be given to the woman before she is induced?
   A Most women will go into labour spontaneously by 42 weeks.
   B Risks associated with pregnancies prolonged beyond 42 weeks include placental insufficiency, increased forceps use and meconium aspiration.

C A membrane sweep involves surgically removing fetal tissue in the event of a stillbirth.

D Induction increases the risk of this woman needing a caesarean.

E If the woman has had a preterm rupture of membranes before 34 weeks, induction of labour should be carried out immediately.

A Caesarean birth.	**G** Forceps birth.
B Oxytocin.	**H** Misoprostol.
C Oral prostaglandins (PGE$_2$).	**I** Castor oil.
D Membrane sweep.	**J** Pessary prostaglandins (PGE$_2$).
E Amniotomy.	**K** Acupuncture.
F Expectant management.	**L** External cephalic version.

Select the most appropriate management option from the above list that corresponds to the following statements. Each answer can be used once, more than once or not at all.

Q3 A 29-year-old, 30 weeks pregnant woman (gravidity three, parity zero), presents with reduced fetal movements and a history of recurrent miscarriages. An ultrasound scan confirms fetal death.

Q4 A 32-year-old mother of three, 38 weeks pregnant, has had a healthy pregnancy until now. She has requested to be induced as she feels very tired, uncomfortably big and is fed up of being pregnant.

Q5 An 18-year-old primigravida with diabetes had a prostaglandin pessary for 24 hours and is reassessed. Her Bishop's score is now 10. What is the anticipated next step?

Q6 A 22-year-old primigravida, 41 weeks and 4 days pregnant, has a confirmed breech presentation. External cephalic version has been attempted twice but has failed on both attempts, and she is apprehensive about having a caesarean section. The midwife has already attempted digital stimulation of the cervix.

Q7 A 37-year-old woman, gravidity four, parity three, is 40 weeks pregnant. Her water broke 24 hours ago, but she has still not felt any contractions.

[Answers on page 396.]

PAIN RELIEF IN LABOUR

Birth is an emotionally intense, life-changing event, and the experience of pain during labour varies greatly. It is essential that compassionate and individualised care is provided to women, most of whom will require one or more methods to manage their pain.

To enable birth of the fetus and placenta, the uterus contracts and the cervix dilates and stretches. This results in pressure on myometrial nerve cells, causing a poorly localised, dull visceral pain. Somatic pain, characterised by sharp pain, is caused by stretching and distension of the pelvic floor, perineum and vagina. As labour progresses, both types of pain become more intense.

Pain in labour can be influenced by many physiological and psychological factors including:

- Position of the baby.
- Strength of contractions.
- The mother's expectations, emotions and psychological well-being at the time of birth.

MANAGEMENT

A variety of pharmacological and non-pharmacological methods can be used to reduce pain in labour, and many women will use a combination of techniques.

Non-pharmacological:
- Support from birth partner and healthcare professionals.
- Breathing and relaxation techniques.
- Immersion in warm water (temperature should not exceed 37.5°C).
- Transcutaneous electronic nerve stimulation (TENS), acupuncture and hypnotherapy.

Pharmacological:
- Paracetamol and/or dihydrocodeine.
- Inhalational analgesia – Entonox©.
- Intramuscular opioids – pethidine or diamorphine.
- Epidural analgesia, including combined spinal-epidural analgesia.
- Intravenous patient-controlled analgesia (PCA) – for example, remifentanil.

INHALATION ANALGESIA

Entonox© (or 'gas and air') is a 50:50 mix of nitrous oxide and oxygen. It works by antagonising N-methyl-D-aspartic acid (NMDA) receptors and has a rapid onset and offset of action, making it ideal for pain that comes and goes. Common side effects are nausea, vomiting and feeling lightheaded.

EPIDURAL ANALGESIA

Epidural analgesia is the most effective form of pain relief in labour. It is also the most invasive, requires additional monitoring and is only available in obstetric units. An anaesthetist sites a small plastic catheter in the epidural space (usually at L1–L4), through which a long-lasting local anaesthetic can be infiltrated. The local anaesthetic blocks sensory nerves to prevent transmission of pain signals from the spinal cord to the brain. The catheter remains in place during the labour, enabling repeated doses to be administered according to the patient's preference.

The epidural space is a potential space between the ligamentum flavum and the dura mater (see Fig. 12.12). A needle is inserted from the skin until the epidural space is reached, and the catheter is passed through the needle. The local anaesthetic then diffuses across the dura mater into the spinal space to exert its effect. This is unlike a 'spinal' (intrathecal) injection, where the needle is passed through the dura mater and drugs are injected into the cerebrospinal fluid in the spinal space (the same space accessed for a lumbar puncture).

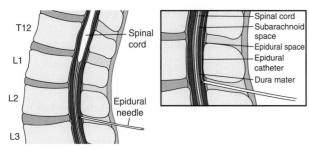

Fig. 12.12 The Anatomy Involved in Epidural Anaesthesia.

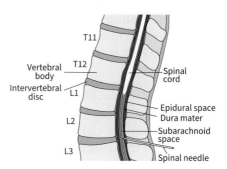

Fig. 12.13 The Anatomy Involved in Spinal Anaesthesia.

Risks:

- Ineffective pain relief – not all epidurals work perfectly and some women may require additional methods for controlling their pain.
- Transient leg weakness – the local anaesthetic can also block motor fibres causing leg weakness which wears off within a few hours of discontinuing use.
- Urinary retention – the epidural blocks sensory and motor fibres to the bladder, which can cause an inability to sense a full bladder or be able to empty it. To avoid bladder over-distension, urinary catheters are routinely sited in women with epidurals.
- Severe headache – the dural space can be accidentally punctured when inserting the needle, causing cerebrospinal fluid to leak from the spinal space. This can cause a characteristic 'low-pressure' headache, which is worse when sitting or standing and improves on lying down.
- Nerve damage – temporary nerve damage (such as a localised area of paraesthesia or leg weakness) is rare, with effects lasting longer than 6 months rarer still. Severe injuries such as paralysis are extremely rare (1/250,000 women).
- Epidural haematoma – at the site of needle insertion is the biggest cause of nerve injuries. Therefore, there are strict guidelines about performing epidurals in mothers with any form of clotting disorder, including heparin injections in pregnancy.
- Infection – epidural abscess or meningitis. Both are very rare as a fully sterile technique is used.
- Hypotension – due to sympathetic block at T4, hypotension can occur suddenly following a dose of epidural medication, with a risk of maternal and fetal circulatory collapse. Women with epidurals require regular blood pressure recordings and CTG monitoring.

REMIFENTANIL PATIENT-CONTROLLED ANALGESIA

Remifentanil is opioid analgesia that has an extremely fast onset and offset, so pain relief can be timed with contractions. It is delivered through a pump attached to an IV drip, with a button for the patient to press to self-administer a dose at the start of each contraction. It requires additional monitoring and can only be given in an obstetric unit. The amount of pain relief experienced varies greatly. Important risks include

drowsiness, respiratory depression and very rarely, respiratory arrest or life-threatening maternal bradycardia. Neonates have an increased risk of transient tachypnoea of the newborn (TTN).

COMPLEMENTARY THERAPIES

There is currently insufficient evidence to say whether hypnotherapy, aromatherapy, acupuncture, massage or TENS are more effective than placebo. However, many women find these techniques effective, especially in the earlier stages of labour, and should be supported in their individual choices.

> ### 💡 Spinal Anaesthesia
>
> Spinal anaesthesia is the injection of a local anaesthetic, usually with an opioid, directly into the spinal space (see Fig. 12.13), causing a block to the spinothalmic nerve tracts (which carry the sensations of sharp pain and temperature). It is the most common choice of anaesthesia for caesarean births. It is also commonly used for difficult assisted vaginal births, where there is a risk of being unsuccessful and then proceeding to caesarean. The risks are similar to those of epidural analgesia, although hypotension is more profound and usually requires treatment with IV medications. In advanced gestations of pregnancy, it is a safer form of anaesthesia than a general anaesthetic.

NSAIDS IN PREGNANCY AND LABOUR

Non-steroidal anti-inflammatories (NSAIDs) are contraindicated in the first and third trimester of pregnancy, as well as during labour. In the first trimester, their use can lead to miscarriage and severe defects in organogenesis. In the third trimester, they can cause premature closure of the patent ductus arteriosus and damage the fetal renal and gastrointestinal systems.

After birth, the mother can be given NSAIDs (assuming no other contraindications or cautions) as the amount passed into breastmilk is not significant.

ANTENATAL PAIN MANAGEMENT

- Paracetamol is not known to be harmful in pregnancy.
- Opioids (including dihydrocodeine and morphine) cross the placenta to the baby but are not teratogenic. Short-term use is considered safe where the mother's pain cannot be controlled with paracetamol alone. However, long-term or recurrent use increases the

risk of neonatal withdrawal. These medications should be used in the lowest doses possible for the shortest length of time.

POSTNATAL PAIN MANAGEMENT

Pain relief should always begin with simple analgesia (paracetamol +/− an NSAID), with weak and then strong opioids added in if pain is not adequately controlled. As with labour, postnatal pain varies amongst women, but most will require regular, simple analgesia for a few days after birth. Surgical procedures (such as assisted vaginal birth, caesarean or repair of perineal injuries) are associated with higher pain scores. If pain is persistent or more severe than expected, a full assessment should be undertaken to look for alternative causes of pain.

Opioids cross in small amounts into breastmilk and should usually only be used in inpatient settings where both mother and baby can be monitored for side effects. Codeine phosphate should not be given to breastfeeding mothers (or children under age 12) as it can cause life-threatening respiratory depression, but dihydrocodeine can be considered.

❓ QUESTIONS

Amy, an 18-year-old primigravida, gestation 41 weeks, has been in labour for 6 hours. She has had a uncomplicated planned pregnancy and is healthy, with a medical history of severe acne only. She initially was planning on having a birth without any pain relief but is now complaining of severe backache and has requested that she be given something soon.

Q1 Answer true or false to the following statements regarding epidural analgesia.
   A Dizziness or shivering may occur.
   B It can increase the length of the second stage of labour.
   C Epidurals are not associated with any adverse effects on the fetus.
   D It is the most effective form of pain relief in labour.
   E It is associated with transient hypotension in 20% of women.

Q2 Answer true or false to the following statements regarding epidural anatomy and analgesia.
   A The epidural space contains spinal nerve roots, the extradural venous plexus, lymphatics and fat.
   B In order to reduce the pain of uterine contractions, an epidural aims to block T10–L1 spinal levels.
   C When inserting a needle, care must be taken to avoid the epidural vessels, as the local anaesthetic can cause maternal seizures.
   D The epidural space contains cerebrospinal fluid.
   E The valves in the epidural venous plexus prevent backflow of blood.

Q3 Which form of analgesia is first line after birth, in the absence of contractions?
   A Paracetamol and ibuprofen.
   B Morphine.
   C Entonox©.
   D Codeine.
   E Nothing should be given until the mother has started skin-to-skin contact.

[Answers on page 398.]

MALPRESENTATION AND MALPOSITION OF THE FETUS

Malposition – positions of the vertex of the fetal head other than OA relative to the maternal pelvis.

Malpresentation – all presentations of a fetus other than vertex at the time of birth (Table 12.7).

The ideal presentation for birth is vertex, with the neck flexed in the OA position. This allows the fetal head to pass through the pelvic outlet with the lowest diameter of the head presenting to the pelvis and allows the fetal neck to extend as the head reaches the perineum to allow birth.

INVESTIGATIONS

The diagnosis can be made clinically during abdominal examination and vaginal examination in labour, and an ultrasound scan can be useful to confirm the diagnosis.

COMPLICATIONS

- Prolonged and obstructed labour.
- Maternal exhaustion.
- Fetal distress.
- Cord prolapse.
- Assisted vaginal birth.
- Need for an unplanned caesarean.
- Shoulder dystocia.

MANAGEMENT

MALPRESENTATION

Continuous CTG monitoring is advised during labour of any malpresentation (Fig. 12.14), along with care in an obstetric labour ward setting (Table 12.8).

MALPOSITION

The fetal skull is not spherical, it is 'rugby ball' or 'egg shaped', meaning that to fit through the space in the middle of the female pelvis, it is easier if the head presents with the smallest diameter possible.

The position of the vertex is determined by the relation of the fetal occiput (at the back of the skull) to the maternal pelvis. For example, the OA position is when the fetal occiput is near the maternal pubic symphysis, and the forehead is closer to the maternal coccyx.

	FACTORS	EXPLANATION
Fetal	Abnormal fetal shape (for example, anencephaly)	Congenital or chromosomal abnormalities may reduce fetal movement. Alternatively, large structural abnormalities may mean that the shape of the fetus is not compatible with a cephalic presentation.
	Polyhydramnios	This means excess amniotic fluid. This allows the fetus to move more, meaning that as the fetus grows it may not engage within the pelvis as it would normally. Any part of the fetus may therefore present at the time of labour.
	Multiple gestation	This may prevent the normal positioning of one or both fetuses. Multiple fetuses will likely obstruct each other's movement, increasing the risk of one or both not presenting as cephalic.
Maternal	Abnormalities of the uterus	This may include lax musculature, presence of masses or deformities such as fibroids or an abnormally shaped uterus, such as a bicornuate or unicornuate uterus. They can all prevent the fetus positioning itself physiologically.
	Abnormally shaped pelvis	This can make it difficult or impossible for the fetal head to engage.
Other	Placenta praevia	With the placenta low in the uterine cavity, it can be difficult for the fetal head to engage in the pelvis due to a physical lack of space.

Table 12.7 Risk Factors for Malpresentation or Malposition

Vaginal examination is the primary method to identify position. The most commonly identified landmark on vaginal exam is the sagittal suture. This can then be followed to the fontanelles to determine fetal position (the posterior fontanelle has three suture lines running into it, whereas the anterior fontanelle is larger and has four suture lines). Identifying the position of the fetal back on abdominal examination can aid diagnosis, as can an ultrasound scan.

The head usually enters the pelvis (pelvic inlet) in the OT position, as the pelvic inlet is widest in the transverse plane. As the head descends, the outlet of the pelvis is widest in the anterior-posterior plane, so the head rotates (most commonly into the OA position) to accommodate this. A vertex presentation, with the head flexed in an OA position is the most likely to result in a spontaneous vaginal birth.

In the OA position, most of the time the fetal head naturally flexes, creating the smallest head diameter as the presenting part. In other positions, the head is not so likely to be flexed. Fig. 12.15 shows clearly that the fetus with the deflexed vertex presentation has a significantly increased presenting diameter compared to the flexed position. This is the reason that a fetus with its head in a malposition is less likely to deliver spontaneously.

The most common malposition is the occipitoposterior (OP) position, where the fetal occiput is closest to the maternal spine (Fig. 12.16). OP position is classically associated with prolonged first and second stages of labour, with pressure and pain felt by the mother in her bottom and back. Women often get urges to push before full dilatation. On abdominal examination the fetal back may be difficult to palpate as it rotates around to the back of the uterus.

On vaginal examination, a classic sign of OP position is delay in first stage, with examination of the cervix showing that as it dilates the anterior aspect (lip) persists longer than the rest of the cervix before becoming fully dilated. These signs should alert the medical staff to the likelihood of an OP position. Positioning can be confirmed on vaginal examination by feeling for the fontanelles and suture lines. Occasionally ultrasound can be used to confirm clinical findings.

The other common malposition is OT. The longest diameter of the presenting part of the vertex is at 90 degrees to the largest diameter of the pelvic outlet, and the head is often deflexed.

Malposition of the fetal head is associated with increased pain and delayed first and second stages of labour, resulting in an increased use of uterotonics to increase frequency and strength of contractions to

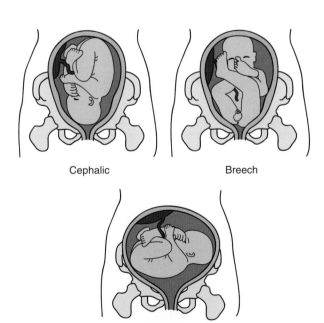

Cephalic   Breech

Transverse

Fig. 12.14 Cephalic, Breech and Transverse Presentation.

Table 12.8 Common Types of Malpresentation, and Associated Management

MALPRESENTATION	MANAGEMENT
Breech (flexed or complete)	<ul><li>To define the position of the fetus in a breech presentation, the position of the fetal sacrum is used.</li><li>External cephalic version (ECV) is often offered prior to labour in an attempt to turn the fetus to cephalic.</li><li>Vaginal breech birth is possible, although it is associated with a higher perinatal mortality. Induction of labour should not be offered.</li><li>Kneeling or footling breeches are not safely deliverable vaginally and should be delivered by caesarean.</li></ul>[See 'Breech' page 280.]
Transverse lie	<ul><li>Caesarean section is required unless spontaneous repositioning occurs. In this position, a shoulder or an arm is likely to be the presenting part and this is impossible to deliver vaginally. Cord prolapse may also occur, which can rapidly cause fetal compromise.</li></ul>
Face	<ul><li>The mentum (chin) is used to define the position in face presentations.</li><li>Vaginal birth is usually possible with an adequate pelvis size and rotation of the head to a mento-anterior position (chin to the maternal front), as the head diameter entering the pelvis is the same as a flexed vertex presentation.</li><li>Head rotation to a mento-posterior position (chin to the maternal back) requires a caesarean. This is because in this position the neck is unable to flex to allow the head to deliver.</li></ul>
Brow	<ul><li>Caesarean is usually required, as the diameter of the head entering the pelvis is large preventing successful delivery. However, it is an unstable presentation, so the neck can occasionally flex to a vertex presentation or extend to a face presentation during labour. In either case, vaginal birth would then be possible.</li></ul>

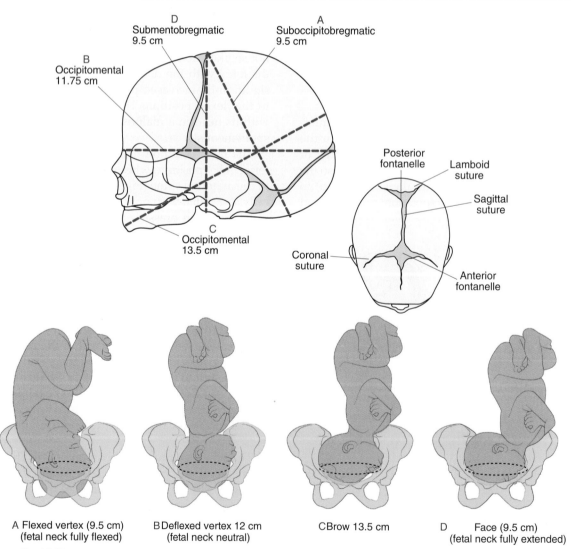

Fig. 12.15 Diagram of fetal skull anatomy and the fetus in different presentations or positions, demonstrating the different presenting diameters of the fetus to the pelvis.

Direct occipitoanterior   **Direct occipitoposterior**   **Left occipitotransverse**

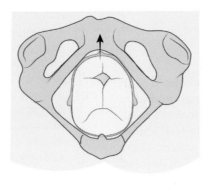
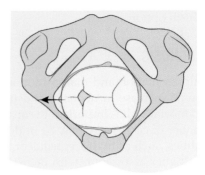

Fig. 12.16 Common Fetal Positions.

augment the labour and encourage movement into the correct OA position. If malposition persists, there is an increased risk of assisted vaginal births and caesarean. Therefore, close maternal and fetal monitoring is recommended (Table 12.9).

- If malposition is identified but there is no delay in labour, then labour can continue as normal. Many malpositions correct without intervention as labour progresses.
- If there is delay in the first stage of labour, an oxytocin infusion will be offered. This increases the frequency and strength of contractions.
  - If delay persists despite oxytocin, caesarean section will be required.
  - If the cervix fully dilates, active pushing in the second stage can commence.
- If there is a delay in the second stage, oxytocin can be commenced if not already done so. Otherwise, obstetric intervention will be required. An epidural or spinal anaesthesia is usually needed prior to

intervention for malposition, as these interventions can be painful, and if they are unsuccessful, a caesarean will be required.

Second stage obstetric interventions for malposition:
- Manual rotation – the obstetrician uses a hand to flex the fetal head and attempts to rotate the head to OA position. If successful, the mother can continue active pushing, or more often, ventouse or forceps are used to deliver.
- Ventouse – the ventouse cup is applied to the flexion point of the head (in front of the posterior fontanelle). Traction by the obstetrician during contractions aims to flex the head and cause rotation to OA position. If this occurs, birth may then occur with traction during subsequent contractions.
- Rotational forceps (Kielland forceps) – the forceps are applied, and then between contractions, the obstetrician attempts to rotate the head into the OA position. If successful, with subsequent contractions,

Table 12.9	Management Summary of Malposition	
MALPOSITION	**MANAGEMENT**	
Occipitoposterior	• Often the woman gets urges to push before fully dilated; this does not help delivery and may cause maternal exhaustion. Discouraging pushing and providing appropriate analgesia, such as an epidural, can be helpful.	
	• Maternal pushing in active second stage may rotate the head to OA position, and a spontaneous birth can occur. Sometimes women can deliver in the direct OP position.	
	• If active pushing is not successful, an obstetrician can attempt manual rotation, vacuum rotation or rotational forceps (Kielland forceps) birth. Occasionally the obstetrician can deliver with forceps in the direct OP position if rotation is unsuccessful, but there is an increased risk of obstetric anal sphincter injury.	
	• If assisted vaginal birth is not successful, a caesarean is required.	
Occipitotransverse	• Head normally enters the pelvic inlet in this position, then rotates as the head descends in the pelvis to the pelvic outlet.	
	• Maternal pushing in the active second stage usually rotates the head to OA position, and a spontaneous birth can occur.	
	• If active pushing is not successful, an obstetrician can attempt manual rotation, vacuum rotation or rotational forceps (Kielland forceps) birth.	
	• If assisted vaginal birth is not successful, a caesarean is required.	

OA, Occipitoanterior; *OP*, occipitoposterior.

the forceps can be used to put traction on the head, causing flexion and hopefully birth.

* If the above are unsuccessful, caesarean is the final birth option.

PROGNOSIS

Malpresentation and malposition are associated with a small increase in neonatal and maternal morbidity and mortality. It is important to consider that in a small number of cases there may be underlying fetal abnormalities, such as hydrocephalus or fetal goitres. There is a higher association with increased use of assisted vaginal birth or caesarean sections.

Prognosis is clearly dependent on each individual case. In experienced, competent hands, the adverse outcomes related to birth of the baby can be reduced, but these can be very difficult labours with risks to the baby which may be long term.

Regardless of the mode of birth, if there are no problems delivering the baby, the presentation and position normally have no long-term impact on either the child's or mother's health. However, vaginal breech births are associated with increased risk of labour hypoxia related to the delayed delivery of the head, which increases perinatal mortality. Choosing the mode of birth depends on various factors that are individual to each case, including the mother's wishes, parity and previous birth histories.

[See 'Breech' page 280.]

❓ QUESTIONS

Lindsay, a 29-year-old primiparous woman at term, presents to the women's assessment unit in the second stage of labour. A vaginal examination is completed, and it is suspected that the baby is OP.

Q1   Which of the following are associated with malpresentation or malposition?
   A Maternal exhaustion.
   B Cord prolapse.
   C Neonatal thyroid mass.
   D High-lying placenta.
   E Shoulder dystocia.

A Transverse lie.	**H** Physiological
B Face presentation.	presentation.
C Left sacrum-anterior.	**I** Sinciput presentation.
D Right sacrum-anterior.	**J** Brow presentation.
E Placenta praevia.	**K** Habitus.
F Oblique lie.	**L** Right occiput
G Footling presentation.	transverse.

Select the most appropriate option from the above list that corresponds to the following statements. Each answer can be used once, more than once or not at all.

Q2   A 23-year-old primigravida of 42 weeks presents with increasing contractions. The midwife who performs a vaginal examination reports a grainy feel and a transvaginal scan is performed.

Q3   A 39-year-old woman, 40 weeks pregnant, gravidity three, parity two, presents with regular contractions. Examination reveals the fetal head engaged in a left OA position.

Q4   A 20-year-old woman, gravidity one, parity zero, is rushed to hospital following complications of an attempted home birth. Ultrasound examination shows the fetal head is against the left side of the pelvis and the buttocks on the right.

Q5   A 27-year-old nulliparous woman has been experiencing contractions for several hours. The midwife examines her vaginally and thinks she finds a heel.

Q6   A 16-year-old girl, gravidity two, parity one, 36 weeks pregnant, comes for an antenatal check-up. The ultrasound scan shows the buttocks lying anteriorly close to the vagina, towards the left. The fetal heart sounds are also heard just above the umbilicus.

Q7   True or false: Which of the following complications are increased with OP deliveries?
   A Increased use of syntocinon
   B Increased risk of obstetric anal sphincter injury
   C Prolonged first and second stages of labour
   D Increased pain
   E Increased risk of shoulder dystocia

[Answers on page 400.]

BREECH

Breech presentation is when the caudal end (the bottom) of the fetus presents to the maternal pelvis. Naming depends on the position of the fetal legs (Fig. 12.17):
* Frank breech – hips flexed, knees extended (also called an extended breech).
* Complete breech – hips flexed, knees flexed (also called a flexed breech).
* Footling breech – hips extended, knees extended (feet coming first).

It is important to determine the type of breech antenatally, as this will help determine whether a vaginal birth can be safely attempted. In a frank and complete breech, the part of the fetus presenting is the bottom which, with the hips flexed, is approximately the same size as the fetal head. Full cervical dilation would have to occur to allow the bottom to deliver, with the cervix needing to remain fully dilated for the after-coming head to be born.

Conversely, in a footling breech, the feet are presenting to the cervix. At the level of the buttocks, the circumference of the fetus is now smaller because the hips are extended rather than flexed. This means the fetus could start to deliver through the cervix without it being fully dilated, and the cervical opening may not be wide enough for the after-coming head. The other

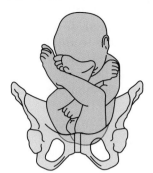
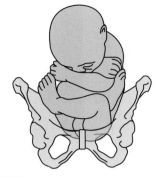
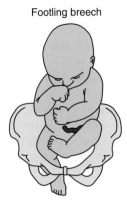

Frank breech / extended breech Complete breech / flexed breech Footling breech

Fig. 12.17 Types of Breech Presentation.

risk is that the umbilical cord can prolapse through the cervix and be compressed by the presenting part of the fetus, causing sudden fetal distress. This occurs in around 15% of footling breeches in labour (compared to 0.5% for cephalic or frank breech presentations). For these reasons, footling breech is an absolute contraindication to vaginal birth.

[See 'Cord Prolapse' page 335.]

RISK FACTORS

The incidence of breech presentation at 28 weeks' gestation is 20%, which falls to 3% at term.

In the first and second trimester, the fetus is small, with a relatively large amount of free space to move and turn in, so it often changes its lie. As the pregnancy moves closer to term, the physical space available for movement decreases. This causes the fetus to become fixed in one lie. Due to the shape of the uterus and pelvis, this is usually longitudinal with a cephalic presentation.

Risk factors for breech presentation can be divided into two groups:
1 Factors that restrict movement – preventing the fetus's head from moving into the maternal pelvis; for example, maternal anatomical abnormality, placentation, fetal anomalies, multiple pregnancies and oligohydramnios.
2 Factors that would promote too much movement – such that the fetus does not fix its lie; for example, preterm or polyhydramnios.

The most common cause for breech presentation at term is idiopathic, with no cause identified. Risk factors are covered more thoroughly in the malpresentation and malposition section of the book.

[See 'Malpresentation and Malposition of the Fetus' page 276.]

DIAGNOSIS OF BREECH

ANTENATAL

A breech presentation may be suspected on clinical examination by a midwife or primary care physician at routine antenatal assessments. Unless there is another indication for a scan, there is little reason to undertake a presentation ultrasound scan before 36 weeks, as the fetus is very likely to move into a cephalic presentation at earlier gestations.

INTRAPARTUM

• Breech presentation may be suspected during labour on:
  • Abdominal palpation.
  • Vaginal examination.
  • If fresh meconium is passed in labour.
• An intrapartum ultrasound scan would be performed if any concerns were raised about presentation.
• If breech presentation is confirmed in labour, birth can be achieved by either an unplanned caesarean, or continuing labour and attempting a vaginal breech birth.

MANAGEMENT

ANTENATAL

If identified after 36 weeks' gestation, a patient can be offered external cephalic version (ECV). This is a procedure whereby obstetricians, under ultrasound guidance, can use their hands on the mother's abdomen to push the fetus around from breech to cephalic presentation. To increase the success rate, guidelines recommend the use of a β-agonist (such as salbutamol or terbutaline) to relax the uterus beforehand. ECV is successful at turning the fetus to cephalic in 50% of cases, although 5% of these spontaneously revert back to a breech presentation after a successful ECV.

The benefit of ECV is that it preserves the opportunity for a cephalic vaginal birth, the safest option for both the mother and baby (compared to a vaginal breech birth).

ECV is offered after 36 weeks in nulliparous women and 37 weeks in parous women. ECV is offered from these gestations because spontaneous version – that is, the fetus spontaneously turning to a cephalic presentation – occurs in only 8% of term breech presentations. If an ECV is done earlier than 36 weeks, there is a high chance that a fetus which was successfully turned by ECV will revert back to breech and then the procedure would need repeating. There is no upper gestation limit for which ECV can be attempted, it is however likely to get more difficult as the fetus gets bigger. If it is felt to be appropriate, a repeat ECV can be attempted if the first effort failed; however, the later the ECV is attempted, the less likely it is to be successful.

ECV is a safe procedure, but there are important risks to discuss prior to undertaking it:

- Pain – it is a potentially painful procedure, so it is important to warn the patient about this prior to doing it and advise them that the procedure can be stopped at any time.
- Feto-maternal haemorrhage – as in any traumatic event, anti-D should be offered after ECV to women who are Rhesus negative.
- Fetal compromise – brief fetal bradycardia and suboptimal CTGs are common during and shortly after ECV, but these normally resolve. Prolonged abnormal CTG could be a sign of placental abruption, cord entanglement or uterine rupture following ECV. In this case, an emergency caesarean section should be performed to deliver the fetus. This occurs in less than 0.5% of ECVs.

Contraindications to performing an ECV:

- Where caesarean birth is required, such as placenta praevia, there is no point in undertaking ECV, as it will not affect management.
- Antepartum haemorrhage within the last 7 days – due to increased risk of causing a significant placental abruption.
- Abnormal CTG – the fetus is likely to become more compromised by the ECV.
- Major uterine anomaly – ECV unlikely to be successful.
- Ruptured membranes – ECV unlikely to be successful due to lack of free space.
- Multiple pregnancy – difficult technically and not easy to monitor both twins.
- Labour.

BIRTH DECISION

If ECV is contraindicated, declined, or fails, a decision needs to be made as to the appropriate mode of birth. The two options available are vaginal breech birth or planned caesarean (usually after 39 weeks to reduce the risk of neonatal breathing difficulties). Vaginal breech birth can be technically challenging, requiring an experienced obstetrician present for birth. The likelihood of a successful vaginal breech birth should be considered when offering the option to the patient. Factors which may contraindicate vaginal breech birth are:

- Footling breech.
- Fetal-pelvic disproportion – nulliparous women have never laboured, so their pelvic anatomy is untested. Concerns would be raised for a woman of very short stature or with an android pelvis. In multiparous women, those with previous delay in labour or shoulder dystocia would be of concern.
- Large baby (more than 3800 g) – fetal pelvic disproportion more likely.
- Growth restricted baby (less than 2000 g or smaller than the 10th centile) – greater risk of compromise during birth and more likely to deliver breech with feet and abdomen passing through a less than fully dilated cervix, resulting in difficulty delivering the after-coming head.

In the UK, 60% of women who attempt vaginal breech birth achieve a successful birth, with the remainder requiring an unplanned caesarean.

Vaginal breech birth has a higher risk of short-term perinatal morbidity (3%) compared with planned caesarean for breech birth (1.5%), but there has been no evidence of a difference in long-term morbidity. The risk of perinatal mortality is 2:1000 cases for vaginal breech birth, compared to 0.5:1000 for a breech caesarean. However, these risks need to be balanced against the increased maternal morbidity associated with caesarean. It is also important to remember that a normal cephalic vaginal birth has a risk of perinatal mortality of 1:1000.

[See 'Caesarean Section' page 286.]

All the above should be discussed with the woman so that they can make an informed decision on their choice of birth. If the woman opts for a caesarean, she needs to be aware there is a 10% chance she may spontaneously go into labour prior to her planned caesarean date, and it is important to discuss whether they would like to continue with a breech vaginal birth or have an emergency caesarean in this scenario.

In the event of a woman wishing to deliver by vaginal breech but not managing to do so spontaneously, a caesarean is required. Induction is rarely offered, as it is associated with an increased risk of birth asphyxia and poor neonatal outcome in breech presentations.

VAGINAL BREECH BIRTH

Vaginal breech birth is a high-risk obstetric event. To manage the risk:

- A senior obstetric and midwifery team skilled in breech birth should be assembled.
- An anaesthetist and obstetric theatre should be available for an emergency caesarean.
- A paediatrician should be present at birth.

- Continuous CTG monitoring throughout labour.
- Early recourse to caesarean if there is:
  - Delay in first or second stage – suggests fetal-pelvic disproportion. Augmentation of spontaneous labour with oxytocin is not recommended in breech presentation, unless contractions have decreased following the placement of an epidural anaesthetic.
  - Suspected fetal compromise

The principle behind the practical procedure of vaginal breech birth is to keep the fetal head flexed.
- Full cervical dilatation should be confirmed prior to active second-stage pushing.
- The delivering obstetrician or midwife should only touch the delivering fetus when necessary. Touching the fetus too much or pulling on the baby to expedite birth (also called breech extraction) can cause the fetus to hyperextend its head, which significantly impairs head delivery.
- The breech should be allowed to deliver without interference. Once the sacrum is delivered, it should be turned so that it is sacro-anterior (fetal back closest to the maternal pubic bone, which is towards the ceiling when the woman is in lithotomy).
- Continuing contractions and maternal pushing will allow the legs and abdomen to deliver.
- The arms may deliver spontaneously; if not, once the level of the scapula is visible, a Lovesets manoeuvre can be undertaken (Fig. 12.18):

- The fetus is held by the pelvic bone and rotated so the shoulders are in the anterior-posterior position relative to the mother's pelvis.
- The anterior arm can then be delivered by inserting a hand, taking hold of the fetal elbow, and pulling the arm gently down and across the fetal chest to deliver it.
- The fetus can then be rotated 180 degrees, and the same technique can be used to deliver the other arm. The fetus is then left in the sacro-anterior position.
- Once the nape of the neck is visible, it is then time to deliver the head. All the manoeuvres listed are intended to flex the fetal head:
  - Suprapubic pressure on the maternal abdomen.
  - Burns-Marshall manoeuvre (Fig. 12.19) – the fetus is lifted by the legs up and over the maternal symphysis. The head is guided out with the other hand, and the baby is delivered by essentially doing a backward roll onto the mother's abdomen (care must be taken not to hyperextend the fetal neck).
  - Modified Mauriceau-Smellie-Veit manoeuvre – one hand is placed above the fetal head and one finger is placed on the occiput (Fig. 12.20). The other hand is placed below the baby, either with a colleague holding the body or the body resting on the lower arm. The lower hand has a finger on each side of the mouth on the maxilla. Both

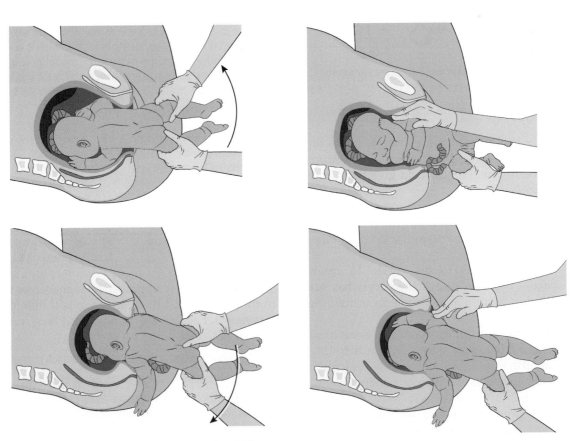

Fig. 12.18 The Lovesets Manoeuvre.

Hold feet up

Guiding the head while lifting the legs

Move the legs over the pubic bone

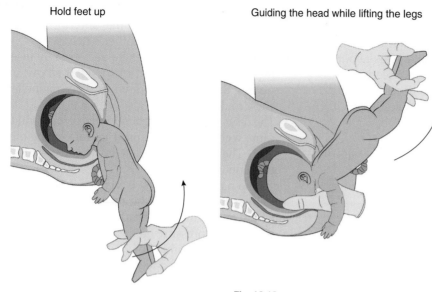
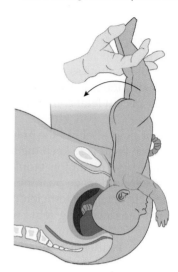

Fig. 12.19 Burns-Marshall Manoeuvre.

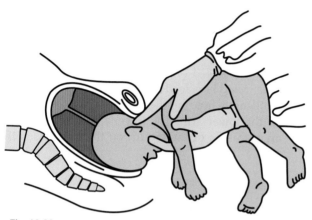

Fig. 12.20 Image of Modified Mauriceau-Smellie-Veit Manoeuvre.

hands then act to flex the fetal head, and pull to deliver.

- Forceps – it is helpful if a colleague holds the body while the forceps are applied. The forceps are pulled to flex the head and give traction to deliver the head.

If these methods fail, emergency measures can be undertaken to deliver the head, but the risk of long-term harm from hypoxia increases the longer it takes to deliver the trapped head.

- Make lateral incisions to the cervix to create more space – this is of use if the cervix has not fully dilated in an unplanned preterm or footling breech.
- Symphysiotomy – cutting open the symphysis pubis to make more space at the pelvic outlet.
- Caesarean birth – technically extremely difficult to replace the whole fetus and deliver it abdominally.

With good preparation and appropriate support, most vaginal breech deliveries occur without incident.

PROGNOSIS

Breech presentation has a higher risk of mortality and morbidity compared to a cephalic presentation. This is partly due to the confounding association of breech presentation with fetal abnormalities and due to the increased morbidity and mortality associated with vaginal breech birth and caesarean.

❓ QUESTIONS

Rachel is 37 weeks pregnant in her first pregnancy, which has been uneventful so far. At her most recent community midwife appointment, the midwife felt the fetus was breech. An ultrasound scan has confirmed the fetal presentation. Rachel and her husband are here to discuss the results of the scan.

A	External cephalic version.	**G**	No birth plan needed.
B	Internal podalic version.	**H**	Either breech vaginal birth or elective caesarean may be appropriate.
C	Planned lower segment caesarean.		
D	Unplanned lower segment caesarean.	**I**	Induction of labour.
E	Vaginal breech birth.	**J**	Fetal blood sampling.
F	Spontaneous vaginal birth.	**K**	Vaginal examination.
		L	Membrane sweep.

Select the most appropriate management option from the above list that corresponds to the following statements. Each answer can be used once, more than once or not at all.

Q1 The ultrasound scan indicates frank breech presentation.

Q2 The ultrasound indicates a cephalic presentation.

Q3 The ultrasound scan indicates frank breech presentation; the woman declines any antenatal intervention.

Q4 The ultrasound scan indicates footling breech presentation; the woman declines any antenatal intervention.

Q5 An attempt is made following ultrasound scan to rotate the fetal lie. After this is performed successfully; the fetus shows prolonged signs of distress.

Q6 What does this illustration show?

A Frank breech.

B Complete breech.

C Footling breech.

D Kneeling breech.

E Cephalic breech.

Q7 Which of the following are risk factors for breech presentation?

A Fetal chromosomal abnormality.

B Maternal BMI.

C Uterine fibroids.

D Male fetus.

E Preterm labour.

Q8 Answer true or false to the following statements regarding breech presentation.

A Breech presentation is the least common form of malpresentation preceding labour.

B For term babies with a breech presentation, there are no long-term health problems associated with either caesarean or vaginal methods of birth.

C ECV should not be attempted before 36 weeks.

D A footling or kneeling breech presentation should not be delivered vaginally.

E The presence of any other additional problems, such as placenta praevia, is an indication for a caesarean.

[Answers on page 402.]

KEY REFERENCES

SPONTANEOUS VAGINAL BIRTH

Birthplace in England Collaborative Group, 2011. Perinatal and maternal outcomes by planned place of birth for healthy women with low risk pregnancies: the Birthplace in England national prospective cohort study. BMJ. 343, 7400.

National Institute for Health and Clinical Excellence, 2014. Intrapartum Care for Healthy Women and Babies. NICE Clinical Guideline (CG 190).

World Health Organisation, 1996. Care in Normal Birth: A Practical Guide. WHO Publication 9624.

MONITORING THE FETUS

Alfirevic, Z., Devane, D., Gyte, G.M., 2006. Continuous cardiotocography (CTG) as a form of electronic fetal monitoring (EFM) for fetal assessment during labour. Cochrane Database Syst. Rev. 19 (3), CD006066.

Grivell, R.M., Alfirevic, Z., Gyte, G.M., Devane, D., 2010. Antenatal cardiotocography for fetal assessment. Cochrane Database Syst. Rev. 20 (1), CD007863.

National Institute for Health and Clinical Excellence, 2021. Antenatal Care. NICE Clinical Guideline (CG 201).

National Institute for Health and Clinical Excellence, 2014. revised 2017. Intrapartum Care: Care pf Healthy Women and Their Babies During Childbirth. NICE Clinical Guideline (CG 190).

INDUCTION AND AUGMENTATION

National Institute for Health and Clinical Excellence, 2021. Inducing Labour. NICE Clinical Guideline (CG 207).

Royal College of Obstetricians and Gynaecologists, 2020. Assisted Vaginal Birth. RCOG Green Top Guideline (GTG 26).

World Health Organisation, 2014. Recommendations for Induction of Labour. WHO Publication, Geneva.

World Health Organisation, 2014. Recommendations for Augmentation of Labour. WHO Publication, Geneva.

PAIN RELIEF IN LABOUR

Jones, L., Othman, M., Dowswell, T., Alfirevic, Z., Gates, S., Newburn, M., et al., 2012. Pain management for women in labour: an overview of systematic reviews. Cochrane Database Syst. Rev. 3 (3), CD009234.

National Institute for Health and Clinical Excellence, 2014. Intrapartum Care for Healthy Women and Babies. NICE Clinical Guideline (CG 190).

National Institute for Health and Care Excellence, 2021. Postnatal Care. NICE Clinical Guideline (NG 194).

Royal College of Obstetricians and Gynaecologists, 2020. Assisted Vaginal Birth. RCOG Green Top Guideline (GTG 26).

MALPRESENTATION AND MALPOSITION OF THE FETUS

Royal College of Obstetricians and Gynaecologists, 2012. Shoulder Dystocia. RCOG Green Top Guideline (GTG 42).

Royal College of Obstetricians and Gynaecologists, 2017. The Management of Breech Presentation. RCOG Green Top Guideline (GTG 20b).

Royal College of Obstetricians and Gynaecologists, 2018. Placenta Praevia. RCOG Green Top Guideline (GTG 27).

BREECH

Royal College of Obstetricians and Gynaecologists, 2017. External Cephalic Version (ECV) and Reducing the Incidence of Breech Presentation. RCOG Green Top Guideline (GTG 20a).

Royal College of Obstetricians and Gynaecologists, 2017. The Management of Breech Presentation. RCOG Green Top Guideline (GTG 20b).

CAESAREAN BIRTH

A caesarean birth involves delivering the baby from the uterus via an abdominal incision. Caesarean births can be classified by the level of urgency (categories 1 to 4) (Table 13.1); this aids team communication and should be documented in the woman's notes.

A category 1 birth should be performed urgently. The main reason for category 1 caesareans is suspected or confirmed fetal compromise, identified with an abnormal CTG or FBS suggesting fetal acidaemia. Other indications include a cord prolapse or a large antenatal haemorrhage. The time between decision for a category 1 caesarean and birth of the baby should be at maximum 30 minutes. These decisions to birth intervals are frequently audited.

 Indications for Rapid Caesarean Section

- Maternal cardiac arrest – after 20 weeks gestation, a perimortem caesarean should be performed immediately if there is no response to cardiopulmonary resuscitation. It should be performed within 5 minutes of arrest to relieve aortocaval compression and improve the chances of maternal survival.
- Prolonged fetal bradycardia – a fetal bradycardia lasting longer than 9 minutes requires immediate birth. An emergency buzzer alerts the team to a bradycardia after 3 minutes. Preparation for delivery and transfer to theatre is often undertaken concurrently alongside assessment and emergency management so that birth can be achieved within 12 minutes if the bradycardia has not resolved. This is often performed under general anaesthesia, as it is the quickest way to give effective analgesia to perform the procedure.

Category 2 caesarean births should be performed within 75 minutes from decision to birth. A common reason for category 2 caesarean is delay in progress in labour.

Category 3 caesareans may be performed for a variety of reasons, including intrauterine growth restriction (IUGR) or breech presentation in early labour, where delay in birth of over an hour is unlikely to affect the outcome for mother or baby. This gives time for the theatre, staff and patient to be adequately prepared for the operation.

Category 4 caesareans are performed when all patient and hospital requirements have been optimised. In most cases, this means that if a caesarean had to be delayed by 24 hours, it would have no effect on fetal or maternal health. Example indications include:

- One previous caesarean birth – increased risk of uterine rupture with vaginal birth. However, vaginal birth is not contraindicated.
- Breech pregnancy (not in labour) – if this is the mother's preference after careful counselling regarding the risks and other options have been explained, including vaginal breech birth and external cephalic version.
- Multiple pregnancy – again, this is up to maternal preference, and all options should be considered. However, in some select cases, caesarean section may reduce the risk of birth-related complications.
- Placenta praevia and/or placenta accreta – unacceptable risk of major haemorrhage with vaginal birth.
- Maternal infection with a risk of transmission to the fetus – for example, high viral load in HIV or active primary genital herpes – ensures that the fetus does not have to traverse the birth canal where the risk of infection is increased.
- Maternal request – after being counselled on the risks and benefits of all birthing options, a pregnant woman can decide that a planned caesarean is the right mode of birth for them and their baby. Depending on the circumstances, additional counselling from midwives, obstetricians, anaesthetists and mental health specialists may be considered to help support the decision-making process.

The shared decision of whether to perform a caesarean is influenced by assessment of risk and benefits, clinical factors and informed patient choice, especially for planned caesarean births. Investigations used to support decision making about caesarean birth may include clinical examination (abdominal and vaginal), ultrasound, CTG and FBS.

Table 13.1 Classification of Urgency of Caesarean Births

CATEGORY	DEFINITION	URGENCY	THE TIME FROM DECIDING A CAESAREAN IS REQUIRED TO DELIVERING BABY SHOULD BE WITHIN:
1	Immediate threat to life of mother or baby	Maternal or fetal compromise	30 minutes
2	No immediate threat to life of either mother or baby, but mother's or baby's health necessitate an expedited birth		75 minutes
3	Requires birth in the next 24 hours	No maternal or fetal compromise	24 hours
4	Birth timed to suit the hospital and mother		Not applicable

PERFORMING A CAESAREAN

PREOPERATIVE PREPARATION

- Informed and documented consent confirmed prior to the procedure. However, verbal consent is valid in an emergency situation (category 1).
- Gain intravenous access and take blood, including FBC and G&S.
- Antibiotic prophylaxis – a single dose before incision.
- Appropriate anaesthesia – this may be via an epidural, spinal or general anaesthesia.
- Bladder catheterisation.

PERFORMING A CAESAREAN SECTION

1. The table should be tilted left laterally by 15 degrees to reduce aortocaval compression and therefore minimise maternal hypotension.
2. Clean and drape the abdomen, check the catheter is draining correctly and check that the anaesthetic is adequate. Complete the WHO Surgical Safety Checklist.
3. An incision should be made cutting through the skin. This is usually a lower abdominal transverse incision 3 cm cranial to the pubic bone (sometimes a curvilinear Pfannensteil is utilised instead), but in some complex cases, a midline incision is preferred for improved access to the abdominal cavity. After the skin, the next layers opened are a layer of fat and the rectus sheath. After cutting through the sheath, the rectus muscles are parted in the midline to reveal the parietal peritoneum, which is then opened to enter the peritoneal cavity.
4. The bladder is freed and pushed down from its usual position in front of the uterus by incising the visceral peritoneum that attaches the bladder to the uterus, which is called the uterovesical fold.
5. An incision that is of an appropriate size to deliver the baby is made in the uterus. Usually this is a transverse lower segment incision, but a vertical uterine incision may be indicated, for example, because of prematurity (sometimes referred to as a classical caesarean).
6. Depending on presentation:
   a. If cephalic, the surgeon's hand is placed under the head, and then the head should be encouraged through the incision followed by firm fundal pressure by the assistant. This may feel strange for the mother. Forceps are sometimes applied to the fetal head to aid delivery where access is limited.
   b. If the baby is breech, then fingers should be placed on the baby's anterior superior iliac spine when the hips are flexed to deliver the baby bottom first. Grasping anywhere else on the trunk risks damage to internal organs. Feet can also be delivered first in footling breech presentations.
   c. If in a transverse position, a foot should be identified and used to turn the baby and deliver it breech.
7. The umbilical cord is clamped and cut. If the baby appears well at birth, this is delayed by 1 to 2 minutes to optimise baby's circulating volume.
8. After birth, syntocinon should be given intravenously to stimulate uterine contractions and encourage placental separation.
9. The placenta should then be delivered by controlled cord traction, and it should be checked that the placenta has been removed whole. The uterine cavity is then checked to ensure it is empty. Blood samples are often taken from the umbilical cord to assess fetal acidosis at birth.
10. The incision is closed with one or two layers of sutures to the uterus, one layer to the rectus sheath and one layer to the skin. Ideally, dissolvable subcuticular stitches are used for the skin incision. However, some clinicians advocate using nonabsorbable interrupted sutures in patients with risk factors for poor wound healing, for example, diabetes or obesity, in an attempt to reduce wound infection and breakdown, but evidence for this is limited.

Impacted Fetal Head

Impacted fetal head (IFH) is diagnosed at caesarean when the fetal head cannot be easily removed from the pelvis, requiring the operator to undertake additional manoeuvres to deliver the baby. The standard technique at a caesarean section is for the obstetrician to pass their hand between the maternal bony pelvis and the fetal head, slide their hand under the head and then lift the head out of the pelvis while flexing the neck to deliver the head through the abdominal incision. IFH is usually diagnosed when the operator cannot pass their hand under the head or struggles to elevate the head to allow birth. This is an emergency situation because once the uterus is open, the blood supply to the fetus is reduced. Experiencing further delay to birth of an already compromised fetus means a higher risk of hypoxic brain injury.

IFH is most common at full dilatation and especially after a failed assisted birth (where an operator may have already pulled the head deeper into the pelvis to attempt vaginal birth), but it can happen at any stage of labour. Other risk factors are low fetal station if labour has been augmented with oxytocin and if features of obstructed labour, such as caput and moulding, are present. Fetal malposition and cephalopelvic disproportion may also increase the risk of impaction.

Complications for the mother include uterine incision extensions, postpartum haemorrhage and damage to surrounding structures, such as the bladder and ureters. Complications for the baby include bony fractures, hypoxic brain injury and, rarely, death.

Management options include:

- Abdominal disimpaction – the operator using their hand to flex and lift baby's head upwards into the maternal abdomen to deliver the head.
- Vaginal disimpaction – an assistant introducing a hand into the vagina to move the baby's head up into the abdomen.
- Reverse breech extraction – the operator introduces their hand into the upper aspect of the uterus, grasps the baby's feet and delivers the baby breech first and then the head. This may need an additional incision in the upper segment of the uterus for the operator to reach the feet.

 World Health Organisation (WHO) Surgical Safety Checklist

Undertaking any surgical operation is a complex process, with each theatre member responsible for executing a myriad of critical and interlinked steps in order to achieve a shared goal. Given the complexity of this system, and in the context of a pressured environment, complications and adverse events can occur, causing avoidable patient morbidity and mortality. The WHO has designed the Surgical Safety Checklist, aimed at improving safety and communication by ensuring key information is shared openly amongst the whole team. By improving teamwork and reducing errors, this simple checklist is proven to reduce surgical morbidity and save lives. It is used in operating theatres across the world.

COMPLICATIONS

The risks (Table 13.2) vary considerably with the health status of the woman and the category of caesarean section performed. The magnitude of these risks varies from case to case and is influenced by a woman's health status, obstetric history, the absence or presence of labour and the category of caesarean birth performed. It is important that a woman is informed if her likelihood of specific risks are higher than those of the baseline population.

[See 'Vaginal birth after caesarean' on page 289.]

Although many of the incidence rates of these risks are low, it is still important that they are outlined to any woman considering a caesarean birth to allow informed decision making. It should be stressed that vaginal birth is also associated with some complications and that these need to be weighed up with the patient, considering her preferences and risk profile before a decision is made.

POSTOPERATIVE MANAGEMENT

- Women should be observed on a one-to-one basis, with monitoring of basic observations, pain, any further bleeding and sedation.
- Pain should be managed using the analgesic ladder, starting with paracetamol and increasing up to opioids as necessary with adjunct therapies where there are no contraindications. NSAIDs, which are contraindicated in pregnancy, can be safely used postnatally and when breastfeeding. Codeine phosphate should not be given to women who are breastfeeding due to the risk of neonatal respiratory depression. Alternative opioids, such as dihydrocodeine or morphine, can be used.
- The catheter should be removed once the woman is mobile.
- Appropriate thromboprophylaxis, such as compression stockings and low-molecular-weight heparin, should be utilised after individualised risk assessment.
- Following significant blood loss, anaemia should be identified and appropriately treated.
- Appropriate discharge from hospital is usually at 24 to 48 hours, depending on the mother recovering well.
- Wound care should include removing the dressing after 24 hours, monitoring for fever and assessing the wound for signs of infection.
- After any caesarean birth, it is good practice to debrief the mother about the procedure and postoperative considerations and to answer any questions. A discussion should be had regarding whether VBAC is an option for a subsequent pregnancy.
- Discussions about contraception should also take place. It is possible for a woman to become pregnant again as soon as 6 weeks following childbirth.

Table 13.2 Risks Following a Caesarean Birth

CAESAREAN BIRTH RISKS		
COMMON OPERATIVE RISKS	**RARE OPERATIVE RISKS**	**ANAESTHETIC RISKS**
• Bleeding • Infection • Pain • Extended hospitalisation • Mild anaesthetic complications risks	• Blood transfusion • Retained placental tissue • VTE • ITU admission • Incidental surgical injuries, for example, injury to bowel, bladder and ureters • Emergency hysterectomy • Amniotic fluid embolus • Maternal death	• Hypotension • Headache • Nerve damage • Insufficient or excessive regional anaesthesia • Local anaesthesia toxicity
LONG-TERM RISKS	**FUTURE PREGNANCY RISKS**	**RISKS TO THE NEWBORN**
• Intraabdominal adhesion formation • Poor birth experience • Chronic pain • Incisional hernia • Reduced fertility	• Repeat caesarean section or VBAC • Uterine rupture • Abnormal placentation – praevia or abnormally invasive placenta • Stillbirth • Hysterectomy	• Respiratory difficulties at birth • Laceration as surgeon opens the uterus • Asthma • Neonatal death

ITU, Intensive treatment unit; *VBAC*, vaginal birth after caesarean; *VTE*, venous thromboembolism.

• After an emergency caesarean, it is important for the mother to be debriefed regarding the events of labour leading up to birth as often, events happen very quickly while in labour, which can lead to the woman having many unanswered questions and a feeling of loss of control. Traumatic birth experiences are more common in these cases and can have long-lasting effects.

PROGNOSIS

Maternal morbidity is higher for emergency caesarean birth than elective operative birth; however, the majority of caesarean births have a good outcome for both the mother and baby.

❓ QUESTIONS

Martha is a 34-year-old primiparous woman; she is 30 weeks pregnant and has asked her midwife about elective caesarean sections, as she is very nervous about childbirth due to her sister's bad experience.

Q1 Which of the following are true regarding the use of a transverse lower segment uterine incision in comparison to a midline, vertical uterine incision?
A It is associated with less postoperative pain.
B It is associated with improved cosmetic effect.
C It is associated with less blood loss.
D There is a reduced risk of postoperative infection.
E There is a reduced risk of uterine rupture in future pregnancies.

Q2 Answer true or false: Which of the following anatomical structures is dissected during a caesarean?
A Cervix.
B Uterovesical fold.

C Rectus sheath.
D Omentum.
E Rectus abdominus.

Q3 Which of the following has an increased risk of occurring following caesarean compared to vaginal birth?
A Difficulties breastfeeding.
B Depression.
C Dyspareunia.
D Urinary tract injury.
E Faecal incontinence.

[Answers on page 404.]

VAGINAL BIRTH AFTER CAESAREAN

VBAC refers to any woman who has had a previous caesarean birth who plans to deliver vaginally. In a VBAC, a woman aims to give birth vaginally, either spontaneously or assisted with instruments. However, if there are concerns about the woman or baby or following maternal request, an emergency caesarean may be required.

For much of the 20th century, most people believed that a woman who had previously undergone a caesarean birth would require an elective caesarean for future pregnancies. From studies done after 1960, we learned that this 'once a caesarean, always caesarean' rule need not apply. Women who have previously undergone caesarean birth can attempt a trial of labour for the purpose of a vaginal birth in subsequent pregnancies if there are no other contraindications with minimal risks.

Most women who have had either one or two caesarean births can be considered for VBAC. If, however, they have had three or more low transverse caesareans or a single high vertical classical caesarean section, they should not be considered for VBAC because there is a significantly increased risk of uterine rupture during labour.

Overall, VBAC is successful in 70%–75% of patients. It is more likely to be successful in patients who:

- Have had previous successful vaginal birth (this is the strongest predictor).
- Labour spontaneously, rather than need induced labour.
- Have a BMI of less than 30 kg/m^2.
- Have an estimated fetal weight of less than 4 kg.

BENEFITS OF A SUCCESSFUL VBAC COMPARED TO ELECTIVE CAESAREAN

- Shorter length of hospital stay and postpartum recovery.
- Fewer neonatal breathing problems.
- Significantly increased chance of successful VBAC in future pregnancies.
- Reduced risk of caesarean-related sequelae, such as placenta praevia, in future pregnancies.

RISKS OF ATTEMPTING VBAC COMPARED TO ELECTIVE CAESAREAN BIRTH

- All of the risks associated with a vaginal birth, for example, pain, assisted vaginal birth or perineal injury.
- A 20–25% risk of requiring an emergency caesarean. Compared to an planned caesarean, there is an increased risk of postpartum haemorrhage, blood transfusion, infection, VTE, internal organ injury, hysterectomy and intensive care admission.
- Increased fetal risks:
  - A 2 to 3 in 10,000 additional risk of birth-related perinatal death.
  - An 8 in 10,000 risk of the infant developing hypoxic ischaemic encephalopathy (HIE). This risk is higher than during a planned caesarean birth, but is very similar to the risk during labour in a primiparous woman.

The main reason for heightened risks is the possibility of uterine scar rupture, which occurs in approximately 0.5%–1% of attempted VBACs. After a caesarean, the scar on the uterus is weaker than the rest of the uterine tissue. When the uterus contracts in labour, a large amount of force is applied to it, which can cause the old scar to pull apart. If this occurs, the fetal blood supply is often disrupted, and the mother bleeds internally. Should this occur, rapid caesarean birth under general anaesthesia and repair of the uterus are required to save the life of mother and baby.

MANAGEMENT

- Antenatally, women and their care providers should have a full discussion regarding the benefits and risks of VBAC and elective caesarean.
  - If planned caesarean is chosen, women need to also be aware they may go into labour before the planned delivery date. They would then need to decide whether to continue with the labour and attempt VBAC, or have an emergency caesarean in this situation.
  - If VBAC is decided upon, a plan for labour should be made.
- VBAC should be conducted in an obstetric unit with resources for immediate caesarean along with advanced neonatal resuscitation.
- There should be continuous maternal and fetal monitoring throughout the labour, including regular maternal observations and continuous CTG monitoring.
- Particular attention should be made to signs of scar rupture and a lowered threshold for unplanned caesarean. Signs include:
  - Maternal tachycardia and hypotension, suggestive of internal bleeding.
  - Antepartum haemorrhage.
  - Scar pain and scar tenderness.
  - Evidence of fetal distress on CTG monitoring.
  - A sudden change in the position of the presenting part.

INDUCTION OF LABOUR

If an induction of labour is required, mechanical methods for induction should be used, as prostaglandins significantly increase the risk of uterine rupture. Once an amniotomy is performed, the majority of women will then require an oxytocin infusion to generate contractions. Oxytocin infusion doubles the risk of scar rupture compared to a woman labouring spontaneously. The mother should be aware of these increased risks and be aware of the alternative option of a caesarean.

PROGNOSIS

Successful VBAC occurs in approximately 75% of attempted cases, with the remaining women requiring a repeat caesarean. The risk of fetal death is extremely low with both VBAC and elective repeat caesarean birth, but the likelihood of fetal death is slightly higher with VBAC than with planned repeat caesarean birth. Maternal death is very rare with either type of birth.

❓ QUESTIONS

Amna is a 32-year-old woman, gravidity two, parity one. She is currently 20^{+6} weeks pregnant. She had planned to have a vaginal birth for her last child. However, after an episode of severe fetal distress, she was rushed for an emergency caesarean section. In this current pregnancy, Amna wants to have a VBAC but is unsure what the risks are. She is otherwise medically fit, and this pregnancy has had no complications.

Q1   Which of the following is the most important concern with a VBAC?
   A Uterine rupture.
   B Uterine dehiscence.
   C Uterine infection.
   D Thromboembolism.
   E Transfusion requirements.

Q2 Answer true or false. Which of the following are contraindications to VBAC?

A One uncomplicated low transverse caesarean section.

B Two uncomplicated low transverse caesarean sections.

C Three uncomplicated low transverse caesarean sections.

D One previous high vertical classical caesarean section.

E Two previous high vertical classical caesarean sections.

Q3 Answer true or false. Which of the following can be used without additional caution during VBAC compared to a spontaneous vaginal birth?

A Prostaglandins.

B Oxytocin.

C Epidural anaesthesia.

D Spinal anaesthesia.

E Continuous electronic fetal monitoring.

[Answers on page 406.]

ASSISTED VAGINAL BIRTH

Assisted vaginal birth refers to the procedure of speeding up the second stage of labour, using instruments to deliver the baby. There are two types of instruments commonly used, forceps and vacuum extractors. An instrument is applied to the fetal head, and then, during a contraction, an obstetrician applies traction while the mother pushes, causing flexion of the fetal head and descent of the head through the birth canal, with the ultimate aim to deliver the fetal head. Forceps are a metal clasping instrument which are applied around the fetal head. A vacuum extractor (ventouse) is an instrument with a small cup which is attached to the fetal head by suction created by using a negative pressure vacuum.

INDICATIONS FOR AN ASSISTED VAGINAL BIRTH

An assisted birth is primarily performed to shorten the second stage of labour and deliver the baby. There are risk factors that increase the likelihood of requiring an assisted vaginal birth. (Table 13.3). Indications for assisted vaginal birth can be divided into maternal and fetal reasons:

MATERNAL

- Fatigue or exhaustion – if the labouring woman can no longer generate effective pushing with contractions, the fetus will not be born without assistance.
- Inadequate progress in the second stage of labour.
- After 2 hours of active pushing in a nulliparous women or 1 hour in a multiparous woman, assisted

Table 13.3 Risk Factors for Requiring an Assisted Vaginal Birth

	RISK FACTOR	EXPLANATION
Maternal	Use of epidural anaesthesia	• Epidurals reduce the sensation of the contractions and the ability of the mother to push effectively during the second stage of labour. After a prolonged second stage, both maternal exhaustion and fetal distress can occur, requiring assistance to achieve birth. The impact of epidurals is however highly debated.
	BMI of more than 30 kg/m²	• Difficulty obtaining the optimum maternal position to generate effective expulsive contractions and the presence of adipose tissue in the myometrium. • Obesity is associated with many other comorbidities in pregnancy such as intrauterine growth restriction, diabetes and pre-eclampsia, all of which can cause fetal distress, requiring birth to be expedited. • Difficulties in safely monitoring the fetus through excess maternal tissue can lead to concerns regarding fetal well-being, leading to expedited birth.
	Primigravida	• Maternal tissues are less compliant and, therefore, more likely to have slow progress in the second stage and then require assisted birth. • Approximately 23% of primigravidas have an assisted vaginal birth compared to less than 5% of multiparous vaginal births.
Fetal	Macrosomia	• Slow progress through the birth canal. • True cephalopelvic disproportion may present as delayed second stage, but when assisted birth is attempted, this fails, necessitating a caesarean.
	Multiple gestation	• Increased risk of maternal exhaustion and abnormal presentation and position with multiple gestations (especially after the first baby has been delivered). • Increased rate of fetal complications leading to fetal distress.
	Occipitoposterior position and other malpositions	• Malposition and lack of flexion of the fetal neck causes a larger diameter of the fetal head presenting to the maternal pelvic outlet, making it harder for the mother to spontaneously give birth with pushing. • Instruments can be used to turn the fetal head to the OA position, where the fetal head can flex and lower the diameter of the presenting part, increasing the likelihood of a successful delivery. These are called rotational assisted births.

BMI, Body mass index; *OA*, occipitoanterior.

vaginal birth should be considered, as maternal exhaustion and fetal distress are likely to occur and spontaneous birth is unlikely.

- Rarely, medical conditions can be exacerbated by prolonged pushing (secondary to Valsalva manoeuvre) which can then endanger the woman. In these women, the time they are advised to push for during the second stage prior to offering assisted vaginal birth is reduced. These conditions include cardiac disease, hypertensive crises, myasthenia gravis, spinal cord injury (if at risk of autonomic dysreflexia) and proliferative retinopathy.

Delay in Second Stage

UK guidance states that all women should give birth within 4 hours of the onset of the second stage (fully dilated). Prior to active pushing in primiparous women, if there are no urges to push, then women can be allowed an hour of passive second stage, allowing the fetus to descend through the birth canal. An hour of passive descent is also advised for anyone with an epidural. The premise is that by allowing the passive descent, active second-stage pushing is more likely to be successful.

FETAL

Fetal distress – birth should be expedited if there is fetal compromise either suspected (abnormal CTG) or confirmed (abnormal FBS).

DECISION FOR AN ASSISTED VAGINAL BIRTH

Where there is no maternal or fetal need to intervene, spontaneous vaginal birth should be encouraged. Where there is an indication to expedite birth, the obstetrician will need to consider whether an instrumental or caesarean should be offered.

CONDITIONS WHICH MUST BE MET FOR ASSISTED VAGINAL BIRTH TO BE CONSIDERED

- Patient consent obtained.
- Fully dilated cervix.
- Ruptured membranes.
- Cephalic presentation.
- Sufficient pain relief.
- Engaged presenting part – the greater diameter of the fetal head should have passed the pelvic brim:
  - On abdominal examination, no more than one-fifth of the fetal head should be palpable.
  - On vaginal examination, the vertex (fetal head) must be at, or lower than, the level of the ischial spines of the maternal pelvis (these are approximately 4 cm from the vaginal opening). This is also called the station of the fetal head, where the ischial spines are 0 station.

CONTRAINDICATIONS TO ASSISTED VAGINAL BIRTH

- If there is a contraindication to assisted vaginal birth, then a caesarean will be the safer birthing option.

- Any contraindication to vaginal birth, such as placenta praevia or transverse lie.
- Cervix is not fully dilated.
- Cephalopelvic disproportion.
- Known or suspected fetal conditions – assisted vaginal births can cause bleeding and trauma to the fetus, including:
  - Fetal bleeding disorders such as haemophilia.
  - Fetal predisposition to fractures.
- Inadequate analgesia.

In addition, vacuum extractors are contraindicated with:

- A face presentation.
- Maternal infection such as hepatitis and HIV– fetal trauma from a ventouse birth could increase the risk of transmission.
- Gestation earlier than 34 weeks – increased risk of neonatal cephalohaematoma, intracranial or subgaleal haemorrhage and neonatal jaundice. Before 34 weeks, forceps may be used, but only after discussion with a consultant, as the risk of trauma is still high, and a caesarean may be safer.

OTHER CONSIDERATIONS FOR ASSISTED VAGINAL BIRTH

- Location for intervention – after examining the patient, the obstetrician will determine how likely an assisted vaginal birth is to be successful.
  - Delivery in room – if the head is at least 1 cm below the ischial spines and in an OA position and appropriate pain relief can be given, then it is very likely that assisted vaginal birth will be successful and can be performed in the labour room.
  - Trial of assisted vaginal birth in theatre – if the fetal head is at, but not below, the ischial spines or the position is not OA, then there is a higher rate of unsuccessful assisted vaginal birth. The patient should be transferred to theatre and pain relief administered by the anaesthetist (epidural or spinal) so that if the assisted vaginal birth fails, a caesarean can then be performed immediately.
- Consent – consent need not be written, as this may delay timely intervention, but appropriate verbal consent should be obtained. Gaining consent can be hindered by maternal exhaustion, pain or the effect of narcotic drugs. Ideally, information should be given between contractions. Good communication skills are essential to be able to fully explain the indication for assisted vaginal birth, the risks and the alternatives so that informed consent is taken.
- A neonatologist should be informed of the decision for an assisted vaginal birth and be in attendance for birth.
- Analgesia
  - Perineal infiltration of local anaesthetic – this numbs the perineum so that episiotomy or a straightforward low cavity (below the ischial

spines) assisted vaginal birth can be carried out in the room.

- Pudendal nerve block – using a long, flexible needle, local anaesthetic is carefully injected medial to the ischial spines to block sensory fibres of the pudendal nerve, which supplies most of the sensation to the vulva and lower third of the vagina. This is often combined with perineal infiltration to optimise pain relief for assisted vaginal births in the labour room.
- Regional analgesia – some women will have an epidural in labour which can be used as analgesia for deliveries in the room. Where a trial of assisted vaginal birth in theatre is required, an extra dose of analgesic can be given through an already sited epidural to 'top it up' sufficiently for a caesarean to be performed if required. If the patient does not have an epidural, then a spinal anaesthetic can be given.

[See 'Pain relief in labour', page 274.

FORCEPS BIRTH

1. Catheterise bladder – this is done to empty the bladder to prevent a distended bladder causing obstruction or trauma.
2. Obtain good analgesic (local or regional).
3. Examine and confirm full dilation along with fetal position and station. For assisted vaginal birth, the vertex must be at or below the ischial spines.
4. Slide each blade of the forceps (Table 13.4) beside the fetal head while using your hands to guide the blade and guard the vaginal wall from trauma. When correctly sited, the handles of the forceps should lock with ease.
5. Apply gentle inline traction with each maternal contraction to help delivery.

6. An episiotomy is often required to protect from severe perineal trauma, such as an obstetric anal sphincter injury.
7. Once the head is delivered to the chin, the blades can be removed and the rest of the baby delivered as per a spontaneous birth.

VENTOUSE BIRTH

1. Catheterise bladder.
2. Obtain good analgesia (local or regional).
3. Examine and confirm full dilation along with fetal position and station. For assisted vaginal births, the vertex must be at least at the ischial spines.
4. The ventouse cup should be placed flat against the fetal head. The suction device is then activated, forming a vacuum. Cup placement is key and should be on the flexion point (3 cm anterior to the posterior fontanelle) so as to aid flexion of the fetal head.
5. Check that no part of the vaginal wall has been trapped by the cup. If so, the suction is stopped and the vaginal tissue released before restarting the vacuum.
6. Apply traction with contractions whilst holding the cup onto the head with the nondominant hand. The correct line of pull is important to prevent the cup from coming off and the head from not flexing properly.
7. Episiotomy may be needed in some cases to prevent severe perineal trauma such as obstetric anal sphincter injury.
8. Once the head is delivered to the chin, the vacuum can be released and the cup removed. The rest of the baby is then delivered as per a spontaneous birth.

The pressure of a vacuum extractor (Fig. 13.1) is set at around 0.8 kg/cm².

Table **13.4** Types of Forceps	
TYPE OF FORCEPS	**DESCRIPTION**
Neville-Barnes/Simpson/Haig Ferguson forceps	The most commonly used types of forceps. They are made with a fetal curve to fit the fetal head and a pelvic curve to follow the angle of the birth canal of the maternal pelvis. They can be used for mid-cavity and low-cavity assisted deliveries, where the fetal head is at 0 station or below. These forceps cannot be used for rotational births, so the fetal position needs to be OA. Occasionally these forceps can also be used to deliver in a direct OP position.
Wrigley forceps	Curved, short forceps used for low cavity extraction, often referred to as a 'lift out', when the maximum fetal head diameter is at +2 station or lower (around 2 cm above the vulva). These forceps are also commonly used to aid in delivery of the head during a caesarean.
Kielland forceps	Rotational forceps made with a fetal curve but with no pelvic curve, which allows the forceps to be applied to the fetal head and rotated without causing maternal trauma. Once a malpositioned fetal head has been rotated to OA, the forceps can be used in the same way as the other forceps, with traction during a contraction to deliver the head.

OA, Occipitoanterior; *OP*, occipitoposterior.

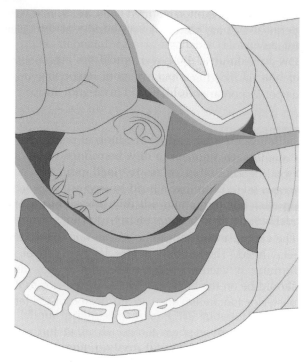

Fig. 13.1 Vacuum extractor attached to fetal head.

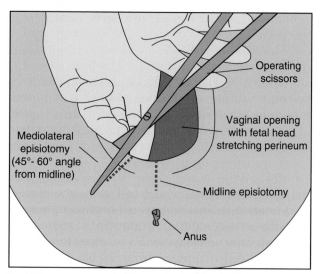

Fig. 13.2 Diagram of an episiotomy. In the UK, right mediolateral episiotomies are performed because they offer significant protection against anal sphincter injury. Midline episiotomies are easier to repair but have a higher rate of extension into the anal sphincter.

MALPOSITION

Performing an assisted vaginal birth can be more challenging when the fetal head is in an occipitoposterior (OP) or occipitotransverse (OT) position. In these positions, delivery of the fetal head is less likely and will need to be corrected first in order to minimise trauma. The obstetrician has three options:

1) Manual rotation – the obstetrician uses their hand to turn the fetal head to an OA position. This can then be managed as a routine assisted vaginal birth.
2) Rotational ventouse – correct cup placement supports rotation of the fetal position during a ventouse assisted birth.
3) Rotational forceps – Kielland forceps can be used to turn the fetus to an OA position.

 Episiotomy

This is a surgical cut made to the perineum (perineal skin and muscles) and posterior vaginal wall during childbirth in order to assist the birth of a fetus and to avoid uncontrolled tearing of tissues (Fig. 13.2). The landmark for this is the fourchette, which is the skin fold where the labia minora meet above the perineum (the frenulum labiorum pudenda).

INDICATIONS FOR AN EPISIOTOMY

- A high risk of third- or fourth-degree perineal tearing.
- Excessively rigid perineal muscles, especially if the perineum appears to be delaying birth.
- Assisted vaginal birth indicated (performed in most forceps and many ventouse births).

- In cases of female genital mutilation (referring to the partial or total removal of the external female genitalia for nonmedical reasons, which is common in some cultures). In these cases, an anterior episiotomy may be performed to cut apart the fused labia to allow delivery.

COMPLICATIONS

The most common complication of assisted vaginal births is a failure to achieve a vaginal birth. Usually, this is anticipated, and the mother is taken to theatre prior to attempting the assisted vaginal birth. If, after three pulls with the instrument, the fetal head is not descending through the birth canal and birth is not imminent, the procedure is abandoned, and the obstetrician proceeds to caesarean.

In experienced hands, the most common minor complication of an assisted vaginal birth is superficial bruising of the neonate, which, in a healthy child, will fade quickly and cause no problems. However, there are more serious complications which can occur.

MATERNAL COMPLICATIONS

- Postpartum haemorrhage with possible secondary anaemia.
- Genital tears.
- Short-term urinary incontinence if bladder or urethral injury.
- Faecal incontinence; if anal sphincters involved, these need careful repair to reduce the chance of long-term symptoms.
- Pelvic organ prolapse in the long term.

FETAL COMPLICATIONS

- Chignon (a temporary benign soft tissue swelling formed on the baby's head by the vacuum extractor).

- Neonatal intracranial (for example, subdural or cerebral) and subgaleal haemorrhage.
- Cephalohaematoma (bruising on the neonatal scalp).
- Temporary facial palsy.
- External eye trauma.
- Skull fracture.
- Seizures.
- Shoulder dystocia leading to brachial plexus injury and/or collarbone fracture.

Vacuum birth, compared to forceps birth, is more likely to result in fetal injuries such as cephalohaematomas or retinal haemorrhages. Conversely, forceps deliveries are more likely to result in maternal injuries such as perineal and vaginal trauma but have a higher rate of successful vaginal birth if used by skilled operators. Both methods have similar rates of reverting to caesarean birth.

Subgaleal bleeding is a rare and particularly feared complication. It occurs when the emissary veins rupture and haemorrhage into the subgaleal or subaponeurotic space (the potential space between the fetal scalp aponeurosis and the skull). It is fatal in up to 20% of cases. Subgaleal bleeding can occur with both vacuum and forceps births and is most likely to occur with excessive force, prolonged cup application times, multiple suction cup pop offs or after serial instrumentation (using ventouse and then switching to forceps) or vice versa.

POSTBIRTH MANAGEMENT

Following assisted vaginal birth, priority should be given to addressing any immediate problems and reducing the risk of any further complications. Care should include:

- Neonatal doctor to review the baby if there are any concerns, to assess the need for resuscitation or transfer to the neonatal unit.
- Cord blood samples should be taken. Blood should be taken from both an artery and the vein of the umbilical cord. The pH of these samples can be checked to assess for fetal hypoxia at the time of birth, which can help guide neonatal management.
- Deliver the placenta.
- A rectal examination should be performed to rule out obstetric anal sphincter injury (OASI). If such injury is identified or suspected, repair should take place in theatres under sufficient lighting, following consent and neuraxial anaesthesia.
- Address any obvious bleeding.
- Suturing if an episiotomy has been performed or other perineal tear has occurred. Proper wound care and the importance of pelvic floor exercises should be discussed once the repair is complete.
- Analgesia in the form of paracetamol and ibuprofen should be given to the mother, assuming there are no contraindications.

- Thromboprophylaxis does not need to be routinely prescribed, but each woman should be individually assessed for risks such as immobility.
- A single dose of antibiotics should be given following an assisted vaginal birth, as this has been shown to decrease likelihood of postnatal maternal infection.
- Bladder care involving a fluid volume chart for the first 24 hours to assess for urinary retention.
- Debriefing the mother and birthing partner on the events. Often, decisions on assisted vaginal birth are made very quickly in a tense situation where there is suspected fetal compromise. Going over events early can help prevent negative emotions and memories of the experience from forming. Proactive and empathetic communication may help to prevent subsequent development of psychological trauma from childbirth.
- Discussions about contraception should also take place. It is possible for a woman to become pregnant as soon as 6 weeks following childbirth.

PROGNOSIS

When performed by experienced clinicians, assisted vaginal births will, at most, inflict only minor trauma to the mother and baby while preventing long-term problems had labour not been expedited and avoiding caesarean associated morbidities. A successful assisted vaginal birth is a good predictor of a spontaneous vaginal birth in a future labour. However, in rare cases, there is potential for serious complications following assisted deliveries.

❓ QUESTIONS

Abi, a 35-year-old woman, gravidity five, parity three, gestation 38 weeks, has just gone into labour with twins. The first fetus has been successfully delivered, but the second twin is showing signs of fetal distress. Abi is becoming exhausted, and a decision is made to assist the delivery using a vacuum extractor.

Q1 Before attempting an assisted vaginal birth, which of the following conditions should be satisfied?
  A The woman should be lying supine.
  B The maternal bladder should be empty.
  C Fetus should be in the occipitoposterior position.
  D The woman should be offered appropriate analgesia.
  E Membranes should have ruptured.

Q2 Which of the following cases would be considered relative contraindications for assisted vaginal birth?
  A A 32-year-old primigravida, gestation 41 weeks, has been in the second stage of labour, pushing for over 2 hours. The crown of the fetal head is at the ischial spines on vaginal examination. She has had a healthy and low risk pregnancy up until her last antenatal ultrasound scan, which showed femoral bowing and a possible long bone fracture.

B A 29-year-old woman, gravidity three, parity zero, gestation 38 weeks, has been in the second stage of labour for nearly 2 hours without analgesia. The mother is known to have HIV; her viral load is undetectable.

C A 42-year-old woman, gravidity two, parity one, gestation 37 weeks, has been pushing in the second stage of labour for 1 hour. The electronic fetal monitor shows a trace with a baseline of 102 bpm and variability of less than 5 bpm for the past hour.

D An 18-year-old primigravida, gestation 40 weeks, has been having regular contractions for 2 hours. The mother has been diagnosed with mitral stenosis. Her cervix is 8 cm dilated.

E A 20-year-old woman, gravida three para two, gestation 41 weeks, has been in the second stage of labour for two hours and is becoming exhausted. Vaginal examination finds the fetal station is above the ischial spines. An antenatal blood test confirmed that the fetus has haemophilia.

Q3 Answer true or false to the following statements regarding assisted vaginal birth.

A Midcavity and rotational births should be exclusively managed with Kielland and Simpson forceps.

B Assisted vaginal birth should be abandoned if there is no descent after three pulls.

C An episiotomy should be performed during fetal traction.

D Forceps should be chosen in preference to ventouse.

E Higher rates of failure are associated with a maternal BMI over 30 kg/m^2.

Q4 Regarding episiotomies, which statement below is correct?

A Episiotomy is associated with a reduced incidence of postpartum haemorrhage.

B A mediolateral episiotomy should be avoided.

C If extensive vaginal tearing appears likely, an episiotomy should not be performed.

D The cuts formed from episiotomies heal better than other tears.

E Having finished suturing, a rectal examination should be performed.

[Answers on page 407.]

KEY REFERENCES

CAESAREAN BIRTH

National Institute for Health and Clinical Excellence, 2021. Caesarean section. NICE clinical guideline (NG192).

VAGINAL BIRTH AFTER CAESAREAN

Fisler, R.E., Cohen, A., Ringer, S.A., Lieberman. E. Neonatal outcome after trial of labor compared with elective repeat cesarean section. Birth. 2003;30(2):83–88.

Royal College of Obstetricians and Gynaecologists, 2015. Birth after previous caesarean birth. RCOG green top guideline (GTG 45).

ASSISTED VAGINAL BIRTH

National Institute for Health and Clinical Excellence, 2014. Intrapartum care for healthy women and babies. NICE clinical guideline (CG190).

Mazouni, C., Porcu, G., Bretelle, F., Loundou, A., Heckenroth, H. Gamerre, M., 2006. Risk factors for forceps delivery in nulliparous patients. *Acta obstetricia et gynecologica Scandinavica*, 85(3), 298–301.

Murphy, D.J., Strachan, B.K., Bahl, R., 2020. On behalf of the Royal College of Obstetricians Gynaecologists. Assisted vaginal birth. BJOG, 127, e70–e112.

Obstetric Complications

Outline

ANTEPARTUM HAEMORRHAGE

Antepartum haemorrhage (APH) is bleeding from the vagina during pregnancy after 24 weeks gestation. Before 24 weeks of gestation, bleeding during pregnancy is known as a threatened miscarriage.

AETIOLOGY

Causes of APH can be divided into uterine, cervical and vaginal causes.

UTERINE CAUSES

- Placental abruption – this occurs in approximately 1% of pregnancies when the placenta partially or completely detaches from the wall of the uterus. The area of the placenta no longer in contact with the uterus is then unable to provide oxygenation and other nutrient transfer for the fetus. The larger the abruption, the greater the risk to the fetus. It typically presents with painful bleeding and a finding of a tense 'woody' uterus on abdominal examination.
- Placenta praevia – in this condition, the placenta is attached in the lower uterine segment, often adjacent to (or covering) the cervical os. As the lower segment extends, or as the cervix dilates, bleeding can occur. This usually presents as painless bleeding, which helps differentiate it from placental abruption. If the placenta is low lying, this will be noted at the 20-week scan. Women with such finding will be advised to have a repeat scan at 32 to 36 weeks. This is because only 10% of women go on to be diagnosed with placenta praevia at more than 34 weeks gestation (approximately 0.5% of pregnancies) because the uterus grows from the lower segment; hence, the placenta effectively 'moves up' the uterus as it grows during the pregnancy.

- Vasa praevia – this occurs when one or more of the umbilical or placental fetal blood vessels is low lying in the womb and covers the cervical os. Often, these are not diagnosed until birth. They are frequently associated with placenta praevia. It is also associated with cases where the placenta has an additional component (a succenturiate lobe) attached to another area of the uterus, which are connected together by unprotected blood vessels. When the mother's cervix dilates during labour, the unprotected blood vessels can become damaged, which results in fetal haemorrhage. The fetus only has a small circulating blood volume, so even a small visible haemorrhage from vasa praevia can quickly cause fetal distress, exsanguination and death.
- Uterine rupture – there is approximately a 1% risk of uterine scar rupture for a woman in labour who has had a previous caesarean section. It can present with abdominal pain, vaginal bleeding and maternal and fetal distress from acute blood loss. Uterine rupture is extremely rare antenatally and for women who have not had uterine surgery.

[See 'Vaginal Birth after Caesarean Section' on page 289.]

CERVICAL CAUSES

- Ectropion – the columnar epithelium in the cervical canal extends out through the external os, resulting in columnar epithelium on and around the external os, which is friable compared to the squamous epithelium which usually covers the ectocervix. It is commonly seen in pregnancy and in patients taking the COCP. This condition often causes bleeding after intercourse but is very rarely treated in pregnancy, as it will likely resolve shortly after birth.
- Cervical cancer.

- Cervical polyp – small, benign tumours which grow inside the cervical canal.
- A 'show' – a plug of mucus from the cervix becomes dislodged and comes away through the genital tract, usually at the end of pregnancy, as the cervix begins to ripen prior to labour. It is common for this plug to contain a small amount of blood.

VAGINAL CAUSES

- Trauma.
- Infection.

The most important obstetric causes to be aware of are placental abruption and placenta praevia (Table 14.1).

INVESTIGATIONS AND MANAGEMENT

LARGE ANTEPARTUM HAEMORRHAGE (MORE THAN 50 mL)

- Resuscitate the patient using an ABC approach, including inserting two large bore cannulae (at which point blood can be taken) during the assessment of the circulation.

Table 14.1 Risk Factors for Placental Abruption and Placenta Praevia

PLACENTAL ABRUPTION	PLACENTA PRAEVIA
Aetiology	**Aetiology**
• The placenta becomes partially separated from the uterus lining, resulting in a haemorrhage. • This occurs because a portion of the placenta separates from its uterine attachment, resulting in a bleed into the decidua basalis of the placenta and causing a haematoma. As the haematoma enlarges, it pushes the placenta farther away from the uterine wall which can worsen the abruption. If the haematoma reaches the edge of the placenta, blood will track down and escape out of the cervix, causing a revealed haemorrhage. If the haematoma fails to reach the placenta edge, it can remain hidden between the placenta and the uterine wall. This is called a concealed abruption, as no bleeding will be seen vaginally (Fig. 14.1). • There is no correlation between how clinically shocked the mother appears and the blood loss seen vaginally, as the bleeding may be concealed within the uterus and therefore not produce visible genital tract bleeding. • In cases of large abruptions, DIC can occur due to a combination of inflammatory processes triggered by the abruption and the consumptive use of clotting factors that occur with any large haemorrhage.	• The placenta is lying in the lower segment of the uterus with partial or full coverage of the uterus opening (internal orifice of the cervix). • In an uncomplicated pregnancy, the placenta lies higher up in the uterus and does not lie in the lower segment or adjacent to (or covering) the cervical os. • Mothers with a placenta praevia need a caesarean because it is impossible for the fetus to be delivered vaginally, as the placenta blocks the cervical opening. • Haemorrhage can occur from a placenta praevia if it is disrupted, for example, during vaginal examination, intercourse, on cervical dilation or as the lower segment of the uterus forms in the third trimester. • There are four types of placenta praevia, depending on its position in the uterus. Types one and two are considered minor and type three, and four are major placenta praevia (Fig. 14.2).
Risk factors	**Risk factors**
• Placental abruption in previous pregnancy (6% reoccur in subsequent pregnancies). • Abdominal trauma (including domestic violence) • Previous caesarean. • Maternal smoking. • Recreational drug use – especially cocaine. • Pre-eclampsia. • Twin pregnancy. • Maternal thrombophilia. • External cephalic version.	• Previous placenta praevia. • Assisted reproduction. • Uterine fibroids causing abnormality in the uterine cavity. • Previous caesarean. • Twin pregnancy (due to large placental size). • Maternal smoking. • Maternal age more than 40 years.
Clinical features	**Clinical features**
• Painful bleeding from the genital tract. • Tense, 'woody', tender uterus. • Dark red blood. • Maternal shock, which may not be in keeping with volume of visible blood loss (blood loss can be concealed). • Distressed fetus, demonstrated by abnormalities on CTG. • Small abruptions may not cause any fetal or maternal compromise.	• Painless bleeding from the genital tract. • Nontender, soft uterus. • Bright red blood. • Maternal shock, in keeping with volume of blood lost. • Low-lying placenta, covering the cervix on ultrasound. • Abnormal lies and malpresentations, for example, breech, are more common. • Fetal heart rate normal, as blood loss is maternal blood not affecting fetal circulation (unless the mother is profoundly shocked, in which case fetus likely to also be distressed).

CTG, Cardiotocography; *DIC*, disseminated intravascular coagulopathy.

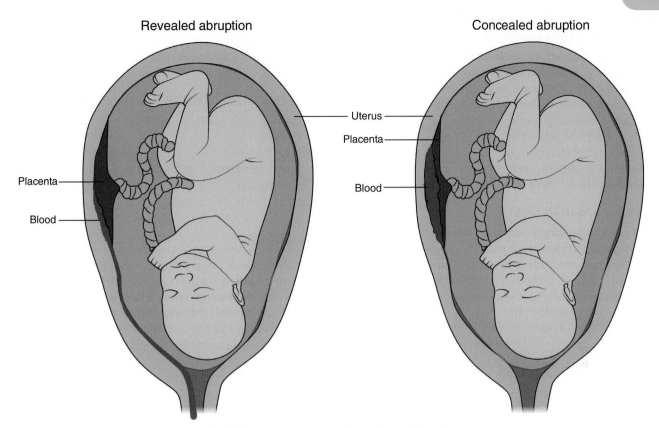

Fig. 14.1 Placental Abruption: Concealed and Revealed.

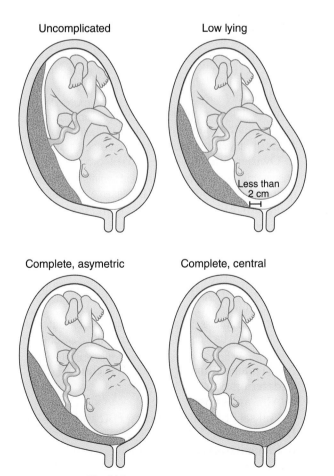

Fig. 14.2 Placenta Praevia Types.

- Regular basic observations – blood pressure, heart rate, temperature, respiratory rate to determine how unwell the woman is and if she is haemodynamically stable after the blood loss.
- CTG to monitor the fetal heart to check for fetal distress.
- Avoid digital vaginal examination until placenta praevia is ruled out, as this can precipitate heavier bleeding. Speculum examination can usually be safely performed to assess blood loss and cervical dilatation.
- Take a full set of blood, including FBC, to check the haemoglobin level, G&S to ensure the mother's blood group and rhesus status are known and a clotting screen to check her blood clotting is optimal. Crossmatch four units of blood in case a blood transfusion is required. If the blood is needed quickly, consider using O-type rhesus-negative blood.
- Kleihauer test if the mother is rhesus negative, to measure how much fetal blood has mixed with the maternal blood; this test is used to determine the amount of rhesus D IgG antibody (anti-D) to give the mother depending on the amount of blood that has mixed.
- Anti-D as prophylaxis if the mother is rhesus negative.
- Consider IM steroids if preterm birth is anticipated; this will aid the lung development of the fetus between 24 and 34 weeks gestation.
- Consider immediate birth of the baby by emergency caesarean if there is profuse haemorrhage and the mother is shocked or the fetus is distressed.

SMALL ANTEPARTUM HAEMORRHAGE (LESS THAN 50 mL, INCLUDING SPOTTING)

Frequently, women attend with a small APH without any maternal or fetal compromise. Even if the bleeding has settled, these women are admitted to the hospital and monitored for at least 24 hours, as a small APH can suddenly proceed to a large haemorrhage compromising both mother and fetus. For this reason, a cannula is still inserted and blood obtained. Steroids may also be given if the fetus is preterm, as there is an increased chance of early delivery, either spontaneous or iatrogenic.

ONGOING MANAGEMENT

- If heavy bleeding continues or there is maternal or fetal compromise, urgent delivery will be advised.
- If bleeding persists but is not causing compromise, a consultant will review to decide whether delivery or continued inpatient monitoring should be advised.
- If bleeding settles, the woman may be allowed home, with advice to return if there is further blood loss, pain or reduced fetal movements.
- If the woman has recurrent (two or more) APHs, regular growth scans and antenatal clinic follow-up may also be arranged, as even small repeat bleeds may result in intrauterine growth restriction (IUGR).
- Some women, such as those who have had a bleed due to a major placenta praevia, may be advised by the consultant to remain in the hospital until delivery even if bleeding has completely resolved due to the risk of sudden heavy bleeding. Even in uncomplicated cases of placenta praevia, delivery by caesarean birth is advised between 36 and 37 weeks.

If the gestation extends beyond 37 weeks, clinicians often have a very low threshold for offering delivery after even a small APH because there are minimal risks to the newborn in terms of prematurity, whereas continuing the pregnancy increases the chance of further heavy bleeding, which could cause fetal or maternal compromise.

If the cause of bleeding is placenta praevia, birth will need to be by caesarean. If the cause of bleeding is unknown after investigation, placental abruption should be presumed, and induction of labour is usually offered with continuous CTG monitoring in labour.

COMPLICATIONS

MATERNAL COMPLICATIONS

- Maternal anaemia.
- Blood transfusion reactions.
- Maternal shock due to hypovolaemia.
- Major haemorrhage requiring hysterectomy.
- Disseminated intravascular coagulation.
- Maternal death.
- Infection in the genital tract or uterus.
- Kidney failure due to renal tubular necrosis from hypovolaemia.
- Prolonged hospital stay and adverse psychological impact.

FETAL COMPLICATIONS

- Fetal growth restriction (FGR).
- Preterm birth.
- Fetal hypoxia due to reduced blood flow.
- Fetal anaemia, possibly requiring a blood transfusion.
- Fetal death.

PROGNOSIS

The prognosis depends on how much blood the woman has lost. Due to multiple factors, including difficulties accessing appropriate care, haemorrhage is the leading cause of maternal death worldwide. The patient is also at a higher risk of postpartum haemorrhage following an APH.

❓ QUESTIONS

Sarah, a 26-year-old, is 32 weeks pregnant. She woke up this morning with severe central abdominal pain. Her pregnancy had been previously uncomplicated. Basic observations revealed a BP of 79/60, pulse rate of 130 and respiratory rate of 22; oxygen saturations on air were 98%, and she was apyrexial. CTG showed fetal distress. Palpation of her abdomen revealed that it was tense and very painful.

Q1   What is the most likely diagnosis for this woman?
  A Placenta praevia.
  B Revealed placental abruption.
  C Concealed placental abruption.
  D Acute pyelonephritis.
  E Ovarian torsion.

Q2   Answer true or false: What signs and symptoms are classically present in an APH caused by placenta praevia?
  A Painful bleeding from the genital tract.
  B Nontender, soft uterus.
  C Bright red blood.
  D Maternal shock in keeping with the amount of blood lost.
  E CTG shows prolonged atypical decelerations of the fetal heart.

Q3   Answer true or false: Which of the following management options would be suitable for a woman with a severe APH (blood loss of more than 1 litre) at 39 weeks gestation?
  A No intervention unless there is clinical deterioration.
  B ABC assessment.
  C Full set of blood, including FBC and G&S.
  D IM steroids.
  E Immediate birth.

[Answers on page 410.]

PRE-ECLAMPSIA AND PREGNANCY-INDUCED HYPERTENSION

Pre-eclampsia is defined as new-onset hypertension and proteinuria after 20 weeks of pregnancy. Pre-eclampsia is a multisystem disorder that is potentially life-threatening to the mother and baby.

The diagnostic criteria for pre-eclampsia are (after 20 weeks of gestation):

- Systolic BP more than or equal to 140 mmHg and/or diastolic BP more than or equal to 90 mmHg.

AND EITHER

- Proteinuria, with a urine protein:creatinine ratio of more than 30 mg/mmol in a single urine sample.

OR

- Signs of end organ damage (such as rise in creatinine, rise in alanine transaminase or fall in platelet count).

Categories of Hypertension in Pregnancy

- Hypertension – systolic BP of 140 to 159 mmHg and/or diastolic BP of 90 to 109 mmHg.
- Severe hypertension – systolic BP of more than 160 mmHg and/or diastolic BP of more than 110 mmHg.

Whenever BP is checked, it is good practice to take three measurements and record the lowest reading. A diagnosis of hypertension should not be made at a single encounter. Outside of pregnancy, women are either sent home with a plan for a follow-up appointment to recheck BP or are given an ambulatory BP monitor to use at home. These can be particularly useful in people suspected to suffer from 'white coat hypertension'.

In pregnancy, due to the significant risk of hypertensive complications, there is a low threshold for close monitoring, and even hospital admission to monitor BP, after just one abnormal reading.

AETIOLOGY

Pre-eclampsia affects up to 5% of pregnancies. Overall, it is more common in a first pregnancy. If pre-eclampsia does not occur in the first pregnancy, it is less likely to occur in subsequent pregnancies. If it does occur in the first pregnancy, depending on severity, the risk of pre-eclampsia occurring in a subsequent pregnancy ranges from 15% to 50%.

MATERNAL RISK FACTORS FOR DEVELOPING PRE-ECLAMPSIA

High Risk

- Past history of pre-eclampsia or pregnancy-induced hypertension.
- Chronic hypertension.
- Chronic kidney disease.

- Autoimmune conditions, such as antiphospholipid syndrome (APS) or systemic lupus erythematosus.
- Diabetes mellitus.

Moderate Risk

- Age more than 40 years.
- Family history of pre-eclampsia.
- BMI of more than 35 kg/m².
- Nulliparity.
- Prolonged interpregnancy interval (>10 years).
- Multiple pregnancy.

Risks If New Male Partner

Paternal genetics appear to play a role in development of pre-eclampsia, but this is not fully understood. Having a different male partner from a previous pregnancy may increase the risk.

Fetal Risk Factors for Developing Pre-Eclampsia

- Unexplained FGR.
- Previous intrauterine death (IUD).
- Previous placental abruption.
- IVF pregnancy (especially if oocyte donation).
- Hydatidiform mole.

It is important to note that pre-eclampsia is a condition where smoking is not a risk factor. Nonetheless, women should be advised against smoking during pregnancy due to other considerable pregnancy-related risks associated with smoking.

PATHOPHYSIOLOGY

The exact pathophysiology of pre-eclampsia is not fully understood but is likely to involve both maternal and fetal factors. Studies have identified the placenta as having a crucial role in the pathophysiology of pre-eclampsia. Normally, the initial key stages of placental development involve adhesion to the uterine wall, after which invasion occurs where cytotrophoblast cells migrate deeper into the decidual layer (Fig. 14.3). These cytotrophoblast cells remodel the maternal spiral arteries, dilating them into a high-flow, low-resistance circulation with a high surface area. This allows a good supply of oxygen and nutrients to reach the fetus. Abnormalities in the placental vasculature development during the early stages of pregnancy have been well documented in pre-eclampsia. As a result of poor trophoblastic invasion, the blood supply to the placenta is less effective, resulting in a high-pressure system. As the fetus grows, it requires increasing amounts of nutrients to support it, but the underdeveloped placenta cannot provide the nutrient transfer required.

In an attempt to improve placental function in this situation, it is believed certain factors are released

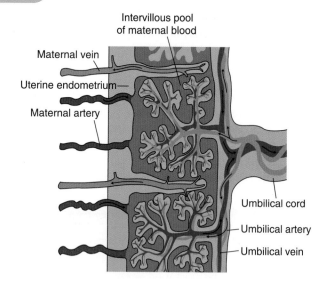

Maternal vein

Uterine endometrium—

Maternal artery

Intervillous pool of maternal blood

Umbilical cord

Umbilical artery

Umbilical vein

Fig. 14.3 Normal Placentation.

either by the fetus or placenta to act on the maternal system. These factors do this by:

- Increasing maternal BP in an attempt to increase blood flow through the placenta, thereby increasing nutrients available for transfer.
- Increasing vascular permeability in an attempt to increase nutrient transfer across the placental vascular bed.

Unfortunately, these effects occur throughout the body, rather than just at the placenta, causing multiple organ dysfunction. Almost all the symptoms and signs of pre-eclampsia can be explained by these changes.

CLINICAL FEATURES

The majority of the signs and symptoms of pre-eclampsia are secondary to hypertension and systemic endothelial dysfunction, occurring in multiple organs in the mother.

SYMPTOMS

- Headache caused by the increased intracranial pressure from the raised BP and exudative oedema.
- Visual disturbances caused by pressure of the oedema on the optic nerve. This can be seen clinically as papilloedema, with the following symptoms:
  - Blurred vision.
  - Floaters – seeing small dark spots moving slowly across the visual field.
  - Less commonly, flashing lights or scotoma.
- Upper abdominal or epigastric pain.
- Vomiting.
- Significant swelling – mild swelling of the hands and feet is common in pregnancy. However, endothelial factors are released in pre-eclampsia which increase vascular permeability throughout the body, causing significant oedema, which may include the face, which is not seen in an uncomplicated pregnancy. In severe cases, oedema can also occur in the abdomen, and in rare cases, the liver capsule can be affected, causing right upper quadrant pain.

- Rarer symptoms associated with severe disease:
  - Confusion.
  - Seizures.
  - Shortness of breath due to pulmonary oedema.

In more severe cases, the increased intracranial pressure begins to affect the routine functioning of the brain. Loss of inhibitory fibres from the brain to the spine results in increased tendon reflexes. If the pressure and oedema worsen, this can cause a decreased conscious level or lead to neuroexcitability, causing the generalised seizure of eclampsia.

SIGNS

- Abnormal bedside observations:
  - Hypertension (systolic BP more than or equal to 140 mmHg and/or diastolic BP more than or equal to 90 mmHg).
  - Proteinuria – endothelial factors disrupt normal renal function, allowing protein to pass through the glomerulus.
- Epigastric or right upper quadrant tenderness.
- Oedema, which can occur externally or internally; the latter causes shortness of breath from pulmonary oedema in severe cases.
- Hyperreflexia and clonus.
- Papilloedema.

FETAL CLINICAL FEATURES

All caused by placental insufficiency:

- Reduced fetal movements.
- Evidence of growth restriction – symphysis fundal height (SFH) measurements or ultrasound.
- IUD – no fetal movement, no heart beat auscultated. Confirmed with an ultrasound scan.

> ### 💡 Eclampsia
>
> If left untreated, pre-eclampsia will lead to eclampsia, which involves new onset of seizures or an unexplained coma. Although rare, it is an obstetric emergency that puts both maternal and fetal life at risk. Usually eclampsia is preceded by worsening pre-eclampsia symptoms and rising BP. Initial management involves an ABCDE assessment, as in any collapse or emergency. The anticonvulsant of choice in eclampsia is IV magnesium sulphate (rather than traditional anticonvulsants such as diazepam). It can also be used in women with severe pre-eclampsia to prevent seizures. Other differential diagnoses for seizures might need to be considered, such as epilepsy or electrolyte abnormality of intracranial pathology.

HELLP Syndrome

HELLP syndrome describes a combination of:
- **H**aemolysis (breakdown of red blood cells)
- **E**levated **l**iver enzymes (specifically alanine transaminase)
- **L**ow **p**latelet count

HELLP can be considered either as a variant of pre-eclampsia (if no hypertension or proteinuria present) or a complication of pre-eclampsia. Just like with pre-eclampsia, the cause is not known, but vasoconstriction and ischaemia may play a role in liver failure, which then may affect clotting.

DIFFERENTIAL DIAGNOSIS

HYPERTENSION DIFFERENTIALS

- Gestational hypertension or pregnancy-induced hypertension – hypertension which begins during pregnancy, after 20 weeks gestation, without proteinuria or signs and symptoms of pre-eclampsia. Hypertension should resolve by 12 weeks postpartum.
- Chronic or preexisting hypertension – hypertension which was diagnosed before pregnancy or before the 20th week of pregnancy. As young asymptomatic women do not routinely have blood tests or BP measurements outside of pregnancy, significant underlying causes of hypertension may be identified in pregnancy. Causes include:
  - Primary renal disease – acute or chronic kidney disease.
  - Renovascular disease such as diabetes mellitus.
  - Primary aldosteronism resulting in excess mineralocorticoid.
  - Cushing syndrome.
  - Hypo-/hyperthyroidism.
  - Hyperparathyroidism.
  - Phaeochromocytoma.
  - Coarctation of the aorta.

Patients with isolated hypertension are at a higher risk of developing pre-eclampsia, so they will be monitored closely throughout pregnancy. They may present later on in pregnancy with worsening hypertension, new proteinuria or symptoms of pre-eclampsia.

PROTEINURIA DIFFERENTIALS

- Exacerbation of pre-existing renal disease.
  - May present as worsening proteinuria or hypertension.
  - Pre-eclampsia is also more likely to develop in these individuals.
  - Careful monitoring is required.
- New renal disease.
  - Likely to present as new proteinuria and may also present with hypertension.
  - Can be difficult to differentiate from pre-eclampsia.

- Examples include:
  - Acute glomerulonephritis – the most common cause in young adults is IgA nephropathy.
  - APS – the presence of antiphospholipid antibodies may help distinguish APS from pre-eclampsia. However, antibodies can be present in healthy individuals in pregnancy.
  - Thrombotic thrombocytopenic purpura haemolytic uraemic syndrome (TTP-HUS) – acute renal failure, thrombocytopenia and neurological abnormalities. May be indistinguishable from severe pre-eclampsia or haemolysis, elevated LFTs, low-platelet (HELLP) syndrome; however, a greater degree of thrombocytopenia and renal failure is associated with TTP-HUS than with pre-eclampsia.

INVESTIGATIONS

- BP – systolic BP more than or equal to 140 mmHg and/or diastolic BP more than or equal to 90 mmHg.
- Urine
  - Urine dipstick to screen for proteinuria. If proteinuria on a dipstick is more than or equal to 1+ (approximately equivalent to more than 0.3 g/L), further quantification is required.
  - Urine protein:creatinine ratio using a single urine sample – more than 30 mg/mmol is significant proteinuria.
- Blood tests
  - FBC – falling platelet count and/or decreasing haemoglobin may suggest haemolysis, both associated with HELLP syndrome.
  - U&Es – monitor for development of renal failure.
  - LFTs – monitor for hepatic dysfunction and development of HELLP syndrome.
  - Coagulation function tests to check the hepatic synthetic function if there is suspicion of hepatic dysfunction.
  - Lactate dehydrogenase (LDH) may be elevated in the presence of miocroangiopathic haemolysis.
- Ultrasound – to measure fetal growth, amniotic fluid volume and umbilical Dopplers in order to monitor the wellbeing of the baby.

Blood Tests in Pre-Eclampsia

Where BP is raised (with or without proteinuria), blood tests should be undertaken to assess for organ dysfunction. When pre-eclampsia has been diagnosed, blood tests should be repeated at least weekly. In cases of severe pre-eclampsia, blood tests might be needed more frequently.

PLACENTAL GROWTH FACTOR TESTING

Placental growth factor (PLGF) is a hormone produced by placenta that can be tested in peripheral blood. In women who have not been diagnosed with pre-eclampsia but are at high risk of developing it (e.g., women with chronic hypertension), levels of PLGF can be measured to help estimate the likelihood of placental dysfunction. Low levels of PLGF are strongly suggestive of placental insufficiency and high risk of preterm birth. On the other hand, high PLGF levels suggest normal placental function and unlikely progression to pre-eclampsia and preterm birth within the next 14 days. This can be used to risk stratify women and plan their care accordingly. PLGF testing should be offered to all women with suspected pre-eclampsia who are between 20 and 35 weeks gestation. PLGF can be particularly useful in women with renal disease who already have raised levels of protein in the urine but are also at higher risk of pre-eclampsia. An abnormal PLGF result can give an indication of whether this is pre-eclampsia or not or potentially worsening renal disease.

COMPLICATIONS

Pre-eclampsia is a potentially life-threatening condition which has significant adverse effects on mother and baby.

MATERNAL

- Death – worldwide, 10% to 15% of direct maternal deaths occur from pre-eclampsia or eclampsia.
- Eclampsia.
- Stroke or cerebral haemorrhage – significant risk with severe hypertension (BP more than 160/110 mmHg).
- Pulmonary oedema.
- Liver failure.
- Renal failure.
- Thrombocytopenia – due to accelerated platelet consumption.
- DIC.
- HELLP syndrome.

 Acute Fatty Liver of Pregnancy (AFLP)

AFLP is not a complication *per se* but presents in a similar way to both severe pre-eclampsia and HELLP. AFLP is associated with more severe liver and renal dysfunction than pre-eclampsia and HELLP syndrome. In addition, AFLP is also associated with a fatty infiltration of the liver, low-grade fever, hypoglycaemia and DIC. It is a rare disease and usually occurs in the third trimester or in the early postpartum period. It can be fatal and diagnosis can be difficult, as it often presents in a similar way to severe pre-eclampsia and HELLP. FBC and LFTs are important tests to track disease severity, while a liver ultrasound scan or other imaging can help to confirm the diagnosis. Management is supportive, with expedited birth of the fetus if necessary.

FETAL

- FGR – due to chronic placental hypoperfusion.
- Oligohydramnios – most liquor is produced by fetal urination, so in the same way as a dehydrated adult reduces urine output; where there is significant placental insufficiency, liquor production reduces.
- Umbilical Doppler abnormalities on ultrasound – associated with poor placental function and FGR.

- Placental abruption – caused by the increased BP.
- Stillbirth – IUD caused by persistent placental insufficiency.
- Preterm birth – mostly iatrogenic to prevent other complications.

MANAGEMENT

ANTENATAL RISK ASSESSMENT AND PREVENTION

As part of routine antenatal care, all pregnant women should have their BP and urine tested during each visit with a healthcare professional. This is because early detection and prompt treatment of cases of pre-eclampsia can minimise maternal and fetal complications.

Women with one high-risk factor or two moderate-risk factors for pre-eclampsia (as outlined earlier in the chapter) should be offered aspirin from 12 weeks gestation until birth. Aspirin has been shown to reduce platelet thromboxane synthesis whilst maintaining vascular wall prostacyclin synthesis. It appears to improve development of the blood vessels of the placenta, improving nutrient supply to the fetus. In the groups at risk, aspirin reduces the chance of developing pre-eclampsia by over 15%. Women should also be informed of the symptoms of pre-eclampsia and who they should contact should they develop them. As well as routine antenatal care, additional appointments may be arranged for those women:
- To check BP and urine protein level.
- Ultrasound scans to monitor fetal growth may be undertaken in patients who have previously had severe pre-eclampsia or a previous small-for-gestational-age (SGA) baby.

Early identification of cases of pre-eclampsia can minimise maternal and fetal complications.

ANTENATAL MANAGEMENT OF CONFIRMED PRE-ECLAMPSIA

Once pre-eclampsia has been diagnosed, the maternal and fetal conditions need to be monitored closely and treatments instigated to optimise their conditions. Often that might mean that the patient should be admitted to hospital, especially if they have severe hypertension (BP is more than 160/110 mmHg).

The definitive management of pre-eclampsia is birth of the baby, as the production of whatever factors drive the condition is halted once the placenta has been removed. Appropriate management can allow for delayed delivery to reduce the complications of preterm birth.

Maternal Monitoring
- BP checks at least four times a day if admitted to hospital and then at least every 48 hours if being managed as an outpatient.
- Monitor for progression of signs and symptoms.
- Blood tests at least twice a week to monitor for organ dysfunction.

Fetal Monitoring

- Patient monitoring of fetal movements.
- CTG – at initial diagnosis, and then repeat if any fetal concerns or change in maternal condition. Auscultation should occur at every antenatal appointment.
- Ultrasound scans to monitor growth every 2 weeks. Liquor volume and umbilical artery Dopplers may also be assessed on scan.

Treatments

- Antihypertensive – should be commenced if BP is more than 140/90 mmHg. The choice of the antihypertensive will depend upon maternal comorbidities. Labetalol is usually the first-choice antihypertensive agent. Labetalol should be avoided in women with asthma, heart failure or heart block. Other agents include nifedipine, methyldopa and hydralazine. The aim should be to keep BP less than 140/90 mmHg. If the BP is more than 160/110 mmHg, IV medication may be required to control the BP. If BP cannot be consistently controlled, this would be an indication for urgent delivery to prevent maternal complications such as stroke and eclampsia.
- Corticosteroids – two doses of antenatal corticosteroids should be given to mothers where there is increased risk of delivery before 34 completed weeks of gestation. Corticosteroids promote fetal lung development, reducing the respiratory complications of prematurity should the child be delivered early.

Planning Birth

The timing of birth is based upon the risk to the baby in delivering preterm, balanced against the risks to the mother and fetus of continuing the pregnancy. Before 34 weeks gestation, the risk of prematurity is significant, so only women with very severe pre-eclampsia would be delivered before this gestation. After 37 weeks gestation, the fetus is defined as full term, so birth is advised in any patient with pre-eclampsia after this gestation. Between 34 and 37 weeks, the decision is individualised, based on the severity of the pre-eclampsia and the patient's wishes.

The pregnancy may be induced with the aim to achieve a vaginal birth, or a caesarean may be performed. This decision will be based on the patient's previous obstetric history, gestation of the pregnancy and the maternal and fetal condition.

> ### Severe Complications of Pre-Eclampsia where Preterm Delivery Would Be Considered
>
> - Severe hypertension of more than 160/110 mmHg, not responsive to medication.
> - Eclampsia.
> - HELLP syndrome.
> - Severe FGR.
> - Fetal compromise.

INTRAPARTUM MANAGEMENT

Birth of the baby may be required if the risks to the mother and baby outweigh the benefits of the continuation of pregnancy.

- Maternal and fetal monitoring – continued monitoring of the clinical status of the mother and baby is essential to identify any signs of complications.
- Fluids – fluid balance should be strictly monitored to avoid iatrogenic overload, as women with pre-eclampsia are at risk of pulmonary oedema. Strict fluid input management, restricting intake to 80 mL/hour, reduces the risk. Inserting a urinary catheter should be considered to assess fluid output.
- Antihypertensives – IV administration may be required in the presence of severe hypertension (more than 160/110 mmHg).
- Seizure prophylaxis – although the mechanism of action is not fully understood, magnesium sulphate can be given to prevent progression to eclampsia (as well as to manage an eclamptic seizure). The efficacy of magnesium sulphate in treatment of eclamptic seizures is superior to any other anticonvulsants.

POSTPARTUM MANAGEMENT

The majority of eclampsia episodes (approximately 50%) occur in the early postpartum period, so vigilance for pre-eclampsia complications should continue. However, the risk of pre-eclampsia complications falls significantly a few days after the baby is delivered. Management includes:

- Maternal assessment with BP and blood tests.
- Antihypertensives often need to be continued after birth if BP does not spontaneously resolve after birth. Note that methyldopa should be stopped or switched to an alternative antihypertensive after delivery, as it has been associated with an increased risk of postpartum depression.
- Magnesium sulphate, if commenced, should be continued for 24 hours following birth.
- Care in the community – a community care plan should be outlined prior to discharge from hospital. This should include:
  - Specified frequency of BP monitoring.
  - Criteria for reducing or stopping antihypertensives.
  - Criteria for referral.
  - The primary care physician should be aware of the need to follow up with these patients. At 6 weeks postnatal, most cases of pregnancy-related hypertension and proteinuria should have resolved. The primary care physician should check both of these and, if they have not resolved, investigate or refer to specialists to investigate for an underlying cause.
- Follow-up – women with pre-eclampsia, especially severe pre-eclampsia or eclampsia, should be reviewed in a postnatal clinic. The obstetrician can debrief regarding events of the pregnancy and birth and discuss the likely risk of recurrence in a future pregnancy.

PROGNOSIS

RECURRENCE

The risk of recurrence in a future pregnancy increases with the severity of the presentation and the earlier the complications developed in pregnancy. The average recurrence risk of pre-eclampsia is approximately 15%. This increases to 25% if complications occurred before 34 weeks gestation and up to 50% if they occurred before 28 weeks. The risk of recurrence can be even higher if HELLP complicated the pregnancy. In addition, it is also important that the primary care physician follows up with this patient after their pregnancy regarding their BP and proteinuria, as pregnancy may have revealed a preexisting condition.

CARDIOVASCULAR DISEASE

Development of pre-eclampsia increases the risk in the mother of future cardiovascular and cerebrovascular disease in later life. The risk can be up to double the background population risk, with a greater risk in those who developed severe pre-eclampsia.

❓ QUESTIONS

Louise, a 41-year-old, 32 weeks pregnant with twins, attends a routine antenatal appointment. She is gravidity five, parity two, and her current pregnancy has been uneventful. Her pregnancy was conceived via IVF treatment, and she received egg donations abroad. Louise feels well and has no other comorbidities. There were no antenatal or postpartum complications with the birth of her two children. All antenatal screening tests in this pregnancy have been normal, including routine growth scans. On examination, her BP is 150/95 mmHg, and urine dipstick reveals 2+ protein. The remaining examination findings and blood tests are unremarkable.

Q1   What is the most likely diagnosis for this woman?
  A Gestational hypertension.
  B Chronic hypertension.
  C HELLP syndrome.
  D Pre-eclampsia.
  E Eclampsia.

Q2   Answer true or false: Which of the following are risk factors for pre-eclampsia?
  A Maternal age of more than 40 years.
  B Preexisting diabetes in the mother.
  C Smoking.
  D Multiple pregnancy.
  E First pregnancy.

Q3   Which antihypertensive agents can be used in treating hypertension during pregnancy?
  A Ramipril.
  B Spironolactone.
  C Labetalol.
  D Methyldopa.
  E Nifedipine.

A Clopidogrel.		**H**	Idiopathic thrombocytopenic purpura.
B Aplastic anaemia.			
C Phenytoin.		**I**	HELLP syndrome.
D Labetalol.		**J**	Lamotrigine.
E Aspirin.		**K**	Nifedipine.
F Eclampsia.		**L**	Hydralazine.
G Magnesium sulphate.			

Select the most appropriate option from the above list that corresponds to the following statements. Each answer can be used once, more than once or not at all.

Q4   A peripheral blood film from a patient with pre-eclampsia is shown below. Successive FBC reveals a falling platelet count. What condition has she developed?

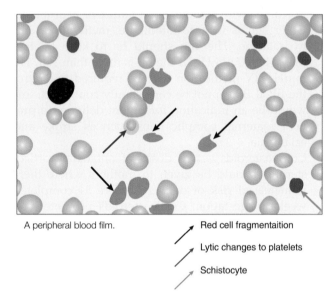

A peripheral blood film.   Red cell fragmentaition

Lytic changes to platelets

Schistocyte

Q5   Which drug is commonly used for seizure prophylaxis during pre-eclampsia?

Q6   Which drug can be used to treat hypertension in pre-eclampsia and also has tocolytic properties?

Q7   Which drug can be offered to patients with moderate or high risk of pre-eclampsia during the antenatal period?

Q8   Which pre-eclampsia complication occurs more frequently postpartum than antenatally?

[Answers on page 411.]

PRETERM LABOUR

Preterm labour is defined as labour occurring before 37 completed weeks of pregnancy. Preterm births can be spontaneous (70%) or iatrogenic (induction or caesarean) (30%), resulting from life-threatening pregnancy complications. The prevalence of preterm birth is about 11% worldwide and accounts for 70% of neonatal death and morbidity.

RISK FACTORS

The pathophysiology of preterm labour is often unknown. The strongest risk factor associated with preterm labour is a history of a previous preterm birth. Other risk factors are:

- Diet/lifestyle – smoking, low BMI of less than 20 kg/m², poor nutrition, alcohol, drug abuse (especially cocaine).
- Infection – UTI, chorioamnionitis.
- Noninfective maternal diseases – pre-eclampsia, diabetes mellitus and APS.
- Maternal inflammatory processes – appendicitis and inflammatory bowel disease exacerbation.
- Bacterial vaginosis.
- Maternal trauma due to injury or surgery during pregnancy.
- Maternal age – less than 17 or more than 35 years old.
- Parity – nulliparous or more than five previous babies.
- Interval of less than 1 year between pregnancies.
- Multiple pregnancy.
- Polyhydramnios.
- IUGR.
- Fetal abnormality.
- Uterine abnormalities.
- Previous cervical surgery.
- Preterm premature rupture of membranes (PPROM) in a previous pregnancy. PPROM often precedes preterm labour. This will be covered in more detail at the end of this section.

CLINICAL FEATURES

SYMPTOMS

Labour should be considered in any pregnant woman presenting with pain. The most common symptoms associated with preterm labour are:

- Regular painful contraction-like abdominal pain.
- Menstrual-like cramping.
- Intermittent nonspecific abdominal pain.
- Lower back pain.
- Pressure sensation in the vagina.

> ### Pertinent History Findings
>
> - Vaginal fluid loss or discharge, which could be preterm rupture of membranes.
> - Vaginal blood loss, which, along with pain, may indicate placental abruption.
> - Infective symptoms, as infection may be:
>   - The cause of preterm labour.
>   - A differential as the cause of the pains.
> - Systematic review to cover the symptoms associated with the differential diagnoses.

SIGNS

- Abdominal examination
  - Palpable uterine contractions support the diagnosis.
  - A tender uterus may suggest the diagnosis of abruption.
  - Other areas of abdominal tenderness may support an alternative diagnosis, such as appendicitis or renal colic.

- Speculum examination
  - Cervical dilatation.
  - Cervical effacement.
  - Clear fluid loss consistent with ROM.
- Vaginal examination
  - Should be avoided when ROM has been identified.
  - Assess cervical dilation; if this is 4 cm or greater, then birth is likely inevitable.
- Maternal observations – to look for signs of infection.

INVESTIGATIONS

- CTG
  - Fetal well-being – if fetal distress is suspected, delivery may need to be expedited.
  - Uterine contraction frequency can be assessed using the tocogram.
- Urinalysis
  - Looking for leucocytes or nitrites as signs of infection.
  - Protein to determine if there is a risk of pre-eclampsia.
- High vaginal swabs – may reveal infection; bacterial vaginosis is associated with preterm labour.
- Blood tests
  - FBC, CRP, blood cultures – identify an infective cause of symptoms.
  - U&E, LFTs, amylase, LDH, lactate – may be requested depending on the presentation to rule out differential causes for symptoms.
  - IV access and G&S – may be considered at the time of blood tests if imminent delivery is anticipated.
- Preterm labour tests.

> ### Preterm Labour Tests
>
> There are two commonly used tests in the UK to assist clinicians with the management of suspected preterm labour. These immunochromatography tests require a swab to be taken from the vagina or cervix. The swab is then placed in a fluid containing labelled antibodies to either fetal fibronectin or phosphorylated insulin-like growth factor binding protein 1. These proteins are not normally present in the vagina but are released from the amniotic membranes when there is a possibility of preterm labour developing. If the protein is present, the antibody binds to it. A test strip is then placed into the liquid. This contains an antibody to the protein that is fixed to the test strip. This fixed antibody binds to the protein antibody complex, and the labelled antibodies in the complex can be visually seen as a blue line indicating a positive result. A fetal fibronectin test gives numerical value, and NICE recommends a cutoff of 50 ng/mL or more to be interpreted as positive result.
>
> The tests are licensed for use between 24 and 34 completed weeks of gestation. These are the weeks where steroids would be administered if a positive result occurs. It is not used if the cervix is dilated to 4 cm or more, as it is likely that birth is inevitable. Recent vaginal examination,

sexual intercourse and vaginal bleeding can also affect the results.

A negative result is very helpful clinically, as there is a 98% chance that preterm labour will not occur within 14 days (high negative predictive value). A positive result does not mean labour will happen but that there is an approximately 30% chance in the following 2 weeks (low positive predictive value).

In most cases, a negative result will reassure both patient and clinician. Other causes for symptoms will be considered, and often the patient is discharged home. If the result is positive, patients are admitted for treatment of preterm labour.

An alternative test to aid clinical diagnosis of preterm labour is measurement of cervical length. This can be done via a transvaginal ultrasound scan. At 30 to 34 weeks pregnant, a cervical length of less than 15 mm is strongly suggestive of preterm labour and warrants admission and treatment.

DIFFERENTIAL DIAGNOSIS

While the initial task of the clinician is to diagnose or rule out preterm labour, in the majority of cases, an alternative diagnosis will need to be made. Hence, the clinician needs to keep in mind the possible differentials when assessing and investigating the patient.

The most common diagnoses for these types of pain in pregnancy are:
- Braxton-Hicks – intermittent uterine tightening that is not as painful as contractions and does not tend to increase in strength or frequency like labour contractions. It does not cause cervical dilation or effacement. However, women, particularly those in their first pregnancy, may not be able to differentiate this from preterm labour.
- Musculoskeletal pain
  - Nonspecific back pain and mild abdominal and pelvic pains are common in pregnancy. These are a diagnosis of exclusion.
    - High progesterone levels cause laxity of tendons, which increases the likelihood of bone pain and muscle sprains.
    - As the uterus enlarges, this causes nonspecific stretching of the peritoneum, muscles and skin.
    - Increased weight and change of centre of gravity also puts increased strain on muscles and joints.
  - Symphysis pubis dysfunction or pelvic girdle pain are terms commonly used to describe the pains caused by laxity of the sacroiliac joints and symphysis pubis in response to progesterone. It is treated with simple analgesia and physiotherapy.
- UTI – reduced immunity of pregnancy and incomplete bladder emptying due to the enlarged uterus pressing on the bladder resulting in urinary stasis contributes to the increased frequency of urinary infections in pregnancy. A UTI can be the cause of the pain but also can precipitate preterm labour.

Severe obstetric differential diagnoses not to be missed:
- Placental abruption.
- Uterine rupture.
- Severe pre-eclampsia or HELLP syndrome.

Any other cause of pain that can occur outside of pregnancy can also occur in pregnancy. They may, however, present atypically in pregnancy. A nonexhaustive list includes:
- Appendicitis.
- Cholecystitis.
- Pancreatitis.
- Gastroesophageal reflux.
- Gastroenteritis.
- Constipation.
- Renal stones.
- Pyelonephritis.
- Ovarian cyst accident.
- Neuropathic pain.

MANAGEMENT

The principles of management of preterm labour are (Fig. 14.4):
- Identify and treat any underlying cause.
- Monitor maternal observations and fetal well-being, and expedite birth if either are compromised.
- Give corticosteroids to mature fetal lungs (advised for pregnancies 24 to 34 weeks gestation).
- Consider tocolysis for 24 to 48 hours (reducing contractions) to delay delivery to extend the time steroids have to take effect or to allow transfer to another hospital.
- Offer IV magnesium sulphate for fetal neuroprotection if gestation is less than 30 weeks; consider for up to 34 weeks.
- Acquire adequate neonatal involvement for the gestation.
  - This will entail the neonatal team discussing with the parents about the likely outcome for the neonate delivered at the current gestation.
  - Prior to birth, transfer to another hospital with higher levels of support for a premature neonate may be required, depending on the gestation and services available at the local hospital.

CORTICOSTEROIDS

Between 24 and 34 completed weeks of gestation, corticosteroids (betamethasone or dexamethasone) are given to enhance fetal lung maturation by increasing surfactant production, which reduces the risk of neonatal respiratory distress syndrome (RDS). Physiologically, lung surfactant production starts from 24 weeks gestation and increases through to 36 weeks. Surfactant is produced by type II pneumocytes. Surfactant increases pulmonary compliance by decreasing the surface tension. Steroids are not recommended after 34 completed weeks because sufficient fetal lung maturity will have been achieved.

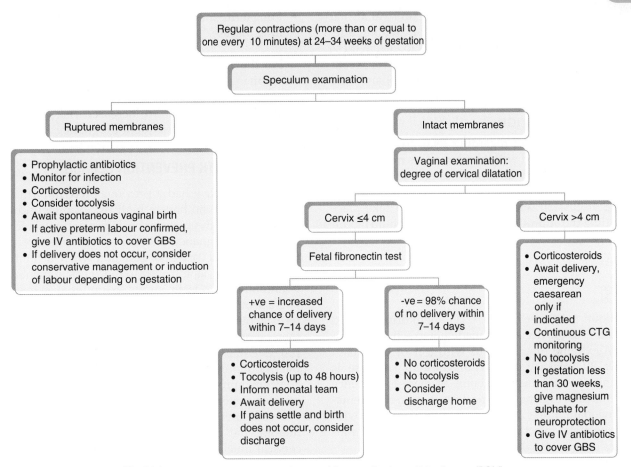

Fig. 14.4 Management of Preterm Labour and Preterm Rupture of Membranes (ROM).

Steroids also reduce the risk of intracerebral haemorrhages in preterm births. Steroids are given to the mother by IM injection, usually in two doses 24 hours apart.

TOCOLYSIS AND TOCOLYTIC DRUGS

If cervical dilatation is less than 4 cm, medications can be used in cases of threatened preterm labour to try to reduce or stop uterine contractions (tocolysis). The aim is to allow additional time for steroids to take effect or to allow safe transfer to a hospital with appropriate neonatal facilities. In the UK, atosiban (oxytocin receptor antagonist) is licensed for the treatment of threatened preterm labour, while nifedipine (calcium channel blocker) is another tocolytic commonly used, but it is unlicensed.

Tocolysis is not normally used for more than 48 hours. Tocolysis does not have a benefit and may worsen outcome if steroids have previously been given in the pregnancy, or if there are signs of infection, bleeding or ROM.

NEONATAL TEAM DISCUSSION

A number of factors will influence the likely outcome for a preterm neonate, including gestation, birth weight, presence of sepsis, evidence of fetal abnormalities and use of steroids. Gestation alone should never be used to give prognosis to a patient, but the information below may be a helpful guide.

- Less than 22 weeks gestation – even in the most specialist centres, neonatal survival to 3 years of age from onset of labour at this gestation is extremely unlikely (less than 1%), with significant neurological dysfunction in the majority of surviving children. For this reason, parents are often advised that no active monitoring of the fetus should occur during labour, and no attempt to resuscitate should be made at delivery. If there are signs of life at birth, palliation will normally be offered.
- 22 to 23 weeks gestation – in specialist centres, neonatal survival is approximately 35% at this gestation, with long-term intact survival (no significant neurological or physical dysfunction) in approximately 70% at 3 years old. However, the specific circumstances of the individual case will be considered before discussing whether active treatment is appropriate.
- 24 to 25 weeks gestation – neonatal survival is around 65%, with long-term intact survival in 85% of cases. Active resuscitation will be offered in the majority of cases where the expected fetal weight is greater than 500 g and there are no other known complications.
- 26 to 29 weeks gestation – neonatal survival increases by about 5% each week, from 80% at 26 weeks to over 95% at 29 weeks. In the vast majority of cases, complete and active obstetric and neonatal treatment will be offered. Intact survival at this gestation is about 95%.
- 30 to 32 weeks gestation – survival rates increase up to 98% at 32 weeks, which is only slightly below the

rate at term, with the rate of intact survival also at a similar rate to term pregnancies, providing adequate neonatal care is available. However, these neonates are likely to require a number of weeks in a neonatal intensive care unit (NICU) and may require long-term hospital follow-up.

FETAL PRESENTATION

Where there is doubt regarding fetal presentation, it should be confirmed with ultrasound, as malpresentations are more likely at earlier gestations. If the fetus is breech, the type of breech will need to be assessed, and a discussion with the mother should take place regarding the appropriate mode of birth, should labour progress.

[See 'Breech' on page 280.]

BIRTH

If labour progresses, fetal CTG monitoring should occur unless the decision is made not to actively monitor an extreme preterm fetus with a poor prognosis. Below 30 weeks gestation, magnesium sulphate is administered IV during labour, as there is evidence that this improves neurological function in the premature neonate. Preterm births are also associated with early neonatal infection, so to reduce this risk, IV antibiotics are given to the mother in labour.

- Fetal blood sampling and the use of vacuum (ventouse) extraction are contraindicated before 34 weeks gestation. Forceps may be used before 34 weeks, but where a difficult assisted vaginal birth is anticipated, there should be a low threshold to offer caesarean. At the time of birth, a senior neonatologist should be available to care for the preterm neonate.

If contractions settle, labour does not progress after 48 to 72 hours of admission and there are no signs of infection, bleeding, ROM or any other medical concerns, the patient may be offered discharge home, with advice to return if further symptoms return.

PROGNOSIS

The later preterm labour occurs in pregnancy, the better the outcome. The prognosis varies depending on the following factors:
- Gestational age and birth weight of the baby.
- The facilities available at the local neonatal unit and whether the baby has to be transferred to a tertiary neonatal centre after birth.
- Health status of the infant at the time of birth.
- Use of antenatal corticosteroids.
- For the neonate, preterm birth may result in:
  - Resuscitation – perinatal mortality.
  - During stay on neonatal unit – infection, RDS, hypoglycaemia, temperature regulation issues, feeding difficulty, hypoxic ischaemic encephalopathy and intraventicular haemorrhage.

- Long term – neurodevelopmental issues and chronic lung disease.

For the mother, the psychological impact of a preterm birth should not be overlooked, and support should be offered as needed. Having had a preterm birth, the patient is at an increased risk of another preterm birth in a subsequent pregnancy.

PRETERM BIRTH PREVENTION CLINICS

Women who have had a previous preterm birth (and other women who have a high risk of preterm birth) can be seen in the preterm birth prevention clinic in a subsequent pregnancy. They are seen a number of times between 16 and 24 weeks gestation where a combination of cervical length ultrasound measurements and quantitative fibronectin swabs are undertaken to calculate a women's individualised risk of going into preterm labour. Where a high risk is identified, women can then be offered treatment with one or both of vaginal progesterones or cervical cerclage. Treatment reduces the risk of preterm birth (<32 weeks) by about 50%.

Vaginal progesterone pessaries are used daily. They prevent preterm labour by relaxing the uterus which prevents uterine contractions from shortening and dilating the cervix. Progesterone also thickens the cervical mucus, which reduces the chance of bacteria entering the cervix and causing inflammation, which can cause preterm labour.

Cervical cerclage is a procedure in which a suture is inserted around the cervix. This provides some structural support to the cervix to prevent shortening and also helps to keep the cervix closed, thereby reducing the risk of an ascending infection causing inflammation. If the cerclage is effective, it is removed at around 36 weeks gestation to allow a vaginal birth to occur. If a woman presents in preterm labour prior to 36 weeks, the stitch is cut to allow the cervix to dilate in response to uterine contractions; otherwise, the cervix will tear.

[See 'Recurrent Miscarriage' on page 63.]

PRETERM PRELABOUR RUPTURE OF MEMBRANES

PPROM is defined as spontaneous rupture of the amniotic sac prior to the onset of regular contractions before 37 weeks gestation. PPROM occurs in 2% of pregnancies but is associated with 40% of preterm births. Approximately 80% of women will labour within 48 hours of rupture and 95% within 7 days.

The risk factors for PPROM are similar to those for preterm labour. If PPROM or preterm labour occurred in a previous pregnancy, first- and second-trimester vaginal swabs are advised to check for bacterial vaginosis, and regular urine dipsticks should be obtained throughout pregnancy to identify a UTI. Treating these infections has been shown to reduce recurrence.

CLINICAL FEATURES

SYMPTOMS

Women usually present with a history of clear fluid loss from the vagina. A large gush with an ongoing loss is a convincing history. The history is less deterministic if only small amounts of fluid have been lost, particularly if a sanitary pad is not required to maintain clothing dryness, if the loss is not ongoing or if the loss only occurs at the time of wishing to pass urine. Alternative diagnoses include an increase in physiological vaginal discharge, which is common in pregnancy; vaginal candidiasis, which may increase discharge or stress urinary incontinence, which is also common in pregnancy.

SIGNS

Visualising clear fluid loss through the cervix on speculum examination is the most convincing evidence of fluid loss. If no fluid is initially seen, asking the patient to cough may cause the fluid to expectorate.

In cases of suspected or confirmed ROM, digital vaginal examination should be avoided, and only essential speculum examinations should be performed. This will avoid introducing an ascending infection.

INVESTIGATIONS

If there is no sign of ROM on examination and the history is not convincing, the clinician may feel no further investigation is necessary. However, if there are negative findings but a convincing history, other investigations may be considered:

- Pad check – ask the patient to wear a pad and to mobilise. The pad can then be checked regularly to see if it becomes damp.
- Vaginal swab – run a bedside immunochromatography test, looking for high concentrations of insulin-like growth factor binding protein 1, which is present in amniotic fluid but not in normal vaginal discharge. A positive test is supportive of the membranes having ruptured, but the limited specificity of these tests may lead to false-positive results.
- Ultrasound assessment of liquor volume – this is rarely done, as it is only able to identify a significant loss of liquor, which is likely to be evident clinically.

If ROM is confirmed, investigations should be performed to identify signs of infection, confirm fetal well-being and prepare for the possibility of preterm birth:

- Maternal observations.
- CTG for fetal well-being.
- FBC, CRP and G&S.
- High vaginal swab.
- Urinalysis.

PATHOPHYSIOLOGY

Once the membranes have ruptured, they cannot reform. This means there is access to the fetus from the external environment, which increases the risk of ascending infection and the development of chorioamnionitis. Fluid may or may not continue to drain after the initial loss, as a fetal part may plug the leak. Liquor is constantly being made by the fetus and the placenta, so liquor volume on palpation and on ultrasound scan may be normal, even after a large loss.

As well as allowing an ascending infection, ROM can be a consequence of an already-established infection.

MANAGEMENT

Once membranes have ruptured, there is a high likelihood of preterm birth. The same management strategies should be employed as described earlier for premature labour, including:

- Steroids – if contractions occur, tocolysis is normally not given when membranes have ruptured, as delaying delivery may be associated with detrimental neonatal outcomes.
- Obtaining appropriate neonatal support for the gestation.
- Review investigation results and monitor maternal and fetal well-being, monitoring for evidence of infection and chorioamnionitis.
- Ultrasound scan to assess presentation if not evident clinically.
- If labour occurs, offer continuous CTG monitoring.

ANTIBIOTICS

In addition to the preterm labour management, there is evidence to support the use of a broad-spectrum antibiotic to reduce the chance of ascending infection and chorioamnionitis. The antibiotic usually offered is a 10-day course of erythromycin, which is stopped earlier if delivery occurs.

When a patient with PPROM is in labour, whether spontaneous or induced, treatment with IV antibiotics to cover group B streptococcus (GBS) should be given (benzylpenicillin or, if allergic, vancomycin).

TIMING OF BIRTH

If labour does not occur spontaneously after 48 to 72 hours, the patient may be allowed home, but a decision has to be made about how to manage the ongoing pregnancy. The longer the pregnancy is allowed to continue, the higher chance there is of an infection developing. This has to be balanced against the risk of prematurity for the neonate if labour is induced.

Gestation Less Than 37 Weeks

The risk of prematurity usually outweighs the risk of infection. Conservative management should be considered. This involves:

- Continuing erythromycin for the 10-day course. There is no evidence supporting prolonging the course, even if conservative management is planned for many weeks.
- Weekly review for maternal observations, CTG, FBC and a vaginal swab to assess for evidence of a developing infection.
- The patient should regularly check her temperature at home, as well as be advised of symptoms of clinical chorioamnionitis (lower abdominal pain, abnormal vaginal discharge, fever, malaise and reduced fetal movements); a woman should attend hospital urgently for review if she develops any signs or symptoms of infection.
- If there are any signs of infection, chorioamnionitis or fetal compromise:
- Broad-spectrum antibiotics should be commenced alongside other routine steps in the treatment of sepsis.
- Delivery should be expedited by the quickest route, often by caesarean.
- If there is no evidence of sepsis, conservative management can be continued. Induction of labour should be planned at 37 weeks gestation, as, at this gestation, the risk of prematurity is very small, and the fetus is full term, whereas the risk of infection persists.

Gestation More Than 37 Weeks

If membranes rupture beyond 37 weeks, this is called prelabour ROM. The fetus is now full term, so there is no risk of prematurity, and there is less likely to be an underlying sinister cause for the rupture. Induction can be offered immediately after membrane rupture, or up to 24 hours can be allowed for labour to establish spontaneously before considering induction of labour.

 Group B Streptococci

GBS is a commensal bacteria within the vagina; it may be present in up to 30% of women. It is associated with neonatal sepsis. Current UK guidance advises antibiotics that cover GBS be offered in labour for any woman who has:
- Confirmed preterm labour.
- Had a previous child affected by GBS infection.
- Had a positive GBS culture in this pregnancy.
  - In cases of prelabour ROM at 34 weeks gestation or more, patients with commensal GBS should be offered immediate induction of labour and antibiotic cover, rather than waiting for spontaneous labour like in the low-risk patient.
- Pyrexia in labour.

If adequate antibiotics are not given in labour, then antibiotic treatment should be considered in the neonate.

PROGNOSIS

The vast majority of pregnancies experiencing PPROM will labour spontaneously within 1 week of membrane rupture. Careful monitoring for infection in both the mother and fetus is required antenatally, intrapartum and postnatally. The outcome for the fetus depends on the gestation at birth and the presence of an infection.

❓ QUESTIONS

Josephine is a 28-year-old nulliparous woman who is pregnant at 31 weeks gestation. Josephine presents with a history of abdominal pain for the past 2 days that seemed to be getting worse. She is mildly overweight, with a BMI of 27 kg/m², and has a past medical history of type 1 diabetes mellitus and hypothyroidism. She has also suffered from recurrent UTIs in the past. She has been trying to quit smoking since the start of her pregnancy and has managed to cut down from smoking 25 cigarettes to 5 cigarettes a day.

Q1   Which of the following would not be a possible cause of the abdominal pain that she is experiencing?
  A Appendicitis.
  B Breech presentation of the fetus.
  C Constipation.
  D Placental abruption.
  E UTI.

Q2   Answer true or false: Which of the following puts Josephine at an increased risk of having a preterm birth?
  A Overweight.
  B Diabetes.
  C Smoking.
  D Vitiligo.
  E UTI.

On further questioning, Josephine admitted to having increased vaginal discharge with a bit of bleeding, together with the onset of abdominal discomfort. There is no leakage of liquor. She now feels that the abdominal pain is intermittent, occurring every few minutes, with no pain at all between episodes. She reported that fetal movements are normal. On examination, Josephine is apyrexic, with a BP of 138/96 mmHg, respiration rate of 19/min and heart rate of 90 bpm. On abdominal palpation, the SFH is 31 cm, with the fetus lying in a breech presentation, and the presenting part feels engaged.

Q3   Answer true or false: Which examinations and/or investigations should now be performed to confirm the diagnosis?
  A Speculum and vaginal examinations.
  B Fetal blood sampling.
  C Fetal fibronectin test.
  D CTG.
  E Maternal blood tests, blood cultures and high vaginal swabs.

Josephine has been diagnosed with preterm labour. Further examination shows that her cervix is 3 cm dilated with intact membranes, and test results suggested that she has a moderate chance of delivering within the next 7 to 14 days. Uterine activity is recorded as 3 in 10, and there is acceleration of fetal heart rate without any signs of deceleration. She is already in a unit with appropriate facilities and professionals to provide optimal neonatal care.

A	Atosiban.	**G**	Discharge home.
B	Progesterone.	**H**	Admit to the delivery unit.
C	Nifedipine.	**I**	Ventouse birth.
D	Betamethasone.	**J**	Caesarean birth.
E	Terbutaline.	**K**	Vaginal birth.
F	Oxytocin.	**L**	Cervical cerclage.

Select the most appropriate option from the above list that corresponds to the following statements. Each answer can be used once, more than once or not at all.

Q4 What should be the first step in management?

Q5 What is the most appropriate drug to be administered to reduce the incidence of RDS?

Q6 What is the most appropriate tocolytic drug for Josephine?

Q7 If Josephine's cervical dilatation does not progress beyond 4 cm at 72 hours and there are no signs of fetal membrane prolapse in the external os on speculum examination, what could possibly be the next treatment option?

Q8 If labour ensues despite tocolysis, what is the best mode of birth for the fetus in vertex presentation?

[Answers on page 414.]

CHORIOAMNIONITIS

Chorioamnionitis (also known as intraamniotic infection) is a pregnancy complication where there is an intrauterine infection of the fetal amnion, chorion membranes, amniotic fluid, placenta or decidua (also known as the endometrium). The infection can occur before or during labour.

RISK FACTORS

- Obesity.
- Impaired glucose tolerance or diabetes mellitus.
- Impaired immunity or immunosuppressant medication.
- Anaemia.
- Vaginal discharge.
- History of pelvic infection.
- History of group B streptococcal infection.
- Amniocentesis and other invasive procedures.
- Cervical cerclage.
- Prolonged spontaneous ROM.
- Group A streptococcus infection in close contacts or family members.

AETIOLOGY

Chorioamnionitis most commonly occurs following ROM which allows the ascent of polymicrobial bacteria from the vaginal flora through the cervix. This causes infection and acute inflammation of the fetal membranes, amniotic fluid, placenta and, ultimately, the fetus. The longer the fetus remains within the uterus after ROM, the higher the risk of ascending infection developing.

[See 'Preterm Labour' on page 306.]

Rarely, chorioamnionitis occurs by haematogenous transplacental spread from the bacteraemic mother and iatrogenic infection through invasive procedures penetrating the amniotic sac (for example, chorionic villus sampling or amniocentesis). Some pathogens are commonly associated with an ascending infection from the lower genital tract, including GBS, *Escherichia coli* and *Chlamydia trachomatis*. The most common pathogen to cross the placenta is *Listeria monocytogenes*.

CLINICAL FEATURES

In many cases of chorioamnionitis, especially in the early stages of infection, there may be no signs or symptoms of an infection (silent or subclinical chorioamnionitis). Symptoms and signs may include:

EVIDENCE OF MATERNAL SEPSIS

- Pyrexia (more than 37.8°C).
- Tachycardia (more than 120 bpm).
- Cold, clammy skin.
- Hypotension.

SITE OF INFECTION

- Presence of discoloured, purulent, offensive-smelling amniotic fluid or vaginal discharge.
- Abdominal pain and uterine tenderness.

FETAL EFFECTS

- Fetal tachycardia (more than 160 to 180 bpm) or decelerating fetal heart rate on CTG.
- Decreased fetal movements.

Where infection is suspected, it is important to complete a thorough examination to assess all possible sites of infection, such as the chest, cannula sites, urinary tract and genital tract. Similarly, where possible fetal distress is identified in isolation, infection should form part of the differential.

INVESTIGATIONS

Chorioamnionitis is commonly investigated using simple blood tests and taking a high vaginal swab during assessment.

- FBC and CRP are used to support the diagnosis of an infection.

- Venous blood gas, including lactate, helps assess the severity of the infection in the mother.
- Blood cultures to identify septicaemia.
- High vaginal swab for culture and sensitivity to identify ascending infections from the vagina to the uterus.
- Midstream urine sample.
- Chest x-ray.
- CTG should be performed if the pregnancy is at an appropriate gestation (usually after 26 weeks) to assess fetal well-being.

DIFFERENTIAL DIAGNOSIS

- Systemic inflammatory response syndrome (SIRS) caused by infection
  - Pneumonia and respiratory tract infections.
  - Pyelonephritis or UTI.
  - Skin infection from prolonged use of IV access.
  - Appendicitis.
- SIRS without infection
  - Peritonitis.
  - Inflammatory bowel disease.
  - Systemic lupus erythematosus.
- Obstetric causes of abdominal pain and fetal tachycardia
  - Abruption.
  - Uterine rupture.
- Other causes of fetal tachycardia
  - Fetal hypoxia and distress due to reduced placental perfusion in labour.
  - Cord prolapse.
  - Fetomaternal haemorrhage.
  - Anaemia.
  - Medications, such as β-agonists used for tocolysis.
  - Fetal cardiac arrhythmia, such as sinus ventricular tachyarrhythmia.

MANAGEMENT

Maternal and fetal clinical status are monitored closely:
- Maternal vital signs and observations at hourly intervals.
- Maternal pyrexia is controlled systematically with paracetamol so as to prevent overheating the fetus within the mother.
- Maternal fluid balance monitoring with consideration of urinary catheter insertion.
- Fetal status is monitored continuously by CTG.

ANTIBIOTICS

When chorioamnionitis is suspected, it should be treated as an emergency, like any source of sepsis. The patient should be started on a combination of broad-spectrum IV antibiotics which cover multiple pathogens, specifically those commonly associated with the vaginal and urinary tracts. The choice of antibiotics will depend on local guidelines and maternofetal condition. Antibiotics can be stopped 48 hours after delivery unless the mother's symptoms do not resolve

following delivery. Starting the baby on antibiotics postnatally should be strongly considered, as they are also likely to have been infected.

BIRTH

- Prolonged fetal infection can cause multiple complications, with the most severe being cerebral palsy and neonatal death. For these reasons, it is very rare for delivery to be delayed, even at extremely preterm gestations.
- If chorioamnionitis is diagnosed in labour, both mother and baby need to be monitored closely. If labour is progressing quickly, then labour may be continued. If there is slow progress in labour or there is any deterioration in the maternal or fetal condition, birth should be expedited (assisted vaginal birth or caesarean).
- When chorioamnionitis is suspected and if an FBS is undertaken, a normal result should be reviewed with caution, as the fetal condition can deteriorate rapidly with sepsis, and significant damage to the fetal brain and other tissues can occur from the inflammatory response to infection or from endotoxins, even without hypoxia. Therefore, most clinicians have a low threshold for expediting birth where there is suspected fetal distress on CTG.
- If chorioamnionitis is suspected prior to labour, several factors need to be considered to decide on the mode and timing of birth, including gestation and degree of fetal and maternal compromise. Usually, birth is expedited to prevent deterioration and long-term fetal complications.
- Steroids are usually offered at preterm gestations to mature the fetal lungs to improve neonatal outcomes. However, they may not be given where infection is suspected, as the steroids can reduce the maternal response to infection, and the delay in delivery waiting for the steroids to take effect may be more detrimental than not using steroids.
- A neonatologist may be present at birth to assess the fetal condition and consider antibiotic treatment.
- After birth, placental swabs are sent for microbiological culture and sensitivity testing.

 Group A Streptococci

Group A streptococcus is a bacteria that often colonises the throat, skin and genital area. It can cause a wide range of infections, including pharyngitis, cellulitis and pneumonia. On rare occasions it can develop into severe sepsis or necrotising fasciitis, leading to ITU admission and potentially death. For that reason, it is an important clinical consideration in cases of pyrexia during pregnancy or in the postpartum period. Young women often look very well in the initial stages of the infection, often presenting with nonspecific or mild symptoms. Subtle signs, such as tachypnoea or a mild tachycardia, may be the only evidence of pathology. If there is not a high clinical suspicion of infection, then these women can suddenly deteriorate. Penicillin-based antibiotics are extremely effective against group A streptococci. Close household contacts of women with group A streptococcal infection should be warned to seek medical attention should symptoms develop, and the situation may warrant antibiotic prophylaxis. Prophylactic antibiotics might also be needed for babies of women who develop group A streptococcus infection in the postpartum period.

PREVENTION

- General advice given to patients to reduce the risks of getting an infection:
  - Practice good self-hygiene, as this prevents vaginal infections, but avoid practices such as douching.
  - Avoid undercooked meat (*Toxoplasmosis gondii*) and unpasteurised dairy products (*L. monocytogenes*).
  - Avoid contact with animals; for example, the faeces of house cats may have toxoplasmosis.
  - Avoid travel to areas where yellow fever, malaria or polio are prevalent.
  - Keep up to date with all scheduled immunisations during pregnancy.
- Speculum examination and especially digital vaginal examinations should be avoided where possible when preterm prelabour ROM has occurred to reduce the risk of ascending infection.
- Use of digital vaginal examinations should be kept to a minimum during labour.

TABLE 14.2	Maternal and Neonatal Complications of Chorioamnionitis
Maternal Complications	
- Unplanned caesarean birth. - Postpartum haemorrhage - Postcaesarean wound infection - Endometritis - Maternal bacteraemia – more common with group A streptococci or *Escherichia coli* - Pelvic abscess - Acute respiratory distress syndrome - Septic shock - ITU admission - Death (very rare)	
Neonatal Complications	
- Pneumonia - Neonatal sepsis – more common in preterm infants - Meningitis - Preterm birth and its associated complications – chronic lung disease, respiratory distress syndrome, intraventricular haemorrhage - Other insults to the neonatal brain – chorioamnionitis increases the risk of cerebral palsy by up to fourfold. If hypoxia is also present, there is an 80 times increased risk - Intrauterine or neonatal death (uncommon in infected term babies). Conversely, preterm babies appear to have a much greater risk of morbidity and mortality in the presence of infection, even accounting for the general risks of prematurity	

ITU, Intensive care unit.

COMPLICATIONS

Chorioamnionitis is considered a medical emergency. However, complications vary, depending on the severity of the infection, as well as the time at which the mother presented and was diagnosed (Table 14.2).

PROGNOSIS

The long-term prognosis for most patients treated early for chorioamnionitis is good. However, sepsis is one of the biggest causes of mortality of pregnant women, often where there has been a delay in diagnosis and treatment of infection. The outcomes of the babies are generally positive, but this is dependent on the gestation and severity of infection.

❓ QUESTIONS

Smruti, a 32-year-old woman, presented at 23^{+6} weeks gestation with a 2-day history of moderate vaginal bleeding and increasing lower abdominal discomfort. Based on her past history of a previous spontaneous mid-second trimester miscarriage, she was given an ultrasound that indicated cervical cerclage 1 week previously. The patient is now distressed, with increasing abdominal pain and vital signs showing a temperature of 38.5°C, a heart rate of 127 bpm, a BP of 95/65 mmHg and a respiratory rate of 24 breaths per minute.

Q1 Answer true or false: Which of the following are likely to be reasonable differential diagnoses?
  A Placental abruption.
  B Uterine rupture.
  C Preterm premature ROM.
  D Chorioamnionitis.
  E Preterm labour pain.

Q2 On abdominal palpation, there is generalised uterine tenderness. An examination of her pad showed fresh bleeding, tinged with foul-smelling discharge. She had leucocytosis with a white cell count of 20×10^9/L and a CRP of 75 mg/L. The consultant has been notified. What is the next best step in management?
  A Perform amniocentesis to obtain amniotic fluid for culture.
  B Start a course of antenatal corticosteroids to enhance fetal lung maturity.
  C Start IV fluids and empirical antibiotics.
  D Remove the cervical cerclage.
  E Give analgesia and prescribe bed rest with tocolysis to allow her pregnancy to continue and reduce the risks of complications of prematurity.

Q3 After the attempt to induce labour failed, the consultant obstetrician performed a caesarean. Assuming that the birth was successful and the baby was born alive, which of the statements about follow-up management are true?
  A The neonate may be admitted to the NICU for close monitoring.

B The placenta and fetal membranes will be sent away for histopathology and microbiology tests.

C The woman should be monitored for the complications of caesarean birth.

D The neonate may be given a septic screen and a course of broad-spectrum IV antibiotics.

E If the woman stabilises after birth, she can be discharged on a course of oral antibiotics with no need for further outpatient follow-up of any sort.

Q4 What is the most appropriate management for a woman known to have vaginal colonisation with GBS?

A Advise delivery by planned caesarean and benzylpenicillin treatment antenatally during any subsequent pregnancies.

B Benzylpenicillin treatment during labour.

C Advise delivery by planned caesarean.

D Benzylpenicillin treatment antenatally.

E Benzylpenicillin treatment antenatally during any subsequent pregnancies.

[Answers on page 415.]

SMALL-FOR-GESTATIONAL-AGE BABIES AND INTRAUTERINE GROWTH RESTRICTION

SGA and IUGR are important obstetric diagnoses, as they can lead to stillbirth (Table 14.3). To monitor for these pathologies in low-risk pregnancies, SFH measurements from 24 weeks gestation onwards are carried out and plotted on customised growth centile charts at every routine antenatal review (Fig. 14.5). These centile charts assess estimated fetal growth at particular gestations. Any value plotted between the 10th and 90th centiles is regarded as normal, but subsequent measurements should continue along the same centile of the chart to demonstrate adequate growth. If either growth is initially measured to be below the 10th centile or the growth velocity reduces (subsequent measurements not following the expected centiles), then low-risk pregnancies should be referred for ultrasound assessment under an obstetrician. In pregnancies known to be high risk for SGA or IUGR, growth is monitored with serial ultrasound measurements plotted on centile charts, as this is more reliable than SFH measurements.

If the repeat ultrasound assessments show that a baby that started with growth below the 10th centile maintains growth on the same centile (following the centiles), then this is SGA. However, if repeat measurements demonstrate that the growth is dropping down centiles, this is IUGR, as demonstrated in Fig. 14.5. In cases where SGA or IUGR is identified, further investigations and monitoring are carried out to optimise the timing of the birth to minimise the risk of prematurity and avoid stillbirth.

SGA is sometimes a physiological variant. IUGR, by comparison, is always a pathological condition, which can occur in normal centiles, although it is

Table 14.3	Key Definitions for Small for Gestational Age and Intrauterine Growth Restriction
TERM	**DEFINITION**
Small for gestational age	Measurement below the 10th centile for abdominal circumference and/or estimated birth weight.
IUGR, also known as FGR	The growth of the baby slows or ceases during intrauterine life.
Prematurity	Birth before 37 weeks gestation. These babies may also be SGA, IUGR or LBW.
LBW	Any baby less the 2.5 kg, regardless of gestational age.
Centile	The position of a measurement within a statistical distribution, demonstrating how it compares with that parameter in other individuals. For example, if an AC of the fetus or the EFW measured was on the 20th centile, this means that for every 100 AC or EFW measurements of that gestation in normal babies, 20 would be expected to be smaller and 80 would be expected to be bigger.

AC, Abdominal circumference; *EFW*, estimated fetal weight; *FGR*, fetal growth restriction; *IUGR*, intrauterine growth restriction; *LBW*, low birth weight; *SGR*, small for gestational age.

more common below the 10th centile. Hence, there is increased monitoring of fetuses estimated to be below the 10th centile. As evidence suggests that both SGA and IUGR fetuses have an increased risk of poor outcomes, they are investigated and treated in the same way. Low birth weight is linked to a worse fetal outcome regardless of aetiology, particularly very low birth weight (less than 1500 g). Babies born at earlier gestations are understandably smaller than those born at term, but growth charts can be used to determine the gestation-specific weight that the baby should have reached to determine if there is an element of SGA or IUGR. It is worth noting that, statistically, 10% of normal babies will always be below the 10th centile, even on customised growth charts, and that centile is not a definitive indicator of the fetal condition.

Concordant and Discordant Growth

Monitoring of fetal growth on ultrasound is performed by measuring the head circumference, abdominal circumference and femur length and then inputting these measurements into an equation to calculate an EFW. In a normally growing fetus, there is concordant growth, where the head and abdominal circumference measurements follow the same centiles, whereas in discordant growth, they follow different centiles. A fetus below the 10th centile with concordant growth is more likely to be SGA. In IUGR, head growth is more likely to persevere, so often the head circumference growth will follow the centiles, whereas the abdominal circumference growth velocity falls.

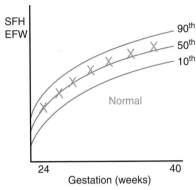

An antenatal centile chart from a low risk pregnancy demonstrating expected SFH measurements throughout pregnancy.

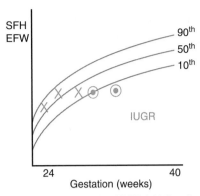

Centile chart demonstrating IUGR. Initially, a low risk pregnancy being monitored with SFH measurements, when growth restriction was suspected ultrasound scans were then conducted.

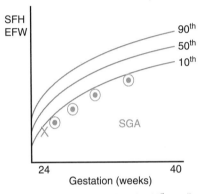

Initial SFH measurement below the 10th centile – ultrasound scanning conducted throughout the rest of the antenatal period. The estimated growth remained below the 10th centile, but the growth velocity follows that expected in an uncomplicated pregnancy (follows the curve of the centile lines). This is supportive of SGA, where the fetus is likely to be one of the 10% of normal fetuses whose growth is normally below the 10th centile.

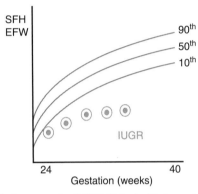

Further example of IUGR. This chart is from a high risk pregnancy, where ultrasound estimation of fetal weight has been used first-line rather than SFH. Growth is initially below the 10th centile, but the growth velocity is less than that of the normal centile curves, and then becomes static.

Fig. 14.5 Examples of Centile Charts Demonstrating Small for Gestational Age (SGA) and Intrauterine Growth Restriction (IUGR). 'X' is usually used clinically to mark a symphysis fundal height (SFH) measurement. A dot with a circle is used to mark an ultrasound measurement of estimated fetal weight (EFW).

PATHOLOGY

PLACENTAL FACTORS

The major cause of IUGR is placental insufficiency. The normal physiology of placental development is trophoblast invasion early in pregnancy, as the extravillous cytotrophoblasts invade into the maternal uterus and into the spiral arteries, transforming them into large vessels of low resistance. Inadequate spiral artery supply or reduced trophoblast invasion into the uterine wall and inadequate vascular function are thought to be the major causes of IUGR. In addition, the placenta can also fail later during the pregnancy, even if it initially formed normally. An issue with the placenta such as this is likely to present as a problem after 28 weeks.

MATERNAL FACTORS

If the placenta itself is normal, maternal conditions such as poor nutrition and severe anaemia may limit the availability of nutrients for the fetus, resulting in decreased growth.

FETAL FACTORS

Fetal factors may also be a causative element such as chromosomal abnormalities, congenital fetal anomalies and intrauterine infection. These are more likely to be the cause of growth restriction if fetal growth is found to be less than expected prior to 28 weeks. In these cases, the fetus has an intrinsic problem with growth, not due to a lack of nutrients, and this is likely to present before 28 weeks with concordant growth between the abdominal and head circumference.

 SGA Detected before 24 Weeks Gestation

Specialist referral is indicated to investigate for cause:

- Structural defects – investigated via a detailed ultrasound scan.
- Chromosomal abnormalities – amniocentesis and free fetal DNA may be performed.
- Infection (for example, cytomegalovirus (CMV), toxoplasmosis and parvovirus) – maternal blood and amniocentesis. Other tests may include culturing, DNA polymerase chain reaction (PCR) or antigen assays.

RISK FACTORS FOR POOR FETAL GROWTH

Maternal prenatal risk factors:
- Diabetes.
- Smoking.
- Age more than 40 years.
- Previous child with IUGR.
- Previous stillbirth or IUD.
- Chronic hypertension.
- Renal disease.
- Systemic lupus erythematosus.

These influences are all independent risk factors for FGR from placental insufficiency. They warrant serial growth scans rather than SFH measurements. Ideally, the modifiable risk factors should be optimised pre-pregnancy or in the early antenatal period to reduce the risk of FGR.

Antenatal risk factors:
- Low PAPP-A – identified during screening for Down syndrome.
- Echogenic bowel – identified during the anomaly scan. Although the pathophysiology of this is poorly understood, echogenic bowel is associated with chromosomal abnormalities, cystic fibrosis and IUGR.
- Pre-eclampsia.
- Unexplained APH or heavy bleeding in early pregnancy.

If any of these are identified in the pregnancy, serial growth scans should also be arranged.

INVESTIGATIONS

Once a fetus has been identified as being at risk of IUGR, increased monitoring is required to optimise the timing of birth. There is a balance between delivering the baby early with the increased risks due to problems associated with prematurity or prolonging the pregnancy where there is a risk of further placental insufficiency and stillbirth.

To help guide management decisions, ultrasound scanning is performed:
- Measurements of fetal growth are performed every 2 weeks.
- Umbilical artery Doppler – if this is normal, it is repeated every 2 weeks. If it is severely abnormal, this may be repeated daily or indicate the need for delivery.

Other investigations are also considered in individual cases to support clinical decision making, but the evidence for their use in reducing mortality in SGA fetuses is less robust:
- Liquor volume assessment on ultrasound scan.
- Computerised CTG analysis (analysis demonstrating normal short-term variability in the fetal heart rate is a reassuring sign of fetal well-being).

UMBILICAL ARTERY DOPPLER IN PREGNANCY

The umbilical arteries are the two arteries which leave the fetus at the umbilicus, carrying deoxygenated blood to the placenta. The single umbilical vein then returns oxygenated and nutrient-rich blood from the placenta to the fetus. In a healthy pregnancy, the blood flow through the umbilical arteries should occur in one direction at all times, just like in an adult. During fetal systole, blood is pushed along the arteries by the fetal heart, and then during diastole, the elastic recoil of the arteries allows blood flow to continue throughout the entire cardiac cycle.

However, when there is a problem with the vasculature of the placenta, there is less surface area for nutrient transfer, and the fetal blood pressure within the placenta increases, which can then reduce blood flow to the placenta along the umbilical arteries. It is at the end of diastole where the BP in the umbilical vessels is at its lowest, so this is where it is first seen.

As the placental function deteriorates and pressure within the placenta increases, the waveform of the umbilical Doppler changes (Fig. 14.6), indicating to the clinician the worsening of the situation, allowing for appropriate timing of birth.
- In the normal waveform, the peak represents blood flow during systole, and the trough is blood flow in diastole.

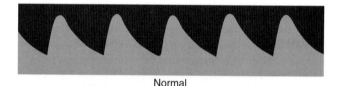

Normal

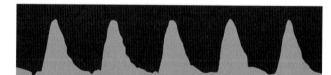

Reduced end diastolic flow (raised resistance index)

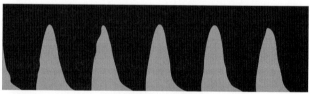

Absent end diastolic flow

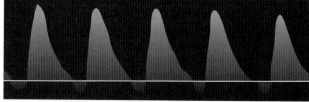

Reversed end diastolic flow

Fig. 14.6 Umbilical Artery Doppler Changes.

- In the second waveform, the trough at the end of the diastole is clearly lower than that in the first picture, indicating that the pressure in the placenta is increased which causes resistance, therefore reducing blood flow in the umbilical artery at the end of the diastole. In clinical practice, visualising a reduced flow is difficult, so a computer calculation is used based on the difference between the peaks and the troughs; this is called the resistance index. If a raised resistance index is found, increased monitoring of the pregnancy is needed (Fig. 14.7).

- The third waveform is the next progression in the deterioration of placental function and increased placental pressure. Here, the pressure in the placenta is equal to that of the umbilical artery pressure at the end of diastole, so there is no pressure differential, and there is no blood flow. It is important to understand the risk of compromise this signifies since diastole represents two-thirds of the cardiac cycle. Specifically in the aforementioned case, the waveform shows that for approximately half of diastole, there is no blood flow, meaning that for one-third of the entire cardiac cycle, there is no blood flow.

- The fourth waveform shows a reverse peak in the waveform at the end of the diastole. This is demonstrating that pressure in the placenta at the end of fetal diastole is now higher than it is in the umbilical artery, so blood is now flowing backward in the vessels. This is a very compromising position for the fetus. Not only is blood not flowing for one-third of the cycle, but now deoxygenated blood that is reverse flowing has to be pumped a second time along the same artery. This is not sustainable and is a clear indication of impending fetal compromise. Birth is usually expedited to prevent IUD.

💡 Other Doppler Investigations

Prior to 32 weeks gestation, where the umbilical artery Doppler shows absent or reversed end diastolic flow, the blood flow through the ductus venosus can also be reviewed. If this is normal, the obstetrician will discuss the option of continuing the pregnancy up to 32 weeks. If it is abnormal, birth will usually be expedited.

The middle cerebral artery Doppler can also be assessed. It is most commonly used to diagnose fetal anaemia but may have some use in aiding delivery timing in the SGA fetus.

MANAGEMENT

STEROIDS

Steroids for fetal lung maturation should be administered antenatally if IUGR is identified prior to 35 weeks gestation, as there is an increased possibility of preterm delivery.

Additionally, if under 30 weeks gestation, magnesium sulphate is given for neuroprotection during labour.

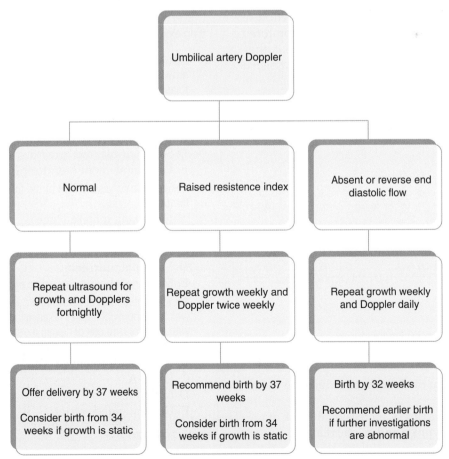

Fig. 14.7 Recommendations by RCOG During Investigation of IUGR.

TIMING OF BIRTH

Balancing the risk of prematurity against the risk of IUD is the key task of the obstetrician, with Doppler abnormalities playing a large role in the delivery decision of the growth-restricted fetus. Once gestation reaches 37 weeks, while there is minimal risk of prematurity, the risk of IUD is still raised in IUGR, even with normal Dopplers. For this reason, birth is offered at 37 weeks. If IUGR is not diagnosed until after 37 weeks, birth is offered at the time of diagnosis. In cases of SGA, birth is advised at 37 weeks for a fetus below the 3rd centile, with birth by 39 weeks advised if below the 10th centile.

UK guidelines also state that if there is no growth on ultrasound scan after 34 weeks gestation, delivery should be offered even in the presence of normal umbilical artery Doppler.

Where there is growth restriction and significant umbilical artery Doppler changes, birth will usually be advised by 32 weeks or sooner if ductus venosus Doppler is abnormal.

MODE OF BIRTH

A growth-restricted fetus is already compromised to a degree. It is therefore less likely to cope with the increased stress of labour. Caesarean should be offered for fetuses with absent or reversed end diastolic flow on umbilical Doppler assessment. Other growth-restricted fetuses can be considered for induction of labour, but they should be continuously monitored with CTG, and there is a higher chance that they will need either an emergency caesarean or assisted vaginal birth due to suspected fetal compromise in labour.

Uterine Artery Dopplers

These Dopplers differ from umbilical artery Dopplers and should not be confused. Where a woman has three or more minor risk factors for IUGR, then uterine artery Doppler exams should be carried out. Evidence has shown that if these are abnormal at 20 to 24 weeks gestation, then the pregnancy is at an increased risk of being complicated by IUGR and further indicates the requirements for intensive investigation and monitoring with more regular growth scans throughout the pregnancy.

COMPLICATIONS

In IUGR, there is an increased risk of:
- Structural or chromosomal fetal anomaly.
- Stillbirth.
- Iatrogenic preterm birth, often to reduce the risk of stillbirth.
- Intrapartum fetal distress, increasing the risk of:
  - Intrapartum hypoxia and acidaemia.

- Assisted vaginal birth.
- Caesarean birth.
- Neonatal complications such as infection, hypothermia, respiratory distress, hypoglycaemia or hypocalcaemia.
- Impaired neurodevelopment.
- Type 2 diabetes mellitus (T2DM) and coronary heart disease in the child's later life.

PROGNOSIS

The prognosis of the baby depends on the extent of FGR and the gestation at which birth is indicated. SGA babies with concordant growth usually have a good outcome. However, babies who have asymmetrical growth restriction (where the head and abdominal circumference measurements are on different centiles) or absent or reversed diastolic blood flow detected on umbilical artery, Dopplers have a worse outcome.

❓ QUESTIONS

Kaitlin, a 24-year-old woman, gravidity two, parity one, is at 28 weeks gestation, and the midwife finds that her SFH is smaller than expected. She is referred for a growth ultrasound scan. Her current pregnancy has so far been uneventful, and she has no significant past medical history. Her previous pregnancy also had no issues, and her son, now aged 3, was born by vaginal birth at term with no complications. During the scan, the obstetrician notes that the EFW is lower than expected.

Q1   Following the abnormalities detected in this ultrasound growth scan, which investigation should now be conducted to assess the well-being of the fetus?
A Fetal CTG.
B SFH measurements.
C Umbilical artery Doppler.
D Serial ultrasound growth scans.
E Fetal movement monitoring.

Q2   Answer true or false: Which of the following are risk factors for IUGR?
A Increasing maternal age.
B Maternal illegal drug use.
C Raised maternal BP.
D Maternal nutrition.
E Maternal rhesus-negative status.

Q3   If Kaitlin opted for first-trimester screening, a low level of which biochemical marker taken is independently associated with an increased risk of having a growth-restricted baby?
A hCG.
B Alpha fetoprotein (AFP).
C PAPP-A.
D Inhibin-A.
E Unconjugated estriol.

[Answers on page 418.]

HAEMOLYTIC DISEASE OF THE FETUS AND NEWBORN

Haemolytic disease of the fetus and newborn (HDFN) is an alloimmune condition where maternal IgG antibodies cross the placenta into the fetal circulation, attach to the corresponding antigen on erythrocytes and destroy fetal red blood cells by haemolysis in the fetal reticuloendothelial system. The rate of haemolysis determines the severity of the disease.

Amongst others, the ABO, rhesus and Kell antigen systems classify blood groups. The maternal immune system can produce IgG antibodies against any of these blood groups and cause HDFN.

PATHOPHYSIOLOGY

SENSITISING

When the immune system comes into contact with a non-self antigen, such as those expressed on a bacteria, virus or a transplanted organ from a donor, antibodies are developed to mount an immune response (Fig. 14.8). The B cell lymphocytes expressing the specific antibody to the non-self-antigen binds to the antigen, activating the B cell. This results in massive reproduction of that type of B cell. These B cells (now called plasma cells) begin producing IgM antibodies. If the antigen is not destroyed by the immune system quickly, T helper lymphocytes will modulate the plasma cells to produce the more specific IgG antibodies. Once the antigen has been removed from the body, the immune response regresses, but some of the plasma cells become memory cells. In the event of the same antigen entering the body again, these memory cells will recognise the antigen and immediately begin producing IgG, producing a faster, larger and more specific response than at the time of the initial antigen presentation. This theory is essential to understand how vaccinations work.

In pregnancy, small amounts of fetal tissue, such as red blood cells, enter the maternal circulation. There are a number of 'sensitising events' which can occur, leading to a significant amount of fetal blood entering the maternal circulation. The maternal immune system can then identify a non-self antigen from fetal red blood cells and then generate an immune response. As described above, the initial response is production of IgM. IgM does not cross the placenta, so it does not affect the fetus. The fetal cells in the maternal blood are destroyed by the immune system, and the immune response subsides. However, memory cells are produced.

In a subsequent pregnancy, if even a small amount of the same type of non-self antigen (fetal blood) enters the maternal circulation, memory cells will identify this and produce large amounts of IgG. IgG crosses the placenta. It then binds to the fetal antigen, which is predominantly on red cells. The primitive fetal immune system then destroys its own red cells, causing fetal anaemia. This is HDFN.

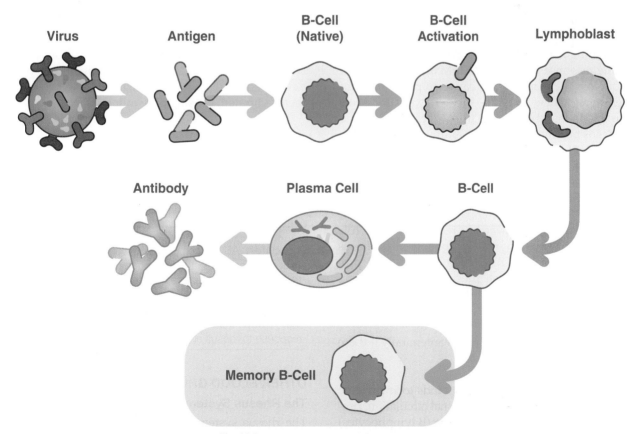

Fig. 14.8 Heamolytic disease of the newborn.

BLOOD GROUPS

As just described, it is fetal red cell antigens that the maternal immune system identifies as non-self, resulting in an immune response in HDFN. Half of the fetal DNA is from the mother, so antigens produced by the fetus of maternal origin will be identified as self by the maternal immune system. However, if the genes passed on by the father produce red cell antigens not present in the mother, these will be identified as non-self by the maternal immune system if there is a sensitising event.

Red cell antigens determine a person's blood group. The ABO blood system is the most significant grouping system for adult crossmatching. This divides blood into type A, B, AB and O, with the type of blood determined by the antigens present on the surface of red blood cells. Additionally, there are many other antigens that may be present in red blood cells. The most important of these additional antigens for HDFN is the rhesus D antigen, otherwise known as the rhesus status of an individual's blood; rhesus positive, where rhesus D antigens are present on the surface of red blood cells and rhesus negative, when they are absent.

RHESUS INCOMPATIBILITY IN HAEMOLYTIC DISEASE OF THE FETUS AND NEWBORN

Approximately 15% of the population lack D antigen and are therefore rhesus negative. If a pregnant woman with rhesus-negative blood group were to come into contact with a foreign rhesus D antigen (sensitising event, for example, rhesus-positive fetal red cells entering maternal circulation), the body forms an immune response initially with IgM antibodies. These do not cross the placenta and cause no problem in the current pregnancy. But if a further exposure event occurs in a subsequent pregnancy, where that fetus is also rhesus positive, the mother's immune system then produces IgG antibodies. These then cross the placenta and cause HDFN.

In the past, as rhesus-negative blood group is so common, HDFN was most commonly caused by rhesus D blood group incompatibilities between the mother and fetus. However, appreciation for the role of previous sensitisation in the pathogenesis of rhesus haemolytic disease has resulted in a successful prophylaxis regimen. Now, all rhesus-negative mothers are offered IM injection of anti-D:

- Antenatally at 28 weeks gestation.
- At birth.
- Further doses may also be given antenatally if there are sensitising events.

The exogenous anti-D antibody binds to any rhesus D antigen (fetal blood) in the maternal circulation, preventing the maternal immune system (B lymphocytes) from identifying the rhesus antigen. Sensitisation does not occur, and the mother's immune system does not mount a response, so memory cells are not produced, preventing HDFN in a future pregnancy.

As a result of this effective prophylaxis program, rhesus D isoimmunisation in the UK now only tends to occur after inadequate doses of prophylactic anti-D are given or there is a missed sensitising event prior to birth.

THE ABO SYSTEM

Following the success of this prophylactic treatment in preventing rhesus haemolytic disease, fetomaternal ABO blood group incompatibility is now the leading cause of immunogenic HDFN.

ABO incompatibility occurs in 20% to 25% of pregnancies, but haemolysis develops in only a minority of cases, and the resulting HDFN is milder than in rhesus incompatibility. ABO haemolytic disease occurs when fetal erythrocytes contain blood group A or B antibodies and the mother is blood group O. Normally, group O humans have large amounts of anti-A and anti-B isohaemagglutinins (antibodies) circulating in their blood, which is predominantly IgM. These IgM antibodies do not cross the placenta and, in most cases, bind to the antigen on the fetal red cells and destroy them before B cells identify the antigen and generate a further immune response. However, a minority of group O women possess IgG antibodies (rather than IgM) against group A or B antigens without previous sensitisation. These can cross the placenta, and therefore, even a woman's first pregnancy can be affected by ABO haemolytic disease. No current treatments exist to prevent ABO incompatibility-mediated haemolytic disease. Fortunately, in the few cases of ABO HDFN, because fetal red cell AB antigens are poorly developed *in utero*, the maternal immune response to them is limited, causing only mild HDFN.

Interestingly, ABO incompatibility is extremely rare in blood group A mothers carrying a B blood group fetus or vice versa. This is because the mother's immune system has circulating IgM antibodies and does not mount a significant IgG response to the blood group antigen.

 Concurrent ABO Incompatibility

Concurrent ABO incompatibility, along with other antigen exposure, prevents the mother from becoming sensitised to these other antigens, as the fetal erythrocytes are swiftly coated by isohaemagglutinins with preexisting anti-A and/or anti-B antibodies found in maternal serum. This results in their removal from the maternal circulation before an immune response to rhesus antigens can be generated.

OTHER BLOOD GROUP SYSTEMS

The Rhesus System

The rhesus system is not just D antigens. It consists of genes of paired alleles (C/c, D/d, E/e) following

Mendelian inheritance. Homozygous dominant (DD) or heterozygous (Dd) individuals express the D-antigen and are rhesus D positive. Homozygous recessive (dd) individuals do not express the D antigen and thus are susceptible to sensitisation if a foreign D antigen is present. C and E antigens cause sensitisation in the same way, with an initial IgM response on first exposure and a rapid IgG response in a subsequent pregnancy. They are, however, less likely to cause significant HDFN.

The Kell System

Anti-Kell antibodies cause the second most common form of severe HDFN. More than 50% of cases are believed to be due to women having developed the IgG antibody following multiple blood transfusions.

Other blood group antibodies, such as Kidd, Lewis, Duffy and P, exist but are very rare, and when they do occur, they usually cause only mild HDFN. Therefore, many countries currently deem it uneconomical to screen for them.

SENSITISING EVENTS

As most sensitising events involve fetal blood entering the maternal circulation, the pregnancy in which the event occurs is not usually affected by the maternal immune response, but any subsequent pregnancy can be. However, first pregnancies can still develop HDFN, as some women naturally have red cell antibodies, while others develop them following blood transfusions (blood is matched to the recipient as best it can be, but there are always small antigenic differences).

The extent of the maternal antibody response depends on the dose of immunising antigen present. Hence, HDFN only develops after a significant transplacental bleed (more than 1 mL of rhesus-positive cells).

Even where none of the sensitising events occur (Table 14.4), fetal erythrocytes can still reach the maternal circulation, as the physical barrier of the cytotrophoblast regresses in the third trimester. This is why anti-D is offered at 28 weeks.

Table **14.4**	Interventions and Pregnancy Events Where Sensitisation Can Occur
Interventions where fetal blood can enter the maternal circulation	Pregnancy events where fetal blood can enter the maternal circulation
• Termination of pregnancy • Evacuation of retained products of conception after miscarriage • Amniocentesis or chorionic villous sampling • External cephalic version	• Antepartum haemorrhage (especially placental abruption) • Abdominal trauma (can cause concealed placental abruption) • Intrauterine death • Fetomaternal haemorrhage during birth

ROUTINE PREGNANCY MANAGEMENT

Management to reduce the chance of rhesus sensitisation is required antenatally (Table 14.5) and postnatally.

ANTENATALLY

Anti-D should be given within 72 hours of any sensitising event. If a large sensitising event is suspected, a Kleihauer blood test can be taken from the mother. This quantifies the amount of fetal blood present in the maternal circulation following a fetomaternal haemorrhage, so further anti-D can be given, if required, to account for all the D antigens and prevent maternal sensitisation.

AT BIRTH

In rhesus-negative mothers, blood is taken from the cord at birth to test the fetal blood group. If the neonate is rhesus positive, maternal blood is taken postnatally and a Kleihauer test performed, measuring the degree of fetal blood mixing with maternal blood. The required dose of anti-D can be calculated (based on degree of mixing) and given to the mother to prevent sensitisation after a potential fetomaternal bleed during parturition.

MANAGEMENT OF HIGH-RISK PREGNANCIES

- If abnormal antibodies are detected in either the 12- or 28- week bloods, then increased monitoring will be required, as the fetus is at risk of the antibodies crossing the placenta and causing haemolysis.
- The risk of haemolysis occurring and to what severity will be determined by the type of antibody and

Table **14.5**	Summary of Routine Antenatal Management to Screen and Prevent Possible Blood Group Incompatibility
WEEKS OF GESTATION	**MANAGEMENT**
6–12 (booking bloods)	Amongst other booking blood tests, expectant mothers have a group and save taken to identify maternal blood group. The blood is also screened for rhesus and the other HDFN-causing antibodies.
28	Along with a full blood count, another group and save is obtained. Maternal blood group and antibodies are checked again, as antibody concentrations can increase in the pregnancy that were not detectable at the time of the booking bloods. A prophylactic dose of anti-D is given to rhesus-negative women (single IM injection).

HDFN, Haemolytic disease of the fetus and newborn; *IM*, intramuscular.

the concentration (titre) in the maternal serum. The frequency of the following antenatal investigations will also be determined by these parameters:

- Maternal antibody titre levels will be monitored regularly (every 2 to 4 weeks).
- Fetal ultrasound monitoring for growth and evidence of fetal haemolytic anaemia (usually performed in the fetal medicine unit).

If fetal anaemia occurs, this can initially be compensated for by increasing the fetal cardiac output. The first sign of this is increased velocity of blood flow in the middle cerebral artery using Doppler ultrasound.

If fetal anaemia becomes more severe, the fetus tries to compensate even more by retaining fluid in an attempt to increase cardiac output (essentially the same process of increasing preload as in an adult). This leads to oedema (caused by a combination of raised hydrostatic pressure and decreased osmotic pressure) that can be in any of the body compartments (cranium, thorax, pelvis, amniotic fluid). This can be seen on ultrasound scan and is called hydrops fetalis. This condition is preterminal. The fetus is in high-output cardiac failure, with no further reserve to increase output. The oedema is damaging and preventing growth of the fetal organs, and the fetal heart is failing to adequately circulate sufficient oxygenated blood for fetal survival.

The management of fetal anaemia will be dependent on severity and gestation:

- Once the fetus is beyond 36 weeks, there is a low risk of neonatal complications following birth due to prematurity. Hence, delivery is advised upon any signs of fetal anaemia.
- Mild anaemia in earlier gestations may be managed expectantly with close observation.
- Severe anaemia in an earlier gestation could be treated in one of two ways:
  - Intrauterine blood transfusion injected into the umbilical vein can be given to correct the fetal anaemia and prolong the pregnancy. The risk of this is fetal haemorrhage, infection and IUD.
  - Deliver the fetus and transfuse. The risk is the morbidity and mortality associated with prematurity.

COMPLICATIONS

If HDFN occurs to a small degree, there will be no intrauterine effects, and it might only be identified after birth. However, if there is a greater degree of haemolysis, this will affect the fetus in utero.

IN UTERO COMPLICATIONS

In utero initiation of immune-mediated fetal erythrocyte lysis causes progressive anaemia leading to intrauterine cardiac failure and peripheral oedema. The resulting intrauterine fluid accumulation can vary from localised oedema to the potentially lethal condition, hydrops fetalis, characterised by progressive, generalised fetal oedema.

NEONATAL COMPLICATIONS

Anaemia can be treated in the newborn with blood transfusions, immunoglobulin or exchange transfusions. Hyperbilirubinaemia may also occur, leading to neonatal jaundice, and if the bilirubin levels are higher than the recommended threshold, phototherapy may be needed. This uses high-frequency blue light to isomerise *trans*-bilirubin to the more water-soluble *cis*-bilirubin, which can be excreted into bile.

Jaundice caused by rhesus disease can be very severe. If phototherapy is unsuccessful, or the bilirubin is very high, exchange transfusions can be performed. This involves the removal of vials of fetal blood and replacement with bilirubin-free donor blood. IV immunoglobulin (IVIG) can also be used. The fetus gradually degrades maternal IgG, and the jaundice resolves. IVIG is used in jaundice that is refractory to phototherapy.

Kernicterus is a rare but serious complication of HDFN. Untreated or unsuccessfully treated neonatal hyperbilirubinaemia can lead to kernicterus. This is bilirubin-induced brain dysfunction, most commonly occurring after a rapid rise in bilirubin levels in the first 24 hours after birth. Bilirubin can cross the blood–brain barrier, accumulate in the basal ganglia of the central nervous system and cause potentially irreversible neurological impairment.

 Hydrops Fetalis

Hydrops is a serious condition defined as abnormal fluid accumulation in two or more fetal compartments, for example, pleural effusion, ascites and skin oedema.

There are two forms:

- Immune hydrops fetalis – this is a complication of severe rhesus incompatibility, leading to severe anaemia and high-output cardiac failure.
- Nonimmune hydrops fetalis – this occurs when a disease or medical condition disrupts the fetus' ability to manage fluid. The main causes for this are severe respiratory or cardiovascular diseases, thalassaemia, genetic defects such as Turner syndrome and certain intrauterine infections such as parvovirus.

PROGNOSIS

Administration of exogenous anti-D to rhesus-negative pregnant women prevents the production of maternal anti-D antibody, reducing isoimmunisation rates in first pregnancies from 1.5% to 0.2%. As a result, the mortality rate from fetal haemolytic disease is now down to 0.02 per 1000 births. With the screening techniques currently available, it is possible to detect fetal anaemia early and treat it before potentially lethal complications such as hydrops fetalis develop. Effective use of phototherapy and exchange transfusion therapy for treating hyperbilirubinaemia in babies has significantly reduced some of the major complications of fetal erythrocyte haemolysis that result from HDFN.

？ QUESTIONS

Pardeep, a 29-year-old woman, gravidity two, parity one, presents to the emergency department after falling over. She is at 20 weeks gestation and is concerned that she may have injured her baby. Her current pregnancy has been uneventful to date, and 2 years ago she gave birth to her first child without complications. She is blood group AB and rhesus negative.

QUESTIONS

Q1 HDFN is due to a hypersensitivity pathophysiology of which type?
   A Type I hypersensitivity.
   B Type II hypersensitivity.
   C Type III hypersensitivity.
   D Type IV hypersensitivity.
   E Type V hypersensitivity.

Q2 Answer true or false: Which of the following increase the chance of alloimmunisation sensitisation for HDFN?
   A Previous birth of rhesus D-positive neonate.
   B Gestational diabetes.
   C Amniocentesis.
   D Maternal nutrition.
   E Trauma.

Q3 At which week(s) of gestation should exogenous anti-D antibody be given to rhesus D-negative women with no history of sensitising events?
   A 12 weeks.
   B 24 weeks.
   C 28 weeks.
   D 32 weeks.
   E 36 weeks.

[Answers on page 419.]

CONGENITAL INTRAUTERINE INFECTIONS

Congenital intrauterine infections are vertically transmitted infections passed directly from the mother to the fetus. They can occur at any time throughout pregnancy, labour and birth and may result in significant long-term sequelae for the neonate. Some of these infections are routinely tested for during pregnancy, but often they are investigated in cases where neonatal death or stillbirth of unknown cause has occurred. This section will cover common infections; however, there are separate sections covering HIV and hepatitis in pregnancy.

[See 'Stillbirth' on page 330.]

[See 'HIV in Pregnancy' on page 244.]

[See 'Hepatitis B in Pregnancy' on page 242.]

The mnemonic TORCH is used to remember the most common pathogens:
- Toxoplasmosis.
- Other – syphilis, varicella zoster, parvovirus B19, hepatitis B and HIV.
- Rubella.
- CMV.
- Herpes infections.

In a healthy pregnant woman, the immune response is physiologically downregulated to prevent rejection of the pregnancy. This makes women more susceptible to pathogens, leading to complications for both fetus and mother.

 Antibodies in Infection

For all infections, maternal IgM antibodies are present in the short period coinciding with the acute phase of the infection, primarily within the first few weeks of most infections, whereby they increase rapidly and then decline. IgG antibodies are produced later in the course of infection, often detected after a few weeks of the initial infection but then persist for life, even if an infection is completely eradicated. If there is clinical suspicion of a particular infection in pregnancy, stored blood samples obtained during appointments throughout the pregnancy (usually the booking appointment bloods, as these are routinely stored for the duration of the pregnancy) can be tested retrospectively for the presence of IgG antibodies. The presence of antibodies in the stored sample indicates previous exposure and acquired immunity. The absence of antibodies in the booking bloods, but presence of IgM or IgG antibodies in a more recent serum sample, suggests a recent infection.

TOXOPLASMOSIS (TOXOPLASMA GONDII)

AETIOLOGY

Toxoplasmosis is classically acquired through exposure to cat faeces (oocysts), farm animals such as lamb or calves and ingestion of undercooked meats. Being immunocompromised is the primary risk factor for acquiring toxoplasmosis. Maternal infection during pregnancy may result in the protozoa crossing the placenta and infecting the fetus.

CLINICAL FEATURES

Maternal – the mother may be asymptomatic or present with flulike symptoms. On physical examination, she may have swollen posterior cervical lymph glands. In complicated cases, ocular toxoplasmosis may present with signs of retinochoroiditis, anterior uveitis and scleritis. Immunocompromised patients are especially susceptible to life-threatening infection and may present with encephalitis.

Fetal – fetal congenital infection results in a triad of chorioretinitis, intracranial calcification and hydrocephalus. Ocular disease normally manifests as persisting visual impairment or blindness. Central nervous system involvement can cause seizures to develop in the neonate. As time progresses, developmental delay and deafness may also be noticed. Toxoplasmosis can also cause miscarriage, IUD and fetal structural abnormalities. Transmission risk and phenotype severity both vary by trimester. While miscarriage is less likely to occur as the pregnancy advances, transmission rates increase. In the first trimester, the risk of transmission is approximately 10% to 15%. By the second trimester, the risk increases to 25%, and by the third trimester, it can be as high as 70% to 80%.

INVESTIGATIONS

- Maternal antibodies – IgM and IgG.
- PCR looking for toxoplasmosis in blood, body tissues and fluids.
- Ultrasound to check for fetal abnormalities in the event of confirmed or suspected vertical transmission.
- Amniocentesis – PCR test can be done on amniotic fluid to detect toxoplasmosis in the fetus.
- CT or MRI head scans may be used to identify ring-enhancing lesions in the mother.

MANAGEMENT

When toxoplasmosis is diagnosed in a pregnant mother, termination may be an option. If the couple opts to continue with pregnancy, treatment with spiramycin is recommended to try and prevent congenital infection.

If congenital infection is confirmed, treatment for mothers and newborns includes pyrimethamine, sulphadiazine and calcium folinate.

Pyrimethamine inhibits the dihydrofolate reductase needed by protozoa for DNA synthesis. It has teratogenic effects and enters breast milk. If pyrimethamine is needed during pregnancy, folic acid supplementation is recommended.

Sulphadiazine also inhibits folic acid synthesis (by a different mechanism), thus inhibiting growth. Breastfeeding is contraindicated, as sulphadiazine also enters breast milk.

Calcium folinate is a form of folic acid that helps supply the body with the cofactors inhibited by the above-described drugs.

Neonates require long-term follow-up from paediatric neurologists for epilepsy and global developmental delay, and from an ophthalmologist for chorioretinitis, as these complications may develop at any time up to the second decade of life.

ERYTHEMA INFECTIOSUM – PARVOVIRUS B19

AETIOLOGY

This viral infection is extremely common, transmitted primarily through respiratory secretions, usually between children in early childhood. It is colloquially referred to as 'slapped cheek syndrome' due to the classical transient facial rash. Mothers will usually have been infected themselves as children and will have developed lifelong immunity (IgG), meaning that they are unlikely to contract it during pregnancy. However, in the rare case where a mother is not immune, vertical transmission across the placenta may occur from mother to fetus. Infectivity begins 10 days before the rash and continues until the rash appears (Fig. 14.9).

CLINICAL FEATURES

Maternal – the classical rash of parvovirus B19 is uniform, maculopapular lesions on the cheeks ('slapped cheek' appearance), more commonly seen in infants than adults. Patients are usually asymptomatic or have minimal flulike symptoms. Rare complications include arthritis, aplastic crisis, myocarditis, meningitis, encephalitis and peripheral neuropathy.

Fetus – parvovirus B19 is associated with high rates of fetal complications. In the first trimester, there is an increased risk of miscarriage. At later gestations, infection can cause intrauterine fetal demise, hydrops fetalis, polyhydramnios, anaemia, myocarditis, hepatomegaly and pancytopenia. Most of these complications occur because parvovirus B19 causes red blood cell destruction, leading to severe anaemia and resulting in high-output cardiac failure, fluid retention and oedema.

INVESTIGATIONS

Serology may be conducted to investigate the presence of parvovirus B19-specific IgM and B19-specific IgG.

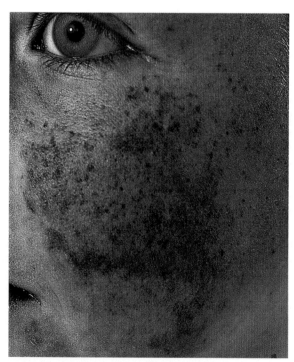

Fig. 14.9 A typical face rash of parvovirus B19 infection.

PCR may also be done to look specifically for parvovirus B19 viral DNA. Most patients will be immune, with IgG present in the booking bloods, meaning no further action is necessary.

MANAGEMENT

If the mother develops parvovirus B19, the fetus should be monitored with regular ultrasound scanning looking for signs of fetal anaemia, polyhydramnios, hydrops and poor growth. Depending on the results and gestation, intrauterine blood transfusion, fluid drainage or early delivery may be considered.

In general, if hydrops fetalis does not occur, there is unlikely to be long-term developmental complications arising from this infection. In mothers, this is a self-limiting infection that does not usually have long-term sequelae.

CHICKENPOX – VARICELLA ZOSTER (HERPES FAMILY)

AETIOLOGY

Varicella zoster virus is primarily transmitted through airborne respiratory secretions and vesicular fluid. For maternal infection with chickenpox to occur, mothers must have had no previous chickenpox infection or vaccination and have close contact with an infected individual, as significant exposure is required. Significant exposure is defined as contact in the same room for 15 minutes or more, face-to-face contact or contact in the setting of a large open ward. Infectivity begins from 48 hours before the classic rash appears and continues until vesicles crust over approximately 5 days later. Reactivation of varicella in mothers causing shingles is of no risk to the fetus.

CLINICAL FEATURES

Maternal – the classic feature of this infection is the pruritic rash. It typically progresses from macules to papules, to vesicles, to crusting lesions. The incubation period is 10 to 20 days, and the most important maternal complication is varicella pneumonia, signs and symptoms of which include cough, fever and tachypnoea. This condition can rapidly progress to hypoxia and respiratory failure. Hepatitis and encephalitis are also maternal complications to be aware of.

Fetus – fetal varicella syndrome (FVS) can develop in the fetus if maternal infection occurs before 28 weeks gestation. Chorioretinitis, cataracts, microphthalmia (small eyes), skin scarring, hypoplasia of limbs and neurological abnormalities (intellectual disability and microcephaly) may occur.

Varicella infection in the newborn can develop if maternal infection occurs after 28 weeks gestation, with the highest risk within 4 weeks of birth. If possible, birth should be delayed for at least 7 days after the onset of maternal rash.

INVESTIGATIONS

Typically, clinical examination is enough for diagnosis. In some cases where additional investigations are needed, a sample via scraping of a lesion may be taken for PCR.

Where there has been possible exposure but no symptoms, serological testing can also be performed. IgM suggests recent infection, whereas IgG suggests previous vaccination or previous infection. The majority of women who do not give a clear history of chickenpox infection will have positive IgG on a booking sample, indicating that they have previously cleared the virus.

MANAGEMENT

Prevention and vaccination – when identified, varicella-naive women planning pregnancy should be vaccinated (two doses, 4 to 8 weeks apart) and avoid becoming pregnant in the first 4 weeks of having the vaccine whilst also avoiding contact with pregnant nonimmune women if a rash occurs postvaccination. Vaccination should be avoided during pregnancy, as the vaccine is live and carries a risk of causing congenital disease.

- Varicella zoster immunoglobulin (VZIg) should be administered to nonimmune pregnant women with significant exposure up to 10 days after the initial contact. Treatment aims to prevent the development of infection. VZIg is of no benefit in symptomatic patients.
- Aciclovir can be given under specialist care if chickenpox begins to develop and presentation is within 24 hours of rash.
- Women who are symptomatic or asymptomatic with significant exposure should be treated away from other pregnant women to avoid spread.
- Neonates should be administered VZIg in the event of significant exposure where a nonimmune mother has signs and symptoms of infection within 7 days of birth or up to 4 days after birth. This is to prevent the development of newborn varicella infection. In a symptomatic newborn, aciclovir may be given.
- Fetal varicella syndrome has a mortality close to 30% despite treatment. Many of those that survive have significant developmental delay. In comparison, maternal outcomes are very good, with mortality rates around 2 to 4 per 100,000.

SYPHILIS – TREPONEMA PALLIDUM (SPIROCHETE)

AETIOLOGY

This spirochete is acquired by the mother through sexual contact and subsequently crosses the placenta to reach the fetus. Transplacental transmission occurs in almost 90% of untreated women. Early detection is important, as it can be treated easily. Syphilis is screened for during the booking appointment as part of the routine antenatal screening in the UK.

CLINICAL FEATURES

Maternal

- Primary – single red indurated painless chancre, which turns into a painless ulcer with a raised border and serous exudate. These ulcers tend to heal spontaneously within 3 to 6 weeks without treatment.
- Secondary – disseminating process that occurs approximately from 6 weeks to 6 months from primary infection. This stage is characterised by symptoms of headaches, chills, fever, myalgia, arthralgia, malaise, photophobia, lymphadenopathy and a rash classically on the palms and soles.
- Latent – asymptomatic infection with positive serology and negative physical examination.
- Tertiary – cutaneous gummatous lesions, aortic aneurysms or insufficiency and neurosyphilis (cranial nerve dysfunction, meningitis and/or altered mental status.)

Fetal

T. pallidum can cross the placenta and infect the fetus as early as 14 weeks gestation. Infection may result in IUGR, hepatomegaly, thrombocytopenia, anaemia and ascites, with a subsequent risk of preterm birth, stillbirth and neonatal death. In neonates, common physical signs are lymphadenopathy, hepatosplenomegaly, bloody rhinitis, jaundice, anaemia, thrombocytopenia and bullous eruptions.

INVESTIGATIONS

Venereal disease research laboratory (VDRL) tests measure the level of antibodies to syphilis.

MANAGEMENT

Maternal – for infection in the first or second trimester, one dose of benzathine penicillin IM. In the third trimester, two doses of benzathine penicillin 1 week apart.

Neonate – the neonate requires a prolonged course of penicillin and further investigations if the mother is inadequately treated or if the neonate is symptomatic. Follow-up is needed for neonatal syphilis infection, with retreatment if necessary.

PROGNOSIS

Treatment is curative with fewer long-term complications the earlier the diagnosis is made.

RUBELLA – SINGLE-STRANDED RNA TOGAVIRUS

AETIOLOGY

Rubella, also known as German measles or 3-day measles, is a viral infection mostly controlled now due to the introduction of vaccination regimens. Within the UK, this virus is a notifiable disease once found or suspected. Transmission of this disease is mostly via infected respiratory secretions. Rubella was routinely screened for at antenatal booking appointments in the UK until 2016 when this was stopped, as the disease has been effectively eradicated from the UK due to the measles mumps and rubella (MMR) vaccination scheme in childhood.

CLINICAL FEATURES

Maternal – mothers may be entirely asymptomatic or have symptoms of a low-grade fever, headache and conjunctivitis. A maculopapular pink rash then begins to appear, starting on the face then spreading to the neck and trunk. In adults, arthralgia may be an accompanying symptom. This is most infectious from 7 days prerash to 5 days postrash.

Fetus – maternal infection within the first 10 to 16 weeks of pregnancy is associated with devastating effects on the fetus, with a 90% rate of congenital rubella syndrome (CRS). CRS can cause miscarriage, stillbirth or IUGR. In other cases, CRS can cause congenital defects, including cataracts and congenital glaucoma, cardiac malformations (for example, patent ductus arteriosus), haemorrhagic purpuric eruptions ('blueberry muffin baby'), hepatosplenomegaly, developmental delay and deafness. Maternal infection between 16 and 20 weeks carries a minimal risk of congenital deafness only, and infection after 20 weeks carries no documented risks.

INVESTIGATIONS

Clinical diagnosis is difficult due to symptoms being short-lived and the rash not being diagnostic. Rubella-specific IgM indicates primary infection, whereas IgG rises over a longer period if the patient is not already immune.

MANAGEMENT

In a woman with suspected infection, the first course of action is to seek specialist advice. Termination may be offered in IgM-positive cases within the first 16 weeks of pregnancy due to the significantly high risk of fetal complications. There have been suggestions in the literature for the use of immunoglobulins, but the efficacy is still uncertain. Currently, the use of immunoglobulins is suggested for women who decline a termination.

Neonates affected by CRS are managed primarily through supportive care and surveillance, as the sequelae of infection are both multifactorial and develop over time. Neonatal outcomes vary in terms of severity and number of defects. If a woman opts for termination after infection, vaccination should be advised and pregnancy avoided for a month after.

CYTOMEGALOVIRUS – DNA VIRUS (HERPES FAMILY)

AETIOLOGY

CMV is a common viral infection that usually causes mild to no symptoms in healthy individuals. This virus is also the most common congenital infection in infants. The virus is transmitted through bodily fluids, most commonly to the mother through sexual contact. Then, from the mother, CMV can be transmitted to the fetus through the placenta at any gestation, during birth or through breastfeeding.

CLINICAL FEATURES

Maternal – mothers typically present with flulike symptoms or are asymptomatic.

Fetus – in congenital infection, the fetus acquires cytomegalic inclusion disease, which causes multisystem dysfunction affecting the neurological, ophthalmological, endocrine and haematological systems. Ninety percent of newborns are asymptomatic at birth but later present with progressive hearing loss. The remaining 10% typically present with jaundice, splenomegaly and petechiae from thrombocytopenia. Other signs on examination may include microcephaly, retinitis and developmental delay.

INVESTIGATIONS

Investigations revolve around isolating CMV while detecting fetal abnormalities that may have been caused by the virus.
- Maternal serology – IgM suggests acute infection.
- Maternal or neonatal – viral cultures, PCR and molecular assays.
- Serial fetal ultrasound scans to look for features of congenital CMV infection. The most typical finding is periventricular calcifications. Other findings include cerebral ventriculomegaly, microcephaly, IUGR, cerebellar hypoplasia, periventricular echogenicity and hydrops.
- Neonates – urine culture and CT scan for central nervous system complications.

MANAGEMENT

In immunocompetent patients and pregnant women, supportive treatment is recommended and education provided on maintaining good hygiene. There is no treatment of proven benefit for congenital CMV, although IV ganciclovir and oral valganciclovir have been studied. The trials were abandoned because of severe maternal side effects.

PROGNOSIS

For congenital CMV, the prognosis depends on the number of complications and extent of involvement. Those born with cytomegalic inclusion disease have a poor prognosis. Between 50% and 60% of newborns born with congenital CMV have severe long-term neurological complications. In contrast, the outcomes for women with CMV are good.

HERPES SIMPLEX VIRUS (HSV-1 AND HSV-2) – DNA VIRUS

AETIOLOGY

This virus is acquired by the mother through mucocutaneous contact. The virus is usually transmitted to the fetus at the time of birth when the fetus comes into contact with active herpetic lesions in the vagina.

HSV infection can be classified into primary and recurrent genital infection. Primary infection close to the time of birth is an indicator for higher risk of transmission, whereas recurrent infection carries a very low risk of transmission with secondary herpes, as the fetus should be protected by maternal IgG.

CLINICAL FEATURES

Maternal – primary infection is characterised by a flu-like prodrome, accompanied by painful vesicular lesions. This initial episode is generally longer than future recurrences.

Fetal – third-trimester infection is associated with the highest chance of transmission to neonates during birth.

Neonatal HSV infection – risk of chorioretinitis, neurological involvement causing lethargy and seizures and vesicular skin lesions. Disseminated infection can quickly lead to jaundice, hepatosplenomegaly and disseminated intravascular coagulation.

INVESTIGATIONS

Maternal – in the mother, it is mostly a clinical diagnosis. Where necessary, viral culture or PCR can be used to confirm the diagnosis.

Neonatal – investigations include a lumbar puncture, FBC, CRP, LFTs, bilirubin, blood PCR and swabs of any cutaneous lesions.

MANAGEMENT
Maternal
- Conservative measures identical to those outside of pregnancy including:
  - Contact tracing and other STI screening in primary infections.
  - Analgesia and hygiene advice.
  - Advise specifically on methods to avoid pain on urination such as passing urine in the bath.
- Aciclovir can be offered to reduce the duration of the infection.
- Where there has been a primary infection in earlier pregnancy or the patient suffers from recurrent outbreaks, aciclovir can be offered prophylactically from 36 weeks gestation onwards through to delivery. This is to reduce reoccurrence at term.
- Primary infection in the last 6 weeks of pregnancy carries the highest risk of transmission during vaginal birth. Planneed caesarean should be offered in these cases to reduce neonatal infection. If primary lesions are present at the time of vaginal birth, the risk of transmission is 40%.

- The risk of transmission with active lesions from recurrent disease at the time of vaginal birth is much lower, around 1%. Women should be counselled on the options of vaginal birth or caesarean section.

Neonate

IV aciclovir is initiated from the moment the diagnosis is suspected. This clinical decision will need to be made by the paediatrics team.

Mortality and morbidity rates for disseminated and central nervous system disease are very high for infants, even if prompt treatment is given.

CHLAMYDIA

Untreated *C. trachomatis* infection has been linked to preterm labour, premature rupture of the membranes and IUGR. The most commonly identified neonatal complication of chlamydia is neonatal eye disease (in up to 50% of neonates born to mothers with chlamydia), which presents as a mucopurulent infective conjunctivitis with copious amounts of discharge. Systemic antibiotics need to be given to the neonate, as there is often a coexisting pneumonia (in up to 20% of neonates). Parents and any other sexual contacts (of the mother) will also need treatment.

[See 'Sexually Transmitted Infections' on page 124.]

LISTERIA

L. monocytogenes is the bacterium that causes listeriosis. Listeria is present in foods, such as soft cheeses, paté and unpasteurised milk. Maternal infection leads to a flulike syndrome or mimics gastroenteritis, and the pregnancy may end in miscarriage, stillbirth or preterm birth. Antibiotics (commonly ampicillin and gentamicin) can be given in a case of listeriosis. The best way to avoid infection is for pregnant women to be counselled regarding which foods to avoid when pregnant. If infection is acquired by the neonate, it manifests with signs of septicaemia and meningitis.

  Zika Virus

The Zika virus has been associated with congenital fetal abnormalities in women infected with the virus before or during pregnancy. The virus is often asymptomatic or causes mild flu-like symptoms in the mother. In contrast, in the fetus, the virus may cause microcephaly and mental retardation. The virus is transmitted by mosquitoes and is not endemic to the UK, but with significant world travel, many women from the UK are at risk of contracting the virus. At present, there are only a few centres set up to test for infection with the virus, so women with risk of exposure to the Zika virus are invited for serial growth scan, paying particular attention to the growth of the fetal head.

? QUESTIONS

Sandra is a 40-year-old woman pregnant for the first time. At her booking visit, the midwife states that they test for infections in the booking bloods. As Sandra became pregnant by IVF, she is very anxious about infections or anything that could negatively impact her pregnancy and has presented to the clinic with her concerns and questions.

Q1 Which antibody, if present in the booking bloods in an asymptomatic woman, suggests previous infection and subsequent acquired immunity?
  A IgA.
  B IgD.
  C IgE.
  D IgG.
  E IgM.

Q2 Answer true or false regarding the following statements related to chicken pox.
  A The incubation period is 10 to 20 days.
  B The classic lesion shape is annular.
  C An individual is only infective until the lesions have crusted over.
  D Reinfection of chickenpox is common after an initial exposure.
  E Shingles can sometimes lead to death if it completely encircles the abdomen.

A	Toxoplasmosis.	H	*Staphylococcus aureus.*
B	Erythema infectiosum.		
C	Listeria.	I	Chicken pox.
D	Rubella.	J	Candida.
E	Lyme disease.	K	Cytomegalovirus.
F	Herpes simplex virus.	L	Chlamydia.
G	Syphilis.		

Select the most appropriate option from the above list that corresponds to the following statements. Each answer can be used once, more than once or not at all.

Q3 A 14-week-pregnant woman presents with flulike symptoms. On examination, you notice animal scratch marks on her forearm.

Q4 A 34-week pregnant woman presents to GUM services for the first time, complaining of painful genital lesions.

Q5 A 28-week-pregnant woman presents with arthropathy, fever, headache and a sore throat.

Q6 A 1-year-old infant is seen in clinic with microcephaly, chorioretinitis and motor delay.

Q7 A newborn presents with jaundice, hepatosplenomegaly and cataracts. In addition, there are purpuric rashes on his body.

[Answers on page 420.]

STILLBIRTH

Stillbirth is broadly defined as the loss of a potentially viable fetus before expulsion from the mother. There is no international consensus on the specific gestational cutoff. In the UK, stillbirth is defined as fetal death in utero after 24 weeks of pregnancy, with fetal death before 24 weeks defined as miscarriage. The World Health Organisation defines stillbirth as fetal death in utero after 28 weeks gestation, and in Australia, the cutoff is 20 weeks. Stillbirth is responsible for 2.65 million deaths worldwide each year; 98% of these deaths occur in the developing world. In the UK, approximately 1 in 200 babies are stillborn.

AETIOLOGY

Many stillbirths remain unexplained, even after investigation. Classification of the cause of stillbirth is based on the clinical history and findings from maternal, fetal and placental examination (Tables 14.6 and 14.7). Whilst some conditions are considered definite causes of death, such as lethal congenital abnormalities and placental abruption, most conditions, such as gestational diabetes, are associated with an increased risk of stillbirth. As a consequence, no international consensus exists on stillbirth classification. Approximately 60% of stillbirths are associated with placental pathology, and the number of unexplained deaths can be reduced by 15% to 20% when the placenta is examined.

DIAGNOSIS

The optimal method for diagnosing stillbirth includes ultrasonography, often augmented with colour Doppler of the fetal heart and umbilical cord to confirm cardiac arrest. A clear four-chamber view of the fetal heart must be obtained and, whenever practically possible, a second ultrasonographer to confirm the findings.

In addition to the absence of fetal cardiac activity, other secondary features may also be seen:
- Collapse of the fetal skull (Spalding's sign).
- Hydrops (accumulation of fluid in two or more fetal compartments).
- Maceration and gross skin oedema.
- Intrafetal gas.

The best practice for discussing the difficult diagnosis of a stillbirth should be to immediately offer any unaccompanied women the option to call their partner, relatives or friends for support. Parents should be offered written information to supplement their decisions, and all discussions should aim to support the parents' choice. Empathy is crucial to determine the emotional feelings and needs of the parents and anyone accompanying them to ensure the best possible outcome out of what is often a very difficult situation.

INVESTIGATIONS

Investigations following a stillbirth have several aims:
1. To assess maternal well-being and reduce the risk of further conception complications.
2. To determine the cause of the stillbirth, which will help assess the chance of recurrence and allow treatment to correct any modifiable risk factors.

If consent is given, investigations to identify a cause may include:
- A detailed history of events during the pregnancy. Clinical examination for pre-eclampsia, chorioamnionitis and placental abruption will also be performed.

Table 14.6   **Antepartum Causes and Conditions Associated with Stillbirth**

	CAUSES	ASSOCIATED CONDITIONS AND RISK FACTORS
Fetal	• Lethal congenital abnormalities (fetal aneuploidy, anencephaly) • Twin-to twin-transfusion • Hydrops fetalis	• Chromosomal abnormalities • Congenital infections • IUGR
Maternal	• Maternal death	• Smoking • Advanced maternal age • Obesity • Gestational diabetes • Hypertensive disorders • Pre-eclampsia • Chronic renal or liver failure • Thyroid disease • Antiphospholipid syndrome • Systemic lupus erythematosus • Thrombophilia
Placental	• Placental abruption • Total placental infarction	• Placental insufficiency • Infarction • Chorioamnionitis • Inflammation • Thrombi and fibrin deposits

IUGR, Intrauterine growth restriction.

Table 14.7 Intrapartum Causes and Conditions Associated with Stillbirth

	CAUSES	ASSOCIATED CONDITIONS AND RISK FACTORS
Maternal	• Uterine rupture	Maternal haemorrhage – abruption or placenta praevia Fetal haemorrhage – vasa praevia
Fetal	• Fetal acidosis • Fetal hypoxia	Obstructed labour Prolonged rupture of membranes Prematurity
Other	• Cord prolapse • Cord obstruction	Cord accidents – knots or compression Cord abnormalities – coiling or abnormal insertion

- Maternal FBC, U&Es and LFTs to support diagnoses of pre-eclampsia, multiorgan failure and obstetric cholestasis.
- Clotting studies, blood platelet count and fibrinogen measurement to assess the risk of maternal disseminated intravascular coagulation.
- Screen for thrombophilias and APS.
- Maternal blood glucose and thyroid function tests to test for an underlying endocrine cause.
- Maternal blood cultures, urine culture, vaginal swabs, FBC and CRP to assess for an underlying infection. Often, serological testing for specific pathogens associated with stillbirth (TORCH screen) is also arranged.
- Kleihauer test to determine if there was maternofetal haemorrhage.
- Placental examination to assess for signs of placental insufficiency and abruption. Swabs may also be taken to assess for infection.
- Postmortem – this can involve a detailed examination of the external features of the baby, x-ray images and macroscopic and microscopic assessment of the internal organs.
- Tissue samples can be sent for karyotyping – if specific genetic disorders are suspected, these could also be tested for. Parental blood can also be taken for karyotyping.

[See 'Congenital Intrauterine Infections' on page 325.]

MANAGEMENT

The management of stillbirth is split into several sections. Each needs to be handled in an empathetic manner using good communication skills. The management of stillbirth is very complicated; hence, only the basics are discussed in this section.

BIRTH

- The mode of birth will depend on the health status of the woman, her previous obstetric history and the maternal or paternal preferences.
- In an uncomplicated case with no uterine scarring, first-line management is induction of labour with mifepristone and prostaglandins. Adequate analgesia will also be required and strong opiates can

be used, as there is no concern regarding placental transfer or neonatal toxicity.
- In an uncomplicated case, where the woman has had one previous caesarean, induction can be done with prostaglandins alone.
- In cases where the woman has had more than two caesareans or has an atypical scar, she should be informed that the safety of her induction of labour is unknown, and the management of these cases need to be decided upon individually with the involvement of a senior obstetrician. An operative birth for a stillbirth is uncommon, as it risks maternal harm with no fetal benefit.
- Immediate delivery is indicated in women who have signs of sepsis, pre-eclampsia, placental abruption or disseminated intravascular coagulation.

A stillborn fetus can cause maternal death when retained in utero. Depending on the length of time that the fetus has been retained, there is a 10% to 30% risk of the mother developing disseminated intravascular coagulation. There is also a risk of maternofetal haemorrhage and maternal sepsis. It is therefore crucial to manage maternal health as a priority when a stillbirth is detected.

LACTATION

Dopamine agonists, such as cabergoline, can be given to suppress lactation, minimising physical discomfort and psychological upset for the woman. They are contraindicated in hypertension and pre-eclampsia.

PSYCHOSOCIAL

The psychosocial effects of a stillbirth should not be underestimated. Mothers, partners and siblings are all at risk of severe posttraumatic stress disorder, and reactions may vary greatly.

Considerations include, but are not limited to:
- Ensuring all key staff members are informed of all events, so the woman does not have to repeat distressing events unnecessarily.
- All existing maternity appointments should be cancelled.
- Counselling should be offered to all women and their partners and considered for other family members.

- Parents should be advised about support groups.
- Bereavement officers should be appointed to coordinate services.
- Parents should be supported if they wish to see, hold, name or keep mementos of their stillborn baby.
- If the baby is named, then this name should be used in future appointments.

MANAGEMENT OF FUTURE PREGNANCIES

The management of future pregnancies is often crucial for women who have had a previous stillbirth, not only for medical reasons but also because of the psychosocial difficulties that this woman may encounter.

- The history of stillbirth should be clearly marked on the case record.
- Women with a previous stillbirth should be recommended to have obstetrician-led antenatal care. Serial ultrasound scans are usually offered throughout pregnancy to monitor fetal growth.
- Previous unexplained stillbirth is an indication to recommend future births at a specialist maternity unit.
- Maternal request for scheduled birth, induction or caesarean on a specific date should take into consideration the gestational age of the stillbirth as well as previous intrapartum history and the safety of induction of labour.
- Caregivers should be aware that there is an increased risk of postnatal depression and bonding difficulties after the next birth.

> ### 💡 Follow-Up After Stillbirth
>
> Patients are generally brought back 12 weeks or so after a stillbirth to see a consultant obstetrician. The aims of this are to:
> - Debrief on antenatal and intrapartum events and answer any questions.
> - Discuss results of any investigations that were performed regarding the underlying cause of the stillbirth.
> - Make a plan for possible further pregnancies to optimise the chance of successful births in the future.
>
> This 12-week time period is in place to allow some of the emotions from the initial situation to pass, allowing a more thorough discussion, and to allow time for any results from investigations to return to give the best chance for closure after the stillbirth.

PROGNOSIS

As explained, there are many underlying reasons or factors resulting in stillbirth. It has, however, been suggested that stillbirth in a woman's first pregnancy does not significantly increase the risk of stillbirth in the second pregnancy after adjusting for confounding factors.

❓ QUESTIONS

Sarah is a 26-year-old primiparous woman who is 31 weeks pregnant. Two days ago, she noticed that her baby was moving less than usual. Sarah called her obstetric unit, and they invited her into the hospital for urgent review. A midwife and registrar examined Sarah and found that the fetus had died, and a consultant confirmed this.

Q1 Which clinical finding is necessary to definitively diagnose stillbirth?
  A Absent fetal heartbeat on CTG.
  B Absent fetal heartbeat on Doppler ultrasound.
  C Absent fetal heartbeat on real-time ultrasound.
  D Absent fetal movement on real-time ultrasound.
  E Absent fetal movement on abdominal palpation.

Q2 Answer true or false: Regarding this case where the woman is well, with her membranes intact and her uterus unscarred.
  A Vaginal birth is most appropriate in this case.
  B Caesarean birth is most appropriate in this case.
  C It is important that the fetus is born as quickly as possible.
  D The value of a postmortem examination decreases the longer the fetus is retained *in utero*.
  E Recommendations about labour and birth should take into account the woman's preferences.

Q3 Answer true or false: Which of the following investigations should be recommended to all women who deliver a stillborn fetus?
  A Maternal blood culture.
  B Kleihauer test.
  C FBC and LFTs.
  D Maternal thrombophilia screen.
  E Postmortem of the baby and placental examination.

[Answers on page 422.]

KEY REFERENCES

ANTEPARTUM HAEMORRHAGE

Royal College of Obstetricians and Gynaecologists, 2011. Antepartum haemorrhage. RCOG Green Top Guideline (GTG 63).

Royal College of Obstetricians and Gynaecologists, 2018. Placenta praevia and placenta accreta: diagnosis and management. RCOG Green Top Guideline (GTG 27a).

PRE-ECLAMPSIA AND PREGNANCY-INDUCED HYPERTENSION

National Institute for Health and Clinical Excellence, 2019. Hypertension in pregnancy: diagnosis and management. NICE Clinical Guideline (BG 133).

National Institute for Health and Clinical Excellence, 2022. PLGF-based testing to help diagnose suspected preterm pre-eclampsia. NICE Diagnostic Guidance (DG 49).

PRETERM LABOUR

National Institute of Health and Clinical Excellence, 2022. Preterm labour and birth. NICE Guidance (NG25).

National Institute for Health and Clinical Excellence, 2021. Inducing labour. NICE Clinical Guideline (NG 207).

Royal College of Obstetricians and Gynaecologists, 2019. Care of women presenting with suspected preterm prelabour rupture of membranes from 24+0 weeks of gestation (GTG 73).

Royal College of Obstetricians and Gynaecologists, 2017. Prevention of early-onset neonatal group B streptococcal disease. RCOG Green Top Guideline (GTG 36).

British Association of Perinatal Medicine, 2020. Perinatal management of extreme preterm birth before 27 weeks of gestation: a framework for practice. Archives of Disease in Childhood - Fetal and Neonatal Edition 105, 232–239.

Royal College of Obstetricians and Gynaecologists, 2017. The management of breech presentation. RCOG Green Top Guideline (GTG 20b).

Royal College of Obstetricians and Gynaecologists, 2022. Cervical cerclage. RCOG Green Top Guideline (GTG 75).

CHORIOAMNIONITIS

National Institute for Health and Care Excellence, 2021. Neonatal infection: antibiotics for prevention and treatment. NICE Clinical Guideline (NG 195).

National Institute for Health and Clinical Excellence, 2021. Inducing labour. NICE Clinical Guideline (NG 207).

Royal College of Obstetricians and Gynaecologists, 2014. Perinatal management of pregnant women at the threshold of infant viability (the obstetric perspective). RCOG Scientific Impact Paper (SIP 41).

Royal College of Obstetricians and Gynaecologists, 2019. Care of women presenting with suspected preterm prelabour rupture of membranes from 24+0 weeks of gestation (GTG 73).

Royal College of Obstetricians and Gynaecologists, 2017. Prevention of early-onset neonatal group B streptococcal disease. RCOG Green Top Guideline (GTG 36).

SMALL-FOR-GESTATIONAL-AGE BABIES AND INTRAUTERINE GROWTH RESTRICTION

Royal College of Obstetricians and Gynaecologists, 2013. The investigation and management of the small for gestational age fetus. RCOG Green Top Guideline (GTG 31).

Royal College of Obstetricians and Gynaecologists, 2022. Antenatal corticosteroids to reduce neonatal morbidity and mortality. RCOG Green Top Guideline (GTG 74).

HEAMOLYTIC DISEASE OF THE FETUS AND NEWBORN

Qureshi, H., Massey, E., Kirwan, D., Davies, T., Robson, S., White, J., Jones, J., Allard, S., 2014. BCSH guideline for the use of anti-D immunoglobulin for the prevention of haemolytic disease of the fetus and newborn. Transfusion Medicine 24 (1), 8–20.

Crowther, C.A., Keirse, M.J., 2015. Anti-D administration in pregnancy for preventing rhesus alloimmunisation. Cochrane Database of Systematic Reviews (2), CD000020.

Royal College of Obstetricians and Gynaecologists, 2014. The management of women with red cell antibodies during pregnancy. RCOG Green Top Guideline (GTG 65).

CONGENITAL INTRAUTERINE INFECTIONS

BMJ Best Practice, 2020. Toxoplasmosis in pregnancy: what treatments work?

BMJ Best Practice, 2020. Toxoplasmosis in pregnancy: what is it?

Public Health England, 2019. Guidance on the investigation, diagnosis and management of viral illness, or exposure to viral rash illness, in pregnancy.

Public Health England, 2017. Parvovirus B19: guidance, data and analysis.

Royal College of Obstetricians and Gynaecologists, 2015. Chickenpox in pregnancy. RCOG Green Top Guideline (GTG 13).

British Association for Sexual Health and HIV, 2015. UK national guidelines on management of syphilis.

Dontigny, L., Arsenault, M.Y., Martel, M.J., 2018. No. 203-Rubella in Pregnancy. Journal of Obstetrics and Gynaecology Canada 40 (8), e615–e21.

Royal College of Obstetricians and Gynaecologists, 2017. Congenital cytomegalovirus infection: update on treatment. Scientific Impact Paper no. 56.

British Association for Sexual Health and HIV, Royal College of Obstetricians and Gynaecologists, 2014. Management of genital herpes in pregnancy.

Public Health England, 2020. Listeria: guidance, data and analysis.

STILLBIRTH

Royal College of Obstetricians and Gynaecologists, 2010. Late intrauterine fetal death and stillbirth. RCOG Green Top Guideline (GTG 55).

Obstetric Emergencies

CORD PROLAPSE

Cord prolapse is the descent of the umbilical cord through the cervix, alongside (occult) or past (overt) the presenting part of the fetus, in the presence of ruptured membranes (Fig. 15.1). It is an obstetric emergency that can have high neonatal morbidity and mortality.

RISK FACTORS

Toward the end of the third trimester, the fetal head engages within the pelvis, fixing it in place, and preventing any other body part from presenting when the woman goes into labour. In any situation where there is not good cephalic engagement, the cord can sit low in the uterus and then prolapse when the cervix dilates and membranes rupture (Table 15.1).

AETIOLOGY

The overall incidence of cord prolapse is approximately 0.3%, with a higher incidence in breech presentation of around 1%.

PATHOLOGY

The umbilical cord contains one vein carrying oxygen and nutrient-rich blood from the placenta to the fetus and two arteries carrying deoxygenated blood and toxic metabolites from the fetus to the placenta. If the blood flow is sufficiently compromised, the fetus only has a few minutes before long-term neurological damage or death can occur.

If a cord prolapses and then the presenting part of the fetus follows it, the cord can be compressed between the cervix and the fetus, occluding blood flow. Even without the fetus descending into the pelvis, the cord can still be compromised. This can occur in response to cold if the cord prolapses out of the vagina, to friction from the vaginal tissues or following repeated touching by a healthcare professional handling the cord. All these events can cause spasm of the umbilical vessels, dramatically reducing blood flow.

CLINICAL FEATURES

Women are unlikely to notice any signs or symptoms themselves except on rare occasions where the cord prolapses out of the vagina. If a cord prolapse is suspected, a vaginal examination should be performed. Usually, there is a history of very recent rupture of membranes just prior to fetal distress. The most common fetal sign of cord prolapse is a prolonged fetal bradycardia, but it can also cause any other CTG abnormality.

COMPLICATIONS

FETAL

- Fetal hypoxia.
- Neurological damage.
- Intrauterine death.

MATERNAL

- Physical trauma associated with rapid assisted vaginal or caesarean birth.
- Psychological trauma.

MANAGEMENT

Cord prolapse is an obstetric emergency requiring delivery by the quickest route. The diagnosis should be considered whenever there is an abnormal CTG trace or bradycardia auscultated in women not on a CTG, particularly after a recent rupture of membranes. Important steps in the management of cord prolapse are described below.

RECOGNITION

In the event of an abnormal CTG trace, a vaginal examination is performed. The cord can be felt, and when it

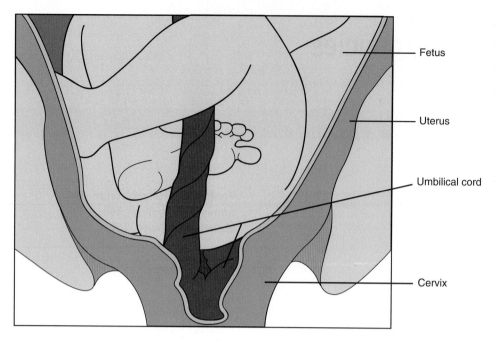

Fig. 15.1 Cord Prolapse.

Table **15.1**	**Risk Factors of Cord Prolapse**
CAUSE	**EXPLANATION**
Premature labour	Presenting part rarely engaged until labour and more likely to present breech.
Breech presentation	Breech presentation fetuses may not be engaged in the pelvis. Cord prolapse is more common with footling breech.
Abnormal/unstable lie	Presenting part is not in the pelvis. Cord prolapse is a significant risk with transverse or oblique lie.
Polyhydramnios	Lots of space for the fetus to move, reducing the likelihood of engagement.
Grand multiparous woman	The head may not engage until labour.
Placenta praevia	Prevents the fetal head from engaging, and if the placenta is not covering the os, the cord could prolapse when the cervix dilates.
Birth of the second twin	After the first twin has delivered, the second twin can lie in any position. When the membranes rupture, the cord can prolapse through the fully dilated cervix.
ARM	Prolapse is rare when the head is engaged, but obstetricians sometimes need to augment labour before good engagement. At the time of ARM, the fetal head may be held via the abdomen to guide the head into the pelvis, reducing the chance of cord prolapse. Once the liquor has drained and the head is in the pelvis and subject to uterine contractions, cord prolapse is then very rare.

ARM, Artificial rupture of membranes.

is identified, the person examining should not remove their hand; they should push the presenting part up off the cord to reduce compression.

CALL FOR HELP

In any case of cord prolapse, help should be called immediately, declaring an obstetric emergency. This will contact an obstetrician who may be needed to expedite birth, an anaesthetist to provide emergency analgesia, a neonatologist to care for the baby after birth and additional midwives and other team members to provide support.

RELIEVE PRESSURE ON THE CORD DURING TRANSFER FOR EMERGENCY DELIVERY

To prevent cord compression, some of the following methods can be adopted. A key aspect to remember is that excessive handling of the cord can cause vasospasm and potentially worsen the condition for the fetus.

- Position the bed so the woman is head down to help lift the presenting part of the fetus off the cord (Fig. 15.2). The examining healthcare professional manually elevates the presenting part to reduce pressure on the cord while being careful not to handle the cord.
- In hospital, birth can be achieved quickly, so no other supportive measures are usually required. If a cord prolapse occurs out of hospital or if there will be a delay going to theatre, further measures can be considered:
  - Catheterising the patient and injecting 0.9% sodium chloride to fill the bladder. This pushes the presenting part of the fetus up and relieves pressure on the cord.

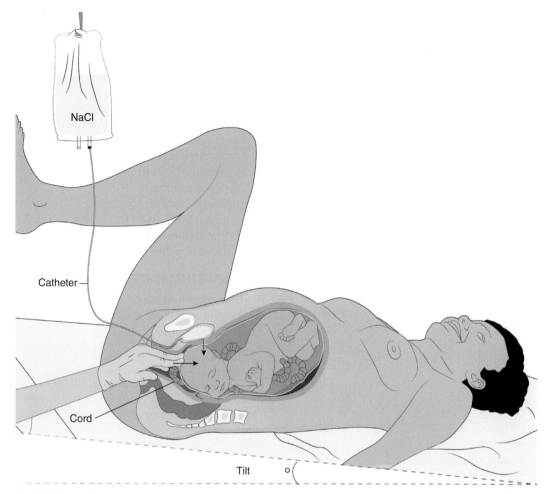

Fig. 15.2 Supportive Measures in the Management of Cord Prolapse. Maternal head down, urinary bladder filled, midwife lifting presenting part off cord.

- Tocolytics, such as terbutaline, can be given to reduce uterine contractions, thereby reducing cord compression.

It is important to remember that although these manoeuvres can potentially help, they must not delay the delivery of the fetus and so may not always be performed.

DELIVER THE BABY AS QUICKLY AS POSSIBLE

The correct mode of birth depends on the individual situation of the mother and baby. If the mother is in the community, rapid transfer to the hospital must be organised. Possible methods include:
- Emergency caesarean is the recommended mode of birth for cord prolapse cases when vaginal birth is not imminent. This is because it is a quick, effective mode of birth that can avert potential fetal hypoxia. This may be performed under general anaesthetic, as it is the quickest way to provide effective anaesthesia, unless the patient has a good working epidural already in place.
- Assisted vaginal birth can be attempted if the mother is fully dilated and it is believed this would be quicker than caesarean.

POSTBIRTH

After birth, it is important that a senior neonatal doctor is present to resuscitate the baby if necessary. Cord gases will be taken to assess for fetal hypoxia. The team and mother will require debriefing regarding the events that have taken place.

PROGNOSIS

A promptly diagnosed and managed cord prolapse generally has a good outcome, as the baby is delivered before compromise can occur. If there is a delay in recognition and/or birth, cord prolapse is associated with high morbidity and mortality.

After an emergency birth for cord prolapse, it is essential to counsel the parents to explain the events that have happened to reduce the risk of psychological trauma and additionally to answer any questions they have.

PREVENTION

Women at risk of cord prolapse are offered admission to hospital so that if it occurs, delivery can be expedited.

The most common admissions for this are patients with transverse or oblique lie at or after 37 weeks. If women with a high risk of cord prolapse decline admission, they are advised, if their membranes rupture, to call 999 to get emergency transfer to a hospital and to lie down with their bottom in the air as an attempt to reduce the chance of cord compression.

❓ QUESTIONS

You have been called to see Sophie, a 29-year-old primigravida. Her pregnancy has been uneventful, with all of the routine scans and investigations normal. She presented to the delivery suite at term and is now 6 cm dilated, and the baby's head is engaged. Her midwife performed an amniotomy to augment uterine activity, as she has been slow to progress. The midwife noticed an abnormal fetal heart rate after performing the amniotomy so commenced CTG monitoring. The CTG shows prolonged and late decelerations.

Q1 What is the average drop in fetal pH for every minute that the umbilical cord is compressed during a cord prolapse?

A 0.01.
B 0.02.
C 0.03.
D 0.04.
E 0.05.

Q2 Answer true or false: Which of the following are risk factors for cord prolapse?

A Raised liquor volume.
B Multiple pregnancy.
C Low-lying placenta.
D Assisted vaginal birth.
E Maternal chronic hypertension.

Q3 Which maternal or fetal features may indicate a cord prolapse?

A Fetal bradycardia.
B Maternal tachycardia.
C Maternal abdominal pain.
D Fetal accelerations on CTG.
E Fetal decelerations on CTG.

[Answers on page 424.]

SHOULDER DYSTOCIA

After the head has been delivered, to complete a vaginal birth, routine traction is applied to the fetal head, usually in conjunction with the next contraction. Shoulder dystocia is defined:
- Clinically – as the failure to deliver the shoulders after one attempt has been made.
- Anatomically – as the impaction of the anterior shoulder on the anterior aspect of the maternal pelvis (pubic bones or symphysis pubis).

RISK FACTORS

Shoulder dystocia is an obstetric emergency that complicates up to 0.5% to 1% of all vaginal births. Although there are several recognised risk factors, in many cases, shoulder dystocia occurs in women with no risk factors. Risk factors for shoulder dystocia can be classified as prelabour or intrapartum factors.

PRELABOUR FACTORS
- Suspected large fetus (macrosomia).
  - Estimated fetal weight of over 4.5 kg.
  - Estimated fetal weight above the 95th centile on a growth chart.
- Induction of labour.
- Diabetes mellitus.
- Previous shoulder dystocia.
- Maternal body mass index more than 30 kg/m².
- Congenital fetal abnormalities.
- Android or platypelloid pelvis.

INTRAPARTUM FACTORS
- Prolonged first stage of labour.
- Prolonged second stage of labour.
- Oxytocin augmentation.
- Assisted vaginal birth.

💡 Pelvis Types in Relation to Birth

The majority of women have a gynaecoid pelvis, which is the most suitable for vaginal birth due to its oval inlet, straight pelvic side walls, wide sacral curve and wide subpubic arch, which all create a large pelvic cavity for passage of the fetus. Conversely, the android and platypelloid pelvis has a prominent sacral promontory, narrowing the anteroposterior (AP) diameter of the pelvis (Fig. 15.3). This is the plane the shoulders need to be in to deliver, so a narrow AP diameter increases the risk of shoulder dystocia.

CLINICAL FEATURES

An important aspect in the management of shoulder dystocia is early recognition that there may be a problem. Several subtle signs can indicate that a problem may exist prior to attempting shoulder delivery. These include difficulty delivering the face, retraction of the head (causing 'turtle neck sign') or failure of restitution.

[See 'Spontaneous Vaginal Birth' on page 258.]

COMPLICATIONS

Delivering a baby with shoulder dystocia needs to be assessed and proceeded with quickly to avoid fetal death or significant long-term neurological disability. When the baby's head emerges from the vagina, due to compression from the maternal tissues, the blood vessels to the head and the umbilical cord have reduced blood flow, which can result in fetal hypoxia. Anaerobic respiration then occurs, resulting in the formation of acidic by-products. For every minute a baby is stuck in this position, the fetal pH is estimated to drop by 0.04. A normal fetal

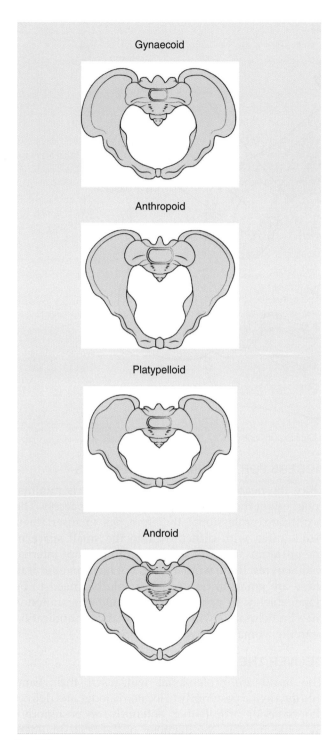

Fig. 15.3 Common Types of Female Pelvises.

head delivery, resulting in less time to conduct a safe birth.

MATERNAL COMPLICATIONS

- Perineal tears.
- Anal sphincter and rectal injury and dysfunction.
- Urethral and bladder injury.
- Postpartum haemorrhage (PPH).
- Emotional and psychological impact.

COMPLICATIONS FOR THE BABY

- Hypoxia, hypoxic ischaemic encephalopathy and death.
- Brachial plexus injuries, for example, Erb palsy.
- Fractured clavicle or cleidotomy (surgical division of the fetal clavicle to allow delivery).
- Fractured humerus.
- Contusions.
- Transfer to NICU and reduced immediate bonding.

Erb palsy is the most common brachial plexus injury and involves nerve routes C5 to C7. This palsy affects the muscles of the upper arm, causing 'winging' of the scapula and the classic 'waiter's tip' posture. These signs arise due to paralysis and subsequent atrophy of the biceps, deltoid and brachialis muscles. Loss of sensation over the related dermatomes can also occur. An Erb palsy (Fig. 15.4) can occur at the time of a shoulder dystocia. This commonly occurs when excessive traction is applied to the fetal head in an attempt to deliver; pulling on the head with the shoulder fixed will cause stretching of the tissues of the neck and upper side of the shoulder, including the C5 to C7 nerve roots.

MANAGEMENT

If there is any suspicion of dystocia, senior help must be called for immediately with an obstetric emergency call. Often, specific manoeuvres (as described here) will be needed. The aim of all the manoeuvres is to disimpact the anterior shoulder from the symphysis pubis. They do this by either increasing the maternal pelvic diameter or reducing the diameter of the fetal shoulders, which then allows delivery of the shoulders and the rest of the baby. The manoeuvres are described here and should be attempted for a maximum of 30 seconds each before moving on to the next manoeuvre.

MCROBERTS MANOEUVRE

This is the first manoeuvre attempted in shoulder dystocia. The mother lies flat on her back, and then her hips are hyperflexed and abducted tight to the maternal abdomen (usually with a member of the emergency team holding each leg to support the manoeuvre). This opens the pelvis by increasing the AP diameter to assist in delivering the baby. Traction is then applied to the

blood pH (venous sample from fetal scalp) is more than 7.25 intrapartum, and a pH of less than 7.0 is associated with long-term neurological impairment. This means that a baby that started with a normal pH must be delivered within 7 minutes to reduce the risk of long-term morbidity. Often, healthcare professionals wait for the next contraction after delivery of the head before even attempting to deliver the rest of the body. Hence, dystocia may not be recognised for a couple of minutes after

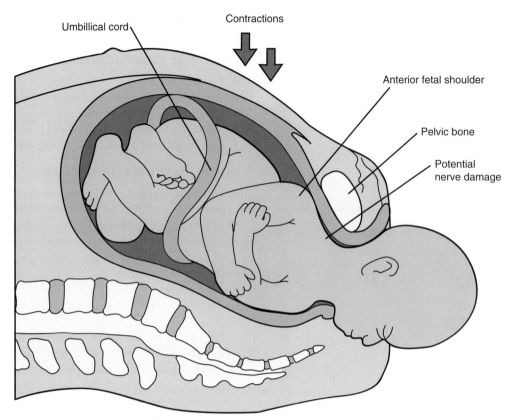

Fig. 15.4 Shoulder Dystocia Causing Erb palsy.

fetal head by the delivering healthcare professional in an attempt to deliver the fetus (Fig. 15.5). In the majority of cases, McRoberts is successful, and the baby is delivered. If unsuccessful, the position is maintained while attempting the following manoeuvres.

SUPRAPUBIC PRESSURE

Suprapubic pressure is performed from the side of the fetal back in a downward lateral direction, using hands in a similar position to cardiac massage in cardiopulmonary resuscitation (CPR) (Fig. 15.6). This works by pushing the shoulder forward, reducing the diameter of the shoulders and also rotating the anterior shoulder laterally, dislodging it from behind the pubic bone. If pressure alone is not effective, a rocking motion can be attempted. If some movement is felt, then the delivering healthcare professional applies traction and attempts delivery.

EPISIOTOMY

This is considered, but not always performed. An episiotomy may help the healthcare professional gain access into the vagina to perform internal manoeuvres but will not directly assist the delivery. Remember, shoulder dystocia is a bone-on-bone impaction and not soft tissue. It is also important to remember that, if required, an episiotomy may have to be performed quickly, without time to give the mother adequate pain relief. Good communication with the mother is vital to reduce panic and subsequent emotional stress.

ACCESS FOR INTERNAL MANOEUVRES

Once the head has been delivered, there is minimal room under the pubic arch for practitioner access. The healthcare professional therefore has to insert their hand (often with difficulty) into the small space in the posterior aspect of the vagina to attempt internal manoeuvres. If the woman does not have an epidural, these are going to be uncomfortable but need to be done quickly to achieve delivery. Offering Entonox may be helpful as will keeping good communication with the woman as to what is happening.

DELIVER THE POSTERIOR ARM

The healthcare professional will insert their hand into the vagina posteriorly to locate, dislodge and deliver the posterior arm (either anteriorly or posteriorly). By achieving this, the diameter of the fetal shoulders reduces by an entire arm width. Space is now formed in the posterior vagina for the baby to drop into, dislodging the anterior shoulder and allowing delivery. If the healthcare professional cannot deliver the arm, they move on to other internal rotational manoeuvres.

OTHER INTERNAL ROTATIONAL MANOEUVRES

If the posterior arm cannot be dislodged or delivered, the healthcare professional should attempt other internal rotational manoeuvres. There are three other ways in which the anterior shoulder could be dislodged, and there is no order to trying these; the healthcare professional will select the method that

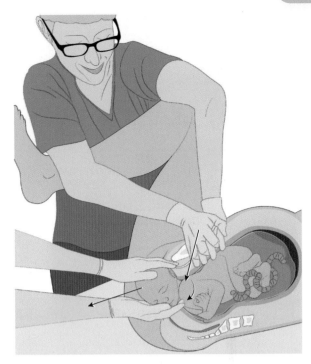

Fig. 15.6 Suprapubic Pressure.

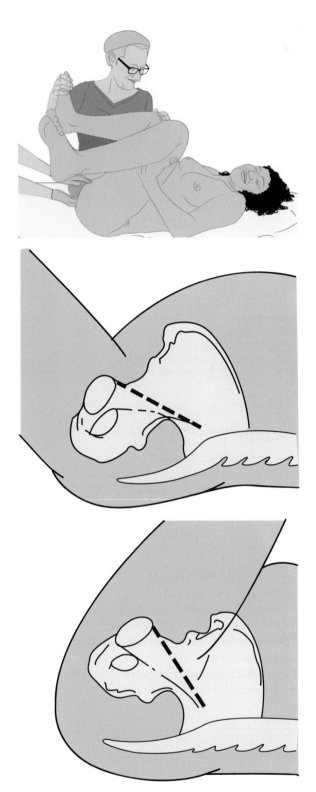

Fig. 15.5 McRoberts Manoeuvre.

most suits the baby and situation in which they are assisting. The first option is for the healthcare professional to run their fingers up to the back of the anterior shoulder. In a similar way to the suprapubic pressure, the obstetrician will push on the shoulder to try to get it to move into the oblique position and dislodge (eponymously called Rubin II). If that does not work, the healthcare professional can try putting their other

hand in the posterior vagina to push on the front of the posterior shoulder at the same time as pushing on the back of the anterior shoulder (formally called Woods screw). If this method also fails, the healthcare professional can push on the back of the posterior shoulder, trying to get the shoulders to dislodge into the oblique position in the other direction (formally called reverse Woods screw). If movement is felt with any of the manoeuvres, traction can be applied to the fetal head to deliver (Fig. 15.7).

ALL FOURS

If the fetus can still not be delivered, the next step is to turn the woman into an all-fours kneeling position and try delivering an arm or internal manoeuvres in this position. The all-fours position can open up the pelvis in a similar way to McRoberts, and the process of moving the woman may dislodge the fetal shoulder.

OTHER RARE MANOEUVRES

Several manoeuvres can be attempted if none of the above is successful. From the options outlined here, the preferred method is a cleidotomy due to low maternal trauma.

- Cleidotomy – fracture or surgical dissection of the fetal clavicle, which reduces the diameter of the shoulders to then allow delivery.
- Symphysiotomy – incision and division of the symphyseal ligament of the maternal pelvis; this will increase the AP diameter of the maternal pelvis. However, it takes time to perform and is a traumatic procedure for the mother and often leaves the mother with long-term pain on mobilising.

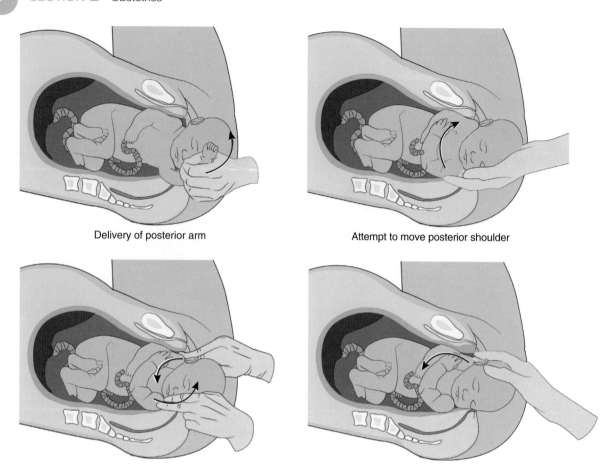

Delivery of posterior arm

Attempt to move posterior shoulder

Try to rotate both shoulders

Try to move the anterior shoulder
from the posterior approach

Fig. 15.7 Internal Manoeuvres.

- Zavanelli manoeuvre – this is undertaken once a toco-lytic has been given. The manoeuvre involves pushing the fetal head back into the uterus, keeping it there by constant pressure and delivery by caesarean section.

It is extremely rare to perform either a symphysi-otomy or Zavanelli manoeuvre, as by the time these options are considered, it is likely the fetus has been hypoxic for a considerable time and is very unlikely to survive, so there is often no benefit in causing the mother the significant physical trauma.

INITIAL CARE FOLLOWING BIRTH
- Neonatal assessment of baby.
  - Immediate assessment of neonatal condition and resuscitation.
  - An x-ray of the clavicle or humerus may be clinically indicated if there is an obvious defor-mity, significant local tenderness or movement limitation.
  - Assessment of movement may indicate periph-eral nerve injury.
  - Further assessment and management may be nec-essary if there has been significant delay in deliv-ery, as the baby may have suffered a profound hypoxia and be at risk of long-term brain injury.

- Cord blood gases to assess the degree of fetal hypoxia.
- Physical assessment of maternal injuries along with measures to prevent PPH.
- Debriefing the mother and birth partner on events to reduce the psychological impact.
- Where possible, allow normal bonding with baby and breastfeeding.
- Debrief staff members present; these situations are psychologically traumatic for staff too.

It is also important to communicate to the mother and birth partner about the possible implications for future pregnancies. It is important that the mother understands that she has an increased risk of shoulder dystocia in a subsequent pregnancy. Nonetheless, with careful monitoring, this risk can be minimised through appropriate birth planning. There may also be a case for offering the option of an elective caesarean section for subsequent pregnancies.

PROGNOSIS

The prognosis of the baby depends on the presence or extent of the injuries (trauma and hypoxic) sustained.

Generally, the sooner the baby is delivered and the quicker any injuries are noted, the better the prognosis. As the majority of shoulder dystocia cases are delivered quickly after the use of McRoberts, outcomes for most are excellent.

PREVENTING A SHOULDER DYSTOCIA

In the UK, if the estimated fetal weight is suspected to be greater than 4.5 kg in a woman with diabetes, or greater than 5 kg in a nondiabetic mother, then birth by caesarean should be offered, as there is significant risk of shoulder dystocia.

Where the estimated fetal weight is greater than the 95th centile or likely to be greater than 4 kg at term, some clinicians advocate early induction of labour to reduce the chance of shoulder dystocia. There is evidence to support this practice; however, national guidelines do not currently advocate this approach.

❓ QUESTIONS

Mundhill, a 32-year-old woman, gravidity two, parity one, is progressing slowly in labour. Her current pregnancy has been uneventful, with all routine scans and investigations normal. During her previous pregnancy, she developed gestational diabetes. There were no complications and her daughter, now 2 years old, was born vaginally at 39 weeks and is fit and healthy. The head of the baby delivers, but with the following contraction, the midwife is unable to deliver the rest of the baby. The emergency bell is pulled.

Q1 If shoulder dystocia is suspected, what is the first position or manoeuvre to encourage the woman to adopt?
  A Left lateral decubitus position.
  B McRoberts manoeuvre.
  C Lithotomy position.
  D Zavanelli manoeuvre.
  E Squatting position.

A Assisted vaginal birth.	**G** Elective caesarean section.
B Gestational hypertension.	**H** Pethidine as analgesia in labour.
C Maternal hypothyroidism.	**I** Epidural as analgesia in labour.
D Gestational diabetes mellitus.	**J** Cervical cerclage.
E Macrosomia.	**K** Multiple pregnancy.
F Maternal obesity.	**L** Oxytocin-induced labour.

Select the most appropriate option from the above list that corresponds to the following statements. Each answer can be used once, more than once or not at all.

Q2 A 26-year-old woman with a BMI of 31 kg/m² had a planned caesarean in her first pregnancy for placenta praevia. She is currently in labour and requires assistance with forceps to aid in the birth of the baby. She has an epidural in place for analgesia. From the options above, which factor is the most important risk factor for shoulder dystocia?

Q3 You have been called to see a woman in active labour. This is her first pregnancy and, despite being diagnosed with gestational diabetes, she has had an uneventful pregnancy. She is asking for an epidural to assist in pain control, as the pethidine she received several hours ago has not been sufficient. From the options above, which factor would most likely increase her risk of shoulder dystocia?

Q4 If a woman with known type 2 diabetes becomes pregnant, based on the options above, what complication can occur that increases the risk of shoulder dystocia?

Q5 Answer true or false: Which of the following are recognised complications of shoulder dystocia for the baby?
  A Bulbar palsy.
  B Brachial plexus injury.
  C Femur fracture.
  D Clavicle fracture.
  E Bells palsy.

[Answers on page 425.]

RETAINED PLACENTA

There are two definitions of retained placenta, varying based on the management of the third stage of labour.
- Active management
  - An IM dose of synthetic oxytocin is given after birth of the baby to increase uterine contractions to cause placental detachment and delivery.
  - At the same time, the healthcare professional gently pulls on the cord to encourage detachment and delivery. This is known as controlled cord traction.
  - Retained placenta is diagnosed if the placenta is not delivered within 30 minutes of the birth of the baby.
  - Active management is encouraged in the UK, as it reduces the incidence of retained placenta and PPH.
- Physiological management
  - Delivery of the placenta is allowed to occur with only maternal effort and natural uterine contractions.
  - Retained placenta is diagnosed if the placenta is not delivered within 60 minutes from birth of the baby.

AETIOLOGY

The incidence of retained placenta is around 3% in high income countries and is rarely associated with mortality. However, retained placentas remain a cause of mortality from infection and PPH worldwide.

There are three main causes of retained placenta:
1. Uterine atony – most common cause.
2. Trapped placenta – placenta detached but unable to deliver due to a closed cervix.
3. Abnormally invasive placenta (placenta accreta or percreta) – more common with previous caesarean

or uterine surgery. The placenta should normally implant into the deciduas basalis of the uterus. In these conditions, the placenta embeds deeper into the uterus and consequently does not easily detach after delivery of the fetus.

INVESTIGATIONS

There is no diagnostic test for retained placenta. It is usually suspected by the midwife looking after the woman and confirmed by the obstetrician following failure to deliver the placenta using controlled cord traction and a vaginal examination to check the placenta is not simply sitting in the vagina.

COMPLICATIONS

- PPH.
- Genital tract infection.
- Lower genital tract trauma.
- Uterine inversion.
- Psychological effects such an emergency would have on both the mother and her family.

 Uterine Inversion

Uterine inversion occurs when the placenta fails to detach and the delivering healthcare professional pulls too hard on the cord. This results in the uterus turning inside out (inversion), often with the fundus protruding through the cervix. This is an obstetric emergency, as it causes acute neurogenic shock, with vagal tone causing profound bradycardia and hypotension. Quickly pushing the uterus back into place resolves the shock; however, there is a risk of atomy leading to PPH after this emergency. Uterine inversion can be avoided by 'guarding' the uterus when applying traction to the cord; this is achieved by placing one hand above the level of the symphysis pubis, applying counterpressure in an upward direction, thus stabilising the uterus as the placenta is being delivered.

MANAGEMENT

- Call for help immediately.
- Assess blood loss – if it is significant, follow the management for PPH.
- IV access and take urgent bloods, including FBC and group and save (G&S).
- Administer IM syntocinon or syntometrine, which can increase uterine tone to aid delivery.
- Ensure the urinary bladder is empty, as urinary retention can contribute to placental retention – consider catheterisation if the patient is unable to pass urine.
- Controlled cord traction is then continued for up to 30 minutes to allow placental delivery as long as the mother remains stable. The evidence for this technique is limited, so it is not always used where theatre is readily available.
- Manual removal of the placenta is the definitive management.

MANUAL REMOVAL OF THE PLACENTA

Manual removal of the placenta should be undertaken in theatre. Following effective analgesia in the form of regional or general anaesthetic, an obstetrician inserts one hand into the vagina and uterus, identifying the placenta and cleaving the placenta off the uterus with their fingers. The delivered placenta and membranes are checked to confirm they appear complete, and the uterine cavity is examined to make sure it feels empty.

Antibiotics are given to reduce the chance of development of an intrauterine infection, and bimanual compression and uterotonics may be used if there is ongoing bleeding. The perineum is also checked for trauma possibly caused during the procedure.

PROGNOSIS

The prognosis depends on the severity, timely recognition and management of the retained placenta. There is a significant risk of PPH and the associated maternal morbidity and mortality. As with any operation, manual removal of the placenta is associated with the risk of infection and genital tract trauma. However, in the UK, most cases of retained placenta are managed uneventfully. The woman is at an increased risk of a retained placenta in a future pregnancy and should be encouraged to accept active management of the third stage.

❓ QUESTIONS

You have been called to see Louise, a 27-year-old primigravida woman. She is a known hypertensive, but her pregnancy has been uneventful. She delivered a healthy baby boy at 19:17. She opted to have active management of her third stage of labour. It is now 19:45, and the placenta has still not been delivered despite the midwife giving syntocinon and using controlled cord traction. The midwife is worried that this could become a case of retained placenta.

Q1 Which maternal conditions contraindicate the use of ergometrine in the active management of the third stage of labour?
   A Severe diabetes.
   B Severe hypertension.
   C Multiple sclerosis.
   D Severe cardiac disease.
   E Sepsis.

Q2 What can cause a retained placenta?
   A Uterine atony.
   B Multiple pregnancy.
   C Placenta accreta.
   D Assisted vaginal birth.
   E Oxytocin use in labour.

Q3 Answer true or false: Which of the following are recognised complications of retained placenta for the woman?
   A Uterine atony.
   B Deep vein thrombosis.
   C PPH.
   D Obstetric anal sphincter injury.
   E Pneumonia.

[Answers on page 427.]

POSTPARTUM HAEMORRHAGE

The WHO's definition of primary minor PPH is any blood loss over 500 mL up to 24 hours after birth, with major PPH defined as blood loss over 1000 mL (Table 15.2). More recently, major PPH has also been defined as more than a 10% drop in haematocrit from admission bloods or bleeding that requires a blood transfusion. Secondary PPH is blood loss between 24 hours and 6 weeks after birth.

PPH is a major cause of maternal mortality worldwide, causing approximately 130,000 deaths each year. While death from PPH is a rare event in the developed world, it still is a significant cause of maternal death and morbidity.

AETIOLOGY

Women who have identifiable risk factors (Table 15.3) in the antenatal period must be counselled so they understand their risk. It is important to remember that in the majority of PPH cases, women have no identifiable risk factors.

There are four main causes of PPH (the 4 Ts):
1. Uterine atony (tone).
2. Lower genital tract lacerations (trauma).
3. Retained placental fragments (tissue).
4. Coagulopathy (thrombin).

By far, the most common cause of PPH is uterine atony (tone). This is where effective uterine contraction is not achieved after birth. There are many causes of this; some relate to overstretching of the uterus during pregnancy,

Table 15.2 Primary Postpartum Haemorrhage Definitions

DEFINITION	BLOOD LOSS
Normal postpartum blood loss	<500 mL
Minor PPH	500–1000 mL
Major PPH	>1000 mL

PPH, Postpartum haemorrhage.

Table 15.3 Risk Factors for Postpartum Haemorrhage

RISK FACTORS – ANTENATAL	RISK FACTORS – INTRAPARTUM
Maternal obesity	Large baby (more than 4 kg)
Maternal coagulation disorders	Pyrexia in labour
Previous PPH	Prolonged labour (more than 12 hours)
Multiple pregnancy	Episiotomy
Pre-eclampsia	Assisted vaginal birth
Placenta praevia	Delivery by caesarean section
Placental abruption	Retained placenta
Antepartum haemorrhage	
Large fibroids	

PPH, Postpartum haemorrhage.

such as multiple pregnancy, whilst others are related to bleeding. The uterine blood vessels run perpendicular to the muscle fibres of the myometrium. When the uterus contracts, the muscle fibres constrict blood vessels. This is why, after birth, good uterine contraction stops bleeding. Without contractions or sufficient tone, uterine atony allows continued bleeding, leading to a PPH. Placental abruption and placenta praevia can also cause significant bleeding into the uterine muscle, leading to the inability of the muscle to contract.

Retained placenta or tissue inside the uterus means the muscle is unable to contract to its full extent. Prolonged retained tissue can also be a source of sepsis, which can lead to disseminated intravascular coagulation (DIC) and secondary PPH.

Trauma during birth can either be iatrogenic or part of a natural birth. It is important that any tear created is assessed and sutured where necessary. The vagina and perineum are highly vascular, which can result in rapid blood loss following trauma.

Maternal coagulation disorders can lead to PPH due to failure of the clotting cascade. Other coagulation problems can occur in pregnancy, leading to an increased risk of PPH; low platelet levels are a classic feature of pre-eclampsia, and sepsis can lead to altered clotting factor levels.

PPH can also be self-perpetuating due to a combination of consumptive coagulopathy and DIC. This means that, for whatever the cause of the blood loss, when a woman loses over about 1500 mL of blood, her clotting factors and platelets will have been significantly consumed. This means that her blood can then no longer form clots effectively, leading to further haemorrhage.

CLINICAL FEATURES

Women with primary minor PPH are likely to have no clinical signs of shock. It is therefore important that their vital signs are regularly monitored.

Women with major primary PPH are likely to have signs of shock in the later stages but may be asymptomatic at first. The first subtle sign of hypovolaemia is pallor. Following this, tachycardia, tachypnoea, sweating, cool peripheries and a widened pulse pressure can be noted. A late sign of hypovolaemia is hypotension; if this is seen, it is a signal of peri-arrest. Other late signs of hypovolaemic shock are oliguria, confusion and reduced responsiveness level, demonstrating failure of end organ perfusion.

It is important to monitor vaginal blood loss. This includes weighing loss on all modalities including sanitary pads, loss on bed sheets and intraoperative and postoperative loss (if during caesarean section).

INVESTIGATIONS

Initial investigations are used to quantify the haematological effect of PPH on homeostasis and preparations for possible treatment with blood products. Key investigations include:

- Haemoglobin – to help quantify blood loss and help decide whether the patient needs a blood transfusion. However, in severe acute blood loss, haemoglobin concentration may not fall initially, so estimated blood loss from what is visible is often used to estimate the need for blood transfusion.
- Platelet count – to assess whether a woman needs a platelet transfusion.
- Coagulation screen – to assess the current clotting ability, check for evidence of DIC and guide replacement of factors (often in the form of fresh frozen plasma (FFP) and/or cryoprecipitate).
  - Prothrombin time (PT).
  - Activated prothrombin time (APTT).
  - Fibrinogen.
- G&S (minor PPH) – to ensure that, if needed, crossmatched red cells can be obtained if needed.
- Crossmatch (major PPH) – to allow replacement of red cells.
  - Ideally, fully crossmatched blood products should be used, which takes about 40 minutes to analyse and assess for all the common red cell antibodies.
  - If blood is required more quickly, a rapid crossmatch can be carried out to give type-specific products. If blood is needed immediately, most obstetric units have O-negative blood within the department.
  - In a major haemorrhage, UK hospitals have protocols in place with their transfusion service to rapidly provide six units of packed red cells, along with replacement platelets and clotting factors, even before blood investigations are back. Optimal management of major haemorrhage is now focused on proactive treatment. Where the estimated blood loss is more than 1500 mL, clinicians assume the patient needs all blood products and administers them, rather than waiting for investigations to confirm anaemia and DIC and then treat.
- Renal and liver function (major PPH) – to help determine the cause of the PPH and to determine the effect on organ function.

COMPLICATIONS

Depending on the degree of blood loss and suitability of the treatment given, complications can include:
- Orthostatic hypotension – this usually is secondary to volume loss and easily reversed by fluids and blood transfusion.
- Anaemia – patients can be asymptomatic, but will usually be pale and complain of shortness of breath, often worse on exertion associated with fatigue. Tachycardia and tachypnoea are common observations.
- Hypovolaemic shock – this is a late complication and a sign that the patient is very unstable. This can lead to the loss of end organ perfusion.

- Sheehan syndrome – this is a rare and serious complication of PPH. Loss of end organ perfusion can lead to anterior pituitary ischaemia, resulting in the need for long-term multiple hormone replacement.
- Transfusion reactions.
- Emotional impact – this is not only on the patient but on any relatives or birthing partners who are present.
- Cardiac arrest and death – fortunately, arrests are rare in the UK, but PPH is the leading cause of death following pregnancy worldwide.

MANAGEMENT

MINOR POSTPARTUM HAEMORRHAGE

For a minor PPH, where the woman is stable and not in shock, the following are the important aspects of management:
- Call for help to ensure that if the woman deteriorates you have assistance close by.
- Start regular monitoring of vital signs and blood loss to assess the woman's stability. Even with a minor PPH, it is still useful to use an airway, breathing, circulation, disability and exposure (ABCDE) assessment method.
- Gain IV access to give fluid or medication as needed.
- Take FBC and G&S to assess haemoglobin and platelet concentration. Having a G&S will allow for crossmatch later if blood products are required. If platelet concentration is low, it would then be sensible to also check clotting, as low platelets may be a marker of a larger-than-estimated blood loss, with significant consumption of clotting factors leading to a coagulopathy.

Further management depends on the cause of the PPH; it is important to recognise the cause as soon as possible.

MAJOR POSTPARTUM HAEMORRHAGE

Communication, resuscitation, monitoring, investigations and bleeding arrest will all need to occur simultaneously, so the more staff on hand, the better.
Immediate actions:
1. Call for help – in most hospitals, this is done by calling the emergency number and activating a PPH emergency call. This usually will alert the senior obstetrician, haematologist on call, anaesthetist, porter, haematology laboratory, blood bank, theatres and obstetric team on call.
2. Rapid assessment – the patient should be laid flat and assessed using an ABCDE approach, with supplementary oxygen and fluids given as necessary. In severe cases, 2 L of warmed fluid are given as a bolus. When IV access is obtained, bloods for FBC, clotting, fibrinogen, crossmatch, U&Es and LFTs should be taken. Ideally, IV access should be with

two large bore cannulae to allow fast infusion of fluid and blood products once they are available.

3. Initial measures to identify the cause and arrest the bleeding (as described later).

It is important to continually reassess the woman via the ABCDE approach to ensure that she remains stable. The degree of haemorrhage must be constantly monitored and assessed, fluid balance maintained (urine output usually monitored hourly by inserting a catheter) and documentation using the maternal early warning chart completed.

BLOOD PRODUCTS

Packed red blood cells are given to replace the loss caused by the PPH to prevent symptomatic anaemia and to assist in maintaining blood pressure:

- O-negative blood – this is used in a dire emergency when there is no time to wait for an emergency crossmatch.
- Emergency crossmatch – this usually takes less than 10 minutes. The lab processes the ABO blood group only.
- Routine crossmatch – this usually takes 40 minutes; the lab processes the ABO blood group and screens for antibodies.

Platelets are given to replace the platelets that are lost during the PPH. They assist in clotting and are part of the clotting cascade. FFP contains many coagulation factors which form part of the clotting cascade. Cryoprecipitate contains coagulation factors and fibrinogen and is given in massive haemorrhage. The blood products are either given once investigations have been reported indicating their need or are given increasingly once blood loss has exceeded approximately 1500 mL without waiting for results, as it is likely that packed red cells, platelets and clotting factors will all be required, and waiting for results delays treatment.

In major obstetric haemorrhage, intravenous tranexamic acid, an antifibrinolytic, is also being used to prevent clot breakdown and decrease blood loss.

MANAGEMENT TO ARREST BLEEDING

While the ABCDE approach of acute management is being followed, the obstetrician in the emergency team can focus on assessing and treating the physical causes of haemorrhage:

- Trauma – assessment of the vagina, perineum and cervix for bleeding tears. Initially, compression can be applied to reduce the bleeding, and once adequate analgesia has been provided, these can be sutured. During initial examination of the vagina, any visible

or palpable retained products or blood clots in the cervix should be removed, as these frequently cause a vasovagal hypotensive response, often causing a profound hypotension and bradycardia, whereas tachycardia is expected in response to hypovolaemic shock. Removal of these can often resolve hypotension rapidly.

- Thrombin – the obstetrician examining would be unable to treat a coagulopathy, but they can certainly monitor the estimated blood loss. They will notice when the blood is no longer forming clots and can alert the rest of the team quickly, so treatment of major haemorrhage and DIC can be expedited.
- Tone.
  - Atony is by far the most common cause of PPH, easily identified on clinical examination of the abdomen, where a soft, lax, large uterus is palpated.
  - A contraction can be 'rubbed up' abdominally by rubbing the uterus.
  - Bimanual compression – the healthcare professional has one hand in the vagina and the other hand on the uterine fundus abdominally, pushing the uterus between their hands to compress it and encourage contraction.
  - Evacuate the uterus of any clots or retained tissue which reduces the capacity of the uterus to contract.
  - Medical management to increase uterine contraction (uterotonics):
    - Oxytocin IV or IM boluses, with or without IV infusion.
    - Ergometrine IV or IM.
    - Synthetic prostaglandin, for example, carboprost and misoprostol.

If the previously described methods fail to stem the haemorrhage, the woman will need to be taken to theatre to further assess under general anaesthetic. A balloon may be inserted into the uterus to compress the vessels within the uterus. If this fails, a laparotomy would be performed. This can identify rare causes of bleeding, such as uterine rupture. If atony is the cause, a 'B-lynch suture' can be inserted to compress the uterus and encourage contraction.

During laparotomy, the internal iliac arteries can be identified and ligated to reduce blood flow to the uterus, stemming the haemorrhage. In some hospitals, radiologists can be called to perform uterine artery embolisation. The radiologist first performs angiography to identify either the internal iliac or uterine arteries and then injects a sclerosing agent. The uterus still has collateral blood supply from branches of the ovarian arteries and vaginal arteries.

At the time of laparotomy, any blood lost can be collected from the abdominal cavity using a vacuum and collected in a cell salvage machine. Here, the collected blood is filtered and centrifuged to leave primarily

- Tissue – examination for completeness of the delivered placenta to check for any missing pieces. If retained tissue is suspected, a digital examination of the uterus can be done under appropriate analgesia.

the woman's own red cells, which can then be infused back into the patient. This reduces the need for blood transfusion. Cell salvage can be used for blood collection from a laparotomy or caesarean section, but not from vaginal blood loss, as this blood is at high risk of bacterial contamination.

If no other technique works, the final method which may be performed is a hysterectomy to save the patient's life.

PROGNOSIS

The prognosis depends on the severity, cause, timely recognition and management of PPH. After a large PPH, a patient requires close monitoring for further blood loss, infection (as they are at increased risk of sepsis) and clinical deterioration. Often, high dependency unit (HDU) or intensive treatment unit (ITU) level care is required initially.

Most PPH cases are minor and easily treated with no long-term sequelae, but the worst cases may lead to emergency hysterectomy or death.

❓ QUESTIONS

Su-Lee, a 28-year-old woman, gravidity three, parity one, has just given birth to twins. Her current pregnancy has been uneventful, with all the routine scans and investigations being normal. Immediately after twin two has been born safely, she becomes tachycardic and tachypnoeic (heart rate of 102 bpm, respiratory rate of 24 breaths/min). The uterus is soft and not firming under uterine massage, and a large amount of blood loss is noted on the sheets.

Q1 For primary PPH to be diagnosed, up to what time after delivery would the haemorrhage have to occur?

   A Less than 4 hours.
   B Less than 24 hours.
   C Less than 72 hours.
   D Less than 4 weeks.
   E Less than 6 weeks.

A Maternal hyperthyroidism.	**G** Maternal low BMI.
B Multiple pregnancy.	**H** Emergency caesarean section.
C Pre-eclampsia.	**I** Polyhydramnios.
D Assisted vaginal birth.	**J** Maternal diabetes.
E Previous menorrhagia.	**K** Elective caesarean section.
F Placenta praevia.	**L** Retained placenta.

Select the most appropriate option from the above list that corresponds to the following statements. Each answer can be used once, more than once or not at all.

Q2 From the options above, which option carries the highest risk of causing a PPH?

Q3 A woman with known type 2 diabetes and trigeminal neuralgia is pregnant with twins. From the options above, which answer carries the greatest risk for PPH for this patient?

Q4 From the options above, which mode of birth carries the highest risk of PPH?

Q5 A 45-year-old woman with a past medical history of hyperthyroidism and menorrhagia has been admitted to the hospital by her midwife. She is at 34 weeks gestation with her first child. Her midwife has noticed that the patient's blood pressure has been increasing over the past few weeks, and now there is protein in her urine. From the options above, which answer is a risk factor for PPH in this patient?

Q6 A 23-year-old woman has just had her first child by assisted vaginal birth. Her obstetrician decided to use forceps to assist in the safe and quick birth of a baby girl. The midwife has noticed that despite the use of synthetic oxytocin, the woman has a retained placenta. From the options above, what answer carries the highest risk of PPH for this patient?

Q7 Answer true or false: Which of the following are causes of PPH?

   A Uterine atony.
   B Coagulopathy.
   C Sepsis.
   D Lower genital tract lacerations.
   E Retained placental fragments.

[Answers on page 428.]

AMNIOTIC EMBOLISM

Amniotic embolism is a rare obstetric emergency where amniotic fluid or fetal cells enter the maternal circulation, causing maternal cardiorespiratory collapse.

RISK FACTORS

Although no risk factors are identified in the majority of cases, several risk factors are considered to be associated with amniotic embolism, including:
- Twin pregnancies.
- Macrosomia.
- Polyhydramnios.
- Intrauterine fetal death.
- Advanced maternal age.
- Trauma.
- Placental abruption.
- Prolonged labour.
- Oxytocin augmented labour.
- Assisted vaginal birth.
- Caesarean section.

AETIOLOGY

The incidence of amniotic embolism is estimated to be 2 cases per 100,000 pregnancies. Approximately half the cases occur within 5 minutes following birth. The pathophysiology of amniotic embolism is poorly understood. It is postulated that amniotic fluid or fetal cells enter the maternal circulation, collect in the lungs and trigger a massive immune response. However, amniotic fluid and/or fetal cells may be found in the blood of women without amniotic embolism. Conversely, not all women who develop amniotic embolism have detectable levels of circulating fetal cells or amniotic fluid.

There are two generally accepted phases to amniotic embolism. Initially, there is a pulmonary embolism, which is an embolus of amniotic fluid in the lungs. This causes direct blockage of the vessels like a thrombus and an anaphylactic type reaction to the fetal antigens, leading to hypoxia and acute respiratory distress syndrome. This is followed by a haemorrhagic phase, caused by activation of complement pathways leading to DIC. This is often fatal.

CLINICAL FEATURES

It is important to remember that amniotic fluid will embolise to the pulmonary circulation. The response to this disruption of homeostasis can be cardiovascular, respiratory, neurological and haematological. Women usually present either with signs and symptoms similar to a pulmonary embolus (Table 15.4) or with acute collapse.

If a woman survives the initial episode, it is likely that her condition will worsen. She will subsequently develop DIC, acute respiratory distress syndrome, neurological impairment or multisystem organ failure.

INVESTIGATIONS

No diagnostic tests are available for this obstetric emergency, but a case of amniotic embolism is considered if the following occur during labour, during caesarean section or up to 30 minutes postpartum:
1. Acute hypotension or cardiac arrest.
2. Acute hypoxia.
3. Coagulopathy or severe haemorrhage.

Radiological investigations, such as a chest x-ray, may help diagnose acute respiratory distress syndrome; however, it is very unlikely that there will be time to perform these investigations.

Unfortunately, due to the high mortality rate, amniotic embolisms are diagnosed postmortem in many cases by identifying amniotic fluid or fetal cells in the maternal circulation.

DIFFERENTIAL DIAGNOSES

Amniotic embolism is often a diagnosis of exclusion, as there is no direct test in the acute situation. Possible differentials include:
- Pulmonary thromboembolism.
- Pulmonary haemorrhage.
- Air embolism.
- Anaphylaxis.
- High spinal anaesthesia.
- Septic shock.
- Uterine rupture.
- Eclampsia.

COMPLICATIONS

An amniotic embolism carries a high level of morbidity and mortality. DIC is a common complication.

If the woman survives, many complications can occur, including:
- Psychological comorbidities.
- Persisting neurological impairment following hypoxia.
- Cardiac arrest.
- Hysterectomy.

MANAGEMENT

Amniotic emboli cannot be prevented. Timely and expert management is the key to ensuring maternal and fetal survival.

This is a major obstetric emergency. Call for help from senior obstetric and anaesthetic staff and from the resuscitation team. The mainstay of management is supportive care, maintaining oxygenation and perfusion of vital organs using an ABCDE resuscitation approach.

OXYGENATION

- This is not only important for maternal survival but also for fetal survival, as they are highly vulnerable to maternal hypoxia.
- One hundred percent supplemental oxygen is advised and mechanical ventilation is usually indicated.

PERFUSION

- To optimise preload and circulating volume, fluid replacement is indicated.
- Inotropic drugs can assist effective myocardial functioning.

CORRECTING COAGULOPATHY

- Discussion with the on-call haematologist is advised.

Table 15.4	Clinical Features of Amniotic Fluid or Fetal Cell Embolism

SIGNS	SYMPTOMS
Tachypnoea	Shortness of breath
Tachycardia	Palpitations
Hypotension	Dizziness
Coagulopathy or severe bleeding	Confusion
Cyanosis	Seizure
Cardiac arrest	Cough
Hypoxia	Pulmonary oedema
Respiratory arrest	Loss of consciousness

- Blood components will assist to combat severe coagulopathy.
- Fresh frozen plasma (FFP), cryoprecipitate or recombinant factors may be indicated.

BIRTH

- Perimortem caesarean section is considered within 5 minutes of acute maternal collapse and cardiac arrest if initial resuscitation is unsuccessful. Delivery will aid maternal cardiac output by reducing blood flow to the uterus, which will improve maternal survival chances.
- If the fetus is at a viable gestation, birth will also improve fetal survival. However, as primary importance is given to maternal survival, delivery may be undertaken even if the fetus may die as a result.

PROGNOSIS

The prognosis is poor for this obstetric emergency, with maternal mortality approaching 40%. Of the survivors, 7% have permanent neurological impairment.

❓ QUESTIONS

Jaspreet, a 24-year-old, is gravidity two, parity one. The rest of her pregnancy has been uneventful, with all the routine scans and investigations normal. She attends for an elective caesarean section after a previous caesarean for her first child. Following spinal anaesthesia, a male baby is born with normal Apgar scores. During placental removal, she begins to cough and complain of shortness of breath. A few minutes later, her oxygen saturation drops, and she progresses to cardiopulmonary arrest. As the junior doctor on the ward, you are called to assist.

Q1 In a life-threatening emergency, when no G&S has been performed, what blood can be given to the woman?
  A B-negative blood.
  B O-positive blood.
  C AB-negative blood.
  D O-negative blood.
  E B-positive blood.

Q2 Answer true or false: Which of the following blood products are typically used in the management of DIC?
  A FFP.
  B Packed red cells.
  C Cryoprecipitate.
  D Platelets.
  E Albumin.

Q3 Which vessels are thought to be involved in carrying amniotic fluid to the maternal pulmonary system?
  A Aorta.
  B Pulmonary veins.
  C Inferior vena cava.
  D Pulmonary arteries.
  E Umbilical veins.

[Answers on page 429.]

MATERNAL COLLAPSE

Maternal collapse is defined as an acute event resulting in reduced or absent conscious level and can be a life-threatening obstetric emergency. This can occur at any point during pregnancy and up to 6 weeks following birth.

AETIOLOGY

The causes of maternal collapse are similar to those that cause shock, loss of consciousness and/or cardiac arrest in any adult, with the addition of specific pregnancy-related disorders such as amniotic fluid embolism and eclampsia. Since pregnancy itself is a significant physiological stressor, it is logical that many conditions exacerbated by stress may present in pregnancy, eventually resulting in maternal collapse. Potential causes of maternal collapse include:

- Sepsis.
- Bleeding – PPH, placental abruption, placenta praevia, aneurysm.
- Pulmonary embolism – thrombotic, amniotic or air.
- Seizures and the postictal state – epilepsy, eclampsia, intracranial bleed.
- Vasovagal collapse.
- Myocardial infarction.
- Cardiomyopathies.
- Hyperglycaemia and hypoglycaemia.
- Hypothermia.
- Drug overdose – such as magnesium sulphate, illicit drugs, local anaesthetics.
- Spinal or epidural complications.

[See 'Amniotic Embolism' on page 348.]
[See 'Pre-Eclampsia and Pregnancy-Induced Hypertension' on page 301.]

The definition of shock is hypotension despite initial fluid resuscitation. Shock often occurs before cardiac arrest, so with rapid assessment and treatment, an arrest can be avoided. Shock is commonly associated with maternal collapse, so it is important to understand the different types and causes of shock (Table 15.5).

MANAGEMENT

Managing a critically unwell pregnant patient involves primarily the same ABCDE assessment approach as is employed with any acutely sick patient in medicine.

AIRWAY

Assess the woman's airway to evaluate if it is compromised. If the woman is able to speak, they have a patent airway. If unable to speak, open the mouth to look for and remove any foreign objects, using appropriate equipment such as suction. If no obvious obstruction or objects need to be removed, use any airway opening manoeuvres, such as head tilt and chin lift or jaw thrust. If cervical spine injury is suspected, always use a jaw

Table 15.5 Classifications of Shock to Consider in a Collapsed Patient

TYPE OF SHOCK	OBSERVATIONS	POTENTIAL CAUSES
Hypovolaemic	• Hypotension. • Tachycardia. • Peripheral pulses weak and thready, with cool and clammy skin – caused by vasoconstriction in attempt to preserve core organ perfusion. • Decreased urine output, drop in GCS – evidence of decreased perfusion to end organs.	Haemorrhage. Dehydration. Diabetic ketoacidosis.

Distributive	• Hypotension.
	• Tachycardia.
	• Warm peripheries – due to vasodilatation increasing the intravascular space.
	• Additional features depend on cause:
	  • Anaphylactic – dyspnoea, and other signs of allergy like pruritus, urticaria and swollen lips.
	  • Septic – tachypnoea, warm and flushed skin, fever.
	  • Vagal – causes bradycardia and vasodilation due to vagal nerve stimulus. Commonly caused by a blood clot in the cervix or pain in obstetric patients.
		Anaphylactic – medication allergy or insect bite.
		Septic – infection.
		Vagal – blood clot in cervical os, pain.

Cardiogenic	• Hypotension. • Tachycardia. • Weak peripheral pulses. • Cool skin. • Decreased urine output. • Decreased consciousness. • Signs of heart failure – tachypnoea, decreased saturations, crackles, raised JVP. • Chest pain.	Cardiac causes: • Cardiac arrest. • Arrhythmias. • Cardiomyopathy. Obstructive causes: • Pulmonary embolism. • Tension pneumothorax. • Cardiac tamponade.
Neurogenic	• Hypotension. • Bradycardia. • Warm, dry skin. • All caused by lack of sympathetic tone causing bradycardia and peripheral vasodilation.	• Trauma, usually acute damage high in the spinal cord. • High spinal or epidural anaesthesia. • Uterine inversion.

GCS, Glasgow Coma Scale; JVP, jugular venous pressure.

thrust. A patient with an altered level of consciousness may need insertion of a properly sized oropharyngeal or nasopharyngeal airway. Patients with significantly reduced conscious levels (GCS less than 8) may need an anaesthetic review and a definitive airway, such as intubation.

BREATHING

Assess for chest wall movements or breath sounds, and feel for breathing by placing your cheek above the woman's mouth.

- If the patient is making no respiratory effort, alert help and start maternal CPR (see below).
- If the woman has some respiratory effort, assist their breathing with 100% inspired oxygen via a non-rebreathe mask and measure their oxygen saturations. Listen to their chest with a stethoscope to assess if any further intervention may be required.

CIRCULATION

Look for signs of circulatory collapse, including cool, pale digits or poor capillary refill, assess the pulse by feeling for the carotid pulse or other central pulse and then take the blood pressure. Look briefly for any obvious life-threatening bleeding, including in the vagina in a patient known to be pregnant.

- If the patient has no pulse, pull the emergency bell and start maternal CPR (see later).
- If the woman has a pulse but is hypotensive, assist by inserting two large-bore intravenous cannulae, and initiate fluid resuscitation. Aggressive fluid resuscitation may be required, and it can be useful to warm the fluid when given. At this point, blood can be taken for FBC, U&E, CRP, clotting, fibrinogen, LFTs, lactate, blood glucose and any relevant blood typing. A venous blood gas can also be performed for immediate information, or an arterial blood gas can be used if a respiratory cause is suspected.
- In a pregnant woman, if there is no suspected head or spinal trauma, it is important to place her in a left lateral position to prevent supine hypotensive syndrome. This is caused by the gravid uterus compressing the vena cava in the supine position, reducing venous return from the lower

half of the body, causing hypotension. By positioning in the left lateral position or by manually displacing the uterus, vena cava patency is maintained.

DISABILITY

Once you feel the patient is stable enough to continue the assessment, it is important to gain some history from the patient (if possible), the healthcare professional looking after them and from the notes. Important points to assess are:

- Conscious level, using GCS or AVPU (alert, responds to voice, responds to pain or unresponsive) scores, with a more detailed neurological exam if necessary.
- Temperature.
- Blood glucose level.

EXPOSURE

This step involves more detailed examination, doing a full 'top-to-toe' assessment, examining for any clues for the collapse. In pregnancy it is essential that this includes:

- A thorough abdominal examination.
- Vaginal examination.

Abdominal and vaginal examination often occurs along with the initial ABCDE assessment where sufficient team members are available, as often the cause of collapse is identified on these examinations.

Concerns regarding the fetus and commencement of fetal monitoring should only occur once the mother is stabilised. The mother is always the priority.

In management of the critically unwell woman, it is vital to constantly reassess the patient before performing further investigation or management steps. Women who are seemingly stable can still deteriorate, so it is important to acknowledge this by constant reassessment and action. Patients should continue to be reassessed every 5 minutes.

> **ABCDE Approach**
>
> The look, listen, feel, measure, treat, reassess approach to the ABCDE assessment is important, as it enables the clinician to have a structured approach when dealing with sick patients.

MATERNAL CARDIOPULMONARY RESUSCITATION

If a patient has collapsed and is showing no pulse or respiratory effort, CPR must take place. The following steps highlight the important aspects of maternal resuscitation. In principle, the steps of resuscitation are the same as an adult resuscitation; however, there are vital adaptations to common steps to consider if a woman is greater than 20 weeks pregnant.

1. If there are no signs of life during ABC assessment, call for help – the adult, obstetric and neonatal (if a viable gestation) cardiac arrest teams should all be called.

2. Apply manual uterine displacement to the left. Historically, women would be moved into a left lateral position to help venous return, but evidence shows that it is very difficult in this position to perform good, productive chest compressions. Therefore, manual displacement is advocated instead. To do this, one person physically pushes on the lower abdomen from the right-hand side to push the uterus over to the left. This is performed because, when lying flat, the pregnant uterus can impinge the flow of the inferior vena cava, causing a reduced cardiac preload and therefore reduced output.

3. Start CPR – this will be basic life support until the resuscitation teams arrive, using a 30:2 ratio of chest compressions to breaths at a speed of 100/minute.

4. Advanced life support commenced once assistance arrives. Important steps here are:
   a. Maintenance of an airway and the use of oxygen.
   b. Good chest compressions.
   c. Accurate timing and documentation, for which someone will be designated scribe.
   d. Defibrillation pad applied and ALS algorithm followed. There is no change in the ALS protocol in pregnancy with regards to the medication given.

5. In cases of unsuccessful CPR for 4 minutes, delivery of the fetus and placenta by perimortem caesarean is necessary if the patient is 20 weeks pregnant or beyond. Delivery should occur within 5 minutes of the maternal collapse to have optimal benefit in the maternal resuscitation effort. It is performed wherever the patient has collapsed, and all that is required is a scalpel. A perimortem caesarean section is performed with the rationale that the uterus and placenta utilise approximately 500 mL/min of blood. By removing this significant blood requirement from the mother, it may benefit venous return of the patient. The reason for delivery is to save the mother and not the baby, although the baby's survival chances may improve as a result.

6. Throughout the CPR process, it is important to identify and correct any reversible causes of the collapse, many of which we have discussed in this section. To aid in remembering important reversible causes, the UK life support algorithm for adults includes the '4 Hs and 4 Ts' reversible causes mnemonic:
   - Hypoxia.
   - Hypovolaemia.
   - Hypothermia.
   - Hypo/hyperkalaemia (plus other electrolyte and glucose disturbances).
   - Tamponade (cardiac).
   - Tension pneumothorax.
   - Thrombus – pulmonary embolus.
   - Toxins – for example drug or alcohol overdose.

Left Lateral Displacement

Left lateral displacement of the uterus enables more venous return of blood to the patient. This is because a pregnant uterus can impinge the flow of the inferior vena cava when the woman is lying flat, causing a reduced cardiac output which can potentially cause profound hypotension and, in severe cases, a cardiac arrest. At the time of cardiac arrest or peri-arrest, left displacement of the uterus can be done by manually pushing on the abdomen. The aim of lateral displacement is to relieve the pressure on the vena cava, improving cardiac output, which increases the chance of a successful resuscitation.

Possible Complications When Resuscitating a Pregnant Woman

Normal physiological and anatomical changes that occur in pregnancy can make resuscitation more challenging. These must be taken into consideration by the anaesthetic team and include:

- Laryngeal oedema – making intubation difficult.
- Excessive breast tissue and weight gain – impairing ventilation.
- Displacement of the diaphragm by gravid uterus – impairing ventilation.
- Decreased functional residual capacity – impairing ventilation.
- Reduced efficiency of the lower oesophageal sphincter – increasing aspiration risk.

POSTCOLLAPSE

If the resuscitation attempt is successful, then the woman will continue to require care in a critical care setting. Once return of spontaneous circulation has occurred and the mother is stable, it is then time to undertake fetal assessment and discuss the delivery plans with senior obstetricians and paediatricians (if birth has not occurred during resuscitation).

If the attempt is unsuccessful, the coroner will need to be informed. Full debriefing and support is vital in such an incident for relatives and all staff members involved.

❓ QUESTIONS

Jane, a 34-year-old woman, is 26 weeks pregnant and was on the day assessment unit because of vaginal bleeding of unknown cause. She has abruptly collapsed in the unit. On assessment, she is unresponsive.

Q1 What is the first action to take?
  A Check for a carotid pulse.
  B Call for your senior clinician.
  C Check the blood pressure.
  D Call for help.
  E Count the respiratory rate.

Q2 If the initial assessment shows she has no respiratory effort, which answer best describes who needs to be called for support?
  A The hospital cardiac arrest team.
  B The obstetric and neonatal teams.

C The hospital intensive care team.
D The cardiac arrest and obstetric teams.
E The cardiac arrest, obstetric and neonatal teams.

A	PPH.	G	Hypoglycaemia.
B	Severe sepsis.	H	Amniotic embolism.
C	Hyponatraemia.	I	Hypothermia.
D	Hyperkalaemia.	J	Hyperthermia.
E	Hypertension.	K	Anaphylaxis.
F	Placental abruption.	L	Eclampsia.

Select the most appropriate option from the above list that corresponds to the following statements. Each answer can be used once, more than once or not at all.

Q3 A 24-year-old woman has consented for a planned caesarean birth. This is her first pregnancy; she has never been in hospital before or had any operations. She has had a spinal anaesthetic and has been prepped for the operation, including having antibiotic cover. Just as the procedure is about to start, she becomes unstable, tachycardic, tachypnoeic and hypoxic. From the options above, which cause of maternal collapse is most likely?

Q4 A 32-year-old woman in her first pregnancy has presented to the delivery suite with abdominal pain and feeling generally unwell. She is 36⁺⁶ weeks pregnant and looks unwell. On initial examination, she is hypotensive and tachycardic and has a tender, firm abdomen. She rapidly becomes unresponsive. From the options above, which cause of maternal collapse is most likely?

Q5 A 27-year-old woman in her third pregnancy with known gestational diabetes has just had a normal vaginal birth. The birth was uncomplicated, with an active third stage and a one-off temperature of 37.9°C. She is feeling generally unwell. She is responding to voice, is pyrexial, tachycardic, hypotensive and tachypnoeic and has normal saturations. From the options above, which cause of maternal collapse is most likely?

[Answers on page 430.]

KEY REFERENCES

CORD PROLAPSE

Royal College of Obstetricians and Gynaecologists, 2014. Umbilical cord prolapse. RCOG green top guideline (GTG 50).

SHOULDER DYSTOCIA

Royal College of Obstetricians and Gynaecologists, 2012. Shoulder dystocia. RCOG green top guideline (GTG 42).
Boulvain, M., Irion, O., Thornton, J.G., 2016. Induction of labour at or near term for suspected fetal macrosomia. Cochrane Database of Systematic Reviews, (5).

RETAINED PLACENTA

Weeks, AD., 2008. The retained placenta. Best practice & research. Clinical Obstetrics and Gynaecology 22 (6), 1103–1117.
National Institute for Health and Clinical Excellence, 2017. Intrapartum care for healthy women and babies. NICE clinical guideline (CG 190).

POSTPARTUM HAEMORRHAGE

Royal College of Obstetricians and Gynaecologists, 2016. Prevention and management of postpartum haemorrhage. RCOG green top guideline (GTG 52).

World Health Organisation, 2009. Guidelines for the management of postpartum haemorrhage and retained placenta [online]. Available from: http://apps.who.int/iris/bitstream/10665/44171/1/9789241598514_eng.pdf. (accessed 10.07.23.).

AMNIOTIC EMBOLISM

Royal College of Obstetricians and Gynaecologists, 2019. Maternal collapse in pregnancy and the puerperium. RCOG green top guideline (GTG 56).

Perozzi, K, Englert, N., 2004. Amniotic fluid embolism: an obstetric emergency. Critical Care Nurse 24 (4), 54–61.

MATERNAL COLLAPSE

Royal College of Obstetricians and Gynaecologists, 2019. Maternal collapse in pregnancy and the puerperium. RCOG green top guideline (GTG 56).

Resuscitation Council UK, 2021. Resuscitation guidelines. Available at: http://www.resus.org.uk/resuscitation-guidelines. (accessed 10.07.23.).

Resuscitation Council UK and Obstetric Anaesthetists' Association, 2021. Obstetric cardiac arrest – quick reference guide. Clinical Guideline.

Postnatal Complications

VENOUS THROMBOEMBOLISM

Venous thromboembolism (VTE) describes a blood clot, or thrombus, forming within a vein before breaking off to travel in the systemic circulation, where it is known as an embolus. This most commonly occurs when a thrombus forms in the deep veins of the lower limb (termed a deep vein thrombosis (DVT)) and embolises to the pulmonary circulation (termed a pulmonary embolism (PE)).

Pregnancy and the postpartum period are associated with an increased risk of VTE, and PEs are the most common direct cause of maternal death in the UK. Importantly, many PEs are preventable with appropriate thromboprophylaxis.

AETIOLOGY

Thrombus formation (Fig. 16.1) occurs as a result of abnormalities in one or more of the components of the Virchow triad:

- The vessel wall – damage or lesions in the endothelium.
- The blood flow – haemostatic changes leading to blood stasis.
- The blood components – hypercoagulability.

Pregnancy increases the risk of VTE for several reasons. Raised oestrogen and other hormones in pregnancy result in an increase in many clotting factors. From an evolutionary viewpoint, this is beneficial, as it limits haemorrhage at the time of birth; however, this hypercoagulable state increases the risk of pathological thrombus formation. In addition to the hypercoagulable state, haemodynamic changes occur as a result of increased intra-abdominal pressure, which can impair venous drainage of the lower limbs, resulting in venous stasis.

RISK FACTORS

Risk assessment scoring systems are used antenatally and postnatally for all patients to identify patients at high risk of VTE and to prescribe appropriate thromboprophylaxis as required (Table 16.1). In the RCOG system, risk factors are associated with a value of one to four, and a total risk score is then generated. The higher the score, the greater the risk.

RISK MANAGEMENT AND PROPHYLAXIS

All women should be assessed for risk of VTE antenatally, usually at the first booking appointment. A risk assessment should be repeated if a woman is admitted to hospital, during early pregnancy, following birth and whenever her obstetric situation changes. This involves scoring risk factors as outlined previously. All patients should avoid dehydration and immobility to reduce risk. Further management depends on the risk score generated, whereby high-risk women (risk score of three or more) are considered for antenatal prophylaxis with low-molecular-weight heparin (LMWH). This is usually continued throughout pregnancy and for 6 weeks postpartum. LMWH is specifically used as it does not cross the placenta, warfarin is teratogenic and newer direct oral anticoagulants (DOACs) have not been studied in pregnancy.

Graduated compression stockings are also recommended:

- In hospitalised women with a contraindication to LMWH.
- In addition to LMWH prophylaxis in hospitalised women who are considered high risk – postsurgery or those with more than three risk factors.
- Outpatient – in women with a prior VTE or undertaking long-distance travel for more than 4 hours.

 Risks of Low-Molecular-Weight Heparin

- Haemorrhage.
- Hyperkalaemia.
- Injection site reactions.
- Rarely, thrombocytopaenia.

Women taking LMWH antenatally should be advised to stop it in the event of signs of labour. LMWH

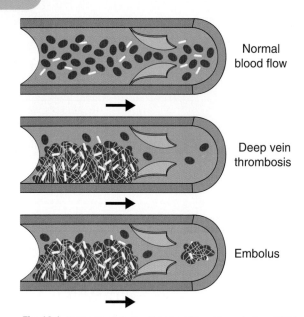

Normal blood flow

Deep vein thrombosis

Embolus

Fig. 16.1 Pathophysiology of Venous Thromboembolism (VTE).

Table 16.1	Risk Factors and Scoring for Venous Thromboembolism in Pregnancy	
RCOG PE RISK FACTORS (WEIGHTED BY RISK CONFERRED)		
4 points	Previous VTE – except for a single event related to major surgery	
	OHSS	
3 points	Previous VTE provoked by major surgery	
	Known high-risk thrombophilia	
	Medical comorbidities, for example, cancer, lupus or nephrotic syndrome	
	Any surgical procedure in pregnancy or puerperium, excluding perineal repair and caesarean	
	Hyperemesis	
2 points	BMI of more than 40 kg/m²	
	Emergency caesarean section	
1 point	Family history of unprovoked or oestrogen-related VTE in a first-degree relative	
	Known low-risk thrombophilia with no VTE	
	Age more than 35 years	
	BMI of more than 30 kg/m²	
	Parity of three or more	
	Smoker	
	Significant varicose veins	
	Pre-eclampsia in current pregnancy	
	Dehydration	
	Multiple pregnancy	
	Assisted reproduction therapy	
	Prolonged labour (more than 24 hours)	
	Assisted vaginal birth	
	Postpartum haemorrhage more than 1 L or requiring transfusion	
	Preterm birth less than 37 weeks gestation in current pregnancy	
	Stillbirth in current pregnancy	
	Immobility including hospital admission	
	Current systemic infection	
	Elective caesarean section	

BMI, Body mass index; *OHSS*, ovarian hyperstimulation syndrome; *PE*, pulmonary embolism; *RCOG*, Royal College of Obstetricians and Gynaecologists; *VTE*, venous thromboembolism.

has to be appropriately timed according to birth, as the risks of labour within 12 hours of LMWH include excessive blood loss and limited analgesic options, as epidural analgesia and spinal anaesthesia are contraindicated due to the increased risk of bleeding around the spine during the procedure, which could cause spinal cord compression.

CLINICAL FEATURES

The classical features of a DVT in the calf are:
- Pain worsened by palpation and dorsiflexion.
- Erythema.
- Swelling – measure the leg circumference with a tape 10 cm below the tibial tuberosity and compare to the asymptomatic leg.
- Warmth.

DVT in pregnancy is much more likely to present in the left leg due to the gravid uterus compressing the left external iliac vein. Atypical DVT presentations are also seen in pregnancy, with proximal vein (femoral or iliac) thrombosis rather than the classic calf pain.

The classical features of a PE are:
- Symptoms
  - Pleuritic chest pain.
  - Shortness of breath.
  - Haemoptysis.
- Signs
  - Tachycardia.
  - Tachypnoea.
  - Mild pyrexia.
  - Pleural rub.

Most presentations with these features are of a minor PE, which are clinically stable. In contrast, an acute massive PE often presents as an acutely unwell patient with severe dyspnoea, cyanosis, as well as signs of circulatory collapse and right heart failure (tachycardia, hypotension, raised jugular venous pressure).

INITIAL TREATMENT

As in general medicine, if a VTE is suspected clinically, presumptive treatment should be commenced while awaiting confirmatory investigations. Note the Well's score is not validated in pregnancy and is therefore not used. Treatment with LMWH should be given until VTE diagnosis is excluded unless strongly contraindicated. These contraindications include threatened or active labour and conditions where there is a high risk of bleeding.

INVESTIGATIONS

Investigations in a woman presenting with a suspected DVT or PE are performed to confirm or exclude VTE and other differential diagnoses, as well as to guide management.

INVESTIGATIONS FOR DVT

- The preferred imaging modality for a DVT is a duplex ultrasound scan of the venous system of the lower limb. Due to occasional false negatives, the scan can be repeated on days 3 and 7 if clinical suspicion persists, while stopping the anticoagulant treatment.
- CT or MRI and contrast venography can also be performed in addition if there is a clinically suspected proximal DVT, where ultrasound has been inconclusive.
- D-dimers are not routinely performed, as they are elevated during pregnancy, independent of the presence of a thrombus.

INVESTIGATIONS FOR PE

Observations

Temperature, blood pressure, pulse, respiratory rate and oxygen saturations should be measured. In addition, an ECG should be performed (Fig.16.2). The most common finding in a PE is sinus tachycardia. Other findings include evidence of right heart strain and the classical S1Q3T3 pattern (S wave in lead I, a Q wave in lead III and an inverted T wave in lead III).

Blood Tests

- Full blood count – low haemoglobin indicates anaemia, which is a differential for shortness of breath. A raised white cell count could support a diagnosis

of a respiratory infection or cellulitis as differentials for a PE or DVT.
- Coagulation screen – this should be included in the baseline blood test prior to starting anticoagulation treatment.
- U&Es and LFTs – the use of contrast for imaging studies and anticoagulant administration are dependent on adequate renal and liver function.
- Arterial blood gas – this may be considered in the acutely unwell patient to guide ongoing ventilation management.

Imaging

Chest x-ray should be performed to exclude differential diagnoses and guide the interpretation of later imaging. Women can be reassured that there is no risk to the fetus with a single chest x-ray.

Options for diagnostic imaging are:
- Computer tomography pulmonary angiogram (CTPA).
- Ventilation/perfusion (V/Q) scan.

> **Imaging in Suspected Venous Thromboembolism**
> - If there is no feature of DVT, but PE is clinically suspected and chest x-ray is abnormal: CTPA or V/Q.
> - If there are clinical features of DVT: compression duplex ultrasound should be done instead of CTPA or V/Q.

The benefits and risks of both modalities need to be discussed with the patient so they can decide which test to proceed with. CTPA is the gold-standard imaging modality for diagnosing a PE and is used first line in the general population. The potential advantages of CTPA include its greater availability, less radiation to the fetus and ability to detect other pathologies such as pneumonia. However, due to radiation exposure

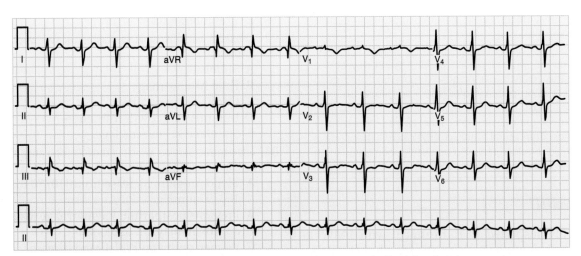

Fig. 16.2 Electrocardiogram (ECG) from a 33-year-old woman who presented with a left main pulmonary artery embolism on chest CT scan. The initial ECG tracing shows an S1Q3T3 (leads I and III) with an S wave in lead I, Q wave in lead III, and inverted T wave in lead III, and incomplete right bundle branch block, with inverted or flattened T waves in leads V1 through V4.

of the breast tissue, which is undergoing physiological hyperplasia in pregnancy, CTPA is associated with an approximately 10% relative risk increase of developing breast cancer (approximately 13% lifetime risk compared to a background population risk of 12%).

While V/Q is safer for the mother than CTPA, including less radiation to the breasts in pregnancy, it exposes the fetus to 10 times more radiation than a CTPA, and a V/Q scan is less likely to give a definitive result, meaning further investigation may be required. Due to fetal radiation exposure, there is approximately a 1:200,000 chance of childhood cancer (the CTPA risk is similar to the background population risk of less than one in a million).

DIFFERENTIAL DIAGNOSIS

DVT

- Musculoskeletal pain.
- Cellulitis.
- Ruptured Baker's cyst.

PE

- Respiratory – bronchitis, pneumonia, asthma, pneumothorax.
- Cardiac – myocardial infarction, pericarditis, cardiomyopathy.
- Musculoskeletal – costochondritis, muscle sprain.
- Psychological – anxiety.
- Physiological dyspnoea of pregnancy.

 Physiological Dyspnoea of Pregnancy

During pregnancy, oxygen consumption is increased by approximately 20%; about 40% of this is to meet the oxygen requirements of the fetoplacental unit. The rest is to satisfy the increased maternal demands for oxygen due to an increase in cardiac output, renal function and other metabolic processes. To achieve this, the mother hyperventilates. The increase in oxygen delivery is largely due to an increase in tidal breathing, meaning the woman breathes more deeply, while her respiratory rate actually changes very little.

The sensation of breathlessness is caused by higher oxygen demands, which increases in later pregnancy as the gravid uterus restricts diaphragmatic movement and deep breathing. The dyspnoea is often more noticeable on exertion, for example, climbing a flight of stairs. It is, however, perceptual for the patient rather than an objective drop in oxygenation. The natural history of physiological dyspnoea is that it should develop gradually over weeks, compared to an acute change associated with a PE.

MANAGEMENT

In clinically suspected VTE, treatment with LMWH should be given until the diagnosis is excluded unless strongly contraindicated.

- Once the diagnosis is confirmed, LMWH should be continued for the duration of the pregnancy (except during labour) and for at least 6 weeks postnatally until at least 3 months of total treatment has been given.
- Postpartum anticoagulation can be with either LMWH or oral anticoagulants such as warfarin. Warfarin is safe in breastfeeding and does not require subcutaneous injections daily like LMWH. Compression stockings should also be worn, and mobilisation should be encouraged. While DOACs are contraindicated if breastfeeding, it could be an alternative anticoagulation postpartum where women are not breastfeeding.

PROGNOSIS

The mortality rate of VTEs associated with pregnancy has declined as the importance of thromboprophylaxis has been stressed and the awareness of DVTs and PEs increased.

❓ QUESTIONS

Anja is a 28-year-old woman, gravidity two and parity two, who gave birth to her second child 2 days ago. Her pregnancy had no complications, but she delivered by emergency caesarean section following evidence of fetal distress. She has presented to accident and emergency with severe pain in her left calf, which is preventing her from walking. On examination, her left calf appears swollen and erythematous and is tender to touch. Her past medical history includes systemic lupus erythematosus and obesity (BMI of 40 kg/m^2). Following a Doppler examination, she is diagnosed as having a DVT in her left leg and is commenced on warfarin, with bridging LMWH until her international normalised ratio (INR) is therapeutic.

Q1 Which of the following factors is considered the most significant predictor of risk of VTE in pregnancy?
  A Immobility.
  B Smoking.
  C Previous VTE following surgery.
  D Previous VTE during pregnancy.
  E Thrombophilia.

Q2 Antenatal warfarin use is associated with which of the following?
  A Stillbirth.
  B Fetal haemorrhage.
  C Cardiac abnormalities.
  D Intrauterine growth restriction.
  E Spontaneous miscarriage.

Q3 Answer true or false: Which of the following are contraindications to using LMWH?
  A Blood pressure increase from 110/70 to 160/90 mmHg.
  B Previous postpartum haemorrhage losing approximately 1 L of blood.
  C Women with von Willebrand disease.
  D Severe liver disease.
  E Severe renal disease.

[Answers on page 431.]

BACTERIAL SEPSIS FOLLOWING PREGNANCY

Sepsis is life-threatening organ dysfunction in which a dysregulated systemic inflammatory response occurs in the presence of an infection. Puerperal sepsis describes sepsis which develops in the period after birth, up to 6 weeks postnatally, and is the cause of approximately 10 deaths per year in the UK.

Septic shock is a subset of sepsis, which occurs when the patient is hypotensive, requiring vasopressors to keep the mean arterial pressure of ≥65 mmHg and have a high serum lactate level of >2 mmol/L despite adequate fluid resuscitation.

RISK FACTORS

Factors which predispose to puerperal sepsis include those which decrease the body's ability to fight infection and those which provide an additional point of entry for bacteria.

GENERAL MATERNAL FACTORS

- Impaired immunity during pregnancy due to alterations in the maternal immune system to prevent an immune response to the fetus.
- Obesity.
- Impaired glucose tolerance or diabetes.
- Anaemia.

ADDITIONAL POINTS OF ENTRY FOR BACTERIA IN OBSTETRICS

- Invasive procedures such as amniocentesis.
- Cervical cerclage (a cervical stitch).
- Prolonged spontaneous rupture of membranes.
- Vaginal trauma, caesarean section or wound haematoma.
- Retained products of conception.
- Prolonged use of intravenous cannulae.

AETIOLOGY

The most common source of infection in the puerperium is the genital tract, particularly the uterus (endometritis).

Other sources include:
- Mastitis.
- Urinary tract infection.
- Pneumonia.
- Skin and soft tissue infection – cannula or injection sites, caesarean or episiotomy wounds.
- Gastroenteritis.
- Pharyngitis.

The major pathogens causing sepsis are:
- *Streptococcus pyogenes* (group A streptococcus).
- *Escherichia coli.*
- *Staphylococcus aureus.*
- *Streptococcus pneumoniae.*
- Methicillin-resistant *S. aureus* (MRSA).

CLINICAL FEATURES

Clinical features of sepsis may be less distinctive than in the nonpregnant population in the initial phase of the disease and are not necessarily present in all cases. A high index of suspicion for sepsis is therefore required for women in the postpartum period. Presence of sepsis should prompt a search for the source of an infection. These signs may be associated with general symptoms such as fever, breathlessness, lethargy, reduced appetite, abdominal pain or a generalised maculopapular rash. It must also be considered that a patient may present initially with very nonspecific symptoms.

Other symptoms and signs may provide clues as to the underlying source of the infection, for example:
- Diarrhoea and vomiting.
- Breast engorgement or redness.
- Abdominal or pelvic pain and tenderness
- Tender uterus on palpation.
- Wound cellulitis or discharge.
- Offensive vaginal discharge.
- Productive cough.
- Urinary symptoms.

Young women are initially able to compensate when septic and appear quite well from the end of the bed. However, their observations (particularly respiratory rate and heart rate) may demonstrate that their bodies are working hard to compensate. If left untreated, the seemingly well-looking patient can suddenly decompensate and become extremely sick very quickly.

Group A streptococci are the typical pathogens that present in this way in pregnancy and early puerperium, with a well-looking patient suddenly deteriorating and often needing intensive care support. However, if identified early, group A streptococcus infection can be easily treated with a penicillin-based antibiotic, potentially avoiding a life-threatening septic shock.

INVESTIGATIONS

Investigations are performed for four main reasons: to confirm the diagnosis of sepsis, to determine the severity of sepsis, to identify the source of the infection and to identify the causative organism.

BEDSIDE

- Regular observations of all vital signs.
- Careful fluid balance monitoring – have a low threshold for catheterisation.
- Appropriate specimens should be sent for urgent microscopy, culture and sensitivity, for example, sputum, throat swab, midstream urine and high vaginal swab.

BLOOD TESTS

- Blood cultures – ideally taken before antibiotics are given, but do not wait for the result before administering.
- FBC and CRP – confirm an inflammatory process.
- U&Es and LFTs – assess end organ function.
- Serum lactate – measure of tissue hypoperfusion.

IMAGING

Relevant imaging studies according to the suspected cause, for example, chest x-ray, pelvic ultrasound or CT may be warranted.

MANAGEMENT

Management should be multidisciplinary, with advice from a senior obstetrician and microbiologist. In more severe cases, input may be required from intensive care and infectious diseases specialists.

INITIAL MANAGEMENT

The most important aspect of management of a septic patient is early treatment with broad-spectrum antibiotics. This should occur within 1 hour of recognition of sepsis ('the golden hour') and should not be delayed whilst investigation results are pending. When these results become available, antimicrobial therapy can then be adjusted according to the sensitivities.

Choice of antibiotic will be guided by local protocols and the breastfeeding status of the mother; therefore, consult with microbiology. Table 16.2 highlights some issues concerning common antibiotics in pregnancy and breastfeeding.

Fluid resuscitation with crystalloids should be performed, guided by the patient's vital signs. Remember, sepsis with hypotension, which is unresponsive to adequate fluid resuscitation, is septic shock. As a junior doctor, you should be seeking advice from seniors and intensive care specialists if they are not already involved. Postpartum women and those diagnosed with preeclampsia are more prone to pulmonary oedema than women in the general population, and careful fluid balance monitoring and examination are necessary.

Patients should also be given oxygen and adequate analgesia. Nonsteroidal antiinflammatory drugs (NSAIDs) should be avoided for pain relief because they impede the immune response to group A streptococcal infections. Infection control issues must also be considered, with single rooms and barrier nursing recommended for women infected with high-risk organisms such as group A streptococcus, MRSA and suspected airborne viral infections.

SUMMARY

As with any form of sepsis, primary assessment with ABC management should be carried out with juniors calling for senior help early.

- Airway – ensure the patient has a patent airway.

Table 16.2   Issues Concerning Prescribing Common Antibiotics in Pregnancy and Breastfeeding

ANTIBIOTIC	USE IN PREGNANCY/ BREASTFEEDING	COMMENTS
Amoxicillin Cephalexin Erythromycin Metronidazole	Safe	Metronidazole can change the taste of milk and may therefore alter the baby's feeding.
Co-amoxiclav	Avoid in third trimester	Can cause necrotising enterocolitis in the neonate if used in third trimester.
Trimethoprim	Avoid in first trimester	Folate antagonist; therefore, can cause neural tube defects if used in first trimester.
Nitrofurantoin	Avoid in third trimester	Can cause haemolytic disease of the newborn if used in third trimester.
Tetracyclines	Avoid in pregnancy and breastfeeding	Tetracyclines deposit in growing bone and teeth by binding to calcium, causing staining and occasionally dental hypoplasia.

- Breathing – note respiratory rate and oxygen saturations, giving oxygen as required, usually high-flow oxygen, 15 L/minute through a nonrebreathe mask.
- Circulation – blood pressure and pulse are crucial before gaining intravenous access by cannulating and taking blood cultures, lactate and relevant blood tests. Fluids should then be given initially as a 500-mL bolus of 0.9% saline. Antibiotics should be given early, often alongside fluids when sepsis is suspected.
- Disability – ensure the patient's GCS and blood glucose levels are closely monitored.
- Exposure – expose the patient to try to find a possible source of infection.

Once the patient is stabilised, assess the site of infection and determine the cause of infection. Take further blood cultures and consider imaging to aid diagnosis. Reassess the response to treatment and ensure senior involvement. Depending on the source of the infection, further treatment may be required, for example, draining of abscesses or uterine evacuation. ITU support may also be required with consideration of central lines, arterial lines, intubation and vasopressors as required; however, these are senior-led decisions.

Sepsis Six

The 'sepsis six' can be a useful way of ensuring key management steps are taken in an emergency:
- Three in – oxygen, fluids and antibiotics.
- Three out – lactate, blood cultures (ideally before antibiotics) and catheterisation to monitor exact fluid output.

MANAGEMENT OF THE NEONATE

If either the mother or baby is infected by group A streptococcus in the postpartum period, treatment with antibiotics for both should be strongly considered. Group B streptococcus (GBS) is also potentially devastating in the neonate. Management of the newborn is guided by both the status of the newborn and the intrapartum antibiotic prophylaxis (IAP) of the mother: which can vary between clinical units therefore ensure that you use local guidelines.

COMPLICATIONS

- VTE – pregnancy, inflammatory responses, dehydration and multiple other factors increase the risk of a VTE.
- Disseminated intravascular coagulation (DIC) – there is an increased risk of DIC where widespread coagulation occurs in the small- and medium-sized vessels, leading to consumption of clotting factors and, ultimately, haemorrhage.
- Permanent organ injury – overwhelming sepsis and DIC can both lead to organ failure.
- Psychological effects – it is important not to underestimate the psychological effects that being ill in the puerperal period and its consequences may have on the mother, particularly bonding with their newborn.
- Death.

PROGNOSIS

Early identification of infection and sepsis is critical to allow prompt treatment and prevent progression to more severe forms. Septic shock is associated with a mortality rate of 60%. Women can decline in a matter of hours in severe cases, and management should therefore be timely and escalated to senior members of the team.

❓ QUESTIONS

Mairi is a 22-year-old woman who gave birth to her second child 3 days ago. She is referred to the emergency department after visiting her primary care physician, complaining of feeling generally unwell. She is a known type 1 diabetic but has no other significant past medical history. Her pregnancy was uncomplicated, and she delivered by elective caesarean section. On admission, her temperature is 35.7°C, heart rate is 102 bpm, respiratory rate is 15 breaths/min and blood pressure is 85/60 mmHg, and she appears drowsy and confused. Her capillary blood glucose level is 9 mmol/L. On further examination, Mairi's caesarean wound is erythematous and warm, and the overlying dressing is soaked with yellow discharge.

Q1 What investigation would be most useful when trying to determine the cause of the infection in Mairi's case?
  A Wound swab.
  B White blood cell count.
  C Serum lactate.
  D Abdominal CT.
  E Tissue biopsy.

A Ampicillin.	**G** Imipenem.
B Clindamycin.	**H** Metronidazole.
C Co-amoxiclav.	**I** Meropenem.
D Daptomycin.	**J** Teicoplanin.
E Erythromycin.	**K** Trimethoprim.
F Gentamicin.	**L** Vancomycin.

Select the most appropriate option from the above list that corresponds to the following statements. Each answer can be used once, more than once or not at all.

Q2 An aminoglycoside antibiotic.

Q3 A glycopeptide commonly used in MRSA-positive patients.

Q4 An antibiotic which is a folate antagonist.

Q5 Only covers anaerobic bacteria and protozoa.

Q6 An antibiotic which should be avoided in penicillin-allergic patients and also in preterm premature rupture of membrane (PPROM).

[Answers on page 433.]

PERINEAL TRAUMA

Trauma following vaginal birth is common. Injured anatomy can include the labia, vagina, urethra, clitoris, perineal skin, perineal muscles, anal sphincter and the rectum (Fig. 16.3). Trauma can occur:
1. Spontaneously, during a vaginal birth.
2. Secondary to trauma during an assisted vaginal birth.
3. Iatrogenically, such as from an episiotomy.

CLASSIFICATION

Damage to the perineum is classified according to the extent of the damage in relation to the anal sphincter:
- First degree – injury to the skin of perineum and or vaginal epithelium only.
- Second degree – involvement of the perineal muscles.
- Third degree – involvement of the anal sphincter muscles.
  - 3A – less than 50% of the external anal sphincter involved.
  - 3B – more than 50% of the external anal sphincter involved.
  - 3C – involvement of the internal anal sphincter.

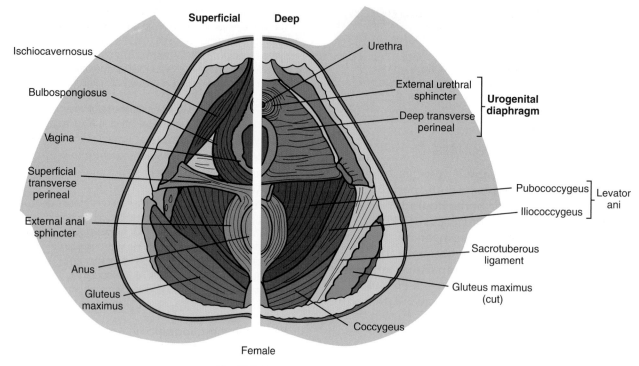

Fig. 16.3 Anatomy Involved in Perineal Tears.

- Fourth degree – involvement of the anal sphincter and the anal epithelium.

The majority of women who have a vaginal birth will sustain some degree of perineal trauma. The overall risk of anal sphincter injury in the UK is around 3% of vaginal births.

RISK FACTORS

Risk factors for obstetric anal sphincter injury (perineal trauma of third or fourth degree) can be considered maternal or neonatal factors.

MATERNAL FACTORS

- Nulliparity.
- Epidural analgesia.
- Induction of labour.
- Forceps birth and, to a lesser extent, vacuum-assisted birth.
- Previous perineal injury from a previous labour.

NEONATAL FACTORS

- Birth weight over 4 kg.
- Persistent occipitoposterior position.
- Shoulder dystocia.

PREVENTION OF PERINEAL TEARS

- There is evidence to support antenatal perineal massage, with the aim to soften the tissues of the perineum, so that during birth they are more likely to stretch rather than tear.
- During the second stage of labour, the application of a warm compress to the perineum may reduce the risk of anal sphincter injury by 50%.
- During birth, the healthcare professional attending the birth can reduce the chance of tearing by controlling the delivery of the head. By guiding the mother to slowly advance the head with gentle pushes at the time of crowning, the perineum is more likely to gently stretch rather than tear. Another way to reduce tears is with perineal protection, where the delivering professional pushes on the perineum with a hand as the head crowns.
- Antenatal and postnatal pelvic floor exercises reduce the risk of perineal, urinary and bowel symptoms following birth in all women, not just women with perineal tears. Indeed, approximately 30% of women have urinary incontinence postnatally, which could be prevented or improved with pelvic floor exercises.
- Where tearing is inevitable or appears likely (such as an assisted vaginal birth), an episiotomy can be performed. This is a cut to the perineal tissues. In the UK this is predominantly a right mediolateral incision, where the vagina, perineal skin, bulbospongiosus and superficial transverse perineal muscles are cut, approximately 45 degrees to 60 degrees from the midline. This cut is the equivalent of a second-degree perineal tear, but by performing the episiotomy, there is more space for delivery of the

head, so this reduces the risk of more complicated or deeper perineal injury, in particular reducing the risk of a tear straight down the midline into the anal sphincter.

[See 'Assisted Delivery and Instrumental Births' on page 291.]

- A planned caesarean avoids the risk of perineal injury. This option may be considered by some women who have suffered an anal sphincter injury during the birth of a previous child.

PERINEAL TRAUMA ASSESSMENT

All women should be examined for perineal trauma following a vaginal birth.

Preparation is extremely important to ensure that this examination is as unintrusive as possible:
- A careful explanation of the purpose and nature of the examination is essential – the initial examination may be immediately after birth, so this should be done gently and with sensitivity.
- The woman is likely to be tender following birth; therefore, steps should be taken to reduce the pain associated with examination – offer inhalation analgesia and position the woman so that she is comfortable.
- Ensure good lighting to improve accuracy and reduce the duration of the examination.
- If genital trauma is identified, an experienced practitioner should perform a thorough assessment – this will be a systematic examination of the vagina and perineum and a rectal examination.

COMPLICATIONS

Perineal damage can have short- and long-term consequences for a woman's physical, psychological and social well-being. These include:
- Chronic perineal pain.
- Sexual dysfunction and dyspareunia.
- Wound dehiscence or infection.
- Increased incidence of postnatal depression.
- Damage to the anal sphincters or rectum can lead to incontinence of flatus or faeces, and, rarely, can lead to a rectovaginal fistula.

It is therefore vital that any damage is accurately identified and managed appropriately.

MANAGEMENT

The management of a woman with perineal trauma is dependent on the degree of the trauma and the preference of the woman. First-degree tears (of the vaginal or perineal skin) are superficial and do not necessarily require suturing, as many will heal effectively on their own. However, many are repaired due to bleeding or to improve cosmetic outcome.

For second-degree tears, a surgical repair is recommended over conservative management; a continuous suture technique is used to appose each layer of tissue. Rapidly absorbable synthetic sutures are usually used to reduce postoperative pain and other complications. The purpose of surgically repairing perineal trauma is to control bleeding and prevent infection. It also assists wound healing by primary intention, which is associated with more rapid healing and less scarring compared to healing by secondary intention. The majority of these repairs can be performed under local anaesthetic in the delivery room.

Repair of third- or fourth-degree tears should be performed by a senior obstetrician in theatre under effective regional or general anaesthesia. Failure to identify and effectively repair these injuries increases the risk of long-term incontinence of flatus or faeces, and, rarely, a rectovaginal fistula.

After the repair, all women should be provided with adequate analgesia and education on hygiene, care of the perineum and pelvic floor exercises.

Women with third- and fourth-degree tears are additionally advised to use laxatives for a short while after birth to reduce the risk of constipation-related strain on the injury. A short course of antibiotics is also prescribed due to the risk of infection caused by the close proximity of faeces to the injury. Early physiotherapy input is beneficial in women with more severe tears. Specialist follow-up at 6 to 12 weeks postpartum is usually arranged to check for full recovery after these tears. Prompt referral should be arranged if complications arise.

PROGNOSIS

Women with low-grade perineal tears or higher-grade tears which have been surgically repaired have a good prognosis. Following an external anal sphincter repair, around 70% of women are asymptomatic at 12 months. The main complication is flatus incontinence or faecal urgency. These symptoms often improve with physiotherapy over time, but if there are ongoing symptoms beyond 12 months, further investigation and repeat surgery may be required.

❓ QUESTIONS

Katherine is a 30-year-old who has just given birth to her first child. Her birth was assisted using forceps, with resultant trauma to her perineum. She is otherwise medically fit, and her pregnancy has been uncomplicated. On examination, Katherine has suffered injury to the perineal muscles, with sparing of the anal sphincter.

Q1 What degree of perineal trauma has the woman sustained?
  A First degree.
  B Second degree.
  C Third degree, classification A.
  D Third degree, classification B.
  E Third degree, classification C.

Q2 Which of the following makes up the bulk of the pelvic diaphragm?

    A Bulbospongiosus muscle.

    B Deep transverse perineal muscle.

    C External anal sphincter.

    D Levator ani.

    E Superficial transverse perineal muscle.

Q3 Answer true or false to the following statements.

    A Women with a previous history of severe perineal trauma should be informed that their risk of perineal trauma is not increased in comparison to nulliparous women.

    B Antenatal perineal massage has been found to reduce the incidence of perineal tears.

    C Postoperatively, laxatives should be administered after a third-degree perineal repair.

    D Women who have had a fourth-degree perineal tear in a previous pregnancy should be offered a prophylactic episiotomy.

    E When episiotomy is indicated, a medial incision should be made.

[Answers on page 433.]

MASTITIS

Mastitis is an inflammation of the breast tissue (Fig. 16.4), which may be due to infective or noninfective causes. Its occurrence is common in breastfeeding women, with an estimated prevalence of one in five women. The most common mechanism of noninfective mastitis is milk stasis due to feeding difficulties, blocked ducts or mild breast trauma. Feeding difficulties include oversupply of breast milk and poor infant attachment or positioning, which leads to increased pressures within the alveoli and duct system. This elevated pressure can force milk into the surrounding breast parenchyma, with resultant local inflammation.

Infective mastitis results from the introduction of bacteria, usually from the infant in a breastfeeding mother. It is more likely if there is a breach in the skin barrier (for example, piercings or cracked or sore nipples), milk stasis or if the mother is more vulnerable to infection (for example, diabetics). The organism most commonly implicated is *S. aureus*, although this may be found in breast milk when there is no clinical evidence of mastitis.

CLINICAL FEATURES

SYMPTOMS

- Pain, swelling, warmth over the inflamed area – normally in a wedge-shaped distribution.
- Painful lump – if the duct is blocked or abscess is present.
- Flulike symptoms – fever, malaise, myalgia.
- Usually unilateral, rare to affect both breasts simultaneously.

SIGNS

- An area of tenderness, erythema and swelling in the breast.
- Pyrexia.
- Purulent discharge may be present in infective mastitis.
- Axillary lymphadenopathy may be palpable.

INVESTIGATIONS

Mastitis is a clinical diagnosis, and the assessment is directed at identifying an underlying cause and possible complications. Feeding should be comprehensively reviewed, including positioning, attachment and pattern. Breast milk cultures should not routinely be done, but should be considered if:

- Mastitis recurs.
- Mastitis is hospital acquired.
- There is a severe or unusual presentation.

Ultrasound may be required to exclude an abscess if there is no improvement following a course of antibiotics. An important differential diagnosis is inflammatory breast cancer, as this can coincide with or mimic mastitis, although this is an unusual presentation. If a lump is present, then both benign and malignant causes of breast masses need to be considered.

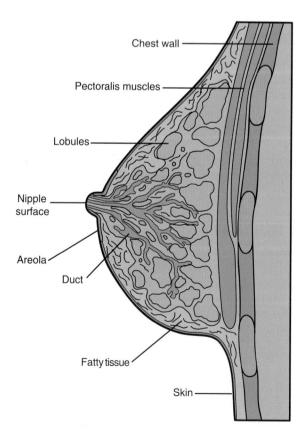

Chest wall

Pectoralis muscles

Lobules

Nipple surface

Areola

Duct

Fatty tissue

Skin

Fig. 16.4 Anatomy of the Breast.

MANAGEMENT

In most mild cases of mastitis, conservative management is all that is needed, with the aim of correcting milk stasis and managing the symptoms. This involves:

- Referral to a health visitor or midwife for help with positioning and attachment if required.
- Frequent effective milk removal.
  - Express milk by hand or pump if necessary.
  - Use a hot compress and gentle massage of the breast to help milk flow.
  - Minimise wearing of a bra and manage other predisposing factors if present.
- Pain management.
  - Oral paracetamol and/or ibuprofen.
- Support recovery.
  - Take adequate fluids, nutrition and rest.
  - Seek additional support at home.

INFECTIVE MASTITIS

Women should be advised to seek medical help if symptoms do not improve after 12 hours of effective and frequent milk removal or if symptoms escalate rapidly, as antibiotic therapy may be indicated. This is usually with a penicillin, for example, flucloxacillin. If the infection persists, antibiotic therapy can then be tailored to the sensitivity results from blood cultures. When considering antibiotic choice, it is imperative to consult local guidelines.

Women should be referred to secondary care if:

- Systemically unwell or signs of sepsis.
- Haemodynamically unstable or immunocompromised.
- Rapid progression of infection.
- A localised area of the breast remains hard, red and tender, suggesting an abscess – which may need ultrasound-guided aspiration or surgical drainage.
- There is an underlying mass, with suspicion of ductal or inflammatory breast cancer (urgent 2-week wait referral).
- Not improving despite conservative management and oral antibiotics.

COMPLICATIONS

Mastitis is usually mild and self-limiting, but it may result in:

- Inhibition of lactation.
- Premature discontinuation of breastfeeding.
- Recurrent mastitis.
- Breast abscess.

PROGNOSIS

With the correct information and support, mastitis can usually be self-managed, as the majority of cases are caused by milk stasis. Cases that become infected can be protected from abscess formation by prompt, effective medical management. Despite treatment, abscesses develop in about 3% of infective mastitis cases.

? QUESTIONS

Sasha is 34-year-old woman who delivered her first child 1 month ago. She is exclusively breastfeeding. She contacts her midwife because over the past 24 hours her left breast has become extremely hot and painful. She is on no medication currently, and she has no significant past medical history. On examination, there is a wedge-shaped erythematous, swollen, tender area of the left breast.

Q1 Which isotype of antibodies is predominantly transferred to the newborn baby in breast milk?

- A IgA.
- B IgD.
- C IgE.
- D IgG.
- E IgM.

Q2 Which organism is most commonly isolated from breast milk in infective mastitis?

- A *S. pyogenes*.
- B *S. aureus*.
- C *Staphylococcus epidermis*.
- D *Neisseria gonorrhoea*.
- E *E. coli*.

Q3 Answer true or false to the following statements regarding mastitis.

- A The risk of mastitis is increased by tight-fitting bras.
- B Women with mastitis should stop breastfeeding.
- C An episode of mastitis following a previous pregnancy increases the risk of mastitis in the current postpartum period.
- D Using only one position to breastfeed increases the risk of mastitis.
- E Mastitis can only develop with broken skin, for example, cracked nipples.

[Answers on page 435.]

POSTNATAL MENTAL HEALTH

During pregnancy, the risk of developing a mental illness is similar to that in the general population. The exception is women with preexisting mental illness, who have an increased risk and particularly those women who stop their medication during pregnancy. During the postpartum period, the risk of serious mental illnesses (SMIs), such as bipolar affective disorder, affective psychoses and severe depression, is significantly elevated for the first 3 months. This is especially the case in women with a previous history of SMI, where the risk approaches 50%.

Specific postpartum conditions include the 'baby blues', postpartum depression and postpartum psychosis (Table 16.3).

Table 16.3 Summary of Specific Postnatal Conditions

POSTNATAL MENTAL HEALTH CONCERNS	BABY BLUES	POSTNATAL DEPRESSION	POSTNATAL PSYCHOSIS
Incidence	500–700 per 1000	10–15 per 100	1–2 per 1000
Clinical features	'Mood swings' Tearful Irritable Low mood Anxiety	Low mood Anhedonia Low energy Sleep disturbance Change in appetite Reduced concentration or memory Reduced libido Negative thought processes (guilt, worthlessness, hopelessness, reduced confidence) Impaired bonding with baby (reluctant to hold or feed, may not feel close to the child or have thoughts of harming the baby)	Rapid mood swings (mania and depression) Confusion Delusions Hallucinations
Onset	3–4 days postnatal	Most common in first few months postnatal	Most commonly in first 2 weeks Onset can be over hours
Duration/prognosis	Lasts less than 2 weeks Increased risk of postnatal depression	Usually lasts for at least 2 weeks	6–12 months to fully recover, with most severe symptoms lasting 2–12 weeks Often followed by a period of depression High risk of SMI in future (pregnancy related or unrelated) High risk of recurrence in future pregnancies High risk of harm to self and/or newborn if diagnosis missed or delayed
Treatment	No specific treatment required as usually self-limiting, but close monitoring for deterioration	Psychological interventions, for example, CBT Antidepressant treatment if necessary	Requires hospital admission (ideally in specialist mother and baby unit) and treatment with antipsychotics, mood stabiliser or both

CBT, Cognitive behavioural therapy; *SMI*, severe mental illness.

Psychiatric disorders can indirectly impact maternal health through physical and social complications and from potential negative effects of treatment.

AETIOLOGY

The greatest risk factors for the development of any mental illness during the antenatal or postnatal period are a personal or family history of mental illness (SMIs, particularly bipolar affective disorder or postpartum psychosis) and stopping medication in a woman with preexisting mental illness. Psychological and social factors also contribute to the risk of postnatal depression. These include:

- Lack of supportive social network.
- Relationship difficulties.
- Stressful life events – related or unrelated to the pregnancy or birth.
- Poor psychological adjustment or coping strategies.

INVESTIGATIONS

Identifying and supporting women who are currently or at risk of suffering from mental illness should ideally begin before they conceive, but it more commonly begins at the antenatal booking visit. This allows for referral to the appropriate services, such as specialised perinatal mental health services for high-risk patients and for a care plan to be made.

Mental health screening questions are asked at the booking visit. If women are positive for any of the following, they are at a higher risk of postpartum psychosis, so they are referred to the joint obstetric and mental health team:

- Previous or current major mental illness.
- Previous postpartum depression or psychosis.
- Previous treatment by mental health services, particularly if inpatient treatment was required.
- Family history of certain psychiatric disorders, particularly postpartum psychosis and bipolar disorders.
- Current treatment with psychotropic medication.

Women are also asked screening questions for symptoms of depression and anxiety:

- Over the past month, have you felt down, depressed or hopeless or had decreased interest or pleasure in doing things?

- Over the last 2 weeks, have you been bothered by feelings of anxiety, nervousness or not being able to stop or control worrying?

If they answer yes to any part of the questions, a more formal review is conducted, using assessment tools such as the Edinburgh postnatal depression score or the generalised anxiety disorder scale. Depending on the results, patients are referred to their GP for ongoing care – or if there are severe concerns, to the mental health team.

Additionally, at booking, social risk factors are often identified which increase the risk of mental health problems, such as domestic violence, sexual abuse, substance misuse, self-harm, a lack of social support or a combination of any of these.

All members of the multidisciplinary team should be aware of the risks surrounding mental illness, and a woman's mental health should be asked about at every contact throughout pregnancy and the postnatal period.

MANAGEMENT

The treatment of mental illness during pregnancy and the postnatal period should follow the same principles and guidelines as in the general population.

Psychological treatments, including 'talking therapies' such as facilitated self-help, cognitive behavioural therapy (CBT), interpersonal psychotherapy (IPT) and couples therapy, can all be used successfully in pregnancy, with evidence supporting their usage to treat depression, anxiety and even the severe mental health conditions such as bipolar disorder and psychosis. Unfortunately, the waiting times to commence treatment (particularly for patients with mild disorders) may be significant.

If medications are required, selective serotonin reuptake inhibitors (SSRIs) are commonly prescribed for depression or anxiety where psychological treatments have not been effective or are not available, the patient declines psychological interventions, or the patient prefers medical treatment. Other medications include tricyclic antidepressants (TCAs) and serotonin and norepinephrine reuptake inhibitors (SNRIs). In order to minimise the risk to both mother and baby, the decision to prescribe (or continue prescribing) psychotropic medication should be made after careful consideration of the pros and cons of pharmacological treatment. The risks of teratogenicity during pregnancy and the risks of withdrawal or toxicity in the neonate should be balanced with the potential risk of harm associated with relapse. Several common antidepressive agents are frequently used in pregnancy and are not considered to have major fetal implications. Women taking medication should be advised to deliver in a consultant unit so neonatal monitoring can be undertaken if needed.

The fetal risks associated with antipsychotic medications are more significant, particularly for treatments such as lithium or carbamazepine. The decision on the choice of medication for these patients requires specialist psychiatric input.

PROGNOSIS

The prognosis for baby blues is usually very good, as often this is a transient response to the hormonal and psychological situation. Postnatal depression, if treated appropriately, also has a good prognosis. Most women with puerperal psychosis go on to make a full recovery. However, this can take 6 to 12 months, and the risk of recurrence is up to 50%. It is also important to remember that puerperal psychosis often occurs in women without any preexisting mental health problems, so vigilance is required in all postpartum women. Missed or poorly treated mental illness can lead to social isolation, relationship breakdown, self-harm and, extremely rarely, the mother killing her child or taking her own life. In the UK, suicide is one of the top 10 causes of maternal death.

❓ QUESTIONS

Sara is a 25-year-old single mother, gravidity one and parity one, who delivered by emergency caesarean section 4 weeks ago. Sara has a past psychiatric history of bipolar affective disorder, diagnosed at the age of 21. Her mental health has been relatively stable on lithium since then. Due to her concerns about teratogenicity, Sara has not been taking any medication since she started trying to conceive. She visits her primary care physician, reporting feeling low for the last 3 weeks. She is tearful during the consultation and admits that she does not feel close to her baby and does not enjoy spending time with him. She reports that he is sleeping well, but she is still struggling with sleep and feeling exhausted. She is afraid that she may harm her baby.

Q1 Which of the following is lithium known to increase the risk of most significantly?
   A Oral cleft.
   B Cardiac abnormalities.
   C Neural tube defects.
   D Gastrointestinal defects.
   E Respiratory defects.

Antidepressants are one of the treatment options for postnatal depression. Match the drug with the corresponding class.

Q2 Fluoxetine.
Q3 Moclobemide.
Q4 Mirtazapine.
Q5 Amitriptyline.
Q6 Venlafaxine.
   A Tricyclic antidepressants.
   B Monoamine oxidase inhibitors.
   C Selective serotonin reuptake inhibitors.
   D Serotonin and noradrenaline reuptake inhibitors.
   E Noradrenaline and specific serotoninergic antidepressants.

Q7 Answer true or false: Which of the following are risk factors for puerperal psychosis?

- **A** Having a sister who developed puerperal psychosis.
- **B** Previous history of bipolar disorder.
- **C** Previous history of schizoaffective disorder.
- **D** Low maternal age.
- **E** Having puerperal psychosis in a previous pregnancy.

[Answers on page 436.]

KEY REFERENCES

VENOUS THROMBOEMBOLISM

Royal College of Obstetricians and Gynaecologists, 2015. Reducing the risk of venous thromboembolism during pregnancy and the puerperium. RCOG green top guideline (GTG 37a).

Royal College of Obstetricians and Gynaecologists, 2015. Thromboembolic disease in pregnancy and the puerperium: acute management. RCOG green top guideline (GTG 37b).

BACTERIAL SEPSIS FOLLOWING PREGNANCY

Royal College of Obstetricians and Gynaecologists, 2012. Bacterial sepsis following pregnancy. RCOG green top guideline (GTG 64b).

Royal College of Obstetricians and Gynaecologists, 2017. The prevention of early-onset neonatal group B streptococcal disease. RCOG green top guideline (GTG 36).

Singer, M., Deutschman, C.S., Seymour, C.W., et al., 2016. The third international consensus definitions for sepsis and septic shock (sepsis-3). JAMA. 315 (8), 801–810.

PERINEAL TRAUMA

NHS Quality Improvement Scotland., 2008. Perineal repair after childbirth [online]. Available from: http://www.nhshealthquality.org. [Accessed 11 July 2023].

Royal College of Obstetricians and Gynaecologists, 2007. The management of third- and fourth-degree perineal tears. RCOG green top guideline (GTG 29).

Royal College of Obstetricians and Gynaecologists. (n.d.) OASI Care Bundle Project. [online] Available from: https://www.rcog.org.uk/about-us/the-rcog-centre-for-quality-improvement-and-clinical-audit/oasi/. [Accessed 11 October 2022].

MASTITIS

National Institute for Health and Clinical Excellence, 2021. Mastitis and breast abscess. NICE clinical guideline.

Guidelines and Audit Implementation Network, 2009. Guidelines on the treatment, management and prevention of mastitis. Clinical guideline.

POSTNATAL MENTAL HEALTH

Royal College of Obstetricians and Gynaecologists, 2011. Management of women with mental health issues during pregnancy and the postnatal period. RCOG good practice guideline (GP14).

National Institute for Health and Clinical Excellence, 2007. Antenatal and postnatal mental health. NICE clinical guideline (CG45).

Royal College of Psychiatrists, 2018. Postnatal depression leaflet.

Royal College of Psychiatrists, 2018. Postpartum psychosis leaflet.

9 ANTENATAL CARE

ORGANISATION AND PRINCIPLES OF ANTENATAL CARE

Q1: Which of the following are suitable for midwife-led care?

The correct answer is A. A nulliparous woman with a family history of diabetes mellitus.

Midwives and primary care physicians should care for women with an uncomplicated pregnancy, providing continuous care throughout the duration of the pregnancy. Obstetricians and specialist teams should only be involved where additional care is needed.

A ✔ **A nulliparous woman with a family history of diabetes mellitus** – Correct. This woman does not herself have diabetes; therefore, at this stage, she can be classed as low risk and is eligible for midwife-led care. She will be offered a glucose tolerance test, and if this is abnormal, then her care may be escalated to obstetrician-led care.

[See 'Diabetes in Pregnancy' on page 251.]

B A multiparous woman with sickle cell disease (SCD) – Incorrect. This patient needs consultant-led care, as she falls within the bracket of haematological disorders. SCD is associated with maternal and fetal complications and an increased incidence of perinatal mortality; therefore, obstetrician input is required.

[See 'Sickle Cell Disease in Pregnancy' on page 245.]

C A multiparous woman with a previous history of pre-eclampsia – Incorrect. This woman needs consultant-led care, as she has previously had pre-eclampsia, a serious obstetric condition known to be more common in women who have previously had a pregnancy affected by the disease. Pre-eclampsia is also associated with growth restriction of the fetus. Increased monitoring of fetal growth may be necessary, and aspirin should be considered.

[See 'Pre-Eclampsia and Pregnancy-Induced Hypertension' on page 301.]

D A primiparous woman with a consistent blood pressure (BP) of above 130/90 mmHg – Incorrect. This patient is more suitable for consultant-led care, as elevated BP could represent chronic or gestational hypertension, which increases the risk of the development of pre-eclampsia. Knowledge of whether the cause of the hypertension is obstetric or nonobstetric is not essential for this question, as both causes fall into categories where obstetrician input is necessary.

E A multiparous woman with well-controlled epilepsy – Incorrect. This patient will need an obstetrician review and will usually be seen regularly in a consultant-led clinic. Epilepsy can be difficult to manage during pregnancy, as many of the medications are teratogenic and therefore require careful risk/benefit analysis, which requires obstetrician and specialist input.

[See 'Epilepsy in Pregnancy' on page 231.]

 Key Point

If a woman has an identified risk factor requiring obstetric input (Table 17.1), this does not mean she has to be managed exclusively by an obstetrician. All patients should still be reviewed routinely by their midwives and primary care physicians.

Q2: Answer true or false: What advice should be given to the woman during antenatal care?

A significant amount of lifestyle advice regarding a number of different factors is given to women during pregnancy.

A ✔ **She should carry her own case notes** – True. Maternity records are structured, standardised, national maternity records, and should be held by the woman. This enables the woman to take her notes with her if she attends appointments with a variety of healthcare professionals. It also includes a lot of important information for the woman to read in her own time and advises her what to do if she has any cause for concern.

B ✔ **If drinking milk, it should be pasteurised** – True. Pasteurised, or ultra-heat-treated milk, is safer for pregnant women to drink, as it has been treated to prevent the risk of infection. Unpasteurised milk and certain cheeses, particularly those with mould, are potentially dangerous due to the increased risk of listeriosis.

C She should be advised that flying is contraindicated during the later stages of pregnancy – False.

Table 17.1	Nonobstetric and Obstetric Example Reasons Why Women Require More Than the Baseline Antenatal Care via Midwives
NONOBSTETRIC	**OBSTETRIC**
Cardiac disease, including hypertension.	Recurrent miscarriage.
Renal disease.	Preterm birth.
Endocrine disorders or diabetes requiring insulin.	Severe pre-eclampsia syndrome or eclampsia.
Psychiatric disorders (treated and untreated).	Rhesus isoimmunisation or other significant blood group antibodies.
Haematological disorders.	
Autoimmune disorders.	Uterine or cervical surgery, including caesarean, myomectomy or cone biopsy.
Epilepsy.	
Malignant disease.	Postpartum haemorrhage.
Severe asthma.	Puerperal psychosis.
Use of recreational drugs such as heroin, cocaine and ecstasy.	Grand multiparity (parity four or more).
HIV or hepatitis B infection.	Previous history of a stillbirth or neonatal death.
Higher risk of developing complications, for example, women aged 40 and older and women who smoke.	A small-for-gestational-age or large-for-gestational-age fetus.
Women who are particularly vulnerable or who lack social support.	A baby with a congenital abnormality (structural or chromosomal).

HELLP, Haemolysis, elevated liver enzymes and low platelets.

Pregnant women should be informed that long-haul air travel is associated with an increased risk of venous thrombosis, which is likely to be compounded by the prothrombotic state of pregnancy. However, in a healthy individual, the risk can be reduced by wearing correctly fitted compression stockings accompanied by adequate hydration and performing gentle in-flight leg exercises. Many airlines will refuse flights for pregnant women beyond 28 weeks gestation due to the potential risk of labour during flight.

D Folic acid should be taken up to 20 weeks gestation – False. In women at low risk of neural tube anomaly, 400 micrograms once daily of folic acid is advised when trying to conceive and at the start of pregnancy. However, it is only until 12 weeks gestation, when the neural tube closes, that folic acid should be taken. Frequently, vitamin D is also provided along with folic acid supplementation for pregnant women in the UK due to a large proportion of the population suffering vitamin D deficiency.

E Regularly wearing compression stockings will prevent the occurrence of varicose veins – False. Varicose veins are a common occurrence in pregnancy. Compression stockings can be worn to reduce existing varicose veins, but they will not prevent them from happening in the first place.

Key Point

Written information can be a useful tool, as pregnant women are often given a lot of information in their antenatal appointments. This is helpful to remember in clinical practice but also in objective structured clinical examinations (OSCEs), as this can be a good way to end a counselling session.

Q3: If this pregnancy continues to be uncomplicated, how many antenatal appointments should she attend?

The correct answer is C. 10.

General guidance for antenatal appointments:
- *Antenatal appointments should take place in a location that women can easily access and that is appropriate to the needs of women.*
- *For an uncomplicated pregnancy in the UK, there should be 10 appointments for nulliparous women and 7 appointments for multiparous women. The WHO advises that, globally, each pregnant woman should be offered at least four antenatal appointments.*
- *Each antenatal appointment should have a structure and a focus.*
- *Appointments early in pregnancy should be longer to provide information and time for discussion about screening so that women can make informed decisions.*
- *Where possible, tests should be incorporated into the appointments to minimise inconvenience to women.*
- *Women should feel able to discuss sensitive issues and disclose problems.*

Key Point

The large number of antenatal appointments attended by women mean that pregnancy is a crucial opportunity for opportunistic screening, not just regarding the medical conditions outlined but also social problems, such as domestic violence, obesity, smoking and alcohol and any other factors that can affect the woman and her family lifelong.

Important Learning Points

- The organisation and implementation of comprehensive antenatal care is labour intensive, as there are multiple components to consider in any pregnancy.
- The level of medical input a woman will require will determine whether she has obstetrician-led or midwife-led care and the number of antenatal appointments.
- Relevant information is given throughout pregnancy; depending on the gestation, this includes communication about screening, routine pregnancy, potential complications, birth and the postnatal period.

OBSTETRIC ABDOMINAL PALPATION

Q1: What is the most important reason for examining a woman in the left lateral position later in pregnancy?

The correct answer is C. It reduces compression of the vena cava.

It is preferred to have a woman lying flat when palpating her uterus, as it enables a more accurate assessment of how the uterus feels and allows a more precise SFH measurement. At the later stages of pregnancy, the gravid uterus may cause a woman discomfort when lying down; thus, during abdominal palpation at later gestations, it may be easier to examine a woman's pregnant abdomen when she is in a semirecumbent position at approximately 30 degrees. At term, examining in the left lateral position may be necessary. This is because the gravid uterus can compress the inferior vena cava, reducing venous return, causing dizziness or occasionally syncope in the woman and sometimes transient fetal distress.

 Key Point

During your exams, it is often important to verbalise to the examiner any aspect of the examination that you are not doing to ensure comfort of the individual being examined. For example, 'ideally, the woman would be lying flat at this stage of the examination to ensure accuracy. However, due to the gravid uterus, this woman is lying in a semirecumbent position for comfort. If I had any concerns, then I could ask her to briefly lie completely flat while I completed the examination.'

Q2: Which of the following could cause her SFH to be larger than expected?

The correct answers are B. Polyhydramnios, **C.** Gestational diabetes and **E.** Raised BMI.

Measuring the SFH should be taken as a blind measurement. This is very important to ensure that the final measurement is not biased. The uterus should grow approximately 1 cm every week of gestation, with the SFH being 2 cm ± gestation. However, this is only a rough guide, and multiple factors can affect how accurate this measurement is (Table 17.2).

A Oligohydramnios – Incorrect. Liquor is a combination of fluid produced by the placenta and fluid excreted through the fetal urinary tract. Oligohydramnios is a reduced volume of amniotic fluid. This can be associated with a history of premature

Table **17.2**	Reasons for a Symphysis Fundal Height Inconsistent with Gestational Age

TOO LARGE	TOO SMALL
• Multiple pregnancy	• Small for gestational age and intrauterine growth restriction
• Fibroids	
• Macrosomia – GDM	
• Polyhydramnios	• Oligohydramnios

GDM, Gestational diabetes mellitus.

rupture of membranes, placental dysfunction and fetal abnormalities. On examination, the SFH may be smaller than expected for the gestational age, and fetal body parts may be easier to palpate due to reduced amniotic fluid surrounding the fetus. The cause of oligohydramnios needs careful investigation and specialist management, as it may be associated with poor fetal outcomes.

B ✔ **Polyhydramnios** – Correct. As well as being produced by the fetus and placenta, to complete a cycle of liquor turnover, the fluid is swallowed and absorbed by the fetus. Excess production is associated with gestational diabetes (from increased fetal urination) and some uterine infections. Other causes include structural abnormalities, such as oesophageal atresia, which are associated with increased liquor due to the inability of the fetus to swallow liquor. On examination, the SFH may be larger than is expected from the current gestation and will also alter how the abdomen feels on palpation, causing the uterus to feel tight and fetal body parts harder to discern. To investigate further, an ultrasound scan and glucose tolerance test are usually performed.

C ✔ **Gestational diabetes** – Correct. Gestational diabetes is associated with both microsomia and macrosomia. It is also associated with polyhydramnios and maternal obesity, which may complicate the pregnancy. Macrosomia is a serious possible complication of gestational diabetes and a significant risk factor for shoulder dystocia; therefore, the diagnosis is important, as its presence may alter how the baby is delivered. Gestational diabetes also increases the risk of prolonged second stage, assisted vaginal birth, emergency caesarean, maternal trauma, brachial plexus injury and neonatal hypoglycaemia. If the baby is macrosomic, then the SFH may be larger than expected.

[See 'Diabetes in Pregnancy' on page 251.]

D Raised BP – Incorrect. A raised BP alone will not cause a larger-than-expected SFH. If a raised BP is part of pre-eclampsia, then it would be more likely that the SFH would be smaller than expected because of associations with growth restriction of the fetus.

[See 'Pre-Eclampsia and Pregnancy-Induced Hypertension' on page 301.]

E ✔ **Raised BMI** – Correct. A raised BMI of the mother makes the SFH difficult to assess, and it also makes abdominal palpation more difficult. Women with a high BMI are at increased risk of gestational diabetes mellitus (GDM), but even if the pregnancy is healthy and the fetal well-being is fine, the SFH may still appear to be larger than expected. Serial ultrasound measurement of fetal growth is used in these women, as SFH measurements in this group are inaccurate.

[See 'The Impact of Maternal Weight on Pregnancy' on page 236.]

Key Point

Scars are an important clinical finding, as they may tell you information about a woman's previous mode of birth or her medical and surgical history in general. The scar from this question is the location of a scar that you would inspect in somebody that has previously had a caesarean.

Q3: What is the name of the scar indicated in the diagram?

The correct answer is B. Pfannenstiel.

A Midline – Incorrect. A midline longitudinal scar may indicate that a woman has previously had a 'classical' caesarean instead of a lower uterine segment caesarean section (LSCS). This type of caesarean is rarely performed today because of the higher rates of complications. These include greater blood loss, longer healing time and greater risk of uterine rupture in future pregnancies. This scar could also indicate previous abdominal surgery requiring a laparotomy.

B ✔ **Pfannenstiel** – Correct. The Pfannenstiel incision is a curved suprapubic incision which can be thought of as a 'bikini line' scar. It is the scar that some women will have after a lower segment caesarean. Most caesarean scars in the UK, however, are not technically Pfannenstiel scars. A Pfannenstiel incision is a curved incision made 1 inch above the pubic symphysis. Most UK obstetricians will make a transverse lower abdominal incision, which is straighter and lower.

C Kocher – Incorrect. The Kocher scar is from an oblique incision made in the right upper quadrant of the abdomen. It is usually used to access the liver, gallbladder and biliary tract.

D Paramedian – Incorrect. Paramedian means that the scar is adjacent to the midline. This is an incision commonly used in anterior rectal resections.

E Lanz – Incorrect. This is the incision used for an open appendicectomy. It is made horizontally over the McBurney point.

 Key Point

Clinical observations of the abdomen during pregnancy:
- Distension of abdomen.
- Linea nigra.
- Striae gravidarum.
- Striae albicans.
- Lumps and bumps.
- Fetal movements.
- Excoriation marks.
- Scars.

🔍 **Important Learning Points**

- Assessing the SFH is an important aspect of an obstetric examination; this should be a blind measurement, and the uterus would be expected to grow approximately 1 cm for every gestational week.

- If the SFH is not as expected, this could be due to maternal reasons such as a raised BMI or fetal issues such as poor fetal growth. Women whose SFH falls outside the expected range should be referred for an ultrasound scan.
- It is important to assess the fetal lie, presentation and engagement, especially during labour, as this will influence the plan for birth.

ANTENATAL SCREENING AND DIAGNOSTIC TESTS

Q1: Answer true or false: At the booking visit, questions are asked about which of the following?

The initial booking visit is a lengthy process, even in a second pregnancy. Many people think that screening questions are only asked to pick up medical problems such as diabetes and hypertension, but many more subtle questions are asked. Antenatal screening also offers the opportunity for a general health review in women who may not have ever seen a healthcare professional before. The booking visit therefore gives a unique opportunity to ask about aspects of the woman's life which may be affecting her and her family.

A ✔ **Mental health issues** – True. Questions are particularly asked related to depression because of the risk of postnatal depression and puerperal psychosis. Other mental health issues, such as schizophrenia and bipolar disorder, are also asked about because of the increased risk of relapse during pregnancy and/or because of concurrent use of medication in pregnancy which may have teratogenic effects.

B ✔ **Social support** – True. Multiple questions are asked about the amount of social support the woman and her family receive, including her employment history, social services involvement and questions related to domestic abuse. One important reason for this is to assess potential child safeguarding concerns so social services and other teams can be involved early.

C ✔ **Diet and nutrition** – True. Diet and nutrition are crucial during pregnancy, so questions are asked regarding this topic and educational information can be given. This may relate to BMI, diet or nutritional supplements such as folic acid. Screening questions related to drug abuse, alcohol intake and smoking are also asked, and health education may be given in the form of verbal information or leaflets or, increasingly, by indicating suitable websites.

D ✔ **Pregnancy intentions** – True. Information is obtained regarding the nature of the conception, for example, whether the pregnancy was planned or unplanned. This may affect alcohol intake and folic acid supplementation. If this was an unplanned pregnancy, the reason for asking about contraception is to initiate the process of arranging appropriate postnatal contraception at the right time to prevent a repeat unplanned pregnancy. Questions are asked related to any fertility treatment, as this may also affect the pregnancy.

E ✔ **Medical comorbidities** – True. Many comorbidities are asked about, particularly diabetes, cardiac disease, BP and any abnormal clotting risk factors.

 Key Point

The rationale behind the screening offered at booking visits is to identify medical, psychological and social risk factors to reduce the risks for both mother and baby for antenatal, intrapartum and postpartum periods.

Q2: Tests for Down syndrome screening are offered between which weeks of gestation?

The correct answers are C. Weeks 10 and 14 and **E.** Weeks 14 and 20.

Screening for Down syndrome is a combination of biochemical blood tests and nuchal translucency on abdominal ultrasound. If the woman books early enough, then this can be done as a combined test at 10 to 14 weeks gestation. However, as the pregnancy progresses past this point, nuchal translucency becomes inaccurate, so the quadruple blood test is performed. This is less accurate than the combined test.

 Key Point

Only 65% of Down syndrome cases are detected antenatally; screening is therefore not optimally sensitive. What this means is that 35% of Down syndrome is diagnosed after birth. In the near future, analysis of free fetal DNA in maternal blood will dramatically increase the sensitivity of screening.

Q3: Which of the following disorders is more common in Afro-Caribbean women than in white Northern European women?

The correct answer is D. Haemoglobinopathies.

Blood tests are offered for all of the answers between weeks 8 and 12 of gestation. However, this question was in direct relation to women of Afro-Caribbean origin. It is important to consider what disorder is the most prevalent in any given patient or group of women, but also recognise that ethnicity does not diagnose or exclude any condition.

A Hepatitis B – Incorrect. Hepatitis B is a bloodborne virus and can therefore be transmitted from mother to baby. Babies affected by hepatitis B may develop liver problems later in life. However, this can be prevented by hepatitis B immunisation and hepatitis B immunoglobulin (HBIG) injection shortly after birth.

[See 'Hepatitis B in Pregnancy' on page 242.]

B Syphilis – Incorrect. Syphilis is a bacterial infection typically spread by sexual contact, intravenous drug use and, historically, blood transfusions. It can also be transmitted from mother to baby during pregnancy. This can lead to stillbirth or death of the baby soon after birth. Syphilis is usually treated with penicillin.

[See 'Congenital Intrauterine Infections' on page 336.]

C HIV – Incorrect. HIV can be transmitted from mother to fetus; therefore, universal screening is suggested for all pregnant women.

[See 'HIV in Pregnancy' on page 244.]

D ✔ **Haemoglobinopathies** – Correct. For genetic reasons, screening for haemoglobinopathies is particularly important to identify pregnancies that are at risk of an affected fetus. Sickle cell anaemia and thalassaemia are the blood disorders particularly screened for by electrophoresis. The prevalence of haemoglobinopathies is significantly greater in the Afro-Caribbean population.

[See 'Sickle Cell Disease in Pregnancy' on page 245.]

E Rubella – Incorrect. The screening test for rubella involves screening for rubella IgG antibodies, not the infection. If IgG antibodies are present, then the patient is immune. Rubella can cause miscarriage, stillbirth and birth anomalies such as hearing loss, brain damage, heart defects and cataracts. Due to the large number of children vaccinated with the MMR vaccine, rubella is now rare in the UK, so routine antenatal screening for rubella has recently been suspended.

[See 'Congenital Intrauterine Infections' on page 336.]

 Key Point

Infectious diseases are a great example of the antenatal screening programme at its best because detection of these bacteria and viruses can lead to management being implemented that improves the health outcomes for mother and baby.

Q4: Answer true or false: In a pregnancy that is progressing normally with no complications, a woman will be offered her first ultrasound scan in the first trimester. What are the primary purposes of this scan?

The first scan, referred to as a booking scan, is undertaken in early pregnancy, ideally between 11 and 14 weeks gestation. This is an important scan for women, socially as well as medically, and expectations of the scan need to be managed appropriately if the outcome is not as expected.

A ✔ **To detect twins** – True. One of the primary purposes of this scan is to detect the fetal number; this may be twins or higher numbers. It is important at this stage, if there is a multiple pregnancy, to determine the chorionicity and amnionicity, as this may affect the rest of the pregnancy. Twin pregnancies are at higher risk, often requiring more regular follow-up and usually obstetrician-led care.

[See 'Multiple Pregnancy' on page 252.]

B ✔ **To date the pregnancy** – True. At least one routine scan in pregnancy to confirm gestational age is found beneficial, especially for reducing the need for intervention for postmaturity. The dating scan is done at this gestation because this is the best time for accurate dating of a pregnancy (performing it later increases the risk that factors like macrosomia and fetal growth restriction may adversely affect the assessment).

C ✔ **To detect miscarriages** – True. At this early stage, determining the viability of the pregnancy is very important, as the symptoms of pregnancy may still be continuing even if the fetus has died. If this is the case, then the woman will need to be managed as clinically appropriate and supported psychologically.

[See 'Miscarriage' on page 181.]

D To detect fetal abnormalities – False. This scan can be used to detect gross fetal abnormalities such as anencephaly. However, the fetal anomaly scan at approximately 20 weeks is the time when there is a more detailed assessment, but the early booking scan may pick up serious anomalies. Terminations may be offered as a result of this earlier scan prior to a detailed anomaly scan.

E ✔ **Down syndrome screening** – True. Nuchal translucency scans are now offered at this time and are used in conjunction with blood tests and aspects of the patient's medical history to calculate a risk of Down syndrome specific to that pregnancy.

 Key Point

Fetal measurements are used to date the pregnancy. Before 13 weeks, the crown rump length (CRL) can be measured accurately. However, after this gestation, the fetus becomes increasingly flexed; therefore, other parameters may be measured, such as the femur length and head circumference.

Q5: At what week of gestation is a woman ideally offered a fetal anomaly scan?
The correct answer is C. 20 weeks.

The timing of the fetal anomaly scan is important since if it is performed too early, it may be difficult to visualise some abnormalities. If performed too late, however, the woman will have reduced management options if a fetal abnormality is detected. The fetal anomaly scan can also be called the '20-week' scan, as, optimally, all women would be offered the ultrasound scan at this week of gestation. If a fetal abnormality is found that could potentially affect the couple's decision of whether to continue with the pregnancy, this allows for some consideration time if they were to decide to have a termination.

 Key Point

The use of ultrasound during pregnancy is interesting when considering the difference between the clinician's and the woman's expectations. Ultrasound is a crucial screening tool, and an abnormality is identified in approximately 1% of pregnancies. However, some pregnant women may view scans as social events without considering the diagnostic implications. It is, therefore, extremely important that the true reason for the scan is explained thoroughly to the woman so that she is prepared for the risk that the ultrasound scan may show abnormalities in the pregnancy.

Q6: Answer true or false: Which of the following, if present, has a greater than 50% chance of being detected by the fetal anomaly scan?

If the woman chooses not to have a booking scan or she finds out that she is pregnant at a later gestation, a '20-week' scan will determine dating information about the pregnancy and diagnose if there are multiple fetuses. The majority of nonviable pregnancies will be lost before the scan at 20 weeks. The anomaly scan is to assess the fetus for structural abnormalities. Each potential abnormality has a different detection rate, which may vary between different scanning centres. Approximately 50% of significant abnormalities can be detected in this scan, and the importance of the timing of this scan is to give parents options about how they might proceed with the pregnancy. The timing is also to allow health professionals time to prepare for antenatal, intrapartum and neonatal management.

A ✔ **Anencephaly** – True. Approximately 99% of anencephaly can be seen on abdominal ultrasound at this stage. Anencephaly is a major anomaly that occurs when the rostral (head) end of the neural tube fails to close, resulting in the absence of a major portion of the brain. All cases detected at this stage will not be compatible with life.

B Cerebral palsy – False. Cerebral palsy cannot be seen on the fetal anomaly scan. Cerebral palsy is an umbrella term for a neurological disorder caused by a nonprogressive brain injury or malformation. It can affect body movement, motor control, coordination, tone, reflex, posture and balance.

C ✔ **Spina bifida** – True. Spina bifida is also a neural tube anomaly caused by incomplete closure of the neural tube. At this stage, approximately 90% of cases will be able to be visualised during the fetal anomaly scan. This is dependent on the degree of spina bifida and how much tissue is herniating through the gap in the spinal vertebrae. It is important that women take 400 micrograms of folic acid before conception until 12 weeks gestation to reduce the risk of neural tube anomalies. Individuals with an increased risk of spina bifida – for example, those with a previous pregnancy affected by spina bifida or women on antiepileptic drugs – are advised to take 5 mg of folic acid until 12 weeks gestation.

D ✔ **Gastroschisis** – True. Gastroschisis is caused by an anomaly in the anterior abdominal wall, allowing the bowel to freely protrude through the wall. It is identified at the anomaly scan in over 95% of cases.

E **Autism** – False. Autism cannot be detected by ultrasound scanning. Autism is a condition that affects social interaction, communication, interests and behaviours of the child.

 Key Point

The exact figures are not necessary to learn here, but it is important to grasp the overarching principle that ultrasound screening has limited sensitivity and specificity.

Q7: At 18⁺⁴ weeks gestation, which diagnostic test is more suitable for this patient?
The correct answer is A. Amniocentesis.

The type of diagnostic tests available and offered to a woman usually depends on the timing of initial screening. Amniocentesis involves the insertion of a needle into the abdominal cavity under ultrasound guidance and drawing off a sample of amniotic fluid. CVS, or placental biopsy, is carried out using a cannula to aspirate or biopsy the placental villi. This can be done by either a transabdominal or transcervical approach. Due to the later gestation of 18 weeks, it is more suitable for this patient to have an amniocentesis. This is because of the lower risk of miscarriage with this procedure and because the results from this invasive prenatal diagnostic test are more accurate. At this gestation, CVS would be more risky to the fetus and is less accurate, so it should not be used in this situation. CVS is more suitable for women at an earlier gestation who have an above-threshold risk of chromosomal abnormality. The other options are screening tools and not diagnostic tests.

 Key Point

Amniocentesis before 15 completed weeks of gestation is referred to as 'early amniocentesis'.

Q8: Julia is told about the risks of miscarriage. Which are the correct percentages quoted for amniocentesis and CVS?
The correct answer is B. Amniocentesis, 1%, and CVS, 2%.

It is extremely important that women are informed of the risk of miscarriage with either of the invasive prenatal diagnostic tests. Women should be informed that CVS carries an additional risk of miscarriage compared to amniocentesis carried out after 15 weeks of gestation. In either case, written consent should be obtained prior to performing an amniocentesis or CVS to confirm that information has been given about national and locally estimated risks of the procedure related to

pregnancy loss. The typical values quoted for risk of miscarriage are 1% for ultrasound-guided amniocentesis and 2% for CVS, although operator and local figures may vary. Women may have to weigh the benefit of being able to know the diagnosis earlier in pregnancy against the higher risk of miscarriage.

 Key Point

Current UK estimates are that approximately 5% of pregnant women are offered invasive prenatal diagnostic tests, with amniocentesis and CVS being the most common. In the near future, with the falling costs of analysing free fetal DNA in maternal serum, these invasive tests will likely become substantially less common.

Q9: She also undergoes a test for Edward syndrome. Which chromosome is a trisomy in this syndrome?
The correct answer is D. 18.

Down syndrome is not the only chromosomal abnormality tested for by amniocentesis or CVS; a variety of other chromosomal abnormalities are also tested for. Edward syndrome affects approximately 1 in 2500 live births and is, therefore, less common than Down syndrome (1:650).

A **13** – Incorrect. This trisomy is Patau syndrome, an even rarer chromosomal abnormality affecting 1 in 5000 live births. Symptoms include growth restriction, severe developmental delay, cleft palate and gastrointestinal atresias. Survival is rare beyond the age of 1 year.

B **21** – Incorrect. Trisomy of chromosome 21 is Down syndrome. Down syndrome can often be recognised in babies with facial features that are typical of the syndrome. Signs include prominent epicanthal folds, flat nasal bridge, Brushfield spots in the eyes, open mouth with protruding tongue and low-set ears.

C **15** – Incorrect. Trisomy of chromosome 15 is a very rare abnormality, as most cases will miscarry in early gestation.

D ✔ **18** – Correct. Edward syndrome is a trisomy of chromosome 18, and most cases are due to nondisjunction. Edward syndrome is often not compatible with life beyond childhood, and 90% of affected babies will die before 12 months.

E **12** – Incorrect. Trisomy of chromosome 12 is also a very rare abnormality. Most cases of this chromosomal abnormality will not survive to term.

 Key Point

Key signs of Edward syndrome:
- Intrauterine growth restriction (IUGR).
- Small elongated head.
- Severe developmental delay.
- Rocker bottom feet.
- Increased risk of gastrointestinal and renal abnormalities.
- Congenital heart disease.

Important Learning Point

- Screening tests are not necessarily diagnostic. They are tools used to identify individuals who would benefit from further testing because they have an increased risk of a disease.
- Screening for Down syndrome is an important aspect of antenatal screening. Two tests are available: the combined test (10^{+0} to 14^{+1} weeks) and the quadruple test (14^{+2} to 20^{+0} weeks). The combined test is more sensitive and more specific than the quadruple test.
- The booking scan is used to date the pregnancy, determine if it is viable, establish the fetal number and perform part of the combined test for Down syndrome screening.
- The fetal anomaly scan is performed at approximately 20 weeks. The timing of this scan is very important to women for decision-making and to healthcare teams for planning care.
- Amniocentesis and CVS are diagnostic tests used to determine the genetic fetal karyotype. CVS is performed from 11^{+0} to 13^{+6} weeks gestation, whereas amniocentesis is usually performed after 15 weeks.
- Miscarriage is the most important complication that patients need counselling for regarding invasive diagnostic tests because it is the most common adverse event.

10 MEDICAL DISORDERS IN PREGNANCY

DIABETES

Q1: Answer true or false: Which of the following risk factors put Emma at increased risk of gestational diabetes?

At the booking appointment, women will be screened for multiple risk factors for GDM. This will inform if an OGTT is required and when in the pregnancy this should be performed. This highlights again the importance of the booking appointment for risk assessing the antenatal care that will be recommended in a person's pregnancy.

A Age >30 years – False. Age >40 years can increase your risk of GDM.

B BMI ≥35 kg/m² – True. A BMI of >30 kg/m² increases your risk of gestational diabetes and therefore is one of the most important modifiable risk factors to counsel anyone considering pregnancy on.

C Multiparity – False. Parity in itself does not increase your risk of GDM. If you had had GDM in a previous pregnancy, then this would be a risk factor. This is an indication for an early OGTT in your pregnancy.

D Family history of diabetes – True. A family history of diabetes (in either your mother, father or grandparents) is a reason to be screened for GDM.

E Glycosuria 3+ on urine dipstick – True. While having glucose in your urine is not necessarily an indication you have GDM, a high level such as >2+ or 2 occasions of 1+ does require investigating.

Key Point

GDM is an increasing problem and can have both short- and long-term consequences for both the pregnant woman and the fetus. It is therefore important to appropriately screen for risk factors and test for GDM so it can be appropriately managed.

Q2: Which of the following statements is correct regarding factors driving increased insulin resistance in pregnancy?

The correct answers are C. Increased placental progesterone, and **E.** Increased weight gain.

Placental hormones, coupled with the effects of increased insulin resistance and increased calorie intake (increased glucose load) for the purposes of fetal development, induce a temporary 'diabetogenic state' in mothers. Growth hormone (GH) controls growth and insulin resistance by regulating insulin-like growth factor-1 (IGF1). GH causes insulin resistance and increases glucose to supply growing tissues. The maternal pancreas must increase insulin production in response to the diabetogenic state induced by the increased insulin resistance. When this is not achieved, GDM results.

A Decreased production of thyroid hormones – Incorrect. Increased production of adrenal steroids (notably glucocorticosteroids) and thyroid hormones (increase basal metabolic rate) also contribute to the diabetogenic state, as the mother needs higher blood glucose levels to support these changes in metabolic activity.

B Decreased placental lactogen – Incorrect. An increase in placental lactogen promotes insulin resistance and leads to maternal hyperglycaemia and subsequent sequelae.

C ✔ **Increased placental progesterone** – Correct. Increased placental progesterone, particularly in the second and third trimesters, leads to an increase in resistance to the actions of insulin. This, combined with the increased placental lactogen (which has a similar function to human GH), glucagon (which increases blood sugar levels to deal with stressors) and cortisol (released in response to stress), results in a 'diabetogenic' state.

D Decreased cortisol and GH – Incorrect. The effects of increased cortisol and GH are additive in terms of increasing insulin resistance in the mother, resulting in maternal hyperglycaemia. Glucose readily crosses the placenta, whereas insulin does not, so maintaining blood sugar levels in the fetus relies completely on the fetus' own endogenous pancreatic insulin production; this production is immature, so fetal hyperglycaemia can result.

E ✔ **Increased weight gain** – Correct. An increase in weight results in adipocyte enlargement and resistance to fat mobilisation due to insulin. This consequently results in higher levels of insulin circulating in the woman's bloodstream. Postprandially, an excess of circulating lipids that would be absorbed by adipocytes is now deposited in other tissues such as skeletal muscle; this deposition is associated with insulin resistance.

> **Key Point**
>
> The insulin-resistant state that develops as pregnancy progresses is thought to be advantageous to the fetus, as it ensures abundant glucose availability for the growing fetus.

Q3: Answer true or false: What antenatal management options could be applied to this woman?

Antenatal management of women with GDM revolves around maintenance of normoglycaemic levels, education and regular review by diabetic nurses under obstetrician-led care. Appropriate diabetic management should be implemented, starting with diet control that includes dietician input and followed by the use of metformin or insulin under supervision of a diabetic clinician. Women are advised to monitor and reattend if they notice decreased fetal movements. Fetal growth is normally monitored by ultrasound every 4 weeks from 28 weeks.

A ✔ **Consistently high blood glucose levels merit the use of metformin or insulin** – True. Consistently high blood glucose levels (more than 7.8 mmol/L), despite adherence to diet, would merit the use of an oral hypoglycaemic agent such as metformin or insulin. Blood glucose levels would be monitored daily, in the morning as well as before and after every meal, using capillary blood glucose. Insulin requirements increase during pregnancy and should therefore be titrated against the requirements of the woman.

B Measurement of glycosylated haemoglobin every 4 to 6 weeks – False. This woman has GDM; therefore, guidelines state that the HbA1c should only be measured at diagnosis. Recent guidelines suggest that if women have had a diagnosis of GDM and have had a negative postnatal diabetes test, they should still be offered an annual HbA1c.

C Ultrasound examinations every 2 weeks in the first trimester – False. Ultrasound examinations in most UK units are carried out every 2 to 4 weeks in the last trimester, based on local protocols. This ensures the monitoring of the fetus of a diabetic mother for abnormal growth trajectories. These growth scans measure the head circumference, abdominal circumference and femur length to calculate weight. In macrosomia, the abdominal circumference increases to a greater extent than the other two measurements. Growth scans can be used in conjunction with obstetric examinations, liquor volume and umbilical artery Doppler to monitor fetal well-being.

D ✔ **Involvement of a dietician in the multidisciplinary team** – True. This woman's BMI categorises her as obese, and a BMI of more than 30 kg/m² is

an independent risk factor for the development of DM. A dietician is an essential member of the multidisciplinary care team in charge of this patient. This person's diet needs to be analysed and modified to return to a healthy weight.

E Regular maternal fundoscopy – False. This patient has GDM and is unlikely to develop *de novo* signs of retinopathy in this short time period. Maternal fundoscopy is performed to look for progression of preexisting diabetic retinopathy in women with preexisting DM during their pregnancy.

> **Key Point**
>
> Diabetes in pregnancy should be managed through a multidisciplinary approach, as several factors need to be monitored and reviewed by specialists. In addition to midwives, members of the joint clinic include:
>
> - The obstetrician – assumes overall responsibility of the woman's care.
> - Diabetic nurse – collects results from diabetes tests and ensures optimum adherence to diabetic care.
> - Endocrinology or diabetic specialist consultant – optimises the patient's diabetic control and medications.
> - Dietician – manages the woman's diet and nutritional aspects.
> - General practitioner – maintains consistent awareness of the patient's pregnancy and GDM and maintains a role, after the pregnancy has ended, for continued care and detection of potential development of T2DM in the future.

Q4: Answer true or false: Which management options could be applied to this woman regarding birth?

The timing and mode of birth are critical with diabetic women, as is their postpartum management, to ensure low complication and mortality rates for the mother and baby. GDM is a risk factor for caesarean birth, given the increased chance of developing macrosomia and shoulder dystocia. NICE guidelines suggest pregnant women with a normally growing fetus should be offered elective birth through induction of labour (or elective caesarean, if indicated) after 38 weeks. The delivery date may need to be brought forward depending on the degree of blood glucose control. GDM women who are not on insulin and therefore are diet controlled with good glycaemic control can birth at term, given no obstetric complications.

A The aim for the mode of birth should always be a caesarean – False. Vaginal birth should be recommended where there are no complications and this is the woman's preference. Vaginal birth avoids surgical and anaesthetic risks associated with caesarean; therefore, this usually leads to better outcomes for the mother and child, mainly in terms of recovery. Note in exams, questions stemming from 'always' or 'never' options tend to be incorrect, as there will likely be cases where the statement does not apply.

B ✔ **The estimated timing of birth in women requiring insulin is 38 to 39 weeks following the absence of obstetric complications** – True. In the absence of obstetric complications, labour should be induced at 38 to 39 weeks gestation for women requiring insulin. This is done to reduce the risks of developing pre-eclampsia, macrosomia, IUGR and stillbirth.

C ✔ **GDM women with blood glucose greater than 7 mmol/L during labour require an insulin sliding scale** – True. In labour, the mother's blood glucose levels need to be carefully monitored and maintained within normal ranges (4.0 mmol/L and 7.0 mmol/L) through the use of an insulin sliding scale to reduce the risk of the fetus developing neonatal hypoglycaemia.

D Women with GDM should have decreased rates of assisted vaginal birth – False. Many labours in women with diabetes are induced, and the baby may also be macrosomic or be growth restricted, so these labours are at increased risk of prolonged second stage and fetal heart rate abnormalities, both of which may be an indication for intervention to expedite birth. Fetal heart rate should be continually monitored for fetal distress.

E There should be a continuation of pregnancy doses of insulin and diabetic medication for a minimum of 6 weeks postpartum – False. Postnatally, medication should be returned to prepregnancy doses in patients with preexisting diabetes because insulin resistance and sensitivity return quickly to pre-pregnancy levels after removal of the hormonal influence of the placenta. At 6 weeks, women with GDM should be seen for a postnatal follow-up with the diabetic team in the hospital and for a fasting plasma glucose measurement.

> 📰 **Key Point**
>
> GDM increases the risk of developing T2DM. Women diagnosed with GDM should be offered lifestyle advice and a fasting plasma glucose measurement at the 6-week follow-up. Primary care physicians should monitor fasting blood glucose annually afterward. Women with diabetes should also be reminded of the importance of preconception care when planning future pregnancies.

Q5: The minimum glucose concentration needed for the diagnosis of GDM with the 2-hour OGTT.
The correct answer is D. 7.8 mmol/L.

In a healthy population, screening for diabetes is undertaken in patients with risk factors at the booking appointment. NICE guidelines recommend the use of an OGTT to test and diagnose GDM. Plasma glucose concentration is measured after a short period of starvation, followed by repeat measurement 2 hours after consumption of 75 g of glucose. Those with a fasting venous glucose concentration of at least 5.6 mmol/L, or 2 hours after the glucose of 7.8 mmol/L or more, are deemed to have GDM.

Q6: Phototherapy is the first-line treatment for this neonatal complication of diabetes.
The correct answer is G. Hyperbilirubinaemia.

Neonatal jaundice may require intensive phototherapy and frequent monitoring of hyperbilirubinaemia to prevent the development of kernicterus. Free bilirubin can cross the blood-brain barrier and cause bilirubin-induced encephalopathy. The following are other notable fetal complications of maternal diabetes:
- *Congenital abnormalities.*
- *Respiratory distress.*
- *Cardiac decompensation.*
- *Polycythaemia.*
- *Neonatal hypoglycaemia.*
- *Neonatal encephalopathy.*
- *Macrosomia.*
- *Fetal growth restriction.*
- *Sudden fetal death.*

Q7: This complication of diabetes causes reduced gastric motility leading to protracted vomiting.
The correct answer is A. Autonomic neuropathy.

Vomiting is the result of the mother experiencing a combination of factors:
- *Gastroparesis due to reduction of enteric nerve function, reducing peristalsis and gastric emptying.*
- *A gravid uterus reducing gastric emptying by physical compression of the abdominal contents.*
- *Progesterone reducing gut motility as well as gastric emptying.*
- *Oestrogen relaxing the oesophageal sphincter and allowing easier reflux of gastric contents.*

Other common effects of poor neuropathy vascular control in pregnancy include orthostatic hypotension, syncope, facial pallor, reduced sweating, poor temperature regulation and paraesthesia in the feet.

Q8: A fetal complication associated with prolonged labour and shoulder dystocia.
The correct answer is B. Macrosomia.

Maternal diabetes is one of the strongest risk factors associated with macrosomia. Macrosomia is a baby with a birthweight more than the 90th percentile (adjusted for race, sex and gestational age) with an increased abdominal weight distribution in comparison to the head. Surplus nutrient delivery to the fetus leads to a unique pattern of macrosomia of increased truncal subcutaneous fat deposition, resulting in an increase in abdominal circumference and shoulder size and an increased risk of shoulder dystocia. However, skeletal growth and head circumference remain normal. A baby weighing more than the 90th percentile, with normal distribution of growth across the head, abdomen and limbs, is generally termed large for gestational age; this is not associated with shoulder dystocia to the same degree as macrosomia from diabetes.

Q9: Women diagnosed with GDM are offered this test at 6 weeks postpartum to assess for T2DM.

The correct answer is J. Fasting plasma glucose measurement.

NICE guidelines state that women diagnosed with GDM should be offered a fasting plasma glucose measurement instead of an OGTT at the 6-week postnatal check and annually afterward. This opportunity should also be used to offer lifestyle advice on weight control, diet and exercise to women who had GDM.

> ### Key Point
>
> The action of placental hormones (hPL, cortisol and placental GH) on muscle is the main factor that increases peripheral insulin resistance. Falling insulin requirements and hypoglycaemia nearing term are an indication to consider birth. Decreased insulin resistance may reflect a failing placenta and, hence, a very high risk of stillbirth. Identifying these babies is important, as they are in danger and need to be born.

Important Learning Points

- Women with previous GDM, or those with known DM, should be offered preconception information on diet, body weight and exercise, as well as on the risks if hypoglycaemia unawareness occurs.
- Women should be educated about the importance of planning pregnancy and maintaining target blood glucose in the preconception period and the reductions in complications by doing so.
- The diagnosis of GDM is made using WHO criteria and the 2-hour 75-g OGTT.
- In the antenatal period, women with preexisting diabetes should be offered monitoring of maternal blood glucose and ketone levels, as well as screening for fetal congenital malformations and evidence of microvascular disease and monitoring of fetal growth and health.
- Neonatal blood glucose should be checked, and infants should not be discharged until feeding well and maintaining normal blood glucose levels.
- Immediately following birth, women with preexisting diabetes should revert back to prepregnancy levels of medication. Women diagnosed with GDM should stop their antiglycaemic medication, and a fasting plasma glucose should be performed at 6 weeks postbirth. These women should be given counselling regarding the increased risk of DM later in life and GDM in future pregnancies.

EPILEPSY

Q1: Regarding the AED sodium valproate, which of the following are correct?

Correct answers include A. Valproate should, if possible, be stopped completely prior to conception, **B.** If on valproate, the woman should have a discussion with an epilepsy specialist regarding an alternate AED prior to conception, **C.** Valproate levels must be monitored at least once per trimester in those taking it during pregnancy and **D.** Adverse effects of valproate may be avoided if the dose is reduced.

Sodium valproate is a widely used drug, primarily taken as an anticonvulsant for the treatment of epilepsy. It also has a role as a mood stabiliser in bipolar disorder. It is often regarded as the first-line treatment in generalised seizures and is also an adjunctive medication for focal and absence seizures. Adverse effects include nausea, confusion, ataxia, tremor, alopecia and weight gain. Its effect on folate metabolism predisposes the fetus to neural tube defects when taken during pregnancy, in addition to numerous other malformations. For these reasons, unless there is no alternative, valproate use should be avoided in women of childbearing age.

A ✔ **Valproate should, if possible, be stopped completely prior to conception** – Correct. This is due to the risk of malformations and neurodevelopmental impairments. However, in some women with difficult-to-control epilepsy (but well controlled on valproate), the risk of stopping or changing antiepileptic medication may be far greater than the risk to the fetus of continuing. In these cases, valproate may be continued with caution. In the case of this woman, whose seizures are not controlled and who has recently required an uptitration in dose, it should definitely not be stopped. The advice here would be to avoid pregnancy until better seizure control is gained.

B ✔ **If on valproate, the woman should have a discussion with an epilepsy specialist regarding an alternate AED prior to conception** – **Correct.** Valproate is known to be associated with neural tube defects, cleft palates and hypospadias. However, uncontrolled seizures will have a greater impact on the pregnancy and health of the pregnant woman. Therefore, it is important to involve an epilepsy specialist in the decision to switch prior to pregnancy in order to gain good seizure control. If valproate works well and other AEDs have been tried, then remaining on valproate with appropriate counselling could outweigh the risks to the fetus.

C ✔ **Valproate levels must be monitored at least once per trimester in those taking it during pregnancy** – Correct. Several studies have shown that levels of valproate may be increased in pregnancy. Monitoring levels once a trimester aims to prevent overdosing, which may increase the risk of teratogenicity and maternal toxicity, or underdosing, which could increase seizures.

D ✔ **Adverse effects of valproate may be avoided if the dose is reduced** – Correct. The risk of teratogenic effects of valproate are particularly high with higher doses (more than 800 mg per day) or as part of polytherapy. The combination of valproate and lamotrigine has been found to be particularly teratogenic.

E Breastfeeding is not recommended for women taking valproate – Incorrect. Breastfeeding has been deemed safe with most AEDs, particularly valproate, carbamazepine and phenytoin, and NICE recommends encouraging all women with epilepsy to breastfeed. Levels of lamotrigine, levetiracetam and gabapentin in breast milk are higher but still considered to be within safe limits.

 Key Point

Although commonly used in epilepsy, valproate is teratogenic and should ideally be discontinued prior to pregnancy if possible. Fetal effects include neural tube defects as well as other malformations. If continued, levels must be monitored regularly throughout pregnancy. The highest risk to the fetus comes from uncontrolled seizures; therefore, optimal seizure control must be balanced against drug toxicity.

Q2: Answer true or false: Which of these statements would constitute appropriate preconception advice for this mother?

Counselling should be offered to all women with epilepsy in advance of conception. This may involve consultations with family or with carers. Risks of malformations, as well as risks and benefits of individual drugs, should be discussed. The woman should be made aware of the limited data available regarding the adverse effects of newer antiepileptic medications.

A ✔ **Stopping the oral contraceptive may significantly alter lamotrigine levels** – True. It has been consistently observed that lamotrigine levels fall with COCP use. On stopping the COCP, levels may rise. In addition, plasma concentrations of lamotrigine in particular fluctuate significantly during pregnancy. Thus, more careful monitoring of lamotrigine levels may be required during pregnancy than with other AEDs.

B Monotherapy should be adopted, as it is always the most appropriate option – False. Monotherapy is the usual treatment aim because of the increased risk of fetal malformations with multiple AEDs. The background low-risk fetal malformation risk is about 1%. In an epileptic patient not on medications, this is 3%. On monotherapy, it is 4%, and on polytherapy, it can be over 6%. With sodium valproate, these rates may be even greater. However, monotherapy may not be sufficient in some patients' cases of refractory epilepsy, and the key is to strike a balance between decreasing the risk of seizure while minimising the risk of fetal malformation. Therefore, monotherapy may not always be appropriate.

C ✔ **Optimising seizure control prior to conception is important because uncontrolled generalised seizures during pregnancy can increase the risk of SUDEP** – True. Most deaths from epilepsy in or after pregnancy are due to SUDEP. Poorly controlled seizures are the main risk factor; therefore, careful counselling and good seizure control are vital for these pregnant women.

D ✔ **Pregnancy itself may lower the seizure threshold, causing increased seizure frequency if not treated adequately** – True. Pregnancy does appear to lower the seizure threshold. In addition to discontinuation or modification of AED use, steroid hormones, sleep deprivation and vomiting may contribute to increased frequency of seizures. Note however, that some individuals show improvement in seizure control.

E ✔ **The patient should be made aware that women with epilepsy are predisposed to a higher risk of complications during pregnancy and labour** – True. It is important that whilst reassuring women with epilepsy that they are likely to have a healthy pregnancy, the risk of complications in pregnancy and labour is greater than for those without epilepsy.

 Key Point

Counselling constitutes an important part of prepregnancy management in women with epilepsy, as it is important that the patient is aware of the risks and benefits of each course of management for both herself and the fetus, particularly in view of the lowered seizure threshold in pregnancy.

Q3: Which aspects of management during the pregnancy would be recommended in this case?

The correct answer is D. Lamotrigine and carbamazepine are largely considered safe to use during pregnancy.

Although the majority of women with epilepsy have healthy and successful pregnancies, care of these women should be shared between the obstetrician and an epilepsy specialist. NICE recommends that the risk of seizures during labour, although low, is sufficient to warrant birth in an obstetrician-led unit with facilities for maternal and neonatal resuscitation and for treating maternal seizures.

A High-resolution ultrasound scan at 12 weeks – Incorrect. A high-resolution scan should take place at 18 to 20 weeks to allow a more detailed assessment of any developing malformations. In most UK hospitals, this scan is the same anomaly scan offered for all pregnancies.

B All AED levels should be routinely monitored – Incorrect. Levels do not routinely need checking. In cases where seizure frequency increases, levels may need to be checked to ensure they are still in the therapeutic range. Levels should be checked once a trimester for sodium valproate and lamotrigine.

C Folate supplementation should not be commenced until a positive pregnancy test – Incorrect. All women with epilepsy should be offered 5 mg folic acid per day before 'any possibility of pregnancy'; i.e., when a couple starts planning to have a baby.

D ✔ **Lamotrigine and carbamazepine are largely considered safe to use during pregnancy** – Correct.

Although data concerning these relatively new drugs are limited, they are the AEDs of choice for pregnant women with epilepsy. Note that polytherapy is consistently associated with higher risk than monotherapy.

E The neonate should not be given 1 mg vitamin K parenterally at birth – Incorrect. Vitamin K should be recommended to be given parenterally to all neonates in the UK. This is particularly important in women taking enzyme-inducing AEDs during pregnancy. The AEDs are thought to induce fetal hepatic enzyme activity, thereby increasing the potential for vitamin K deficiency and the risk of neonatal bleeding.

> ### 💬 Key Point
>
> Lamotrigine and carbamazepine are considered the safest antiepileptics in pregnancy. Lamotrigine levels may be monitored antenatally, especially if seizure frequency increases. Carbamazepine level monitoring is rarely required. Folate supplements should be started before conception, and fetal vitamin K administration is particularly important for patients who have been exposed to AEDs.

> ### 🔍 Important Learning Points
>
> - Epilepsy can be diagnosed as a primary condition, often congenital, or it can result from reversible causes of lowered seizure threshold, such as drugs, hypoglycaemia, infection and pregnancy.
> - If seizures occur after 24 weeks gestation, it is necessary to consider eclampsia.
> - Counselling constitutes an important part of prepregnancy management in women with epilepsy.
> - All women with epilepsy should be offered 5 mg folic acid per day before conception.
> - Lamotrigine and carbamazepine are largely considered relatively safe to use during pregnancy.
> - Valproate is teratogenic and should ideally be discontinued prior to pregnancy, if possible.

CARDIAC DISORDERS

Q1: Answer true or false: Which of the following could be considered normal when investigating a pregnant woman?

Pregnancy results in increased cardiac output and decreased peripheral vascular resistance. Cardiac output increases approximately 40% due to increases in stroke volume and cardiac rate. Peripheral vascular resistance is mainly mediated by vasodilatation, allowing maternal BP to fall by as much as 5 mmHg systolic in the second trimester. However, BP will increase again in the third trimester and stabilise to normal after birth.

A ✔ **Enlarged cardiac borders on chest x-ray** – True. Due to increased workload, the heart can increase in size and shift in the mediastinum. Other than abdominal and pelvic x-rays, x-ray films can be obtained with minimal risk of radiation to the fetus by using lead-lined protective sheets.

B ✔ **Changing cardiac axis on ECG** – True. The changes in cardiac output can also be reflected in left axis deviation on an ECG. The shift is partly due to the change in mediastinal position of the heart following hypertrophy.

C ST wave elevation on ECG – False. There is no physiological reason for ST wave elevation on ECG during pregnancy. This should therefore be investigated further and managed in an appropriate manner.

D ✔ **Palmar erythema** – True. Red palms and warm extremities are common in pregnancy due to increased oestrogen levels and peripheral vasodilatation. Spider naevi can also be more noticeable or increased in number during pregnancy for the same reasons.

E ✔ **Flow murmurs** – True. The hyperdynamic circulation of pregnancy can often reveal harmless flow murmurs; however, valvular pathologies may also be picked up for the first time during pregnancy. These may have significant implications for maternal health antenatally, during labour and in the postpartum period.

> ### 💬 Key Point
>
> Cardiac examination during pregnancy:
> - After midgestation, many women have a third heart sound.
> - Diastolic murmurs should be considered potentially pathological.
> - Systolic flow murmurs are common.

Q2: Answer true or false: Which of these factors is a risk factor for developing a cardiac disorder in pregnancy?

The physiological and haemodynamic changes that take place in the body during pregnancy affect the cardiovascular system. Therefore, the risk of developing a cardiac disorder increases when pregnant. There are, however, multiple other risk factors.

A ✔ **Increased age (more than 35)** – True. In high income countries across the world, women are waiting until later in life to bear children. This is a major reason why the incidence of cardiac disorders during pregnancy has increased. Pregnancy puts a huge strain on the human body, and the body may not be able to cope or recover well from these changes as it ages. This can result in poor functioning of the cardiac muscle.

B ✔ **Smoking** – True. Other lifestyle choices that may have adverse effects include consumption of alcohol, lack of exercise or a diet rich in fat, salt, sugar and cholesterol. This can lead to deposition of fatty plaques in blood vessels, increasing BP and resulting in an increased amount of strain put on the heart. This can lead to many types of cardiac disorders and complications, such as arrhythmias or even heart failure.

C ✔ **Pre-existing cardiac disorder** – True. This factor can increase the chance of other cardiac disorders developing or complications of the preexisting condition arising. As the heart is already in a compromised state, the physiological changes that take place in pregnancy can worsen the preexisting heart condition.

D Pre-existing diagnosis of asthma – False. There is no evidence that suffering from asthma increases your risk of cardiac disease in pregnancy. However, women with asthma may have an increased risk of adverse perinatal outcomes if their disease is moderate to severe and is poorly controlled.

E Busy lifestyle – False. This is not a risk factor. Nonetheless, it is advised that a pregnant woman remains relatively relaxed, as unnecessary stress can lead to poor physical health and worsen preexisting heart conditions.

 Key Point

Those with pre-existing severe cardiac disease need to be monitored closely, often in a joint cardiac and obstetric clinic. Those with severe disease may be advised not to become pregnant in the first place due to the significant risk of cardiovascular compromise.

Q3: Which of these blood tests, when there are increased levels, indicate possible myocardial damage?
The correct answer is B. Troponin I.

Some of the changes that occur in pregnancy strongly resemble the changes that occur in a person with a cardiac disorder, such as physiological breathlessness and peripheral oedema. Hence, it may be difficult to diagnose a cardiac disorder antenatally.

A Thyroid hormones – Incorrect. An imbalance of these levels and potassium levels can result in arrhythmias, but they are not an indication of myocardial damage during pregnancy.

B ✔ **Troponin I** – Correct. Increased levels are not seen in a healthy pregnant woman, so increased levels are an indication of a cardiac disorder.

C Iron level – Incorrect. Iron levels normally relate to anaemia rather than cardiac problems. However, anaemia can worsen a preexisting cardiac disorder due to the increased workload of the heart to compensate for the reduced haemoglobin level.

D Carbon dioxide – Incorrect. An increase in carbon dioxide level is usually a result of a primary respiratory problem, not cardiac.

E Potassium – Incorrect. An imbalance of potassium levels can result in arrhythmias, but they are not

an indication of myocardial damage. Changes on an ECG with hyperkalaemia include flattened or absent P waves, widening of the QRS segment, tented T waves and slurring of the ST segment.

 Key Point

Increased troponin I levels are not seen in healthy pregnant women and could indicate a cardiac disorder.

 Important Learning Points

- Pregnancy is a risk factor for developing cardiac disease.
- Physiological and haemodynamic changes that take place in the body begin in the first 8 weeks of gestation and continue into the later stages of the second trimester.
- The most likely complications to arise from cardiac disease during pregnancy are arrhythmias and heart failure.

MATERNAL WEIGHT

Q1: Which of these BMI calculations and classification pairings is correct for Rachel (160 cm tall and 92.5 kg)?
The correct answer is B. 36.1 kg/m²; obese class 2.

BMI is a way of expressing numerically whether a patient's weight is appropriate for their height and, if not, the extent of the problem. BMI = weight (kg) ÷ height² (m). Rachel's height is 160 cm (1.6 m), and her weight is 92.5 kg. Therefore, Rachel's BMI can be calculated using the following formula: $92.5 \div 1.6^2 = 36.1$ kg/m².

 Key Point

People often underestimate or overestimate their height and weight, especially if it hasn't been measured for a while. Therefore, healthcare professionals need to take accurate measurements themselves rather than relying on the information given by the individual.

Q2: Using the correct BMI for Rachel, select what additional monitoring or treatment should be offered throughout her pregnancy.

The correct answers are A. OGTT between 24 and 28 weeks, **C.** Birth in a consultant-led unit and **E.** Monitoring for pre-eclampsia every 3 weeks from 24 to 32 weeks and every 2 weeks thereafter.

Numerous conditions, such as gestational diabetes, are associated with obesity during pregnancy. The patient should be screened for these conditions so that treatment can be offered at the earliest stage to minimise harm.

A ✔ **OGTT between 24 and 28 weeks** – Correct. All obese women should have this test due to the increased risk of gestational diabetes. If the disease is detected early enough, then the complications such as fetal macrosomia can be minimised by effective control of blood glucose levels. Most women recover from this condition after birth, but a number of women continue to have poor blood sugar control. Therefore, a fasting glucose level should be checked around 6 weeks after birth in women who developed gestational diabetes.

B   Seven days of thromboprophylaxis following birth – Incorrect. This is reserved for patients with a BMI above 40 kg/m^2 or with additional risk factors, such as smoking or a previous VTE. Rachel has neither of these, as she is within obese class 2 and is otherwise fit and well. Therefore, she does not require this treatment.

C   ✔ **Birth in a consultant-led unit** – Correct. Rachel's BMI is above 35 kg/m^2, so the recommendation is that she should birth in a consultant-led unit rather than at home or in a midwife-led suite because of the increased risk of complications.

D   Routine measurement of maternal weight at every midwife and medical consultation – Incorrect. Maternal weight should not be checked unless it will affect the clinical management of the woman, such as in the planning of equipment that may be required during birth. Repeat measurements may also be necessary in order to confirm that the mother is not gaining an excessive amount of weight during the pregnancy. Keeping the weight gain within an optimum range (5 to 9 kg for obese women) improves outcomes for both mother and baby.

E   ✔ **Monitoring for pre-eclampsia every three weeks from 24 to 32 weeks and every two weeks thereafter** – Correct. Rachel's BMI is above 35 kg/m^2, so she is at a higher risk. Therefore, she should have more intensive monitoring for signs of pre-eclampsia. Pre-eclampsia is a condition where the patient will develop hypertension and proteinuria. If this develops into eclampsia, then the mother will have seizures, which may be life-threatening to her and the baby. Treatment with aspirin from 12 weeks gestation throughout pregnancy reduces the chance of developing pre-eclampsia.

[See 'Pre-Eclampsia and Pregnancy-Induced Hypertension' on page 301.]

> **Key Point**
>
> Knowing the patient's BMI, and therefore the extent of her obesity, is essential in determining which interventions are necessary during pregnancy and labour. All obese women requiring a caesarean should be given prophylactic antibiotics to prevent wound infection. Early venous access during labour is necessary in those with a BMI over 40 kg/m^2. This is because cannulation is likely to be difficult in morbidly obese women should an emergency arise.

Q3: Answer true or false: Obese women are likely to be at risk for which of the following obstetric complications?

Identifying the complications for which an obese woman is likely at increased risk is important in order to educate her appropriately and manage her treatment effectively.

A   ✔ **Seizures** – True. This is a life-threatening consequence of pre-eclampsia. Obese women are more likely to develop pre-eclampsia, and subsequently eclampsia, so they are more likely to experience seizures. Women with a BMI over 35 kg/m^2 are in the highest risk category and should have regular monitoring.

B   ✔ **A large baby** – True. Macrosomia is a common complication of maternal obesity, particularly in diabetic patients. The child is at risk of obesity and metabolic abnormalities, but birth can also be difficult for macrosomal babies. Fetal growth scans using ultrasound can estimate the weight of the baby to help plan birth. Conversely, obesity is also associated with IUGR.

C   ✔ **Pulmonary embolism (PE)** – True. An obese patient is more at risk of VTE, including PE. She should have a thorough VTE risk assessment at her booking appointment with her midwife. If she is deemed to be at high risk, thromboprophylaxis may be given throughout the pregnancy and/or after birth. Low-molecular-weight heparin (LMWH) is the most suitable agent for these at-risk women.

D   A baby with a flat philtrum – False. This is a birth defect that most commonly occurs as part of fetal alcohol syndrome. It is not associated with obesity. Congenital abnormalities can be associated with obesity, but these are typically neural tube defects or cardiac abnormalities rather than facial anomalies.

E   ✔ **Requirement of ventouse for birth** – True. Obese women are more likely to require an assisted vaginal birth (ventouse or forceps) or caesarean. A myriad of causes exist for this, including macrosomia, fetal distress caused by IUGR, difficulties monitoring in labour and difficulties with optimum positioning in pregnancy.

> **Key Point**
>
> Obesity can have serious consequences for both the mother and baby throughout the pregnancy and birth and after birth. The risks associated with obesity should always be considered when making care plans for pregnant women.

> **Important Learning Points**
>
> • Obesity during pregnancy is defined as a BMI of 30 kg/m^2 or higher at the patient's booking appointment. Patients with a BMI of 25.0 to 29.9 kg/m^2 are classed as overweight, and those with a BMI of less than 18.5 kg/m^2 are classed as underweight.

- Women who are at either end of the BMI spectrum may have problems conceiving, and they should be advised to normalise their weight prior to conception where possible.
- Obesity carries significant risks to the mother's health throughout pregnancy and the birth, in addition to predisposing the baby to diseases such as childhood obesity.
- An obese pregnant woman should have regular monitoring and a thorough plan for birth. This may be in a consultant-led unit where appropriate.
- Low BMI causes an increased risk of preterm birth and low birth weight. An increase in maternal weight during the pregnancy is believed to improve outcomes.

THYROID DISEASE

Q1: Answer true or false regarding the following statements concerning hyperthyroidism in pregnancy.

Hyperthyroidism occasionally presents as a new diagnosis in pregnancy, most commonly due to Graves disease. More often, women may experience a relapse of previously well-controlled hyperthyroidism. It is important that all affected women are fully informed regarding the maternal and fetal effects of hyperthyroidism. Thyroid gland hypertrophy is a normal occurrence during pregnancy and reverses postpartum.

A Thyroid function is routinely screened for in the antenatal booking visit – False. Despite the increased rate of presentation of thyroid disease during pregnancy and the puerperium, evidence does not currently support the routine screening of thyroid function in pregnancy. Nevertheless, thyroid testing should clearly be performed in those with the relevant symptoms.

B Free T4 is the active thyroid hormone exerting the main physiologic effect – False. Over 99% of thyroid hormone is bound to carrier protein, usually thyroid binding globulin (TBG), with only the free hormone being active. T4 is converted peripherally to T3, which contributes the majority of thyroid action.

C ✔ **Free T4 is the most useful investigation in diagnosing hyperthyroidism in pregnancy** – True. Free T4 is used to biochemically diagnose hyperthyroidism due to the alterations in total T4 and TBG that occur during pregnancy.

D Carbimazole is the first-line treatment for hyperthyroidism in the first trimester – False. Propylthiouracil is the first-line antithyroid medication in pregnancy due to reduced placental transfer in comparison with carbimazole. Although a small amount does cross the placenta, propylthiouracil is not thought to be teratogenic. Carbimazole is not absolutely contraindicated in pregnancy, but it has rarely been associated with an increased risk of congenital malformations.

E ✔ **Graves disease is the most common cause of hyperthyroidism in pregnancy** – True. The vast majority of presentations of hyperthyroidism in pregnancy are due to Graves disease. The IgG antibodies responsible for Graves disease are known to cross the placenta. Less common causes would include toxic nodules or viral, granulomatous or autoimmune thyroiditis. It should be noted that these causes should be differentiated from transient gestational hyperthyroidism, which is usually milder and rarely requires antithyroid medications. It is thought to result from high levels of human chorionic gonadotropin (hCG) and is often associated with hyperemesis gravidarum.

 Key Point

Although T3 is the physiologically active thyroid hormone, free T4 levels are the most useful for diagnosis.

Q2: During pregnancy, levels of which of the following would be expected to increase?

In the first trimester, fetal thyroxine is entirely derived from maternal sources prior to development of a functional thyroid gland. Increased glomerular filtration and loss of iodine through the fetoplacental unit result in a state of maternal iodine deficiency during pregnancy. Nevertheless, pregnancy is associated with increased total T3 and T4 and largely unchanged free T3, free T4 and TSH.

A TSH – False. Overall, TSH levels remain unchanged in pregnancy, although they are often at the lower end of the normal range. There is an initial decrease in TSH in the first trimester due to stimulation of TSH receptors by increased hCG (structurally similar to TSH), but this subsequently normalises for the remainder of gestation.

B Free T4 – False. Although the total level of thyroid hormone appears elevated due to increased TBG, levels of free circulating T4 and T3 are not significantly altered overall.

C ✔ **Total T4** – True. There is an initial rise in TBG in the first fortnight of pregnancy, induced by increased oestrogen. This causes a rise in total T4 and T3, but the level of free thyroid hormone remains unchanged.

D Maternal iodide – False. Pregnancy is a state of relative iodine deficiency, secondary to both renal loss and fetal thyroid activity. Iodine supplementation may be required in those with deficiency.

E ✔ **TBG** – True. TBG increases in the first trimester, reaching a plateau by 20 weeks.

 Key Point

TBG shows an initial rise in pregnancy, with associated rises in total T3 and T4. Levels of free thyroid hormones and TSH remain largely unchanged throughout pregnancy.

Q3: Answer true or false: The risk of which of the following are increased with hyperthyroidism in pregnancy?

Although routine screening of thyroid function is not recommended in guidelines, those with known thyroid disease should be given appropriate counselling to address any concerns and referred to a specialist for monitoring of thyroid function and medication.

A ✔ **Fetal growth restriction** – True. Severe uncontrolled hyperthyroidism during pregnancy increases risk of fetal growth restriction.

B Deep vein thrombosis (DVT) – False. Risk of DVT is not increased by maternal hyperthyroidism or hypothyroidism. There is, however, a significant increase in risk of DVT secondary to pregnancy itself.

C ✔ **Neonatal hypothyroidism** – True. Maternal hyperthyroidism can result in both neonatal hyperthyroidism and hypothyroidism.

D ✔ **Miscarriage** – True. Hyperthyroidism increases the risk of miscarriage.

E Congenital malformations – False. Congenital malformations are not known to be associated with hyperthyroidism itself. Antithyroid medications, such as carbimazole, have been associated with such malformations, albeit rarely.

 Key Point

Hyperthyroidism induces an increased risk of miscarriage, pre-eclampsia and neonatal thyroid disease.

Important Learning Points

- Hyperthyroidism in pregnancy is most commonly due to Graves disease.
- Free T4 is the most useful investigation in diagnosing hyperthyroidism in pregnancy.
- Propylthiouracil is the first-line antithyroid medication in pregnancy.
- Hyperthyroidism induces an increased risk of miscarriage, pre-eclampsia and neonatal thyroid disease.
- Routine screening of thyroid function is not recommended. Nonetheless, those with known thyroid disease should be given appropriate counselling on pregnancy risks.

HEPATITIS B

Q1: Which option is the most appropriate immediate step in Rose's management?

The correct answer is D. Refer to a hepatologist or relevant specialist and arrange further tests.

The presence of HBsAg indicates a current hepatitis B infection, but it does not provide adequate information about its stage, so further investigations are required. If found to be HBsAg positive, the patient should be referred to a specialist within 6 weeks. Further testing is indicated to detect:

- *HBeAg/anti-HBe status.*
- *HBV DNA level.*

- *Anti-HBc IgM.*
- *Tests to identify infection with other common hepatitis viruses (A, C, D and E).*
- *Additional tests, including alanine transaminase (ALT), gamma-glutamyl transferase (gamma GT), alkaline phosphatase (ALP), serum albumin, total bilirubin, total globulins, FBC, prothrombin time and hepatic ultrasound.*

A Lamivudine, zidovudine and lopinavir – Incorrect. Treatment may or may not be needed, depending on further testing. The current recommendation is to treat those at high risk with tenofovir disoproxil, not lamivudine.

B Commence tenofovir disoproxil at 28 weeks – Incorrect. This is a recommended treatment for HBV that has been determined to pose a very high risk of vertical transmission. In this case, the infection stage has not yet been determined, nor is it clear whether this will persist until the third trimester.

C Ribavirin and PEG-IFNα-2a – Incorrect. This has previously been a standard treatment for HCV infection. However, a significant risk of harm to the baby arises with ribavirin or ribavirin combination therapy with any interferon.

D ✔ **Refer to a hepatologist or relevant specialist and arrange further tests** – Correct. Therapy may be indicated in women with raised ALT and HBV DNA of more than 2000 IU/mL. However, treatment within these parameters can be delayed until after birth.

E Sofosbuvir oral medication and referral to specialist – Incorrect. Sofosbuvir is a second-generation direct-acting antiviral treatment for the treatment of hepatitis C.

 Key Point

HBsAg indicates an infection; however, it does not reveal infectivity. HBeAg and HBV DNA indicate current viral replication and high infectivity. Antiviral therapy should be discussed with pregnant women and offered to those at the highest risk.

Q2: Answer true or false to the following statements regarding this woman's results.

HBV serology is a frequently examined topic, and the markers of infection can be used to determine the stage of infection. A chronic infection is characterised by the presence of HBsAg more than 6 months after the initial infection and may be HBeAg positive or HBeAg negative. HBeAg and HBV DNA are markers of active viral replication.

A She was vaccinated against HBV when training as a nurse – False. It can never be assumed that an adequate vaccination series has been administered to anyone. Anti-HBs indicate immunity following vaccination where all other serum markers are absent. The presence of HBsAg confirms the patient has a hepatitis B infection.

B ✔ **She may need to commence antiviral treatment in the third trimester to prevent transmission** – True. The objective of treatment in pregnancy is to reduce the risk of mother-to-child transmission. Both HBeAg and HBV DNA of more than 2000 IU/mL are markers of viral replication. The lowest rate of transmission occurs where anti-HBe is detected. If these results persist and maternal viral DNA titre reaches 1.0×10^7 IU/mL, tenofovir disoproxil is recommended after 28 weeks gestation.

C ✔ **She was probably infected with hepatitis B early in life** – True. The presence of anti-HBc IgG indicates that she has a chronic infection. The majority of infections in adults clear spontaneously. By contrast, there is a 95% chance of the infection becoming chronic if transmitted perinatally. The fact that she was born in a region where HBV is more common increases the likelihood of perinatal transmission. Areas of high endemicity include most of Asia and Africa, some South American and European countries and the Pacific islands, although infections can occur anywhere in the world, and there is risk variation even within high risk regions.

D ✔ **Her baby requires the hepatitis B vaccine at birth** – True. All infants born to those who are HBsAg positive in pregnancy must receive a full vaccination series commencing at birth. In this case, there appears to be an acute exacerbation of a chronic infection. In the absence of anti-HBe, the risk of transmission is high, and the infant should receive hepatitis B immunoglobulin within 12 hours of birth in addition to the full vaccination series.

E ✔ **She is likely to be a chronic carrier of HBV** – True. Chronic infection is characterised by the presence of HBsAg more than 6 months after the initial infection. A chronic infection may be HBeAg positive or HBeAg negative.

> **Key Point**
>
> The rate of mother-to-child transmission is 90% in the highest-risk cases of active viral replication, indicated by a positive HBeAg and/or high HBV DNA. In total, 95% of those infected in the first year of life develop chronic HBV.

Q3: The presence of this indicates a markedly lower likelihood of vertical transmission of HBV.

The correct answer is G. Anti-HBe.

Both HBV DNA and HBeAg are markers of viral replication and high infectivity. Vertical transmission is very likely to occur in cases where one or both of these are present. Anti-HBe will not always be present, but in cases where it is detected, it has a protective effect and is associated with the lowest incidence of mother-to-child transmission, where a mother has hepatitis B.

Q4: Chronic infection is identified by its persistence past 6 months.

The correct answer is D. HBsAg.

Chronic infection is identified by the presence of HBsAg for more than 6 months following the initial infection. A chronic infection can be HBeAg positive or HBeAg negative, and anti-HBc IgG positive. In the 'window phase' of a resolving infection, targeting the immune complex of HBsAg and HBeAg can prevent their serological detection. The appearance of anti-HBs indicates a resolved infection, or, if present in isolation, it indicates immunity from vaccination.

Q5: The most reliable predictor of infectivity and viral replication in HBV.

The correct answer is K. HBV DNA.

Vertical transmission occurs in 90% of highest-risk pregnancies, with up to 95% of the infants infected in utero or within the first year developing chronic HBV infection. HBeAg is a strong indication of replication and infectivity, with its antibody anti-HBe associated with a lower risk of transmission. HBV DNA titre detected by PCR is a more accurate measure of the current viral load, replication and infectivity, whereas HBeAg titres can be falsely negative as a result of a common viral mutation.

Q6: A significant elevation of this enzyme is commonly associated with viral hepatitis.

The correct answer is J. ALT.

The serum transaminases ALT and, to a lesser extent, AST, are most likely to be raised in a setting of viral hepatitis. ALT is a more sensitive and specific marker of liver injury than AST. Mild or moderate elevation of ALT can occur in chronic viral hepatitis, with a marked rise observed in acute viral or autoimmune hepatitis and an extreme rise indicative of a severe acute viral hepatitis, drug injury, necrosis or acute liver failure. Abnormal elevations of ALP or GGT indicate an alternative or overlap aetiology such as a chronic cholestatic liver disease.

> **Key Point**
>
> Understanding the liver function tests and the hepatitis screen is fundamental to determining what is wrong with the patient.

> **Important Learning Points**
>
> - Viral hepatitis is the most common cause of non-pregnancy-related hepatic dysfunction. Common pregnancy-related causes include pre-eclampsia and intrahepatic cholestasis of pregnancy.
> - Acute viral hepatitis is frequently characterised by a marked increase in ALT, occasionally accompanied by raised AST and mild elevation of GGT and ALP. Significantly raised levels of ALP, GGT and serum bilirubin are suggestive of an alternative (cholestatic) cause.
> - Hepatitis B carries a very high risk of vertical transmission when there is high viral load with or without detectable HBeAg and a high risk of chronic infection in the infant. The primary goal of any treatment in pregnancy is to minimise the rate of transmission to the infant.
> - Antiviral medication may be used in late pregnancy.
> - Ensuring timely administration of HBIG and administration of a full vaccine series in the neonate dramatically reduces the risk of infection.

HIV

Q1: Answer true or false: Which of the following would represent correct advice to the woman?

The current recommendation is that all pregnant women in the UK undergo screening for infection with HIV in addition to hepatitis B and syphilis. It is important that pregnant women with HIV are managed holistically with appropriate input from a multidisciplinary team experienced in management of patients with HIV. Pregnant women should receive early assessment of social circumstances and an offer of counselling.

A ✔ **Screening for hepatitis B and C should be performed** – True. All pregnant women are screened for hepatitis B, as neonatal immunisation may reduce transmission rates. There is currently no universal antenatal screening of UK women for hepatitis C, as no intervention has yet been shown to reduce vertical transmission. The exception to this applies to women with HIV, whose risk of hepatitis C transmission increases from 5% to 15% with HIV co-infection. It is important that these women be informed that a planned caesarean will reduce risk of transmission of hepatitis C together with HIV. Universal screening of hepatitis C in the UK remains a topic of considerable debate.

B ✔ **Smoking should be discontinued, as it may increase risk of vertical HIV transmission** – True. Although not considered one of the major risk factors for vertical transmission of HIV, several studies have shown a significant association with smoking, in addition to insights on the effects of smoking on fetal growth and development.

C ✔ **Antiretroviral therapy (ART) should be continued pre- and postpartum** – True. The RCOG guidelines are clear that those who require ART prior to pregnancy should continue to take it throughout its duration, as well as postpartum. For those who do not require ART for their own health, it should be commenced between 20 and 28 weeks and stopped after birth. Those who do not take ART, who have a viral load less than 10,000 copies/mL and who opt for a planned caesarean may be offered zidovudine monotherapy in place of the standard multiple-medication ART regime for pregnancy.

D ✔ **Birth by planned caesarean is advisable depending on viral load** –True. Caesarean birth provides reduced vertical transmission rates compared with vaginal birth. The RCOG guidelines suggest that those women with a viral load of less than 50 copies/mL can be offered a planned vaginal birth, minimising undue risk.

E Pneumocystis pneumonia (PCP) prophylaxis should be discontinued due to its teratogenicity – False. Concerns have been raised about the teratogenicity of PCP prophylaxis in the past, particularly regarding co-trimoxazole. As co-trimoxazole contains trimethoprim, a folate antagonist, the risk of congenital malformation is significantly higher for women taking co-trimoxazole in the first trimester. Effects include neural tube defects and cardiac and renal tube malformations. This risk is negated by co-administration of high-dose folate (5 mg daily), and it is now considered of overall benefit to continue PCP prophylaxis in women requiring it prior to pregnancy.

 Key Point

Effects of folate deficiency in pregnancy:
- Low birth weight.
- Prematurity.
- Neural tube defects.
- Cardiac malformations.
- Renal tubule malformations.

Q2: This woman decides to continue taking antiretroviral medications and undergoes a planned caesarean. They also choose not to breastfeed. What is the approximate risk of vertical HIV transmission in this case?
The correct answer is A. 1%

Risks to the fetus from maternal HIV infection are numerous, and it is important that both parents are given the opportunity to make informed decisions regarding the pregnancy and to receive support as necessary. They should be aware that, if opting for vaginal birth, some procedures, such as assisted vaginal birth, may increase the risk of transmission. Those who have not taken antiretrovirals during previous pregnancies should be informed of the benefits of intrapartum regimens.

A ✔ 1% – Correct. The combination of appropriate ART, elective caesarean neonatal zidovudine and avoidance of breastfeeding reduces the risk of vertical transmission to less than 1.4%.
B 8% – Incorrect. Antiretrovirals alone, with a vaginal birth, reduce transmission to approximately 8%.
C 15% – Incorrect. This is the approximate risk of vertical transmission of hepatitis B in those who are surface antigen positive.
D 25% – Incorrect. This is the risk of HIV transmission in the absence of any intervention.
E 40% – Incorrect. This is the risk of maternal cytomegalovirus (CMV) transmission.

 Key Point

Women in the UK and other high income countries who are HIV positive are advised not to breastfeed in order to reduce the neonatal transmission risk. However, in other regions, care should be taken regarding giving the same advice, as a lack of access to formula, sterilising equipment and clean water may mean that not breastfeeding could actually place the neonate at a high risk of death from malnutrition and infection other than HIV.

Q3: Answer true or false: Which of the following are risks to the fetus posed by maternal HIV infection?

Despite the evidence for methods of reducing vertical transmission, the sequelae of maternal HIV infection for the neonate are seen. These are wide-ranging but often treatable. Overall, 25% of HIV-infected neonates develop acquired immune deficiency syndrome (AIDS) by 1 year of age and 40% by age 5.

A ✔ **IUGR** – True. Maternal HIV infection has been estimated to double the risk of low birth weight. Some studies suggest that this relationship is at least partially due to maternal weight during pregnancy. These studies emphasise the need for dietary education and counselling during pregnancy.

B ✔ **Prematurity** – True. HIV infection is consistently linked with preterm rupture of membranes and preterm labour. For each hour that membranes are ruptured, risk of vertical transmission increases by approximately 2%. The risks of stillbirth are also significantly higher in women with HIV.

C **Neonatal bradycardia** – False. No significant association has been recognised between HIV and neonatal bradycardia. Administration of certain antiretroviral medications, such as ritonavir, is believed to cause neonatal cardiotoxicity; therefore, the effects may include bradycardia, but this is not due to the HIV infection itself.

D ✔ **Neonatal acute respiratory distress syndrome (ARDS)** – True. HIV increases the risk of neonatal ARDS, as well as neonatal pneumonia, conjunctivitis and sepsis. Usually, due to insufficient production of surfactant, the alveoli are relatively collapsed. Therefore, symptoms related to tachypnoea develop.

E ✔ **AIDS dysmorphic syndrome** – True. This rare syndrome describes several craniofacial abnormalities associated with HIV infection. In addition to growth restriction, these include a small head, prominent forehead, wide-set eyes, flattened nasal bridge and pronounced philtrum.

> **Key Point**
>
> Counselling is of particular importance in women with HIV in order to impart awareness regarding management of the condition during pregnancy and regarding factors that reduce transmission. Patients on ART should continue this therapy during and after pregnancy. Women need to be counselled on the risks and complications related to the neonate as a result of their HIV status.

> **Important Learning Points**
>
> - Risk of HIV transmission is highest during labour, although antenatal intrauterine transmission and breastfeeding transmission may also occur.
> - All pregnant women in the UK should be offered screening for HIV (as well as hepatitis B and C) at 8 to 10 weeks.

- CD4 count and viral load must also be established if the mother tests positive for HIV.
- If there is detectable HIV viral load (more than 50 copies/mL), appropriate ART should be started.
- Women with a viral load of more than 50 copies/mL should give birth at 38 weeks by caesarean.
- Women taking ART who have a viral load less than 50 copies/mL may be offered vaginal birth.
- Maternal HIV infection confers several increased risks to the fetus, including IUGR, prematurity, neonatal ARDS and AIDS dysmorphic syndrome.

SICKLE CELL DISEASE

Q1: At what stage in a pregnancy could this woman first know whether their baby has inherited SCD?
The correct answer is C. At the end of the first trimester, following CVS.

Knowing the haemoglobinopathy status of both parents will only give a probability of the baby having inherited the disorder. Therefore, further investigations are required to confirm whether the baby has SCD or sickle cell trait, which would result in very different outcomes.

A ✔ **After conception, following haemoglobinopathy screening of the father** – Correct. If the mother has SCD and the father does not have the trait, then the baby will have sickle cell trait. If he also has SCD, then the chance that the baby will be affected and have SCD is 100%. However, if he is a carrier, then the chance of SCD in the baby is 50%, so further testing such as CVS would be needed. So in this scenario, depending on the result of the screening of the father, the fetal SCD status could be known at this stage.

B During the first trimester, following blood testing of the mother – Incorrect. As explained above, knowing the sickle cell status of the mother is not enough information to determine how the baby is likely to be affected. The father's haemoglobinopathy status is also needed.

C At the end of the first trimester, following CVS – Incorrect. Invasive diagnostic techniques can confirm the fetus's status *in utero*. The methods commonly used are CVS (usually between the 11th and 14th weeks of pregnancy) or amniocentesis (usually between the 15th and 20th weeks of pregnancy). In this scenario, if the father had sickle cell trait, then this would be the earliest that the SCD status of the fetus could be ascertained.

[See 'Antenatal Screening and Diagnostic Tests' on page 223.]

D During labour, following fetal blood sample (FBS) from the baby – Incorrect. FBS is normally performed to assess for fetal distress in labour by taking a small sample of blood from the fetal scalp. The technique is not used for any other diagnostic tests, as there are safer and more reliable methods to do so.

Fetal blood could be taken from the umbilical cord after birth for diagnostic purposes.

E After the birth of the baby, following the heel prick test – Incorrect. Again, this is an option, and SCD is tested for in the heel prick test, as some pregnancies will not have had this additional surveillance. However, this can only be done after conception, much later than CVS or amniocentesis.

Key Point

All pregnant women in the UK are screened for SCD in early pregnancy. Those with haemoglobinopathies are urged to find out the status of their partners. Expectant parents wishing to know the status of their child can have invasive diagnostic procedures carried out during pregnancy or wait until after the baby is born.

Q2: At the antenatal clinic, Ifemelu has a medication review. Which of the following changes does not need to be implemented?

The correct answer is B. Commencement of iron tablets.

Iron supplements are only given if there is evidence of iron deficiency. Otherwise, there is a risk of iron overload. Iron overload is associated with cardiomyopathy and endocrinopathies (particularly diabetes mellitus, hypothyroidism and hypoparathyroidism) in the mother, as well as IUGR.

A An increase in folic acid dosage – Incorrect. Folic acid is often given at an increased dose of 5 mg/day. Evidence regarding this is conflicting, and drawing definitive conclusions is difficult in a small patient group. However, often, an increased dose will be given to protect against megaloblastic anaemia.

B ✔ **Commencement of iron tablets** – Correct. Starting iron supplementation does not occur as part of an antenatal medication review unless indicated by laboratory results stating low iron.

C Commencement of low-dose aspirin – Incorrect. Low-dose prophylactic aspirin is advised from 12 weeks onward to reduce the risk of developing pre-eclampsia. A dose of 75–150 mg should be prescribed. In addition, women should be advised to receive prophylactic LMWH during antenatal hospital admissions.

D Stopping of hydroxycarbamide – Incorrect. Hydroxycarbamide does not need to be stopped during pregnancy. Hydroxyurea, in comparison, should be stopped, as it is thought to be teratogenic. This has been demonstrated in animal models where it was found to be embryotoxic and cause fetal abnormalities, including hydrocephaly and missing lumbar vertebrae.

E Stopping of ramipril – Incorrect. In most clinical settings, when it is known that a woman is pregnant, ramipril should be stopped. This is because ACE inhibitors affect the renin angiotensin aldosterone system, which has been shown to reduce fetal renal function and increase the risk of fetal and neonatal morbidity and mortality. However, in SCD, ramipril may be continued where the benefit of the medication outweighs the risk.

Key Point

Ideally, medication should be reviewed 3 months prior to conception, but in reality, a number of reasons result in many women presenting at the antenatal clinic still taking the medications they were on prior to conception. Potentially teratogenic medications should be stopped, where possible, immediately.

Q3: Ifemelu attends the emergency department at 28 weeks, presenting with worsening shortness of breath, a cough and feeling generally unwell over the past 48 hours.

The correct answer is B. IV antibiotics, oxygen, blood transfusion and involvement of haematology.

ACS is the second most common complication in pregnancy for women with SCD (7% to 20% of pregnancies). ACS is thought to be due to vaso-occlusion within the pulmonary vasculature, leading to triggering of an inflammatory response. There is normally a triggering event such as fat embolus or infection, but not always.

A IV antibiotics, analgesia and nebulisers – Incorrect. Nebulisers do not make up part of the treatment of ACS. ACS presents similarly to pneumonia, and therefore, this needs to be treated in conjunction with ACS.

B ✔ **IV antibiotics, oxygen, blood transfusion and involvement of haematology** – Correct. These management strategies make up the basis of treatment for ACS. Treatment needs to be commenced promptly, as it can be life-threatening. Oxygen, antibiotics, blood transfusion and inclusion of the haematologist are the basis of treatment. ITU may be required if the patient deteriorates.

C Oxygen, treatment-dose LMWH and involvement of haematology. – Incorrect. Although SCD does increase the risk of stroke and VTE, this does not require treatment-dose heparin.

D Oxygen, IV antibiotics, treatment-dose LMWH and analgesia – Incorrect. Analgesia is important for ACS, and patients with SCD need to be carefully managed regarding their analgesia requirements; however, this option misses some of the key components of management of ACS.

E Involvement of ITU, oxygen and IV antibiotics. – Incorrect. ITU may sometimes need to be involved, especially if the patient is deteriorating. They will need input from haematology also and an MDT approach. In this case, however, Ifemelu is not unwell enough to merit involving ITU at present.

 Key Point

ACS is the second most common complication (after acute pain syndrome) of SCD in pregnancy. It is characterised by a fever, shortness of breath and new lung infiltrates on chest x-ray. It requires rapid recognition and treatment whilst looking for other possible causes for the symptoms such as PE or infection.

Q4: The results of a heel prick test show that a newborn does not have SCD, nor is he a carrier. His parents had been concerned because the condition exists on both sides of the family. After testing the parents antenatally, the obstetrician had told the parents that there had been a 50% chance of the baby not carrying sickle cell genes. What are the most likely statuses of the baby's parents?

The correct answer is E. One parent is a carrier, and one parent has normal haemoglobin.

A Both parents occasionally suffer from sickle cell crises – Incorrect. Regardless of clinical severity, both parents will be homozygous for HbS. This means there is a 100% probability of their children also having SCD.

B Both parents have SCD, and a spontaneous mutation has occurred – Incorrect. A spontaneous mutation would be extremely rare, and the chance of this rectifying a condition from homozygous HbS to normal is near impossible.

C One parent has SCD, and one parent is a carrier – Incorrect. In this case, there would be a 50% chance of a child having SCD and a 50% chance of a child being a carrier.

D Both parents have sickle cell trait – Incorrect. In this case, there would be a 25% chance of a child having normal haemoglobin, a 50% chance of being a carrier and a 25% chance of having SCD.

E ✔ **One parent is a carrier, and one parent has normal haemoglobin** – Correct. In this case, there would be a 50% chance of a child not have any HbS genes and a 50% chance of being a carrier.

 Key Point

A parent with sickle cell anaemia will only have children who either are carriers or have the disease (depending on the partner's haemoglobinopathy status).

 Important Learning Points

- All women are offered screening for haemoglobinopathies (less than 10 weeks gestation) and are often given a card stating their haemoglobinopathy status.
- A medication review should take place 3 months before conception, or as soon as possible, to stop all potential teratogens.
- Pregnant women with SCD can minimise the likelihood of crises by remaining warm and hydrated and avoiding unnecessary exertion. Pethidine should not be given during labour, as it can cause seizures in those with SCD.
- Thromboprophylaxis is important postnatally for all haemoglobinopathies: LMWH, compression stockings, keeping mobile and good hydration.
- Invasive diagnostic techniques are needed to confirm the fetus's haemoglobinopathy status. Postnatally, SCD is tested for in the heel prick test. Newborns are not tested for thalassaemia unless indicated.

INTRAHEPATIC CHOLESTASIS

Q1: The main hepatic duct joins with which other duct to form the common bile duct?

The correct answer is B. Cystic duct.

Cholestasis during pregnancy and outside of obstetrics, is a condition where bile from the liver (Fig. 17.1) is prevented from passing to the duodenum. Cholestasis can be obstructive or nonobstructive.

 Key Point

The ampulla of Vater is formed by the union of the pancreatic duct and the common bile duct. It is an important landmark midway across the duodenum, marking where the foregut becomes the midgut, the point where the coeliac artery stops supplying the gut, and the superior mesenteric artery takes over. Multiple sphincters control flow through the ampulla of Vater, particularly the sphincter of Oddi, which controls the flow of bile and pancreatic juices into the duodenum.

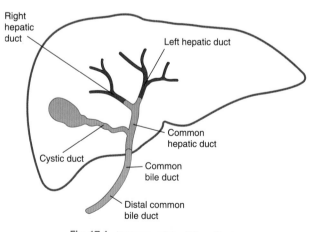

Fig. 17.1 Anatomy of the Biliary System.

Q2: Which of the following liver function test components are increased during pregnancy as part of a normal physiological response?

The correct answers are B. ALP and **E.** Serum cholesterol.

Normal pregnancy is characterised by a mildly cholestatic state. This may affect the absorption of fat-soluble vitamins and increase the likelihood of gallstone development. The placenta secretes ALP, causing its levels to almost double during pregnancy. Oestrogen causes an increase in serum cholesterol, which causes an increase in bile salt production. This makes bile more salt saturated, increasing the risk of gallstone formation. In addition, increased levels of progesterone relax smooth muscle, thus making gallbladder emptying less efficient.

 Key Point

It is important not to disregard abnormal LFTs in pregnancy as physiological. They can be a sign of pre-eclampsia or incidental liver diseases presenting during pregnancy, which include:
- Nonalcoholic steatohepatitis.
- Cholangitis.
- Viral hepatitis.
- Primary biliary cirrhosis.
- Primary sclerosing cholangitis.
- Budd-Chiari syndrome.
- Autoimmune hepatitis.

Q3: Answer true or false: Which of the following aspects of this woman's case are risk factors for intrahepatic cholestasis of pregnancy (ICP)?

Pruritus can have many potential causes in pregnancy; therefore, it is important to be able to recognise risk factors for obstetric cholestasis. However, this can be difficult because the underlying aetiology remains poorly understood.

A Primiparous – False. The parity of the woman is not a risk factor for ICP.

B ✔ **Family history** – True. There may be a positive family history in up to 50% of cases. Both personal and family history increase the risk.

C Maternal age more than 30 – False. Maternal age has not been linked to ICP.

D Male fetus – False. ICP is not related to the gender of the pregnancy.

E Previous history of smoking – False. Smoking has not been linked to ICP. However, smoking is harmful to the mother and fetus, and it has been linked to several other pregnancy disorders. Hence, pregnant women should be especially encouraged to quit.

 Key Point

There is a high chance that a woman who has ICP in one pregnancy will be affected by it again in future pregnancies. Studies give a broad recurrence rate of 45% to 90%. It is important to ask about ICP in multiparous women, as a previous history of ICP is a risk factor in itself.

Q4: What is the primary reason for considering induction of labour before 36 weeks gestation in a woman with known ICP?

The correct answer is D. Total bile acids >100 umol/L.

[See 'Preterm Labour' on page 306.]

A Fetal distress – Incorrect. Although fetal distress is associated with ICP and is something for women and clinicians to be aware of, it is not the primary reason for which induction may be considered.

B Fetal growth restriction – Incorrect. Fetal growth restriction is not thought to be a complication of ICP.

C Maternal sleep deprivation – Incorrect. There are no serious long-term health risks for the mother. Antihistamines, emollient creams and other drugs can be prescribed for symptomatic relief. Nonetheless, it is important to note the psychological impact that constant itching and poor sleep may have on a woman.

D ✔ **Total bile acids >100 umol/L – Correct.** Bile acids at this level indicate severe disease and increase the level of stillbirth to higher than the general population background risk, and therefore, it is recommended to plan birth between 35 and 36 weeks.

E Meconium – Incorrect. Sometimes on ultrasound, scan particulate liquor can be seen on ultrasound. If all other markers of fetal well-being are normal, the suggestion of meconium would not be a reason for induction in a case of ICP.

 Key Point

Women who have had ICP are advised to meet 6 to 8 weeks after birth with a health professional with knowledge of the condition. This is to ensure the woman's pruritus has resolved and her LFTs have normalised. If this is not the case, it will be necessary to look for an alternative cause of the woman's symptoms.

Q5: Answer true or false regarding the following management options.

Treatment options are limited, and risks and benefits need to be clearly explained to women.

A Emollient creams are both safe and highly effective – False. Emollient creams are safe in pregnancy, but they usually only mildly and temporarily provide relief from pruritus.

B Dexamethasone is the first-line treatment option for ICP – False. Results from trials of its effectiveness are currently conflicting. Also note that dexamethasone crosses the placenta, and the effect of its recurrent use on the fetus needs further investigation.

C Activated charcoal improves pruritus – False. Activated charcoal does not improve pruritus. However, it has been found to lower the serum bile acid concentrations in small trials.

D Ursodeoxycholic acid improves pruritus but has no effect on liver function – False. Ursodeoxycholic acid has been found to improve both pruritus and liver function in women with ICP. However, its effect on fetal outcome, if any, is unknown.

E ✔ **No treatment options have been found to improve fetal or neonatal outcomes** – True. The poorly understood pathophysiology of ICP complicates the determination of a therapy that treats the disease. Therefore, no treatment options have yet been found to improve the outcome for the fetus, and drugs can only be prescribed for maternal benefit.

> **Key Point**
>
> Women with ICP may benefit more from lifestyle advice. Some women find that having cool baths and wearing loose-fitting cotton clothing helps to reduce the irritation. Cutting nails short may help to prevent excoriation, though women should be encouraged to avoid scratching in the first place.

> **Important Learning Points**
>
> - ICP is characterised by pruritus and abnormal LFTs with no alternative cause, and the condition resolves after birth.
> - The clinical importance of ICP is the potential negative outcomes for the fetus, particularly stillbirth.
> - The pathology of ICP is unknown, rendering disease-modifying treatment ineffective.
> - Symptomatic management of ICP may include topical emollients, antihistamines and ursodeoxycholic acid.
> - Many women experience pruritus during pregnancy, but only a very small proportion of these will have ICP.

11 MULTIPLE PREGNANCY

TWIN PREGNANCY

Q1: If the two fetuses have separate membranes but share the same placenta, how is this pregnancy described?

The correct answer is B. Monochorionic diamniotic (MCDA).

The fetuses are sharing the same placenta (monochorionic) but have separate membranes (diamniotic). The nature of chorionicity and amnionicity make them risk factors during pregnancy and birth. In the case of monochorionic twins, due to the shared placental mass, they are susceptible to complications including feto-fetal transfusion syndrome (FFTS), twin anaemia polycythemia sequence (TAPS) and twin reversed arterial perfusion (TRAP). This leads to an increased risk of perinatal morbidity and mortality. Identification of the chorionicity of the fetuses early in pregnancy is therefore essential so that correct monitoring for related complications can be instigated.

> **Key Point**
>
> Determining chorionicity and amnionicity allows assignment to the correct management and any additional care needed for the pregnancy and birth

Q2: Which structure gives rise to the placenta during embryological development?

The correct answer is A. Trophoblast.

To understand the answer to this question, it is best to go back to the early development of the embryo.

- *Day 0 – the gametes fuse in the fallopian tube to form a zygote.*
- *Day 1 – the first cleavage occurs, leading to the two-cell stage and, later, the four-cell stage on day three.*
- *Day 3 – a further division occurs to form the uncompacted morula.*
- *Day 4 – development into compacted morula, followed by the entering into the uterine cavity.*
- *Day 5 – formation of early blastocyst.*
- *Day 6 – hatching of the blastocyst to become a late-stage blastocyst.*
- *Day 8 – implantation of blastocyst into the uterine wall, where the cells differentiate into an inner cell mass growing on the interior of the blastocyst cavity and an outer cell mass of trophoblast cells. The latter develops into the placenta.*

A ✔ **Trophoblast** – Correct. The trophoblasts are the cells that form the outer layer of the blastocyst. They develop into the placenta, which provides nutrition for the developing fetus. During implantation, the trophoblast differentiates into two layers: the cytotrophoblast and syncytiotrophoblast. These both play an important role in invading the uterine wall.

B Morula – Incorrect. A morula consists of a ball of cells called blastomeres surrounded by the zona pellucida. The morula is formed by cleavage divisions of the original zygote. At approximately 5 days after fertilisation, the morula undergoes cell differentiation and structural changes, forming the blastocyst that implants into the uterine lining.

C Blastocyst – Incorrect. The blastocyst is made up of the surrounding trophoblast and inner cell mass. Implantation into the uterus is usually completed by day 9 or 10 after fertilisation. Some of the cells from the trophoblast develop into an outer layer of membranes, the chorion, which surrounds the developing blastocyst, and the other cells develop into the inner membranes, the amnion. When the amniotic sac forms from this, between days 10 to 12, the blastocyst is considered an embryo.

D Inner cell mass – Incorrect. The inner cell mass is what will ultimately become the fetus. It is the inner cell mass that will give rise to the ectoderm, mesoderm and endoderm to allow embryological development.

E Zona pellucida – Incorrect. The zona pellucida is the glycoprotein membrane surrounding the oocyte, providing nutrition for the oocyte. When a spermatozoon binds to this structure, it initiates the acrosome reaction, preventing further sperm from entering the oocyte. On day 5 after fertilisation, the blastocyst undergoes zona hatching, where the zona pellucida degenerates to be replaced by the underlying layer of trophoblastic cells.

Key Point

The clinical significance of the trophoblast is its invasion into the maternal uterus, which marks a critical stage in the establishment of a pregnancy. Diseases where this is particularly relevant include:

- Pre-eclampsia, where the trophoblast does not invade sufficiently.
- Placenta accreta spectrum, where the trophoblast may invade too deeply.
- Gestational trophoblastic disease, where there is overproliferation of trophoblastic cells.

[See 'Molar Pregnancy' on page 49.]

[See 'Pre-Eclampsia and Pregnancy-Induced Hypertension' on page 301.]

Q3: If Dheepa's pregnancy was diagnosed with FFTS, what is the best management at this gestation?

The correct answer is B. Laser ablation.

Untreated FFTS can lead to perinatal mortality of more than 90%. Hence, the focus of scans in monochorionic pregnancies between 16 and 24 weeks is the detection of FFTS. Both fetuses are at risk of morbidity and mortality. However, the recipient is at a higher risk than the donor. Women with monochorionic pregnancies should be asked to report sudden increases in abdominal size or breathlessness, as these may be manifestations of FFTS.

A Conservative management – Incorrect. Due to the high risk of mortality with FFTS, this is the not the management of choice. Some women may request termination of pregnancy when severe FFTS is diagnosed, and this should be discussed. In the case of stage one disease, the patient may be managed with close observation in hope of spontaneous resolution, but this would not be the best management option in significant cases of FFTS.

B ✔ Laser ablation – Correct. Management of FFTS should be according to local trust guidelines, and treatment will always be offered at a tertiary specialist centre. Although it is difficult to determine the difference in outcome between laser ablation, amnioreduction and septostomy, laser ablation is the most commonly offered, as it appears to have a reduced mortality rate. Approximate figures for treatment of FFTS by laser ablation are: one third likelihood of both twins surviving, one third likelihood of one twin surviving and one third likelihood of both twins dying.

C Amnioreduction – Incorrect. While this is possible, current data suggest that there are fewer deaths of both babies, fewer neonatal deaths and fewer perinatal deaths with laser ablation.

D Septostomy – Incorrect. Septostomy is the deliberate creation of a hole in the dividing septum with the intention of improving amniotic fluid volume in the donor sac. Although research is also still ongoing comparing amnioreduction, septostomy and laser ablation, current data suggest laser ablation as the best option.

E Bipolar diathermy – Incorrect. Bipolar diathermy is used to selectively terminate one of the fetuses by coagulating the vessels in the umbilical cord supplying that fetus, effectively sacrificing it in the hope that the other baby will live. Though it is possible to perform this on live fetuses, it is generally avoided in preference for attempting to save both. Bipolar diathermy may be used in cases when one of the twins has died *in utero* to prevent toxins formed during necrosis from reaching the other twin via the shared fetal-placental circulation.

Key Point

FFTS is a possible complication of monochorionic twins, affecting 10% to 15% of these pregnancies.

Important Learning Point

- Determining the chorionicity and amnionicity is important to determine the amount of surveillance required in a twin pregnancy and to predict complications that may arise.
- Multiple pregnancies can be diagnosed via ultrasound scans; however, it is notable that they are most commonly diagnosed worldwide by an increased SFH.
- There are multiple fetal and maternal complications that have an increased risk of occurring in a multiple pregnancy in comparison to a singleton pregnancy. Hence, their antenatal care should be more comprehensive.
- Management involves careful planning of the birth and intensive intrapartum care to minimise the risk of harm to the babies or mother.
- Even when uncomplicated, multiple pregnancies have a marginally worse outcome than singleton pregnancies.

12 MANAGEMENT OF LABOUR

SPONTANEOUS VAGINAL BIRTH

Q1: Answer true or false: How is progress in the first stage of labour measured?

It is often said that the diagnosis of labour is easy in retrospect; however, diagnosing it at the time can be much more difficult. There is no normal length of time expected for labour, and it can be lengthened or shortened by many factors. In this clinical case, the fact that this woman is having her third vaginal birth could lead to the expectation of a shorter length of labour. Nonetheless, each woman should be clinically assessed on an individual basis.

A ✔ **Descent of the fetal head** – True. Descent of the fetal head is an important marker of the progression of labour. This is measured in fifths of the head palpable above the pelvic brim when felt abdominally, and it is compared to the position of the ischial spine of the maternal pelvis if examined vaginally.

B Pain scales – False. Pain during labour is a very individual experience. Some women experience very little discomfort, and other women report severe pain; this is not an accurate marker of the progression of labour.

C ✔ **Cervical dilatation** – True. As labour progresses, the cervix dilates. It is important that you know how many previous vaginal births the woman has had, as this affects the appearance of the cervix. A primigravida usually has a cervix with a circular os; however, multiparous women who have had a previous vaginal birth may have an external os that is more slit-like, and the cervix may no longer completely close. Vaginal examinations should be performed every 4 hours, and ideally this should be by the same person to minimise subjective interindividual variation. NICE guidance advises that, in the first stage of labour (from 4 cm dilated onward), the cervix should dilate at a minimum rate of 0.5 cm/hour for primigravidous women and 1 cm/hour for multiparous.

D Fetal heart rate – False. Although monitoring the fetal heart in labour is essential to confirm fetal well-being, this is not a method of monitoring the progress of labour. In a low-risk pregnancy, fetal heart rate monitoring is in the form of intermittent auscultation. The use of a CTG is restricted for high-risk pregnancies.

E Rate of contractions – False. Although it is expected that the rate of contractions will increase during labour, and this is recorded on a partogram, it is not a reliable sign of the progress of labour.

> **Key Point**
>
> Descent of the fetal head and cervical dilatation are reliable ways to monitor progress of labour.

Q2: What is the definition for established labour?
The correct answer is D. Regular, painful contractions and cervical dilatation of 4 cm or more.

It is clinically important to know when a woman has entered into established labour because it helps indicate when a woman should be admitted to the labour ward and the extent of clinical management that should be provided.

A Regular contractions and cervical dilatation of 3 cm or more – Incorrect. Although some hospitals may use cervical dilatation of more than 3 cm as the definition of established labour, it is important that contractions are painful as well as regular since this demonstrates that the uterus is contracting in a manner required for birth of the fetus.

B When the fetal head descends below the ischial spines – Incorrect. This is purely a measure of the degree of fetal engagement, not labour.

C When the mother feels the urge to push – Incorrect. This is important in the second stage of labour. Progress of the second stage of labour is monitored in terms of descent of the fetal head and rotation of the fetal head through the birth canal. It can be split into two phases, passive (before pushing) and active (active maternal pushing with contractions).

D ✔ **Regular, painful contractions and cervical dilatation of 4 cm or more** – Correct. This is the definition of established labour.

E Regular, painful contractions and cervical dilatation of 5 cm or more – Incorrect. Although the contractions are correct in this answer, when the cervix is dilated more than 5 cm, the woman is likely to have been in established labour for some time already.

> **Key Point**
>
> Women should be supported in their labour and given confidence in following their own urge to push whilst also ensuring they do not push before they are fully dilated to prevent maternal exhaustion. Breathing throughout pushing is very important, as breath holding during direct pushing has been found to be harmful. Women should adopt whatever position they find most comfortable during labour.

Q3: What can be given to 'actively manage' the third stage of labour?
The correct answer is E. Oxytocics.

When understanding which drugs are given when during pregnancy, it is very important to consider what factors are pro-pregnancy (keeping the baby in the uterus) and which are pro-labour (therefore increasing the chance of birth).
Pro-pregnancy factors:
• *Progesterone.*

Pro-labour factors:
- *Oestrogens.*
- *Oxytocin.*
- *Prostaglandins.*

[See 'Induction and Augmentation' on page 270.]

A Oestrogen – Incorrect. Oestrogen is a pro-labour hormone, and levels increase in the buildup to labour as the gestation increases. Oestrogen, however, does not directly affect contractility of the uterus required for delivery of the placenta; instead, it increases oxytocin receptor expression in the uterus. Therefore, oxytocics are more suitable drugs for administration.

B Vitamin K – Incorrect. Vitamin K is given to the baby, not the mother, soon after birth if there is parental consent. Vitamin K is given as an injection to prevent haemorrhagic disease of the newborn, but it is not used in the management of the third stage of labour.

C Progesterone – Incorrect. Progesterone is a pro-pregnancy hormone which dampens down uterine activity. This is therefore the opposite of what you want in this situation.

D Nitric oxide – Incorrect. Nitric oxide is thought to have an important role in vessel reactivity in the placenta. However, it is a pro-pregnancy hormone and therefore not suitable to aid in delivery of the placenta in the third stage of labour.

E ✔ **Oxytocics** – Correct. Oxytocin should be given for active management of the third stage of labour. It is not just the administration of this drug that is important in an actively managed third stage of labour; gentle cord traction is also important. Oxytocics increase uterine contractions, thereby aiding delivery of the placenta.

 Key Point

Syntocinon and syntometrine are the most common oxytocics used in the UK. They are administered as an intramuscular injection in the mother's thigh. Many women may opt to have a physiological third stage of labour, and this decision should be taken after weighing the pros and cons of both options. The most common risk of oxytocics to manage the third stage of labour is nausea and vomiting. but the benefit is of reducing the risk of excessive blood loss and the need for a blood transfusion.

Q4: What is the term for the fetal head descending into the maternal pelvis?

The correct answer is C. Engagement.

Engagement is when the lowermost part of the fetus descends into the mother's pelvis. In this case, that part of the fetal body is the head. Engagement typically occurs 2 to 3 weeks before labour, although multiparous women may not experience engagement until labour begins. The degree of engagement is determined by the lowermost part of the fetus being assessed in relation to the ischial spines of the mother's pelvis on vaginal examination or by fifths of the head palpable on abdominal palpation.

Q5: What action of the fetal head is caused by the contracting uterus above to ensure that the minimum head diameter is presented for birth?

The correct answer is F. Flexion.

Flexion of the head occurs to ensure that the occipital part of the fetal skull enters first into the birth canal. This is the smallest diameter of the fetal head and minimises moulding by the maternal pelvic bones.

Q6: What movement of the fetal neck enables the fetal head to be delivered completely?

The correct answer is D. Extension.

Extension of the fetal neck allows the fetal head to be completely delivered from the birth canal.

Q7: What is the name of the action describing the fetal head realigning with the shoulders?

The correct answer is L. Restitution.

Restitution is when the head rotates to realign with the shoulders after the shoulders have turned 45 degrees. This movement is crucial to allow the delivery of the anterior shoulder.

Q8: What change in the cervix is required to enable birth of the fetus vaginally?

The correct answer is B. Effacement.

During birth, the role of the cervix changes from keeping the fetus within the uterus during pregnancy to facilitating delivery of the fetus at birth. The cervix dilates in response to the contracting uterus, which causes the cervix to shorten as the os becomes wider. Effacement describes the shortening of the cervix from approximately 4 cm long when not pregnant to fully effaced during birth, where there is no length and the cervix is flush with the vagina.

Key Point

Many key steps are required during a vaginal birth, and a problem at any stage can cause a delay in the birth, resulting in midwife or obstetrician input.

Important Learning Points

- Descent of the fetal head and cervical dilatation are used to measure the progression of labour.
- Established labour is defined as regular, painful contractions causing cervical dilatation when the cervix has been dilated to at least 4 cm.
- Active management of labour with oxytocics reduces the risk of postpartum haemorrhage (PPH).
- The mechanism of labour can be briefly summarised as follows: head at pelvic brim, neck flexes, head descends and engages, internal rotation of head. The head delivers by extension, descent continues and shoulders rotate. The head restitutes, the anterior shoulder is delivered, the posterior shoulder is delivered and the body follows.

MONITORING THE FETUS

Q1: You have been asked to review the CTG. What is the most appropriate management?

The correct answer is B. Call for obstetrician review immediately and stop oxytocin.

The trace described is 'abnormal' due to the presence of late decelerations of 30 minutes duration. The woman requires an obstetric review in order to determine further management. The cause of the abnormal CTG trace is likely to be hyperstimulation from the oxytocin infusion, so stopping the infusion should improve fetal oxygenation and normalise the CTG. If this occurs, the infusion may then be restarted at a lower rate aiming to produce approximately four contractions in 10 minutes to allow labour to progress. If the CTG does not improve, an obstetrician will make a decision to offer either FBS or expedite birth.

Key Point

Intravenous synthetic oxytocin, in the absence of contraindications, may be used if delays in labour are experienced. It mimics the action of endogenous oxytocin, secreted by the posterior pituitary gland, by increasing the frequency and intensity of uterine contractions. This can precipitate uterine hyperstimulation, and if a pathological trace is detected, the oxytocin infusion should be stopped, pending obstetrician review. This will allow uterine relaxation and restoration of optimum uteroplacental blood flow.

Q2: What are late decelerations?

The correct answer is D. Episodes of decreased FHR for 15 seconds of at least 15 bpm from the baseline heart rate, which occur during the middle of the contraction's peak and end after the termination of the contraction. It is associated with poor neonatal outcome.

Persistent, repetitive late decelerations are indicative of uteroplacental insufficiency, which may be secondary to a number of causes, for example, pre-eclampsia, uterine hyperstimulation, maternal hypertension and diabetes mellitus.

Key Point

When hypoxia develops more slowly, the first signs to note include reduced baseline variability, absent accelerations and increased baseline rate. If the clinical picture deteriorates further, this may be reflected by the increased depth and width of decelerations. Always look at every feature of a CTG and categorise each as 'reassuring', 'nonreassuring' or 'abnormal'. Consider the clinical context of the case, and ask for senior help if unclear about the type and significance of the deceleration patterns.

Q3: At what time point does a bradycardia become abnormal by NICE classification?

The correct answer is D. A bradycardia is an ongoing deceleration lasting 3 minutes or more. Remember that a deceleration needs to last at least 15 seconds.

A bradycardia is a deceleration that is prolonged. Important differentials to be considered for a fetal bradycardia include placental abruption and uterine rupture (usually in the context of previous caesarean or uterine surgery), as these can be catastrophic events for the mother and baby. There are, however, many other causes of bradycardia that are less life-threatening.

Key Point

A bradycardia is a time-critical CTG finding that requires immediate recognition and appropriate management. If the fetus is compromised, the longer the bradycardia, the greater the risk for the baby.

Important Learning Points

- CTG is a form of electronic fetal monitoring which is used to identify fetal compromise and intrapartum hypoxia, with the aim of reducing fetal death and disability.
- CTG is not recommended in low-risk pregnancies but is currently an integral component in the management of high-risk pregnancies during the antenatal and intrapartum periods.
- CTGs can be interpreted systematically by the use of the mnemonic 'Dr C BRaVADO', with appreciation of the clinical context of the case. Once interpreted, the CTG can then be classified as 'normal', 'suspicious' or 'pathological'.
- A pathological trace needs to be reviewed by an obstetrician and may indicate the need for immediate birth or use of an adjunctive investigation.
- Evidence has shown CTG does not result in a statistically significant improvement in rates of cerebral palsy, infant mortality or other standard measures of neonatal well-being.

INDUCTION AND AUGMENTATION

Q1: Which of the following are indications for induction?
The correct answer is A. Pre-eclampsia.

Multiple methods are proven to induce labour, but the standard approach is to begin by doing a membrane sweep. Next, if spontaneous contractions do not occur, pessary or gel prostaglandin is administered, again with the aim of initiating spontaneous contractions and/or cervical dilation sufficient to attempt an amniotomy (artificial rupture of membranes (ARM)). Once an amniotomy has been carried out, intravenous oxytocin infusion generates regular uterine contractions.

A ✔ **Pre-eclampsia** – Correct. Pre-eclampsia is both a maternal and fetal problem which would indicate induction. There is a risk of developing eclampsia, which could be life-threatening to the baby and the mother, as well as complicate the onset of labour. It is also associated with IUGR and potentially intrauterine death. Birth would be indicated if the condition of the mother or fetus deteriorates, with risks of continuing the pregnancy outweighing the risk of ending the pregnancy for mother or fetus.

[See 'Pre-Eclampsia and Pregnancy-Induced Hypertension' on page 301.]

B Breech presentation – Incorrect. Breech presentation is not an indication for induction. Instead, external cephalic version (ECV), spontaneous breech vaginal birth or elective caesarean should be discussed with the patient. Induction and augmentation should be performed with extreme caution and involvement of senior clinicians in the case of breech presentation.

C History of precipitate labour – Incorrect. Induction of labour should not be routinely offered to women with a history of precipitate labour (labours that happen very quickly) to avoid birth unattended by healthcare professionals.

D Maternal request – Incorrect. Only in exceptional circumstances – for example, the partner is due to go overseas in the armed forces soon – would this be considered and usually only after 40 weeks of pregnancy.

E History of previous caesarean – Incorrect. This is not an indication for induction on its own; however, it is not a contraindication either. For women who have had a previous caesarean, giving birth vaginally carries a higher risk of uterine rupture because the scar tissue from the caesarean may be more prone to dehisce. This risk is raised when they are induced. Although this means the approach toward induction is more cautious, vaginal births after caesarean, with and without induction, are still encouraged in the absence of other contraindications.

[See 'Vaginal Birth after Caesarean' on page 289.]

 Key Point

Induction of labour is usually performed via vaginal prostaglandin administration, which aims to ripen the cervix, and then followed by an amniotomy. During amniotomy, an amniohook is used to break open the membranes surrounding the fetus.

Q2: Answer true or false: Which of the following statements include accurate information that should be given to the woman before she is induced?

The decision of whether to induce is often influenced by the gestation of the fetus. Below 34 weeks gestation, the risks associated with prematurity are often great enough that it is beneficial to attempt to prolong the pregnancy to allow fetal maturity in utero. However, if the risks to the fetus or the mother are thought to be greater if the pregnancy continues, delivery would then be the preferable option.

A ✔ **Most women will go into labour spontaneously by 42 weeks** – True. A spontaneous labour is one which starts naturally without any artificial intervention. For most women, if left long enough, spontaneous labour will occur. However, pregnancies continuing past 42 weeks are associated with an increased risk of stillbirth and fetal compromise. Therefore, induction is usually offered to all women whose pregnancies look set to continue beyond this time.

B ✔ **Risks associated with pregnancies prolonged beyond 42 weeks include placental insufficiency, increased forceps use and meconium aspiration** – True. Placental insufficiency refers to an inadequate supply of oxygen and nutrients for the growing fetus, which increases the risk of a stillbirth. Prolonged intrauterine growth is associated with cephalopelvic disproportion and complications during labour and increased risks during assisted vaginal or caesarean birth. Meconium is more likely to be produced the longer the fetus remains in utero, as the neurological system of the bowel matures enough to begin peristalsis. This means the fetus is more likely to produce meconium and subsequently aspirate it. This can lead to neonatal respiratory problems.

C A membrane sweep involves surgically removing fetal tissue in the event of a stillbirth – False. A membrane sweep involves inserting a finger into the cervix and stretching it a bit. This releases prostaglandins, which can cause labour without the need for induction. You may hear this referred to as a 'stretch and sweep' on the wards.

D Induction increases the risk of this woman needing a caesarean – False. Evidence suggests that for women being induced for postdates, the rate of caesarean is not increased compared to expectant management. However, at earlier gestations, induction does increase the risk of caesarean. Induction of labour has other additional risks compared to natural onset of labour; these should be balanced against the risks of prolonging the pregnancy. Others include uterine rupture, umbilical cord prolapse, shoulder dystocia, uterine hyperstimulation, infection, fetal bradycardia, uterine atony and PPH.

E If the woman has had a preterm rupture of membranes before 34 weeks, induction of labour should be carried out immediately – False. Unless there are additional obstetric complications (for example, infection or fetal compromise), induction of labour should be delayed until after 34 weeks. Before 34 weeks, the risk of prematurity outweighs the risk of maintaining the pregnancy. In this case, this would be the development of an intrauterine infection, which could cause maternal sepsis and fetal death. Continuing the pregnancy allows for further intrauterine growth of the baby, thereby reducing the risks associated with premature birth, which include low birth weight, increased infant mortality, respiratory problems and poorer health throughout childhood. After 34 weeks, the risk of problems associated with prematurity are reduced, and considering labour induction is appropriate. However, if no signs of infection develop, there may also be a benefit in prolonging the pregnancy until approximately 37 weeks. Nonetheless, note that the longer a pregnancy continues with ruptured membranes, the greater the risk of development of an intrauterine infection.

[See 'Congenital Intrauterine Infections' on page 336.]

> **Key Point**
>
> Postterm pregnancies are associated with higher risks, such as placental insufficiency, increased forceps use and meconium aspiration. Therefore, induction of labour should be considered.

Q3: A 29-year-old, 30 weeks pregnant woman (gravidity three, parity zero), presents with reduced fetal movements and a history of recurrent miscarriages. An ultrasound scan confirms fetal death.

The correct answer is H. Misoprostol.

Misoprostol is a synthetic prostaglandin analogue, which should only be used as an induction method in the event of intrauterine fetal death. This is because it is associated with a risk of uterine hyperstimulation, which may be harmful to a live fetus. Earlier in pregnancy, it may also be used in terminations. Mifepristone is a progesterone receptor antagonist, which is often used along with misoprostol, as progesterone is one of the hormones which maintains the pregnancy and aids in uterine relaxation.

Q4: A 32-year-old mother of three, 38 weeks pregnant, has had a healthy pregnancy until now. She has requested to be induced as she feels very tired, uncomfortably big and is fed up with being pregnant.

The correct answer is F. Expectant management.

Induction of labour is inappropriate in this case. The woman should be reassured that these symptoms are common and normal in pregnancy and that a spontaneous labour is safest for her and her child. If a mother does experience severe psychological distress associated with being pregnant, additional support can be given, and on rare occasions where there is severe distress, a clinician might consider induction of labour.

Q5: An 18-year-old primigravida with diabetes had a prostaglandin pessary for 24 hours and is reassessed. Her Bishop score is now 10. What is the anticipated next step?

The correct answer is E. Amniotomy.

Amniotomy, or ARM, involves breaking the membranes that contain amniotic fluid either surgically with a sterile hook or digitally. Frequently, prostaglandin administration will merely dilate the cervix enough to allow amniotomy (based on the Bishop score), rather than establishing labour directly. If the onset of labour has still not started after ARM, an oxytocin drip would be used to stimulate contractions.

Q6: A 22-year-old primigravida, 41 weeks and 4 days pregnant, has a confirmed breech presentation. ECV has been attempted twice but has failed on both attempts, and she is apprehensive about having a caesarean. The midwife has already attempted digital stimulation of the cervix.

The correct answer is A. Caesarean birth.

Expectant management is not advised, as continuing the pregnancy increases the risk of intrauterine death due to postmaturity. Induction is contraindicated because of breech presentation, and the fetus is extremely unlikely to turn spontaneously. A caesarean is therefore the safest option for the fetus. The woman should be fully counselled about the risks and benefits of each option, clearly explaining why alternative options are not advised. Most women will follow medical advice; however, some women, after reflecting on the information given, will opt for an alternative management. As long as she has been correctly counselled and the woman has capacity, her choice must be respected.

Q7: A 37-year-old woman, gravidity four, parity three, is 40 weeks pregnant. Her water broke 24 hours ago, but she has still not felt any contractions.

The correct answer is B. Oxytocin.

The management decision before 24 hours is slightly controversial, as some centres would advocate a membrane sweep, while others believe examining the patient increases the risk of ascending infection. However, by 24 hours, oxytocin would be appropriate to induce this woman, rather than augment, as she is not in labour.

> **Key Point**
>
> It is important to consider the psychological impacts of inducing a labour. Many women may feel that they have 'failed' by not going into labour themselves or may be adverse to any drugs being administered during labour and birth. They may also be scared that oxytocin could bring on their contractions too quickly. It is therefore important to communicate the importance of inducing the labour for mother and baby and stress that oxytocin will be used with utmost caution, titrating the amount of drug given to ensure optimal contractions.

> **Important Learning Points**
>
> - Induction of labour artificially initiates contractions, cervical ripeness and dilatation, rather than waiting for them to start naturally. Augmentation of labour hastens childbirth by increasing the strength and frequency of contractions.
> - Induction is usually carried out after 39 weeks but can be performed earlier if the mother or the fetus is deemed at risk.
> - The most common method is to administer prostaglandins in the form of a gel or pessary, which ripens and dilates the cervix and initiates contractions.
> - Membranes surrounding the fetus can then be artificially ruptured.
> - Oxytocin can be used for induction or to augment the contractions once labour has begun.

PAIN RELIEF IN LABOUR

Q1: Answer true or false to the following statements regarding epidural analgesia.

Epidural analgesia provides safe pain relief and tends to be more effective than other methods. Levobupivacaine is the most common local anaesthetic used, normally in combination with a low-dose opioid such as fentanyl. Usually, the catheter is inserted between L1 and L5. The level of nerve block required needs to be higher than this, and this is achieved as more volume of local anaesthetic is given, causing it to move upwards in the tight epidural space. For labour analgesia, a block height of T8 to T10 is aimed for, which reduces sensation from the uterine contractions and cervical stretching. Later in labour, pressure from the fetal head descending is transmitted by the pudendal nerves (S2 to S4). Some epidurals will provide analgesia to this area as well.

A ✔ **Dizziness or shivering may occur** – True. Other side effects of epidurals include hypotension, discomfort at the injection site, loss of bladder control and pruritus.

B ✔ **It can increase the length of the second stage of labour** – True. It can increase length by around 15 to 30 minutes and is associated with increased incidence of assisted birth and oxytocin infusions. This is because epidurals may block the pelvic autonomic nerves, preventing the normal rise in oxytocin during the second stage.

C Epidurals are not associated with any adverse effects on the fetus – False. Epidurals can cause maternal hypotension. Women with epidurals must have regular BP monitoring and continuous electronic fetal monitoring. Epidurals are also associated with increased rate of assisted birth. However, overall, epidurals are considered safe.

D ✔ **It is the most effective form of pain relief in labour** – True. It is a very effective method of relieving pain in labour, with a better evidence base than Entonox, intramuscular opioids and TENS.

E ✔ **It is associated with transient hypotension in 20% of women** – True. This is due to the blocking of sympathetic nerve fibres in the epidural space, which causes dilation of the blood vessels (hence reduced pressure). Some women may require intravenous fluids to help counteract this effect. Hypotension can also cause fetal distress due to reduced blood supply to the placenta, which may necessitate urgent birth if not corrected promptly.

> 🗨 **Key Point**
>
> Maternal side effects from epidurals include dizziness, shivering, hypotension, pain, loss of bladder control, and pruritus. Important complications include severe headache, nerve injury and infection.

Q2: Answer true or false to the following statements regarding epidural anatomy and analgesia.

It is important to understand the anatomy of the epidural and spinal space in order to understand the complications that can occur. Although rare, some risks are serious, and women must receive informed consent before having an epidural.

A The epidural space contains spinal nerve roots, the extradural venous plexus, lymphatics and fat – False. The epidural space does not contain spinal nerve roots; local anaesthetic must cross the dura mater to exert its effect on nerves.

B ✔ **In order to reduce the pain of uterine contractions, an epidural aims to block T10-L1 spinal levels** – True. T8 to 10 is particularly important for blocking nerve conduction regarding pain generated from the uterus and cervix during labour. Most epidurals will also provide some pain relief to the S2 to S4 pudendal nerves (see Q1).

C When inserting a needle, care must be taken to avoid the epidural vessels, as the local anaesthetic can cause maternal seizures – True. The epidural venous plexus lies on the ventral floor of the vertebral column and can be penetrated by the needle. On threading the catheter, blood will be visible, and it should be resited. Injection of levobupivacaine or ropivicaine into blood vessels can cause seizures as well as life-threatening arrhythmias.

D The epidural space contains cerebrospinal fluid – False. The epidural space is a potential space (like the pleural space and peritoneal space) containing no fluid. This potential space creates a 'loss of resistance' when the epidural needle is inserted, which is utilised to find the epidural space. Cerebrospinal fluid is contained within the spinal space, deep into the epidural space and separated by the dura mater.

E The valves in the epidural venous plexus prevent backflow of blood – False. There are no valves in the epidural venous plexus. This means that blood from any of the connected systems can flow into the epidural vessels. This feature is important during pregnancy, where the gravid uterus causes compression of major vessels, resulting in engorged epidural veins, which increases the risk of an epidural needle or catheter entering the vein.

> 🗨 **Key Point**
>
> The epidural space is a potential space which contains blood vessels, lymphatics and fat. Local anaesthetic crosses the dura mater into the spinal space to exert its effect, unlike spinal injections where the injection is direct into the cerebrospinal fluid in the spinal space.

Q3: Which form of analgesia is first line after birth, in the absence of contractions?

The correct answer is A. Paracetamol and ibuprofen.

Postnatally, a woman may still experience considerable pain. This may occur for several reasons. There may also be back pain or pains from postnatal uterine contractions as the uterus involutes back to prepregnancy size over a number of weeks. Treating pain is extremely important in enabling the mother to care for her newborn, rest and recover. For perineal pain, topical cooling therapy can help, for example, crushed ice or gel pads. If oral analgesia is needed, paracetamol is first line. Escalation of pain relief should then follow the WHO analgesic ladder.

A ✔ **Paracetamol and ibuprofen** – Correct. Regular paracetamol should be offered after all births unless contraindicated. Ibuprofen should also be offered but may be withheld if there was a significant PPH or diagnosis of pre-eclampsia.

B Morphine – Incorrect. Oral morphine syrup is an opioid and therefore is not first line in acute pain management. It may be required postnatally, especially after assisted vaginal and caesarean births, and can be given safely to breastfeeding women in hospital.

C Entonox – Incorrect. Gas and air used during the first and second stages of labour to relieve painful contractions. It provides rapid pain and anxiety reduction but is very short acting so not suitable after birth other than during procedures such as repair of minor perineal injuries.

D Codeine – Incorrect. Codeine is metabolised in the liver by cytochrome CYP2D6 into the active form (dihydrocodeine). The rate of this metabolism varies between people, with some people metabolising to the active form very quickly. These ultrafast metabolisers will have more of the active drug available to use in their body, which can result in life-threatening opioid toxicity. Codeine is therefore contraindicated in breastfeeding and children under the age of 12.

E Nothing should be given until the mother has started skin-to-skin contact – Incorrect. Skin-to-skin contact care is a technique used between neonates and another person, usually the mother, to encourage physiological and psychological warmth and bonding. The baby is held skin to skin against an adult to help regulate the baby's temperature and allow for accessible breastfeeding. Skin-to-skin contact is encouraged as soon as possible after birth but does not interfere with giving analgesia.

> **Key Point**
>
> Most women will require analgesia after birth, with more required where they have undergone a surgical procedure. Adequate pain relief is essential to allow the woman higher-quality time with their newborn.

> **Important Learning Points**
>
> • Labour pain can be treated in various ways. Entonox, paracetamol, opioids and epidurals are the main pharmacological options.
> • Epidural analgesia is the most effective method of analgesia, although important complications include severe headaches, infection and nerve injury.
> • Postnatal pain relief should be prescribed according to the WHO pain ladder. Opioids should be used with caution, as they can pass into breastmilk, whilst codeine should not be given.

• The psychological aspects of pain should be sufficiently acknowledged, and nonbiomedical therapies, such as a supportive atmosphere, water immersion and complementary therapies should be considered.

MALPRESENTATION AND MALPOSITION OF THE FETUS

Q1: Answer true or false: Which of the following are associated with malpresentation or malposition?

The correct answers are **A.** Maternal exhaustion, **B.** Cord prolapse, **C.** Thyroid mass and **E.** Shoulder dystocia.

A ✔ **Maternal exhaustion** – True. This is associated with prolonged labour, which often occurs in complicated births such as those involving malpresentations and malpositions. Prevention of exhaustion can be helped by allowing the mother to eat small amounts, drink plenty and try and stay calm and restful between contractions. This can be further supported by offering adequate analgesia. Breathing techniques can also help conserve energy and allow pushing to be more efficient.

B ✔ **Cord prolapse** – True. This can particularly be a concern in footling breech presentations and transverse lies. The cord can slip down ahead of the presenting part of the fetus, becoming prolapsed. It can subsequently become compressed as the fetus is pushed upon it when the uterus contracts, restricting oxygen supply to the fetus and potentially causing neurological damage if birth is not expedited quickly, usually by caesarean.

C ✔ **Neonatal thyroid mass** – True. Face presentations are often associated with neck masses or hydrocephalus in the fetus. These cases present with a hyperextended fetal head and neck.

D High-lying placenta – False. In most pregnancies, the placenta will lie high in the uterus, away from the cervix, and should not affect the presentation or positioning of the fetus. However, if the placenta lies low or near the cervix (placenta praevia), this can increase risk of malpresentation.

E ✔ **Shoulder dystocia** – True. Shoulder dystocia refers to the need for additional obstetric manoeuvres to deliver the fetus after the head has delivered. It occurs when the fetal shoulder impacts the maternal symphysis pubis and is associated with neonatal brachial plexus injury, which can be a lifelong condition. Prolonged second stages and assisted vaginal birth, both of which can occur in cases of malposition, are associated with increased incidence of shoulder dystocia.

[See 'Spontaneous Vaginal Birth' on page 258.]

Key Point

It is important to remember that many labours with malposition or malpresentation occur where no risk factors are apparent. This is a common factor in many complications during labour and highlights the importance of careful observation.

Q2: A 23-year-old primigravida of 42 weeks presents with increasing contractions. The midwife who performs a vaginal examination reports a grainy feel, and a transvaginal scan is performed.
The correct answer is E. Placenta praevia.

In known cases of placenta praevia, vaginal examination should be avoided due to the risk of haemorrhage. Placenta praevia is a complication where the placenta is attached to the lower segment of the uterus; in most severe cases, it completely obstructs the internal os of the cervix. As the placenta is very vascular, damage can cause massive haemorrhage, often indicating the need for a caesarean, complete with blood products immediately available. It is usually picked up during antenatal screening via ultrasound scanning. If the placenta is felt vaginally, it can have a 'grainy' feel.

[See 'Antepartum Haemorrhage' on page 297.]

Q3: A 39-year-old woman, 40 weeks pregnant, gravidity three, parity two, presents with regular contractions. Examination reveals the fetal head engaged in a left occipitoanterior (OA) position.
The correct answer is H. Physiological presentation.

This is a description of a normal progression of labour. Most fetal heads, when engaged, will lie to the left, but it is also normal for some to lie to the right. At birth, most will rotate to the direct OA position.

Q4: A 20-year-old woman, gravidity one, parity zero, is rushed to hospital following complications during an attempted home birth. Ultrasound examination shows the fetal head is against the left side of the pelvis and the buttocks on the right.
The correct answer is A. Transverse lie.

This malpresentation is usually impossible to deliver vaginally (unless the membranes are intact and ECV can be attempted). It typically has a shoulder presentation. It is not always known why a physiological longitudinal lie is not reached, but it can be associated with an abnormally shaped pelvis, lax uterine musculature and pelvic or uterine masses.

Q5: A 27-year-old nulliparous woman has been experiencing contractions for several hours. The midwife examines her vaginally and thinks she finds a heel.
The correct answer is G. Footling presentation.

This presentation is classed as breech. Footling presentations are more common in preterm babies. One or both hips are extended, with a foot presenting first. Footling breech presentations should be delivered by caesarean.

[See 'Breech' on page 280.]

Q6: A 16-year-old girl, gravidity two, parity one, 36 weeks pregnant, comes for an antenatal checkup. The ultrasound scan shows the buttocks lying anteriorly close to the vagina, toward the left. The fetal heart sounds are also heard just above the umbilicus.

The correct answer is C. Left sacrum anterior.

This is also known as a breech presentation, which remains in about 3% to 4% of term babies. ECV should be attempted after 37 weeks, by which time around 50% of these attempts will be successful.

 Key Point

It is useful to remember the approximate diameter of the fetal head in different presentations to understand why malpresentation can cause a more problematic labour. When the occiput is delivered first, this is usually about 9.5 cm; however, a deflexed presentation is about 11.5 cm in comparison, while a brow presentation can be 13 cm.

Q7 True or false: Which of the following complications are increased with occipitoposterior (OP) deliveries?

All of the options are true. OP labours are more likely to be more painful, with delay in the first and second stages of labour. This may lead to increased use of oxytocics and a higher chance of assisted vaginal birth or caesarean. This is due to the increased diameter of the fetal skull in the OP position (11.5 cm versus 9.5 cm in an OA position). Due to this increased diameter, there is a higher risk of obstetric anal sphincter injury. Malposition is associated with shoulder dystocia for the reason that the fetus has not traversed the maternal pelvis in the optimum direction, which may also affect delivery of the shoulders.

 Key Point

Evidence of malposition on vaginal examination can include an asymmetrically dilated cervix. On the labour ward, you may hear healthcare professionals refer to examination findings as anterior lip, and this is where, posteriorly, the cervix is fully dilated, but anteriorly, maternal tissue remains overlying the presenting part of the fetus. This is more likely to happen in malposition because the occiput is not being evenly applied to the cervix as in a flexed OA position.

 Important Learning Points

- Presentation refers to which anatomical part of the fetus is leading during birth. Malpresentation occurs when another aspect of the fetal body, other than the top of the head (vertex), is the presenting part.
- Position of the baby refers to where the fetal head lies in relation to the mother's pelvis. Malposition refers to any abnormal position of the fetal head as it engages in the pelvis. Ideally, the fetal head should be positioned in the maternal pelvis with the face facing the maternal spine (OA).
- Malpresentation will usually be picked up on ultrasound and/or manual palpation of the abdomen or on vaginal examination before or around the time of birth.

- Either malpresentation or malposition can prolong and complicate labour, increasing both maternal and fetal risks.
- Alternative presentations, of which breech presentation is the most common, may have a number of potential causes and can potentially endanger maternal and fetal life during labour.

BREECH

Q1: The ultrasound scan indicates frank breech presentation.
The correct answer is A. ECV.

ECV is a technique where obstetricians place their hands on a patient's abdomen and push the fetus around from breech to cephalic presentation. If successful, the fetus remains cephalic, and the patient can then aim for a vaginal birth. If the patient declined ECV or the ECV failed, then a planned caesarean would be another management option. If the patient declined caesarean, the only other way to deliver is a vaginal breech birth. However, the woman should be informed that vaginal breech birth is associated with increased perinatal morbidity and mortality.

Q2: The ultrasound indicates a cephalic presentation.
The correct answer is F. Spontaneous vaginal birth.

This fetus is presenting head first to the cervix. This is unlikely to change past 37 weeks gestation, so no intervention is required, and this woman can prepare to deliver vaginally.

Q3: The ultrasound scan indicates frank breech presentation; the patient declines any antenatal intervention.
The correct answer is H. Either breech vaginal birth or elective caesarean may be appropriate.

As stated earlier, ECV (which, if successful, allows for a cephalic vaginal birth), planned caesarean and vaginal breech birth are the three management options for breech presentation. This woman has declined ECV. This woman would need to be counselled on the risks and benefits of the other two options. With the fetus presenting as a frank breech (hips flexed, knees extended), a breech vaginal birth is not contraindicated, but there is a higher risk of perinatal morbidity and mortality than for elective caesarean.

Q4: The ultrasound scan indicates footling breech presentation; the woman declines any antenatal intervention.
The correct answer is C. Planned lower segment caesarean.

As in the previous question, the woman has declined ECV. However, this case presentation is a footling breech. Attempting labour (and a vaginal birth) would be hazardous for the fetus because there is a significantly increased risk of cord prolapse, which can cause fetal compromise and death very

quickly. There is also an increased risk of difficulty in delivering the fetal head because the limbs and body can potentially deliver without dilating the cervix fully, trapping the head. Planned caesarean would be the safest method of birth.

Q5: An attempt is made following the ultrasound scan to rotate the fetal lie. After this is performed successfully, the fetus shows prolonged signs of distress.
The correct answer is D. Unplanned lower segment caesarean.

This woman has just undergone a successful ECV. It is common during the procedure for the fetus to have a brief bradycardia, believed to be caused by compression of the cord during rotation. However, occasionally the cord can become persistently compressed, or other complications can occur, such as placental abruption, which can compromise the fetus, causing either a prolonged bradycardia on ultrasound scan or a prolonged abnormal CTG. In the case where a fetus is showing signs of distress that are not resolving, an emergency birth is needed to prevent any long-term morbidity or stillbirth. This is done by caesarean, as no other method is possible since the woman is not in labour.

> ### 💬 Key Point
>
> A breech fetus may be delivered by breech vaginal birth or by caesarean. If appropriate, ECV should be offered to turn the fetus to a cephalic presentation, improving the chances of achieving a safer vaginal birth.

Q6: What does this illustration show?
The correct answer is A. Frank breech.

Breech presentation is common, with 3% of term babies being breech. Both maternal factors and fetal factors, including the type of breech presentation, will influence management of birth.

A ✔ Frank breech – Correct. This is characterised by a bottom-first presentation to the pelvic outlet with hips flexed and knees extended. If a woman so wishes and labour progresses well, this breech presentation is potentially deliverable vaginally. This position is also known as extended breech.
B Complete breech – Incorrect. This is characterised by a bottom-first presentation to the pelvic outlet with hips flexed and knees flexed. Like a frank breech, this presentation is potentially deliverable vaginally.
C Footling breech – Incorrect. This is characterised by one or both feet presenting (hips in neutral position, one or both knees extended). If labour occurs with this presentation, there is a high risk of complications for the fetus, including cord prolapse and difficulty delivering the head, both of which can result in fetal hypoxaemia. Footling breech presentations are much safer delivered by caesarean section.

D Kneeling breech – Incorrect. This is characterised by at least one hip extending with the knee on that leg flexed so that the part of the fetus presenting to the pelvic outlet is the knee (of one or both legs). This carries similar risks to footling breech.

E Cephalic breech – Incorrect. This is not a real term. Cephalic presentation is characterised by the head presenting to the pelvic inlet, usually with the vertex (top of the head) presenting. This is the safest presentation to achieve a successful vaginal birth.

 Key Point

It is important to recognise the different breech presentations, as these can affect decisions regarding the safest mode of birth.

Q7: Which of the following are risk factors for breech presentation?

The correct answers are A. Fetal chromosomal anomaly, **C.** Uterine fibroids and **E.** Preterm labour.

In the majority of cases, breech presentation at term is idiopathic. When possible, identifying a cause is useful for managing the current pregnancy and to give sensible advice to the patient on the likelihood of recurrence in a future pregnancy.

A ✔ **Fetal chromosomal anomaly** – Correct. Fetal anomalies can restrict movement structurally if the fetus has a large mass preventing movement. Movement can also be restricted if the fetus has a neuromuscular condition resulting in fewer or no fetal movements. Without movement, the fetus is less likely to naturally move around into the correct presentation.

B Maternal BMI – Incorrect. Raised BMI increases the risk of many obstetric complications but does not appear to have an effect on the incidence of breech presentation.

C ✔ **Uterine fibroids** – Correct. Physical structural abnormalities such as fibroids, a septate uterus or bicornuate uterus can prevent the movement of a fetus into the correct presentation. If the placenta is low (placenta praevia), this prevents the head from engaging in the pelvis, making it more likely to have a breech or other noncephalic presentation.

D Male fetus – Incorrect. There is no gender bias with regard to breech presentation.

E ✔ **Preterm labour** – Correct. At 28 weeks gestation, 20% of fetuses are breech compared to 3% at term. This is because the fetus is relatively small compared to the amount of fluid and potential space it has to move around in compared to later gestations. Closer to term, a bigger fetus now has less space to rotate, meaning the presenting part tends to be pushed down into the pelvis and fixed. Therefore, a preterm labour is more likely to have a breech presentation.

 Key Point

The majority of breech presentations occur with no cause identified; however, a number of factors increase the risk of breech presentations, including:
- Factors allowing excess movement.
  - Preterm birth.
  - Polyhydramnios.
- Factors restricting fetal movement.
  - Maternal variant – pelvic bone, uterus.
  - Fetal variant – hydrocephalus, neuromuscular abnormality preventing the fetus from being able to move into the correct cephalic presentation.

Q8: Answer true or false to the following statements regarding breech presentation.

Breech presentation is the most common form of malpresentation. Unless there are contraindications, such as the presentation of macrosomia, a spontaneous vaginal birth can be attempted. Prognosis following breech presentations is similar, regardless of method of birth.

A Breech presentation is the least common form of malpresentation preceding labour – False. Breech presentation is the most common form of malpresentation preceding labour, with 3% to 4% of fetuses in this position at term. Before 34 weeks, fetuses are relatively small and are able to constantly change their lie. Therefore, they are often in breech lies during earlier stages of pregnancy. After 34 weeks, as the fetus grows, the shape of the uterus encourages the fetus to fix in one lie, usually head down.

B For term babies with a breech presentation, there are no long-term health problems associated with either caesarean or vaginal methods of birth – False. Breech presentation is associated with a higher perinatal mortality and morbidity compared to cephalic presentation. This is principally because preterm births and fetuses with congenital malformations are more likely to deliver breech. There is also an increased risk of birth trauma or asphyxia compared with cephalic presentations.

C ✔ **ECV should not be attempted before 36 weeks** – True. It is more likely before this time that the fetus will turn back around to breech position; therefore, it should not be attempted. After 36 weeks, if ECV is successful, the fetus is likely to remain cephalic.

D ✔ **A footling or kneeling breech presentation should not be delivered vaginally** – True. If possible, a footling or kneeling presentation should be delivered by caesarean because these presentations can begin to deliver before the cervix is fully dilated. This means that whilst the legs and body can deliver, the head can be stuck in a partially dilated cervix – with the umbilical cord compressed between the fetal abdomen and the maternal pelvis. This severely deprives the fetus of oxygen and requires a very swift birth to avoid neurological damage, which can additionally pose a significant risk of fetal and maternal trauma.

E ✔ **The presence of any other additional problems, such as placenta praevia, is an indication for a caesarean** – True. A breech presentation is considered unfavourable for vaginal birth in cases including the following:

- Other contraindications to vaginal birth, for example, placenta praevia or compromised fetal condition.
- Footling or kneeling breech presentation.
- Babies weighing more than 3800 g or clinically assessed that the baby is too large relative to the maternal pelvis.
- Growth-restricted baby, usually defined as smaller than 2000 g.
- Hyperextended fetal neck in labour, diagnosed with ultrasound.
- Lack of presence of a clinician trained in vaginal breech birth.
- Previous caesarean.

> **Key Point**
>
> Breech presentation is common at term. Women should be counselled on the risks of the different modes of birth so that appropriate management decisions can be made.

> **Important Learning Points**
>
> - 3% of term babies and 20% of preterm babies present breech.
> - Maternal and fetal factors can increase the chance of breech presentation; however, most breech presentations are idiopathic.
> - The three management options to be aware of for breech presentation are ECV, planned caesarean and vaginal breech birth.
> - Vaginal breech birth is associated with higher short-term perinatal mortality and morbidity compared to cephalic vaginal birth or planned caesarean.

13 MODES OF BIRTH

CAESAREAN BIRTH

Q1: Which of the following are true regarding the use of a transverse lower segment uterine incision in comparison to a midline, vertical uterine incision?

Caesareans are usually performed using a transverse skin incision and a transverse incision to enter the lower segment of the uterus. A Joel Cohen entry technique is usually used (a straight skin incision, 2 to 3 cm above the symphysis pubis; subsequent tissue layers are opened bluntly and, if necessary, extended with scissors and not a knife). This

is because it is associated with shorter operating times and reduced postoperative infection.

A ✔ **It is associated with less postoperative pain** – True. The transverse uterine incision is associated with less postoperative pain than a midline, vertical uterine incision. This has been demonstrated through reduced postoperative analgesic requirements, as well as individual pain scores.

B It is associated with improved cosmetic effect – False. The cosmetic appearance after a caesarean birth is not affected by the direction of the uterine incision but by the skin incision. It is important to remember that the direction of the incision of the skin does not always correspond to the direction of the incision on the uterus. Lower transverse skin incisions are thought to have a better cosmetic appearance in comparison to a vertical skin incision, which would be easily visible along the abdomen. A transverse skin incision can usually be hidden by most items of clothing and is often hidden by pubic hair.

C ✔ **It is associated with less blood loss** – True. Vertical uterine incisions are associated with more blood loss. However, advantages of vertical uterine incisions include faster entry, reduced risk of nerve injury and the ability to extend the incision farther if required. Vertical incisions are of particular use in preterm births where the lower segment of the uterus has not formed. In this situation, transverse incisions risk extension into large blood vessels, therefore causing severe haemorrhage.

D There is a reduced risk of postoperative infection – False. The risk of postoperative infection is not affected by the direction of the uterine incision. However, postoperative infection is a very important consideration for all women who have had a caesarean.

E ✔ **There is a reduced risk of uterine rupture in future pregnancies** – True. Transverse uterine incisions are associated with a lower risk of uterine rupture in future pregnancies than midline uterine incisions.

> **Key Point**
>
> One of the main determinants of whether a transverse or vertical incision is whether the lower uterine segment has formed. During the second half of pregnancy, the lower uterine segment (located between the internal cervix os and the body of the uterus) becomes more distinct. This part of the uterus stretches and develops as pregnancy advances and thins during the course of labour.

During a caesarean the lower uterine segment can be approximately identified as the portion of uterus beneath the uterovesical fold. If a transverse lower segment incision is proving insufficient to birth a baby, this can be extended into either a 'J' shape or a 'T' shape.

Q2: Answer true or false: Which of the following anatomical structures is dissected during a caesarean?

A   Cervix – False. During a caesarean, an incision is made to the lower segment of the uterus, which is located just above the cervix. Incorrect placement of the incision to the uterus may injure the cervix, causing potential complications in future pregnancies such as increased risk of preterm birth. This is more likely when the cervix has been stretched and is close to full dilatation.

B   ✔ **Uterovesical fold** – True. The uterovesical fold is the fold of visceral peritoneum overlying the bladder and uterus. Dissecting this allows the surgeon to move the bladder down away from the site of the uterine incision, minimising the risk of bladder injury. It also allows access to the lower uterine segment, the thinnest part of the uterus. There is no evidence to support closure of visceral or parietal peritoneum layers during caesarean.

C   ✔ **Rectus sheath** – True. The rectus sheath is the aponeurosis of fibres from the external obliques, internal obliques and transversus abdomimus muscles. The rectus sheath is disected during caesarean birth. It is repaired during closure to restore core muscle strength and minimise the risk of a postoperative hernia.

D   Omentum – False. The omentum is a fatty apron overlying intraperitoneal organs. During pregnancy, the gravid uterus pushes this structure cephlad within the abdomen. It is unlikely to impede during a routine caesarean.

E   Rectus abdominus – False. Pressure from the expanding uterus often causes the rectus abdominal muscles to separate at the linea alba. This allows birth of the baby during caesarean. This separation may need to expand during a caesarean, but this is dissection in the traditional sense. There is no evidence to support recuts abdominus repair during closure, and this would likely significantly increase postoperative pain.

> 💬 **Key Point**
>
> Often when in the operating theatre, students are asked the anatomical layers that a surgeon dissects to get to the uterus.
> These are:
> 1. Skin.
> 2. Subcutaneous tissue.
> 3. Superficial fascia – fatty (Camper) and membranous (Scarpa).
> 4. Anterior rectus sheath.
> 5. Rectus abdominis muscle.
> 6. Transversalis fascia (rarely seen separate from muscle).
> 7. Parietal peritoneum.
> 8. Visceral peritoneum (uterovesical fold).

Q3: Which of the following has an increased risk of occurring following caesarean compared to vaginal birth?
The correct answer is D. Urinary tract injury.

The risks following caesarean and vaginal birth are different. Overall, caesarean is known to have higher rates of maternal morbidity and mortality compared to vaginal birth. Recovery after surgery can be prolonged. It is important that if caesarean is planned, women are aware of these risks and difficulties, especially if the decision for caesarean is due to maternal choice with no other medical factors making an impact.

A   Difficulties breastfeeding – Incorrect. This is a common misconception – that breastfeeding can be harder for women who have had a caesarean birth – but it is incorrect. In both modes of birth, skin-to-skin contact should occur as soon as possible, and women should be supported regarding breastfeeding.

B   Depression – Incorrect. Postnatal depression has not been linked more strongly to caesarean or vaginal birth. However, there are many other factors that may impact the mental state of a woman who has just given birth. Emergency births, either vaginally or by caesarean, may increase the risk of a mental health condition such as depression. Bonding between mother and baby does not have to be impaired due to caesarean, as skin-to-skin contact can still usually occur soon after the baby is delivered as long as the caesarean has not been performed under general anaesthesia.

C   Dyspareunia – Incorrect. Dyspareunia is increased with vaginal birth because of the damage that can happen to the birth canal during the traversal of the fetus through the birth canal. Women who have had a caesarean may have a relatively unchanged genital tract. For example, their cervical os will still be a small hole instead of an enlarged slit. However, if the caesarean was carried out during labour, the cervix may have already dilated and therefore will be permanently changed.

D   ✔ **Urinary tract injury** – Correct. Due to the invasive nature of a caesarean, the risk of bladder and ureteric injury is increased in comparison to vaginal birth. Other increased risks include postoperative adhesions, haemorrhage and infection.

E   Faecal incontinence – Incorrect. The risk of faecal incontinence is increased in women who have had a vaginal birth, particularly if the birth was assisted, a water birth or complicated by shoulder dystocia because of physical trauma to the perineum. If perineal trauma extends into the anal sphincters, it can cause long-term incontinence of faecal matter and flatus.

Key Point

It is important to consider a woman's social situation and the effect this will have on recovery from a caesarean when making a decision regarding mode of birth. If, for example, she looks after young children, this will be very difficult while the abdominal incision heals.

Important Learning Points

- Caesareans may be planned or unplanned.
- Elective caesareans have lower rates of morbidity and mortality than emergency caesareans.
- The primary reasons for an emergency caesarean birth include failure to progress and fetal distress.
- The main risks of caesarean birth include haemorrhage, infection, damage to anatomical structures during the operation and the increased risk of VTE.
- The main stages in a caesarean birth following preoperative preparation are gaining access to the uterus, birth of the baby, removal of the placenta with the aid of syntocinon, ensuring that the uterine cavity is empty, haemostasis and closing appropriately.
- It is important to remember that the majority of caesareans are relatively uneventful and have a good outcome for mother and baby.

VAGINAL BIRTH AFTER CAESAREAN

Q1: Which of the following is the most important concern with a vaginal birth after caesarean (VBAC)? The correct answer is A. Uterine rupture.

The biggest risk during VBAC is uterine rupture. There is also a very small risk of uterine rupture throughout pregnancy, not just in labour, so patients need to be aware that they should present if they get scar tenderness at any point in their gestation.

A ✔ **Uterine rupture** – Correct. Although uncommon, uterine rupture is associated with significant maternal and perinatal morbidity and possible perinatal mortality. Uterine rupture is disruption of the uterine muscle extending to the uterine serosa or extending to the bladder or broad ligament. Uterine rupture is extremely rare in patients without previous uterine surgery. A caesarean scar on the uterus is not as strong as an unscarred uterus, so during labour, this area can be torn open during contractions. This often causes severe pain, and both mother and baby can become quickly compromised by massive haemorrhage. An emergency caesarean birth is required in this event to deliver the baby and stop the bleeding.

B Uterine dehiscence – Incorrect. Uterine dehiscence is when there is disruption of the uterine muscle. However, the uterine serosa remains intact. This is diagnosed at the time of caesarean. Dehiscence is essentially the thinning of the layers of the uterus, but the uterus remains intact. There is no pain or

bleeding, and neither mother nor baby is compromised by this. However, it is a marker for the clinician that if this patient had continued in labour, then there would have been an increased risk of scar rupture. It may affect the management of future pregnancies.

C Uterine infection – Incorrect. Compared to an elective caesarean, the risk of uterine infection is decreased with a successful VBAC but increased with an unsuccessful VBAC.

D Thromboembolism – Incorrect. The difference in risk of thromboembolism is not statistically significant in women undergoing VBAC in comparison to elective repeat caesarean.

E Transfusion requirements – Incorrect. Although during VBAC, there is a higher overall risk of needing a blood transfusion (170/10,000) in comparison to uterine rupture during VBAC (22 to 74/10,000), the risk of requirement for a blood transfusion is still present with elective repeat caesarean, and therefore, the comparative morbidity and mortality associated with blood transfusion are much smaller than those associated with uterine rupture.

Key Point

The presentation of uterine rupture is classically nonspecific and inconsistent, making the diagnosis difficult. It should therefore be considered in any woman in labour who presents with pain, fetal distress or signs of shock. The diagnosis can often be delayed, as it is an uncommon clinical event resulting in worse outcomes for the mother and baby.

Q2: Answer true or false: Which of the following are contraindications to VBAC?

Women who have had one or two lower segment transverse caesarean sections are not contraindicated for VBAC as outlined in RCOG guidelines. Women who have had three or more previous caesarean births, even if they were uncomplicated, should not be considered for VBAC because the risk of rupture is not known. Any previous high vertical classical caesarean is a contraindication to VBAC, especially if the uterine incision has involved the whole length of the uterine corpus.

A One uncomplicated low transverse caesarean section – False.

B Two uncomplicated low transverse caesarean sections – False.

C ✔ **Three uncomplicated low transverse caesarean sections** – True.

D ✔ **One previous high vertical classical caesarean section** – True.

E ✔ **Two previous high vertical classical caesarean sections** – True.

> **Key Point**
>
> The risk of uterine rupture may be related in part to the type of uterine incision made during the first caesarean birth. A previous lower segment transverse uterine incision has the lowest risk of rupture (0.2% to 1.5% risk). Vertical or T-shaped uterine incisions have a higher risk of uterine rupture (4% to 9% risk). It is important to remember that the direction of the skin incision does not indicate the type or direction of the uterine incision; a woman with a transverse skin incision may have had a vertical uterine incision.

Q3: Answer true or false: Which of the following can be used without additional cautions during VBAC compared to a spontaneous vaginal birth?

There is an increased risk of rupture in women undergoing an induction or augmentation of their labour in comparison to spontaneous labour during VBAC because of the effects that induction agents have on uterine activity.

A Prostaglandins – False. Induced or augmented labours increase the risk of uterine rupture during VBAC, so prostaglandins should be used with caution. Women should be informed that there is a higher risk of uterine rupture with their use. Prostaglandins work by softening the cervix, causing dilatation to make it possible for artificial rupture of the membranes. As well as softening the cervix, it also softens the rest of the uterus, including an existing scar, making it more prone to rupture. Prostaglandins also increase the force of contractions, so again, this can increase the risk of rupture.

B Oxytocin – False. Oxytocin augmentation also increases the risk of uterine rupture because it increases the force and frequency of contractions. Therefore, it needs to be used with caution, correctly titrating the oxytocin so that contractions do not exceed a maximum rate of four contractions in 10 minutes. The duration of use of oxytocin also increases the risk. For this reason, there is more caution regarding how long oxytocin is used for. When delay occurs in the first stage of a spontaneous labour, caesarean may be offered instead of using syntocinon.

C ✔ **Epidural anaesthesia** – True. Previously, concerns existed that epidural anaesthesia might mask the signs and symptoms associated with uterine rupture. However, a study has found that epidural anaesthesia is safe and actually makes the patient more comfortable to facilitate intervention if needed.

D ✔ **Spinal anaesthesia** – True. Spinal anaesthesia is not often used in labour, as it is a one-off injection which cannot be topped up like an epidural. There are, however, no contraindications to it being used in a VBAC labour, although this would be very uncommon.

E ✔ **Continuous electronic fetal monitoring** – True. An abnormal CTG is the most consistent finding in

uterine rupture. Therefore, women are advised to have continuous electronic fetal monitoring following the onset of uterine contractions for the duration of a planned VBAC.

> **Key Point**
>
> Approximate risk of rupture in VBAC:
> - Spontaneous labour, 1:200.
> - With oxytocin, 1:100.
> - With prostaglandin, 1:50.

> **Q Important Learning Points**
>
> - A successful VBAC refers to any woman who has had a previous caesarean and who subsequently births vaginally, either spontaneously or assisted.
> - Benefits of VBAC include an easier recovery with fewer complications and fewer admissions for the baby to the neonatal unit.
> - The major concern is uterine rupture. Therefore, it is important that the risks and benefits of VBAC are carefully weighed up.
> - In general, delivering by VBAC in an obstetrician-led unit with CTG monitoring and continuous intrapartum care can reduce the risks of adverse outcomes.

ASSISTED VAGINAL BIRTH

Q1: Before attempting an assisted vaginal birth, which of the following conditions should be satisfied?
The correct answers are B. The maternal bladder should be empty, **D.** The woman should be offered appropriate analgesia, and **E.** Membranes should have ruptured.

An assisted vaginal birth may be considered in the second stage of labour, particularly for labours which are prolonged or have complications requiring birth to be expedited, such as fetal distress or maternal cardiac disease.

A The woman should be lying supine – Incorrect. This is not a prerequisite for assisted vaginal birth. However, most obstetricians are more comfortable delivering the mother lying supine with her legs in stirrups in the lithotomy position.

B ✔ **The maternal bladder should be empty** – Correct. This is to reduce the risk of puncturing or otherwise damaging the bladder when using instruments and to prevent a full bladder from obstructing and preventing birth. It may be done via catheterisation, in which case the catheter should be removed or the catheter balloon deflated before carrying out assisted birth. Despite this, urinary incontinence is more prevalent following assisted vaginal birth than following spontaneous vaginal birth (forceps more than ventouse).

C Fetus should be in the OP position – Incorrect. OA presentations are preferred for an assisted birth. However, this is not absolute, and it will depend on the individual case, including experience of the clinician.

D ✔ **The woman should be offered appropriate analgesia** – Correct. Adequate pain relief is important when carrying out an assisted vaginal birth. Nerve blockage should make the woman more comfortable and therefore more likely to push effectively with contractions, which improves the likelihood of successful birth. Also, in many assisted vaginal births, an episiotomy reduces the incidence of complicated perineal tears so analgesia in place before this cut is beneficial. A minimum of a perineal nerve blockage is recommended, as it is effective pain relief in the areas most likely to sense further pain. More effective analgesia can be given in the form of a higher nerve blockage, for example, pudendal nerve block, epidural or spinal.

E ✔ **Membranes should have ruptured** – Correct. This is a prerequisite for assisted vaginal birth and is to allow proper placement of instruments on the fetal head. It should be confirmed on vaginal examination if this has not already been done, and if membranes remain intact in an otherwise indicated assisted birth, they should be artificially ruptured.

Q2: Which of the following cases would be considered relative contraindications for assisted vaginal birth?

Assisted vaginal birth can be associated with significant maternal and fetal mortality and morbidity. Clinicians with less experience tend to have more complications, and each case is individual when deciding whether or not to offer an assisted birth. A maximum of three pulls with forceps, if there is insufficient descent, should be carried out before reverting to a caesarean. For a vacuum birth, if birth of the fetal head has not been achieved after three pulls but birth appears imminent, a further three gentle pulls may be utilised in this situation. The latest RCOG guidelines give no absolute contraindications for assisted vaginal birth, but there are clinical situations when the consideration for caesarean may be weighed more favourably.

A ✔ **A 32-year-old primigravida, gestation 41 weeks, has been in the second stage of labour, pushing for over 2 hours. The crown of the fetal head is at the ischial spines on vaginal examination. She has had a healthy and low risk pregnancy up until her last antenatal ultrasound scan, which showed femoral bowing and a possible long bone fracture** – Correct. Any known fetal predisposition to fractures (for example, osteogenesis imperfecta) is a relative contraindication, as forceps and vacuum extractors may cause further problems. In this case, a caesarean birth would be the best management option but should be carried out by a senior obstetrician.

B A 29-year-old woman, gravidity three, parity zero, gestation 38 weeks, has been in the second stage of labour for nearly 2 hours without analgesia.

The mother is known to have HIV; her viral load is undetectable – Incorrect. Bloodborne viruses are not a contraindication to assisted vaginal birth if the viral load is undetectable. Assuming there are no other contraindications and the correct conditions are met, it would be appropriate to offer this woman an assisted vaginal birth (as she has been in the second stage of labour for 3 hours).

C A 42-year-old woman, gravidity two, parity one, gestation 37 weeks, has been pushing in the second stage of labour for 1 hour. The electronic fetal monitor shows a trace with a baseline of 102 bpm and variability of less than 5 bpm for the past hour. – Incorrect. The fetal electronic monitor trace is abnormal, and she is in the second stage of labour; hence, expediting birth is the most appropriate step, either by assisted vaginal birth or caesarean.

D ✔ **An 18-year-old primigravida, gestation 40 weeks, has been having regular contractions. The woman has been diagnosed with mitral stenosis. Her cervix is 8 cm dilated** – Correct. The cervix should be fully dilated before an assisted vaginal birth is attempted. This is to allow maximum space for the fetus to be delivered through, and spontaneous birth may be possible with a fully dilated cervix. In a case of known cardiac problems, an appropriate birth plan should have been previously prepared to inform both the woman and clinical staff of preferences. These preferences may include mode of birth, length of time for safe pushing and minimum amount of analgesia required for safe delivery. This is to avoid unnecessary cardiac strain from Valsalva manoeuvres.

E ✔ **A 20-year-old woman, gravidity three, parity two, 41 weeks, has been in the second stage of labour for 2 hours and is becoming exhausted. Vaginal examination finds the fetal station is above the ischial spines. An antenatal blood test confirmed that the fetus has haemophilia** – Correct. Known or suspected fetal blood disorders (haemophilia or alloimmune thrombocytopaenia) are contraindications for assisted vaginal birth. This is because assisted vaginal birth increases these risk of trauma to the fetus and woman. These complications can range from minor cuts and bruises to intracranial haemorrhages, which may be fatal, especially if there are clotting problems in the fetus. Separately in this case, the fetal head is above the ischial spines, which is itself another relative contraindication for assisted vaginal birth.

 Key Point

Assisted vaginal birth is relatively contraindicated when there is an already increased risk of fetal bleeding or fractures, a face presentation, gestation under 34 weeks or if the cervix is not fully dilated. Experienced obstetricians are less likely to cause maternal or fetal trauma when assisting labour.

Q3: Answer true or false to the following statements regarding assisted vaginal birth.

The rate of assisted vaginal birth is around 13%. Although there are significant risks associated with rotational and midcavity assisted vaginal births, caesareans in the second stage of labour are also associated with considerable morbidity. Assisted vaginal births are usually performed using vacuum extractors or forceps to deliver the fetus, depending on the situation and experience of the operator.

A Midcavity and rotational births should be exclusively managed with Kielland and Simpson forceps – False. A midcavity birth can be managed with several options, which include use of Kielland and Simpson forceps. Nonetheless, ventouse or caesarean may also be appropriate. It is undertaken when the fetal head is in line with the ischial spines. Fetuses which are not lying in the physiological OA position may necessitate a manual or instrumental rotation. However, independent of the type of instrument used, rotations demand a high level of clinical and technical skill, requiring the operator to have received adequate training.

B ✔ **Assisted vaginal birth should be abandoned if there is no descent after two pulls** – True. If there is no descent after two pulls of an instrument that has been correctly applied and used, birth is unlikely to be achieved with a third pull. The obstetrician should opt for a caesarean birth in this situation. Sequential instrumentation to birth the baby could result in serious fetal and maternal trauma, so it is felt to be safer to convert to caesarean.

C An episiotomy should be performed during fetal traction – False. Traction refers to the pulling of the fetus with forceps or vacuum extractors. Episiotomies should be performed when the perineal region is under the least strain, and care should be taken not to harm the fetus whilst performing an episiotomy. Timing of episiotomy is also important and should only be performed following confirmed fetal descent. Converting to a caesarean after performing an episiotomy is an undesired and often avoidable outcome. Episiotomies should not be performed in traction to reduce risk of making unnecessarily deep cuts or harming the fetus. However, episiotomies are usually performed during maternal contractions, as stretched muscle is easier to cut. Bleeding is also reduced since the raw edges are compressed.

D Forceps should be chosen in preference to ventouse – False. Both forceps and ventouse have different merits and risks, for example, vacuum extractors are easier to place but more likely to dislodge. The choice of which to use depends on a combination of the clinical situation and the experience of the operator.

E ✔ **Higher rates of failure are associated with a maternal BMI over 30 kg/m² – True.** Higher failures rates are also associated with:
- Estimated fetal weight more than or equal to 4 kg.
- OP position.
- Midcavity births.

 Key Point

Assisted vaginal birth has a high risk of trauma to the mother or fetus. An episiotomy is usually performed to increase the size of the space available for the birth of the baby if perineal tears are likely otherwise.

Q4: Regarding episiotomies, which statement below is correct?
The correct answer is E. Having finished suturing, a rectal examination should be performed.

An episiotomy is a surgical cut made to the opening of the vagina to assist the birth of a baby and to avoid uncontrolled tissue trauma. Although routine episiotomies for childbirth are less common now in the UK, they are still widely practised in certain parts of the world. It may make the baby's birth easier whilst attempting to prevent tears which may be difficult to repair. After the birth, the cut is repaired with sutures.

A Episiotomy is associated with a reduced incidence of PPH – Incorrect. The opposite is true. The purpose of the episiotomy is to prevent uncontrolled perineal trauma and rectal injuries.

B A mediolateral episiotomy should be avoided – Incorrect. In the UK, a mediolateral position is generally used, as it has a reduced risk of causing third- and fourth-degree tears, which is the principal aim of episiotomies. In the United States, however, a midline approach is taken. Cutting in the midline is done because it is relatively avascular and incises the muscle aponeuroses rather than the muscle bodies. It should be noted that a midline cut is more likely to extend backward into the rectum and increase the chance of a third- or fourth-degree tear.

[See 'Perineal Trauma' on page 361.]

C If extensive vaginal tearing appears likely, an episiotomy should not be performed – Incorrect. An episiotomy is performed to control tearing, reduce the chance of anal sphincter tears and widen the opening of the vagina to allow the baby to pass more easily. If extensive tearing looks likely, a controlled cut can be preferable.

D The cuts formed from episiotomies heal better than other tears – Incorrect. There is no evidence to support either cuts or tears as healing faster. Tears are often more superficial than deliberate surgical cuts and may not need repairing, but may be more complicated and deep and may be hidden. In both cases, the cut or tear should be sutured and properly cared for postbirth to optimise healing and minimise infection risk.

E ✔ **Having finished suturing, a rectal examination should be performed** – Correct. A finger should be inserted into the rectum prior to repair to assess for anal sphincter or mucosal injuries. Failure to identify and repair these can result in long-term faecal incontinence or rectovaginal fistulas. After repair, a further rectal exam should be performed to check again for trauma and for stitches incorrectly placed into the rectum. If sutures are felt in the rectum, they should be removed and replaced. If not replaced, there is a risk of a rectovaginal fistula forming. If a fistula occurs, it can cause significant morbidity, including faecal incontinence and vaginal infection.

 Key Point

An episiotomy is a surgical cut made to the vaginal opening to widen the space for the fetus to pass and to attempt to control tissue trauma. If a fistula is formed between the vagina and the rectum, drastic long-term incontinence problems may develop if it is not found and repaired.

Important Learning Points

- Assisted vaginal birth involves using forceps or vacuum extraction (ventouse) to help deliver the fetus.
- It can be carried out during the second stage of labour if the labour is prolonged or complicated.
- It should only be attempted by an experienced obstetrician or a closely supervised trainee.
- It significantly increases risk of maternal and fetal trauma, and depending on individual circumstances, a caesarean may be a less risky option.

An episiotomy is often performed to aid birth and control perineal trauma. The episiotomy requires suturing and appropriate wound care afterward.

14 OBSTETRIC COMPLICATIONS

ANTEPARTUM HAEMORRHAGE

Q1: What is the most likely diagnosis for this woman?
The correct answer is C. Concealed placental abruption.

The set of observations for this woman is typical of a person who is haemodynamically shocked. She is hypotensive, tachycardic and tachypnoeic, with a normal oxygen saturation and temperature. This woman is very unwell; she needs to be assessed in an ABC approach and managed according to these findings.

A Placenta praevia – Incorrect. Placenta praevia presents with painless bleeding from the genital tract. The blood is often a bright red colour, and when the abdomen is palpated, it is nontender and soft.

B Revealed placental abruption – Incorrect. A revealed placental abruption presents with painful dark red bleeding from the genital tract. The palpated abdomen is tense and tender. Maternal shock may not be in keeping with the amount of blood loss seen. The fetus is often distressed. Revealed placental abruption is caused by a placenta where the edge comes away from the uterus wall, allowing blood to track down into the genital tract. This woman does have a tense and tender abdomen and fetal distress and is shocked, but she does not have genital tract bleeding.

C ✔ **Concealed placental abruption** – Correct. This patient has all the signs of placental abruption but not genital tract bleeding. This case fits the diagnosis of concealed placental abruption. This woman's placenta has come away from the uterus wall, causing a tense, tender abdomen. The blood has not been able to track down into the genital tract but has become concealed between the placenta and the uterus wall. This has caused severe pain and maternal shock due to the blood loss.

D Acute pyelonephritis – Incorrect. If the woman has this condition, she would have pain on one side, a high temperature and rigors; she would feel very weak and tired and would have lost her appetite.

E Ovarian torsion – Incorrect. This woman would have presented with one-sided lower abdominal pain, feeling nauseated and vomiting, and the uterus would not be tender.

 Key Point

Exam questions often discuss the colour of blood to help distinguish between placenta praevia and placental abruption. The concept is that the blood in abruption becomes darker since it is older as it is slowly built up rather than blood from the edge of a placenta praevia immediately leaving the uterus, which is bright red. In practice, blood colour is unhelpful, as blood from an acute placental abruption can also appear bright red.

Q2: Answer true or false: What signs and symptoms are classically present in an APH caused by placenta praevia?

The clinical features of placenta praevia are very important both clinically and for exams. In addition, it is important to ask about previous ultrasound scan findings, as placenta praevia is usually identified at the 20-week scan.

A Painful bleeding from the genital tract – False. Placenta praevia results in painless bleeding from the genital tract. The placenta is low lying in the uterus. If bleeding was to occur, it can track out from the uterus without causing pain. There is no pain because the blood can leave the uterus without irritating the uterus wall.

B ✔ **Nontender, soft uterus** – True. This is because the placenta is low lying in the uterus, and the blood which is lost can flow easily out, so it does not irritate the uterus wall. In abruption, blood present against the uterine wall would cause a tense, hard uterus because the blood irritates the wall of the uterus.

C ✔ **Bright red blood** – True. Blood can easily escape the uterus because of the placenta lying over the internal os, resulting in fresh bright red blood being seen. The blood can leave the genital tract before it has a chance to become clotted and dark brown in colour, which is more commonly seen in placental abruption.

D ✔ **Maternal shock in keeping with the amount of blood lost** – True. In placenta praevia, no blood loss is concealed, as all of the blood loss can easily flow out of the genital tract. Medical staff can therefore estimate how much blood has been lost.

E CTG shows prolonged atypical decelerations of the fetal heart – False. The fetus does not often become distressed from a bleed from placenta praevia, as the placenta is still functioning normally, providing nutrients. The blood lost in placenta praevia is maternal blood. However, if the mother becomes compromised by the blood loss, then maternal hypotension would compromise the fetus. Where there is a small amount of painless bleeding and fetal compromise, the diagnosis of vasa praevia should be considered.

> **Key Point**
>
> When taking a history, especially in OSCEs, it is crucial to determine if the bleeding is painful or painless, to distinguish between placenta praevia and placental abruption.

Q3: Answer true or false: Which of the following management options would be suitable for a woman with a severe APH (blood loss of more than 1 L) at 39 weeks gestation?

A No intervention unless there is clinical deterioration – False. This is inappropriate management (also known as watch-and-wait management). If the woman is pregnant and haemorrhaging, she needs to be assessed fully. This should include a full ABC assessment, basic bloods, crossmatch two to four units and to be reviewed and seen by a senior for advice. A small haemorrhage in a pregnant woman can quickly become severe. Even with a small haemorrhage, at 39 weeks gestation, there is no risk of prematurity, so most obstetricians would advocate delivery rather than waiting.

B ✔ **ABC assessment** – True. This method of assessment allows a systematic approach to a patient and also stops you from missing key information. It ensures basic observations are combined with clinical examination to ensure you make an informed assessment.

C ✔ **Full set of bloods including FBC and group and save (G&S)** – True. The FBC allows you to look at the haemoglobin level of a woman; it can quickly tell you if an individual has lost a significant amount of blood and needs a blood transfusion. Haemoglobin concentration does not drop immediately following a haemorrhage, so it should be repeated once the patient has been fluid resuscitated. G&S is needed to determine the woman's blood group. Hence, if blood is needed for a transfusion, it is quicker to crossmatch the woman. It is common practice to insert two large bore cannulae and to crossmatch at least four units of packed red cells when a woman presents with a large haemorrhage.

D Intramuscular steroids – False. The woman is 39 weeks pregnant; her baby's lungs would have developed at this point. Intramuscular steroids are given to women who are 24 to 34 weeks gestation to help their lungs mature by increasing surfactant production.

E ✔ **Immediate birth** – True. Senior review is needed to determine this, but if she was haemorrhaging significantly and because the baby is 39 weeks gestation, it is likely they would perform an emergency caesarean.

> **Key Point**
>
> Blood loss during pregnancy is dangerous for the mother and fetus. If the mother has insufficient blood circulating, her BP may drop, resulting in poor blood flow through the placenta to the fetus. If poor blood supply to the fetus is prolonged, it may result in cerebral palsy caused by hypoxia (due to lack of oxygen to the fetal brain).

> **Important Learning Points**
>
> - APH is bleeding during pregnancy after 24 weeks gestation.
> - Placental abruption occurs when the placenta comes away from the uterus partially or completely, typically resulting in painful dark red bleeding from the genital tract. The mother has a tense, tender uterus, and fetal heart monitoring often shows signs of fetal distress.
> - Placenta praevia is where the placenta is in an abnormal position in the uterus, covering the internal cervical os. In contrast, this condition typically presents with painless, bright red bleeding from the genital tract. The uterus of the mother is nontender and soft.
> - Management should be via an ABC approach.
> - Haemorrhage is the leading cause of maternal death worldwide and needs to be identified and managed early.

PRE-ECLAMPSIA AND PREGNANCY-INDUCED HYPERTENSION

Q1: What is the most likely diagnosis for this woman?

The correct answer is D. Pre-eclampsia.

Hypertensive disorders in pregnancy can occur in women with preexisting hypertension (either primary or secondary), or they can newly arise after 20 weeks gestation. Hypertensive disorders in pregnancy can increase the risk of maternal and/or fetal mortality or morbidity. Overall, 5% of stillbirths in infants without congenital abnormalities occur in mothers with pre-eclampsia.

A Gestational hypertension – Incorrect. Although this patient has new-onset hypertension and is asymptomatic, proteinuria would not be expected in gestational hypertension. The presence of more than 1+ protein on urine dipstick should alert you to a more serious underlying cause of her hypertension in pregnancy.

B Chronic hypertension – Incorrect. From this history, the patient is not known to have hypertension. Whilst it is possible she may have some underlying hypertension prior to the pregnancy, one should assume she has developed new-onset hypertension. Chronic hypertension can be defined as a systolic BP more than or equal to 140 mmHg or diastolic BP more than or equal to 90 mmHg prior to pregnancy or the 20th week of pregnancy (on at least two occasions). Chronic hypertension would be expected to persist beyond 12 weeks postpartum (when gestational hypertension should have resolved).

C Haemolysis, elevated liver enzymes and low platelets (HELLP) syndrome – Incorrect. HELLP syndrome may represent a severe form of pre-eclampsia. From this case, we are told that the blood tests are unremarkable. Although the details of the tests are not specified, it would be acceptable to assume that this patient did not have HELLP syndrome.

D ✔ Pre-eclampsia – Correct. This woman meets the criteria for the diagnosis of pre-eclampsia. She is a previously normotensive person presenting with new-onset hypertension and proteinuria after 20 weeks gestation. She also has several risk factors that increase the risk of her developing pre-eclampsia such as: more than 40 years old, triplets and egg donation.

E Eclampsia – Incorrect. Eclampsia refers to the development of generalised seizures and/or coma in a woman with pre-eclampsia. In addition, there must be an absence of other neurological conditions that may account for the seizure. The case history does not describe any active seizures. Hence, the woman's condition cannot be characterised as eclampsia.

> **Key Point**
>
> Hypertensive disorders in pregnancy can have potentially serious consequences for mother and baby. Proteinuria and hypertension in pregnancy should prompt further assessment.

Q2: Answer true or false: Which of the following are risk factors for pre-eclampsia?

The woman in this case has several risk factors for pre-eclampsia, which can be grouped into maternal and fetal. The magnitude of risk depends on the specific risk factor, whereby certain factors confer a higher chance of developing pre-eclampsia. For instance, a past history of pre-eclampsia increases the risk of developing pre-eclampsia in a subsequent pregnancy by sevenfold compared with women with no history of pre-eclampsia.

A ✔ **Maternal age more than 40 years** – True. Advanced maternal age (more than 40 years old) is associated with an increased risk of developing pre-eclampsia. Advanced maternal age may be confounded by the presence of other comorbidities, such as chronic hypertension, which are more likely to be present at this age group.

B ✔ **Preexisting diabetes in the mother** – True. Vascular disease as a result of diabetes may affect placental perfusion, leading to pre-eclampsia. Other factors caused by diabetes which may contribute are renal disease, insulin resistance and abnormal lipid metabolism.

C Smoking – False. Interestingly, smoking is associated with a decreased risk of pre-eclampsia. Nonetheless, the multiple fetal and maternal risks of smoking far outweigh this beneficial effect.

D ✔ **Multiple pregnancy** – True. The risk of developing pre-eclampsia is increased with multiple-order pregnancies. It is believed that it is the larger placenta that is responsible for the increased risk.

E ✔ **First pregnancy** – True. It is unclear why, but nulliparity is associated with an increased risk of developing pre-eclampsia.

> **Key Point**
>
> Antenatal clinics assist in identifying women who have risk factors for developing pre-eclampsia. Women at risk of developing pre-eclampsia will be offered low-dose antenatal aspirin and will have increased monitoring throughout pregnancy.

Q3: Which antihypertensive agents can be used in treating hypertension during pregnancy?

The correct answers are C. Labetalol, **D.** Methyldopa and **E.** Nifedipine.

The definitive treatment of pre-eclampsia is birth of the baby. If the mother has ongoing pre-eclampsia, she is at increased risk of complications such as eclampsia, cerebral haemorrhage and HELLP. In addition, the baby is at increased risk of complications, such as IUGR and stillbirth. The decision to deliver the baby has to be balanced between the potential risks of a preterm baby and the clinical state of the mother and fetus.

A Ramipril – Incorrect. Angiotensin-converting enzyme (ACE) inhibitors, angiotensin II receptor blockers and renin inhibitors are contraindicated in all stages of pregnancy. ACE inhibitors have a significant adverse effect on fetal and neonatal BP control and renal function. Furthermore, skull defects and oligohydramnios have been reported with ACE inhibitors.

B Spironolactone – Incorrect. The diuretic spironolactone is not recommended in pregnancy. Animal studies revealed feminisation of male fetuses with spironolactone.

C ✔ **Labetalol** – Correct. This beta-blocker is usually the first-line antihypertensive for gestational hypertension or pre-eclampsia. Labetalol has an advantage that it can be given orally or intravenously and has a rapid onset of action (within 2 hours). As a drug class, beta-blockers have been reported to cause IUGR, neonatal hypoglycaemia and neonatal bradycardia.

D ✔ **Methyldopa** – Correct. This centrally acting alpha-2 adrenergic agonist has been widely used in managing hypertension in pregnancy due to its long-term safety in the fetus. However, it has a mild hypertensive effect with a slower onset of action than labetalol. It is also associated with postnatal depression and hence is not recommended in the postnatal period.

E ✔ **Nifedipine** – Correct. The calcium channel antagonist is recommended as an alternative to labetalol for the management of hypertension in pregnancy. It is also used to try and inhibit labour in specific situations. Nifedipine's tocolytic action arises from the blockade of calcium entry into smooth muscle cells, thereby preventing uterine contractions.

> 💬 **Key Point**
>
> The definitive treatment of pre-eclampsia is birth of the baby. The timing of delivery needs to be balanced between the risks of a preterm baby and the mother and fetus' clinical state. Antihypertensives, such as labetalol and nifedipine, can be used in the conservative management of pre-eclampsia.

Q4: A peripheral blood film from a patient with pre-eclampsia is shown below. Successive full blood counts reveal a falling platelet count. What condition has she developed?
The correct answer is I. HELLP syndrome.

The peripheral blood film demonstrates microangiopathic haemolytic anaemia, which can occur in HELLP syndrome. The blood film demonstrates marked red cell fragmentation (large black arrow) and helmet cells or schistocytes (small black arrow), which can occur during haemolysis. The red arrow shows lytic changes to the platelets. Blood tests such as FBC, LFTs and U&Es should be done regularly in confirmed cases of pre-eclampsia to detect the presence of any haematological, hepatic or renal complications that may develop. Progression to complications may be gradual or rapid.

Q5: Which drug is commonly used for seizure prophylaxis during pre-eclampsia?
The correct answer is G. Magnesium sulphate.

Magnesium sulphate is commonly used for seizure prophylaxis during pre-eclampsia. The exact mechanism of action of magnesium sulphate in seizure prophylaxis is not fully understood. However, it has a good safety profile in pregnancy and has been shown to be more effective in seizure prevention than any other anticonvulsant.

Q6: Which drug can be used to treat hypertension in pre-eclampsia and also has tocolytic properties?
The correct answer is K. Nifedipine.

Nifedipine is a calcium channel antagonist that can be used to treat hypertension in pre-eclampsia. Nifedipine also has tocolytic properties (i.e., it inhibits labour) by preventing uterine contractions by blocking calcium entry into uterine smooth muscle cells.

Q7: Which drug can be offered to patients with moderate or high risk of pre-eclampsia during the antenatal period?
The correct answer is E. Aspirin.

Current guidelines recommend aspirin daily from 12 weeks until 36 weeks for moderate- to high-risk patients to reduce the risk of developing a hypertensive disorder in pregnancy. Factors that carry a high risk, according to NICE guidelines, are: past history of pre-eclampsia, chronic kidney disease, autoimmune diseases, diabetes and chronic hypertension. Aspirin has been shown to reduce platelet thromboxane synthesis whilst maintaining vascular wall prostacyclin synthesis. The theoretical result of this is improved placental function. Randomised trials with aspirin have demonstrated a modest reduction in the risk of pre-eclampsia by 10% to 15% and a reduction in adverse pregnancy outcomes, such as preterm birth and fetal growth restriction.

Q8: Which pre-eclampsia complication occurs more frequently postpartum than antenatally?
The correct answer is F. Eclampsia.

Eclampsia is defined as generalised seizures and/or coma in a woman with pre-eclampsia, with no other neurological cause of the seizure. Eclampsia occurs in about 1 in 2000 pregnancies. Eclamptic seizures are usually self-limiting. When they occur, it is important to investigate to rule out other causes for seizures.

> 🔍 **Important Learning Points**
>
> - Pre-eclampsia is a serious hypertensive disorder in pregnancy that is potentially life-threatening to mother and baby.
> - It is defined as hypertension and proteinuria after 20 weeks of gestation.
> - Symptoms include headache, visual disturbances and upper abdominal pain. Signs may include hyperreflexia, clonus, hypertension and peripheral oedema.

- Multisystem complications can arise in the mother or baby. Maternal complications include stroke, eclampsia, pulmonary oedema, liver and renal failure. Fetal complications include growth restriction, preterm birth and stillbirth.
- Birth of the baby is the definitive treatment of preeclampsia. The timing of delivery depends on the severity of the pre-eclampsia and the gestation of the pregnancy.
- Antihypertensives such as labetalol can be used in the conservative management of pre-eclampsia.
- Although the risk of pre-eclampsia complications falls after delivery, the majority of eclampsia episodes occur postpartum.
- Pre-eclampsia can be a predictor of cardiovascular and cerebrovascular disease in later life.

PRETERM LABOUR

Q1: Which of the following would not be a possible cause of the abdominal pain that she is experiencing?
The correct answer is B. Breech presentation of the fetus.

Fetal presentation during pregnancy does not normally cause pain. Appendicitis, constipation and UTI can cause abdominal pain. Women who have placental abruption normally present with vaginal bleeding, abdominal pain and uterine contractions.

 Key Point

When formulating the differential diagnoses for abdominal pain, remember that the causes of abdominal pain that could happen during pregnancy also include all causes of abdominal pain outside of pregnancy, some of which may present atypically.

Q2: Answer true or false: Which of the following put Josephine at an increased risk of having a preterm birth?

Early identification of risk factors for preterm labour facilitates appropriate counselling and management of any risk factor that might be modifiable.

A Overweight – False. Low BMI, rather than high BMI, increases the risk of preterm birth. Obesity does not directly cause preterm delivery but may be associated with gestational diabetes, which leads to premature births.

B ✔ **Diabetes** – True. The hyperglycaemic environment from maternal diabetes (both type 1 and type 2 diabetes) could result in polyhydramnios leading to preterm labour.

C ✔ **Smoking** – True. Smoking is known to be associated with preterm premature rupture of membranes (PPROM) and poor placental development. The latter could result in placental abruption or poor placental exchange leading to fetal developmental abnormalities, ultimately causing preterm labour.

D Vitiligo – False. Vitiligo is a dermatological condition where areas of the skin lose their pigmentation. Vitiligo

often occurs in patients with other autoimmune conditions, such as type 1 diabetes and hypothyroidism. These conditions have been found to be linked to preterm birth, but vitiligo itself is not a risk factor.

E ✔ **UTI** – True. UTIs are a known risk factor for preterm labour, as there is a strong association between UTI and PPROM.

 Key Point

The most important risk factor for preterm birth is a previous preterm birth. An important risk factor to remember for many obstetric conditions is a previous history of that condition.

Q3: Answer true or false: Which examinations and/or investigations should now be performed to confirm the diagnosis?

To confirm the diagnosis of preterm labour:
- *Speculum examination to look for any pooling of liquor – evidence that membranes have ruptured.*
- *Digital vaginal exam to further assess cervical dilatation unless rupture of membranes has occurred.*
- *CTG to monitor uterine activity and contractions, as well as fetal heart monitoring.*

A ✔ **Speculum and vaginal examinations** – True. Although more technologically advanced investigations are available, a speculum and vaginal examination is still crucial to determine the state of the maternal cervix. The need for other investigations generally depends on these examination findings.

B Fetal blood sampling – False. Fetal blood sampling is used intrapartum where the CTG has demonstrated abnormal findings, but urgent caesarean is not warranted. This is to determine the pH of the fetal blood to elucidate the degree of hypoxia. A contraindication for fetal blood sampling in this setting is prematurity, less than 34 weeks gestation.

C ✔ **Fetal fibronectin test** – True. A fetal fibronectin test is indicated in this case, as the patient has presented at 32 weeks with intact membranes. It is a protein found at the interface of the chorion and decidua. Fetal fibronectin is like the D-dimer of pregnancy. If negative, this is extremely useful and, when plotted alongside cervical length, can reassure women that they are very unlikely to go into premature labour. However, positive results have a poor sensitivity and specificity.

D ✔ **CTG** – True. CTG is an important noninvasive investigation that can be performed quickly to examine both the activity of the uterus and fetal well-being.

E Maternal blood tests, blood cultures and high vaginal swabs – False. Maternal blood tests, blood cultures and high vaginal swabs help in the investigation for signs of infections in chorioamnionitis but do not confirm whether preterm labour will occur.

Key Point

It is important to establish the following factors for a woman with suspected preterm labour, as these will determine the subsequent management plan:

- Presence of membrane rupture – PPROM should be treated with antibiotics.
- Degree of cervical dilatation – tocolysis is only effective if dilatation is less than 4 cm.
- Signs of fetal compromise – expedited birth with labour augmentation or caesarean.

Q4: What should be the first step in management?
The correct answer is H. Admit to the delivery unit.

Admission to the delivery unit is important for monitoring both maternal and fetal condition. It will allow the team to investigate potential causes of preterm labour, such as infection, and optimise treatment in case of delivery. The patient is in the correct place with neonatal support, steroids can be administered in a timely manner and tocolysis can be given to increase the time for steroids to take effect, reducing the risk of RDS.

Q5: What is the most appropriate drug to be administered to reduce incidences of RDS?
The correct answer is D. Betamethasone.

Corticosteroids should be prescribed at this stage of threatened preterm labour to help mature fetal lungs and reduce the incidence of RDS. Although corticosteroids cause hyperglycaemia as a side effect, it is not an absolute contraindication in women with diabetes, as long as their blood glucose is monitored closely. Betamethasone is the only corticosteroid option available on the list. Corticosteroids are given by intramuscular injection, in divided doses, usually 24 hours apart.

Q6: What is the most appropriate tocolytic drug for Josephine?
The correct answer is A. Atosiban.

As the cervix has dilated to only 3 cm in Josephine's case, tocolysis is indicated to delay birth and generate time for corticosteroids to work. Atosiban is an oxytocin receptor antagonist licensed for use in threatened preterm labour. Terbutaline is a β-agonist used to relax the uterus prior to performing ECV but is not commonly used for this indication. There is no evidence for progesterone preventing preterm labour. Nifedipine is used in the UK for tocolysis, but it is not licensed for this indication, so the licensed option, atosiban, is preferable. Oxytocin is contraindicated, as it induces labour.

Q7: If Josephine's cervical dilatation does not progress beyond 4 cm at 72 hours and there are no signs of fetal membrane prolapse in the external os on speculum examination, what could possibly be the next treatment option?

The correct answer is G. Discharge home.

While it can be disconcerting at times to be able to do relatively little for a patient, if they have been assessed for a prolonged period and labour is not established, it would be better to allow the woman to go home, with the counselling to come back in if anything changes.

Q8: If labour ensues despite tocolysis, what is the best mode of birth for the fetus in vertex presentation?
The correct answer is K. Vaginal birth.

Spontaneous vaginal birth should be awaited in an uncomplicated preterm vertex presentation. Ventouse assisted vaginal birth is absolutely contraindicated in the delivery of babies less than 34 weeks gestation, as it increases the risk of neonatal cephalohaematoma.

Key Point

As preterm births are a major cause of perinatal mortality, the main principles of managing a woman in preterm labour are as follows:

1. Prolong pregnancy to prevent RDS and complications associated with early gestational ages.
2. Decide on the mode of birth.
3. Plan for immediate continual postnatal care – this involves ensuring that the centre where delivery is going to take place has facilities to support the premature neonate and the paediatricians are aware of the imminent delivery.

Important Learning Points

- Preterm labour is defined as the onset of labour occurring before 37 completed weeks of pregnancy.
- PPROM is defined as ROM occurring before 37 weeks of gestation and before the onset of labour.
- Diagnosis can be confirmed by clinical examination. The presence of vaginal bleeding is a cause for concern and should be investigated thoroughly.
- In preterm labour cases not complicated by infections or ROM, tocolysis can be considered to prolong gestation for up to 48 hours, during which time antenatal corticosteroids can be administered to accelerate the maturation of fetal lungs.
- Where there are no other contraindications, aim to deliver premature babies vaginally, with careful use of forceps where needed.

CHORIOAMNIONITIS

Q1: Answer true or false: Which of the following are likely to be reasonable differential diagnoses?

It is important to know the differential diagnosis for a pregnant woman coming in with increasing abdominal pain and moderate vaginal bleeding. These signs often indicate an emergency, and the outcome is highly dependent on prompt diagnosis.

A ✔ Placental abruption – True. The usual presentation of placental abruption is pain and bleeding, although about 20% may not have vaginal bleeding (concealed abruption).

B ✔ **Uterine rupture** – True. As the woman had a previous caesarean, the presence of a uterine scar increases her risk of having a uterine rupture. The typical clinical features of uterine rupture include abdominal pain, vaginal bleeding, fetal distress and maternal shock.

C PPROM – False. PPROM does not cause pain and vaginal bleeding. Most women present only with a sensation of a 'gush' of fluid coming through. In uncomplicated PPROM, the mother should have normal vital signs, unlike those described in this scenario. Bleeding may occur if placental abruption occurs secondary to the loss of amniotic fluid in PPROM. It is not necessary for ROM to precede chorioamnionitis. ROM merely increases the risk of ascending infections.

D ✔ **Chorioamnionitis** – True. The patient's vital signs indicate that it is likely that she is suffering from sepsis. Although chorioamnionitis does not necessarily present with abdominal pain and vaginal bleeding, the overall clinical picture should raise suspicions of chorioamnionitis. Furthermore, the insertion of a foreign object (cervical cerclage) further increases her risk of developing chorioamnionitis.

E Preterm labour pain – False. Some women can confuse labour pains with abdominal pain. While vaginal bleeding is possible in preterm labour, however, signs of shock are not.

> ### Key Point
>
> These clinical features should raise suspicions of chorioamnionitis, or other systemic inflammation, as these reflect clinical signs of sepsis. Chorioamnionitis can be 'silent' initially, however, not causing any symptoms or signs in the mother or fetus. In addition, it can occur even with intact membranes, as infection may spread via the transplacental route.

Q2: On abdominal palpation, there is generalised uterine tenderness. An examination of her pad showed fresh bleeding, tinged with foul-smelling discharge. She had leucocytosis with a white cell count of 20 × 10⁹/L and a CRP of 75 mg/L. The consultant has been notified. What is the next best step in management?
The correct answer is C. Start IV fluids and empirical antibiotics.

Chorioamnionitis, particularly with clinical signs of sepsis, should be managed and treated as an obstetric emergency. In this case, the woman has become septic secondary to suspected chorioamnionitis. The offending pathogen was likely to have been introduced when the cervical cerclage was placed.

A Perform amniocentesis to obtain amniotic fluid for culture – Incorrect. Based on the clinical picture, it is quite likely that the diagnosis is chorioamnionitis. Although amniocentesis is the 'gold' standard in diagnosing chorioamnionitis, it is invasive and unlikely to add value to the diagnosis in this case. High vaginal swabs and maternal blood culture sent for microbiology, culture and sensitivity tests would be sufficient enough in determining the prescription of the appropriate antibiotics.

B Start a course of antenatal corticosteroids to enhance fetal lung maturity – Incorrect. Antenatal steroids to prevent RDS are contraindicated in this case, as the patient is already septic, and it may increase the severity of infection.

C ✔ **Start IV fluids and empirical antibiotics** – Correct. IV fluid resuscitation is an appropriate step in management of a septic obstetric patient. Ideally, before broad-spectrum IV antibiotics are given, bloods and a high vaginal swab should be taken for culture. However, antibiotics should not be delayed in a clinically septic patient to enable cultures to be taken if this is proving difficult. The empirical antibiotic therapy given should provide broad-spectrum Gram-negative, Gram-positive and anaerobic cover.

D Remove the cervical cerclage – Incorrect. In this case where cervical cerclage is thought to be the cause of chorioamnionitis, removal of the cerclage would be undertaken when the woman was clinically stable and after basic investigations and the administration of antibiotics has occurred.

E Give analgesia and prescribe bed rest with tocolysis to allow her pregnancy to continue and reduce the risks of complications of prematurity – Incorrect. Paracetamol is given regularly to bring down the maternal temperature and to relieve abdominal pain. However, tocolysis is contraindicated, especially in a case of sepsis such as this.

> ### Key Point
>
> Septic chorioamnionitis can be life-threatening to the mother. It is a major cause of morbidity and mortality in both the mother and fetus. The only 'curative' management is to stabilise the woman and either birth the baby or remove all products of conception in the event of a miscarriage.

Q3: After the attempt to induce labour failed, the consultant obstetrician performed a caesarean. Assuming that the birth was successful and the baby was born alive, which of the statements about the follow-up management are true?

This question requires an understanding of the follow-up management of preterm birth in the context of a complication (chorioamnionitis). The patient has undergone an unplanned caesarean because she is septic and her fetus was deemed to be in distress. Prior to birth, the obstetrician would have discussed her options with her regarding the subsequent care for her baby, as she is giving birth to an infant at the threshold of viability (23⁺⁰ to 24⁺⁶ weeks' gestation).

A ✔ **The neonate may be admitted to NICU for close monitoring** – True. Most babies under 34 weeks are admitted, as they may require feeding support, temperature control, antibiotics and respiratory support. However, at this gestation, resuscitation may not be started at all, particularly if the baby is very small, and the parents do not want resuscitation. If the baby is resuscitated, advanced interventions like giving adrenaline would be deemed not in the baby's best interest, as by that stage, the prognosis would be so poor.

B ✔ **The placenta and fetal membranes will be sent away for histopathology and microbiology tests** – True. Subsequent antibiotic treatment of the baby will be dependent on the results of these placental swabs and microscopic analysis of the fetal membranes.

C ✔ **The woman should be monitored for the complications of caesarean birth** – True. For a caesarean carried out in the context of systemic infection, women should be monitored carefully in the postpartum period, observing for factors such as bleeding, uterine atony and disseminated intravascular coagulopathy.

D ✔ **The neonate may be given a septic screen and a course of broad-spectrum IV antibiotics** – True. Empiric broad-spectrum IV antibiotics are given as first-line treatment to protect the baby against both aerobic and anaerobic organisms, for example, benzylpenicillin and gentamicin. Thereafter, the regimen of antibiotic therapy can be tailored according to the results obtained from the babies' blood cultures and the placental swabs.

E If the woman stabilises after birth, she can be discharged on a course of oral antibiotics with no need for further outpatient follow-up of any sort – False. Based on the RCOG guidelines, there is currently no evidence on the optimum postnatal follow-up management for the mother. However, a follow-up appointment with an experienced obstetrician should be offered to parents whose infant is born at the threshold of viability. This is to address issues such as the risk of recurrence and the management of a future pregnancy, as well as any other questions that the parents might have.

> 💬 **Key Point**
>
> The woman should be counselled that the outcome is likely to be poor, particularly as she is septic. If the baby does survive, they will be in hospital for several months. There is also a high risk of long-term morbidity, such as chronic lung disease, neonatal sepsis, cerebral palsy and other complications associated with prematurity. The woman will ideally have the opportunity to make an informed decision prior to delivery to consider whether her baby should be resuscitated and given intensive care, only a trial of treatment to see if the baby responds to it or to be provided with palliative care.

Q4: What is the most appropriate management of a woman known to have vaginal colonisation with group B streptococcus?

The correct answer is B. Benzylpenicillin treatment during labour.

GBS are common bacteria, found in the vagina and gut, which can rarely be transmitted to the neonate during birth with potentially devastating consequences.

GBS are usually commensal bacteria, found in up to 3 in 10 women in the UK and transmitted by skin-to-skin contact. They are not normally pathological but can be associated with UTIs and chorioamnionitis. Women with diabetes, cardiovascular disease and renal disease are at increased risk of pathological, symptomatic GBS infection. In most cases, pregnant women who are GBS carriers are able to carry and birth their babies without any adverse consequences. The bacteria can, uncommonly, be transmitted to the neonate in utero and during birth, which rarely can lead to early labour, stillbirth or neonatal sepsis. This risk is increased in premature babies if the mother is febrile during labour or with premature rupture of membranes.

A Advise birth by planned caesarean and benzylpenicillin treatment antenatally during any subsequent pregnancies – Incorrect. GBS infection is not an indication for either elective caesarean or antenatal antibiotics.

B ✔ **Benzylpenicillin treatment during labour** – Correct. GBS is not screened for in pregnancy in the UK, but women who are known to be GBS carriers are offered antibiotic treatment during labour.

C Advise birth by planned caesarean – Incorrect. GBS infection is not an indication for elective caesarean.

D Benzylpenicillin treatment antenatally – Incorrect. GBS infection is not an indication for antenatal antibiotics.

E Benzylpenicillin treatment antenatally during any subsequent pregnancies – Incorrect. GBS infection is not an indication for antenatal antibiotics in this or subsequent pregnancies.

> 💬 **Key Point**
>
> Women should be reassured that GBS infection is common and, in the majority of cases, is not associated with any adverse consequences for either mother or baby.

> 🔍 **Important Learning Points**
>
> - Chorioamnionitis is an infection of the fetal membranes or amniotic fluid that can occur before or during labour.
> - Symptoms include maternal pyrexia, maternal and fetal tachycardia, uterine tenderness or excess vaginal discharge that is purulent and/or discoloured.
> - Chorioamnionitis may result in complications that could affect both the infant and the woman. Early recognition and treatment of infection is important in reducing the risk of these complications.
> - Chorioamnionitis does not usually significantly affect the future fertility of the mother.

SMALL-FOR-GESTATIONAL-AGE BABIES AND INTRAUTERINE GROWTH RESTRICTION

Q1: Following the abnormalities detected in this ultrasound growth scan, which investigation should now be conducted to assess the well-being of the fetus?

The correct answer is C. Umbilical artery Doppler.

Multiple methods are used to detect SGA fetuses, of which a proportion will have IUGR. For monitoring the fetal well-being, umbilical artery Doppler should be the primary surveillance tool. Note that one individual test alone does not tend to be predictive of outcome in IUGR. Therefore, multiple tests are generally used, and a collection of abnormal results may indicate pathology. It is the overall growth trend that is of more importance in diagnosing IUGR.

A Fetal CTG – Incorrect. Use of CTG is not specific to IUGR fetuses, and its use in the antepartum period to assess fetal condition has not been found to be associated with better perinatal outcome.

B SFH measurements – Incorrect. SFH measurements are regularly taken to attempt to identify possible IUGR pregnancies to refer for ultrasound scan. The sensitivity and specificity of this test are increased with serial measurements and when using a customised growth chart. However, this does not monitor the well-being of the fetus.

C ✔ **Umbilical artery Doppler** – Correct. For monitoring fetal well-being, umbilical artery Doppler should be the primary surveillance tool. It has, in fact, been found that umbilical artery Doppler is the only test that has significant value in predicting poor perinatal outcomes in IUGR fetuses. The most concerning findings on Doppler are absent or reversed end diastolic flow, as this demonstrates that there is no fetal blood moving to the placenta to exchange nutrients and toxins with the maternal circulation during the end of the fetal diastolic phase.

D Serial ultrasound growth scans – Incorrect. AC and EFW are the most accurate diagnostic measurements used to diagnose IUGR. Conversely, this is a biometric test which does not assess the well-being of the fetus. Serial growth scans are commonly undertaken for IUGR fetuses to aid decisions regarding the appropriate timing of birth.

E Fetal movement monitoring – Incorrect. Although women are often asked to monitor fetal movements, this is a very crude measurement of fetal well-being. If a mother reports decreased fetal movements, this should be taken seriously and investigated further, initially with CTG monitoring and in recurrent cases of reduced movements with ultrasound scan. While it was generally believed that a poorly nourished fetus may move less to conserve energy, multiple studies have failed to demonstrate correlations in routine fetal movement counting.

 Key Point

There are biometric tests, which measure the size of the fetus, and biophysical tests, which are used to assess fetal well-being. This is an important difference, as biometric tests are used to imply a diagnosis of SGA (though serial measures can imply growth restriction), whereas biophysical tests are used to indicate whether the fetus is at risk of compromise.

Q2: Answer true or false: Which of the following are risk factors for IUGR?

As outlined, risk factors for IUGR can be divided into maternal, fetal and placental. Fetal growth is determined largely by the genetic makeup of the fetus; however, maternal factors also play a role.

A ✔ **Increasing maternal age** – True. Maternal age of 35 years or above has been associated with an increased risk of IUGR, with a further increased risk after 40 years.

B ✔ **Maternal illegal drug use** – True. Drugs such as cocaine and amphetamines may cause a decrease in fetal growth. Tobacco and alcohol have also been linked to IUGR babies, and the effects of cigarette smoking are dose dependent. Cocaine use during pregnancy is the most significant illegal drug associated with IUGR.

C ✔ **Raised maternal BP** – True. Chronic hypertension has an odds ratio of 2.5 for SGA. BP alone is also a risk factor for pre-eclampsia, which has been strongly linked to IUGR. Hypertension, when associated with severe renal impairment, has also been associated with an increased risk of IUGR.

D ✔ **Maternal nutrition** – True. Small variations in diet are not likely to have an effect on fetal growth. However, extreme starvation does cause significant growth impairment. This is also thought to be a factor in teenage pregnancies, where the mother is still growing so there may be some competition for available nutrients for growth.

E Maternal rhesus-negative status – False. The rhesus status of the mother is not linked to IUGR pregnancies. However, rhesus disease can cause severe fetal and neonatal anaemia and fetal hydrops which may lead to IUGR, but this is rare.

 Key Point

The most important factor considered by many clinicians is how the placenta is functioning. In IUGR, the fetus is the end organ, and therefore a pathological or poorly functioning placenta may be recognised by insufficient fetal growth.

Q3: If Kaitlin opted for first-trimester screening, a low level of which biochemical marker taken is independently associated with an increased risk of having a growth-restricted baby?

The correct answer is C. PAPP-A.

As part of routine antenatal care, all women in the UK are offered screening to assess their chance of having a baby with Down, Edward or Patau syndrome (trisomies 21, 18 and 13). This is usually done during the dating scan (10 to 14 weeks) in a form of a combined test. The nuchal translucency measurement from the ultrasound, as well as levels of two biochemical markers – bHCG and PAPP-A – together with maternal age are used to calculate the chance of baby having any of the mentioned three syndromes. After 14 weeks, nuchal translucency cannot be measured accurately; therefore, a combined test cannot be offered. Instead, a quadruple test can be done to assess chances of trisomy 21 in the baby only. Quadruple test consists of levels of four markers: alpha-fetoprotein (AFP), hCG, inhibin-A and unconjugated oestriol (uE3). Due to their placental origin, several of those biochemical markers have been investigated as screening tests for a growth-restricted fetus.

A   hCG – Incorrect. In the largest study of use of first-trimester markers to predict SGA fetus, there was no association between low levels of hCG and SGA risk. hCG is highly used in early pregnancy to monitor women with pregnancy of unknown location.

B   AFP – Incorrect. Second-trimester markers (used in quadruple test) have not been shown to have a strong association with risk of growth restriction. AFP is a major plasma protein produced by the yolk sac and the fetal liver during fetal development. It can also be used as a tumour marker of germ cell tumours and hepatocellular carcinoma.

C   ✔ PAPP-A – Correct. Low levels (<0.415 MoM) are considered a major risk factor for having a growth-restricted baby. Women with low PAPP-A levels should be offered additional growth scans during their pregnancies.

D   Inhibin-A – Incorrect. Second-trimester markers (used in quadruple test) have not been shown to have a strong association with growth restriction risk. During the menstrual cycle, inhibin-A inhibits the release of FSH from the pituitary to inhibit folliculogenesis.

E   uE3 – Incorrect. Second-trimester markers (used in quadruple test) have not been shown to have a strong association with growth restriction risk. Low levels of uE3 may indicate the presence of trisomies 13, 18 and 21.

> ### Important Learning Points
>
> - IUGR refers to the failure of the fetus to reach its genetically predetermined size. This can therefore occur at any centile but is significantly more common below the 10th centile.
> - Monitoring fetal growth on a customised growth chart is crucial when making the diagnosis.
> - Poor placental function is thought to be the most important risk factor for IUGR.
> - Umbilical artery Doppler is the gold standard for monitoring fetal well-being.

- IUGR has been linked to immediate and lifelong complications, such as diabetes and cardiovascular disease. Hence, appropriate antenatal management is important, as it can have long-term effects.
- However, currently, the only management strategy is timely delivery of the baby, with antenatal corticosteroids.

HAEMOLYTIC DISEASE OF THE FETUS AND NEWBORN

Q1: HDFN is due to a hypersensitivity pathophysiology of which type?
The correct answer is B. Type II hypersensitivity.

Immune responses are normally protective but are capable of causing tissue injury in hypersensitivity reactions. Hypersensitivity reactions are divided into four types, each with a different underlying immune mechanism responsible. Types I, II and III are antibody mediated, with type IV being T cell mediated.

A   Type I hypersensitivity – Incorrect. This is due to the production of IgE antibodies in response to allergens and is more common in atopic individuals.

B   ✔ **Type II hypersensitivity** – Correct. This is due to IgG or IgM antibodies directed against target antigens on the cell surface, resulting in the activation of complement or phagocytosis.

C   Type III hypersensitivity – Incorrect. This is due to circulating IgG or IgM antibodies which form immune complexes with antigens in the blood and deposit it in the blood vessels of various organs, triggering complement activation and acute inflammation.

D   Type IV hypersensitivity – Incorrect. This is due to T cell-mediated cytotoxicity and is also known as delayed-type hypersensitivity, as T cell responses can take up to 12 to 48 hours to occur.

E   Type V hypersensitivity – Incorrect. This is an additional type of hypersensitivity not recognised in all countries; it is a variation of type II. Type V impairs cell signalling by antibodies that bind to cell surface receptors, for example, in Graves disease or myasthenia gravis.

> ### Key Point
>
> Circulating fetal phagocytes express receptors for the Fc component of the maternal IgG antibody and for complement protein breakdown products. Once the target cell (fetal erythrocyte in HDFN) becomes coated in the antibody (opsonisation), it becomes vulnerable to phagocytosis or complement-mediated lysis.

Q2: Answer true or false: Which of the following increase the chance of alloimmunisation sensitisation for HDFN?
Sensitisation is the process by which the maternal immune system detects the presence of a 'foreign' antigen on the fetal

red blood cells and mounts a humoral immune response. This can result in the production of IgG antibodies against the fetal antigen, which may cross the placenta and destroy fetal erythrocytes.

A ✔ **Previous birth of a rhesus D-positive neonate** – True. Fetomaternal haemorrhage can occur in previous pregnancies, causing sensitisation.

B Gestational diabetes – False. Gestational diabetes does not increase the risk of fetomaternal haemorrhage.

C ✔ **Amniocentesis** – True. This invasive uterine procedure carried out at 15 to 20 weeks gestation detects genetic variants in the fetus such as Down syndrome, spina bifida and sickle cell anaemia. A needle is used to aspirate a sample of amniotic fluid, which contains cells shed by the fetus. CVS is an alternative diagnostic test used from 10 to 13 weeks gestation. Both procedures carry a small risk of fetomaternal haemorrhage.

D Maternal nutrition – False. Maternal nutrition can modulate the immune response of the mother and child and affect fetal development, but nutrition does not increase the risk of fetal and maternal blood mixing.

E ✔ **Trauma** – True. Trauma can be mild and induce small tears in the placenta that allow small amounts of fetal blood to enter the maternal circulation, or it can be severe enough to cause placental abruption and threaten the pregnancy entirely.

> **Key Point**
>
> HDFN due to rhesus incompatibility can only occur in rhesus-negative mothers. There is, however, a small risk of severe HDFN occurring due to other more rare antibodies, but this is not a clinical event that can commonly be predicted.

Q3: At which week(s) of gestation should exogenous anti-D antibody be given to rhesus D-negative women with no history of sensitising events?

The correct answer is C. 28 weeks.

Prevention of HDFN is achieved by giving exogenous anti-D antibody to the woman. This binds to the rhesus D antigen on fetal erythrocytes that have entered the maternal circulation, preventing sensitisation and therefore the production of maternal anti-D IgG, which can cross the placenta and cause HDFN.

> **Key Point**
>
> There are two regimens for prophylactic anti-D immunoglobulin. In one regimen, a dose of anti-D IgG is given at 28 weeks and 34 weeks gestation. The more common regime in the UK is a single larger dose at 28 weeks. The iatrogenic anti-D IgG can cross the placenta but does not have any detrimental effect on fetal well-being.

> **Important Learning Points**
>
> - HDFN is an alloimmune response mediated by the production of maternal antibodies against fetal erythrocyte surface antigens in the ABO, rhesus or Kell antigen systems.
> - Sensitising events during pregnancy are required for rhesus disease to occur and involve the mixing of rhesus-positive fetal blood with rhesus-negative maternal blood.
> - Rhesus-negative mothers are given prophylactic anti-D immunoglobulin during pregnancy to mask the rhesus D antigens on fetal erythrocytes that may have entered the maternal circulation. This prevents the mother from mounting a type II hypersensitivity reaction against the fetal antigen.
> - At birth, a Kleihauer test is performed to titrate the amount of anti-D immunoglobulin to give the woman. This prevents sensitisation from potential fetomaternal haemorrhage during parturition, reducing the risk of HDFN in subsequent pregnancies.

CONGENITAL INTRAUTERINE INFECTIONS

A good understanding of the presenting symptoms is essential in identifying the correct cause and treatment of infections. A delay in identifying the cause can lead to serious long-term complications for both the woman and baby.

Q1: Which antibody, if present in the booking bloods in an asymptomatic woman, suggests previous infection and subsequent acquired immunity?

The correct answer is D. IgG.

Understanding the physiology underlying the order that antibodies are produced during the immune system's response to an infection is crucial for determining whether this is an active infection or previous infection that resulted in acquired immunity. IgM immunoglobulins are the first antibodies to be produced in response to a foreign antigen and can reappear, to a lesser extent, if there is further exposure to that pathogen. IgG antibodies then form part of the secondary immune response, and these either suggest past infection or can suggest acquired immunity, as they persist after the infection has resolved. It is important, therefore, to be able to compare the presence of antibodies in previous blood samples to determine this. Only IgG antibodies are capable of crossing the placenta.

> **Key Point**
>
> Passive immunity of the neonate is supplied by IgG antibodies which crossed the placenta *in utero* and IgA antibodies which are present in breast milk. Relatively little is known about IgD in comparison to the other classes of immunoglobulin. IgE has important roles in allergy and in diseases such as asthma and atopic dermatitis.

Q2: Answer true or false regarding the following statements related to chickenpox.

Chickenpox during pregnancy is only an issue for women who have never been exposed to the varicella zoster virus or had chickenpox themselves. As soon as a woman is immune, there is no further risk to the pregnancy or the fetus in the long term. It is therefore important to know any pregnant person's immune status to determine if they are at risk of complications.

A ✔ **The incubation period is 10 to 20 days** – True. The incubation period of the herpes zoster virus is 10 days to 3 weeks, which can be remembered simply as 10 to 20 days. The incubation period is defined as the time between initially acquiring the virus and the first presentation of symptoms.

B The classic lesion shape is annular – False. A typical description of the rash in chickenpox is erythematous papular lesions that start on the trunk and spread to the face and extremities, often described as rose petal shape. The lesions evolve to develop a clear fluid-filled vesicle that becomes cloudy and then breaks, leading to a crusty lesion. This can then form a scar over time. Annular lesions are ring-shaped.

C ✔ **An individual is only infective until the lesions have crusted over** – True. It is the fluid in the vesicles that is highly contagious in varicella. Therefore, once a crust has formed, the lesion is no longer infective. However, new lesions often crop up every few days; thus, the individual is only considered to be noncontagious when all lesions have crusted over.

D Reinfection of chickenpox is common after an initial exposure – False. Individuals will usually only be affected by chickenpox once in their lives. Reactivation of Herpes zoster can occur in shingles, but reinfection is usually only seen in severely immunocompromised patients, such as those undergoing chemotherapy.

E Shingles can sometimes lead to death if it completely encircles the abdomen – False. It is possible for shingles to form a circle around the trunk because it affects dermatomes due to its pathophysiology in the distribution of the sensory nerve root ganglia, but this in itself will not lead to mortality.

🗨 Key Point

Ninety percent of women in the UK are immune to chickenpox, most commonly because they had the disease when they were children. However, women from other countries in the world, are less likely to be immune, which can be a greater issue not only for pregnancy but also because chickenpox affects adults more severely than children. It is therefore important to consider the mother's birthplace and location history.

Q3: A 14-week-pregnant woman presents with flulike symptoms. On examination, you notice scratches on her forearm.

The correct answer is A. Toxoplasmosis.

With the patient presenting with such vague symptoms, toxoplasmosis, erythema infectiosum and CMV could all be possibilities. However, the scratch marks are a risk factor for toxoplasmosis, as feline-related faeces exposure could transmit the disease.

Q4: A 34-weeks-pregnant woman presents to GUM services for the first time, complaining of painful genital lesions.

The correct answer is F. Herpes simplex virus.

Painful genital lesions are most likely to be caused by HSV. Since this is her first presentation, the patient should be referred to an obstetrician for further management. Women contracting primary HSV within 6 weeks of estimated delivery should be offered a caesarean.

Q5: A 28-week-pregnant woman presents with arthropathy, fever, headache and a sore throat.

The correct answer is B. Erythema infectiosum.

Erythema infectiosum accounts for the presentation of these symptoms. This disease has typically an almost biphasic clinical course, where patients experience flulike symptoms for the first week. In the following week, patients may begin to experience arthralgia. Erythema infectiosum is associated with high complication rates during the first trimester; however, even after pregnancy has progressed beyond that point, fetal complications like hydrops fetalis may still occur. Therefore, serial ultrasound scans are required for close follow-up.

Q6: A 1-year-old infant is seen in clinic with microcephaly, chorioretinitis and motor delay.

The correct answer is K. CMV.

CMV is the most common congenital infection. After infection during pregnancy, infants born with the infection may not show symptoms immediately. Long-term sequelae may develop, such as chorioretinitis, developmental delay, microcephaly and motor impairment, but may not be seen until after the neonatal period.

Q7: A newborn presents with jaundice, hepatosplenomegaly and cataracts. In addition, there are purpuric rashes on his body.

The correct answer is D. Rubella.

More specifically, the newborn has presented with congenital rubella syndrome (CRS). The appearance of the purpuric rash can be described as a 'blueberry muffin baby'. This appearance is from a combination of lesions caused by extramedullary haematopoiesis and hyperbilirubinaemia. Infants with CRS must be monitored closely for the first 12 months of life, primarily for signs of hearing impairment and developmental abnormalities.

 Key Point

'Blueberry muffin baby' was a term used originally to describe rubella, but other diseases can also cause this cutaneous manifestation. It is usually associated with a pathological process starting in utero. Other causes include infection, haemolysis, malignancy and hereditary spherocytosis.

Important Learning Points

- TORCH can be a useful mnemonic – toxoplasmosis, other (syphilis, varicella-zoster, parvovirus B19, hepatitis B and HIV), rubella, CMV and herpes infections.
- These diseases may present similarly, so it is important to consider subtle differences in the symptoms and signs to direct your investigations.
- It is important to consider the mother's vaccination history and history of previous infections to determine what infections she may be at risk of. If in doubt, check the booking bloods for previously acquired immunity by examining presence of specific IgG antibodies.

STILLBIRTH

Q1: Which clinical finding is necessary to definitively diagnose stillbirth?

The correct answer is C. Absent fetal heartbeat on real-time ultrasound.

It is crucial to have a definitive diagnosis of stillbirth. Although certain clinical signs, such as absent fetal movement or absent heartbeat on auscultation, are useful for identifying a possible fetal death, these findings must be confirmed using real-time ultrasound. It is also preferable to seek a second opinion to confirm the diagnosis.

A Absent fetal heartbeat on CTG – Incorrect. Although CTG is a useful tool for identifying fetal distress, the accuracy of this test is insufficient to give a definitive diagnosis of fetal demise. There is a risk that CTG can record maternal heart rate rather than fetal, so potentially a normal appearance of a CTG can be from the mother in the presence of intrauterine death. Conversely, the absence of heart rate on CTG can be caused by incorrect placement of the CTG probe or maternal obesity.

B Absent fetal heartbeat on Doppler ultrasound – Incorrect. Doppler ultrasound may give inaccurate findings, suggesting fetal death in viable fetuses. However, it is often used as a precursor to real-time ultrasound if the patient reports reduced fetal movements.

C ✔ Absent fetal heartbeat on real-time ultrasound – Correct. Real-time ultrasound allows the clinician to visualise the fetal heart and thereby confirm the absence of fetal heartbeat. This can be augmented with colour Doppler, which helps to identify fetal blood flow through the heart chambers and umbilical cord.

D Absent fetal movement on real-time ultrasound – Incorrect. Absent fetal movements give an indication of fetal death and are useful for determining whether there are no signs of life, but identification of absent fetal cardiac activity is crucial for a definitive diagnosis.

E Absent fetal movement on abdominal palpation – Incorrect. Reduced fetal movements are associated with fetal growth restriction and stillbirth. The number of fetal movements a woman experiences per day can vary considerably between different patients. Women should be advised to contact their midwives or maternity units if they are concerned about a reduction in fetal movements. Two or more episodes of reduced fetal movements are associated with poor perinatal outcomes, such as stillbirth and prematurity. Reduced or absent fetal movements provide insufficient evidence to diagnose stillbirth. In contrast, some women may still report feeling movements after fetal death. These factors should be considered in making a diagnosis and communicating with the woman.

 Key Point

Real-time ultrasound can give an indication of how long a fetus has been retained in utero after death. There may be signs of maceration, skull collapse and oedema. Certain causes of fetal death can also be identified by ultrasound, such as hydrops fetalis, which is where fluid accumulates in multiple fetal compartments, such as the brain, lungs and pericardium.

Q2: Answer true or false: Regarding this case where the woman is well, with her membranes intact and her uterus unscarred.

In this case, it would be suitable for a consultant obstetrician to confirm the diagnosis and deliver the bad news. If the woman was well and her membranes were intact, management options would be discussed, including the potential to induce labour, if this was her preference. If this was the case, she would be given a combination of mifepristone and a prostaglandin preparation, as this particular woman has not had a previous caesarean. A meeting with a bereavement counsellor would be arranged, and at the woman's request, the team could arrange for her to hold her baby after birth.

A ✔ Vaginal birth is most appropriate in this case – True. This is the case of an otherwise well woman with no uterine scarring or other medical issues; therefore, vaginal birth is appropriate. Guidelines state that vaginal birth is the recommended mode of birth for most women. Vaginal birth can usually be achieved within 24 hours of induction of labour. The first-line intervention for a woman with an unscarred uterus is a combination of mifepristone and a prostaglandin preparation.

B Caesarean birth is most appropriate in this case – False. There are no indications in this case for caesarean and caesarean birth would increase the time needed to recover and slow the woman's return home. However, women may request caesarean because of previous experiences or because of a desire to avoid the vaginal birth of a dead baby.

C It is important that the fetus is born as quickly as possible – False. As this woman is otherwise well, a more flexible approach can be discussed. It has, however, been shown that an increased time between diagnosis and birth has been linked to increasing levels of anxiety. Although immediate management is not necessary, if labour is delayed for more than 48 hours, then the woman should be advised to have testing for disseminated intravascular coagulation twice weekly.

D ✔ **The value of a postmortem examination decreases the longer the fetus is retained *in utero*** – True. It should also be taken into consideration for women who are willing to have a postmortem that if they prolong expectant management, then the value of postmortem may be reduced. In this time, the appearance of the baby may also deteriorate, which can be very distressing for the woman.

E ✔ **Recommendations about labour and birth should take into account the woman's preferences** – True. Stillbirth is a very emotionally traumatic time for women and their families. It is therefore important that, wherever medically possible, the woman's preferences are taken into consideration, as well as her medical conditions and previous intrapartum history.

> **💬 Key Point**
>
> Recommendations about how to deliver a stillborn baby should take into account the mother's preferences, as well as her medical condition and previous intrapartum history. This decision does not always need to be rushed. However, if there is sepsis, pre-eclampsia, placental abruption or membrane rupture, then women should be strongly advised to take immediate steps towards birth.

Q3: Answer true or false: Which of the following investigations should be recommended to all women who deliver a stillborn fetus?

Certain clinical investigations, such as fetal karyotyping, are useful for determining the cause of fetal death, whilst other investigations, such as an FBC, are used to assess maternal health. A stillborn fetus can cause maternal death when retained in utero; therefore, managing maternal health is a priority. Although the majority of women will want to know the cause of fetal death, the decision to investigate is at the couple's discretion. Many investigations, including postmortem examination of the fetus, require written consent from the parents.

A Maternal blood culture – False. Maternal blood culture is only recommended when there is evidence of maternal sepsis, such as fever and hypovolaemia, purulent or offensive liquor or prolonged rupture of membranes.

B ✔ **Kleihauer test** – True. A Kleihauer test measures the amount of fetal haemoglobin in maternal serum and is used to quantify maternofetal haemorrhage. Severe maternofetal haemorrhage can result from placental abruption, which causes approximately 10% of all stillbirths. In a rhesus-negative woman, a Kleihauer test is vital for calculating the optimal dose of anti-rhesus D gamma globulin to prevent a sensitising reaction, which can be potentially life-threatening. Guidelines recommend that all women should receive a Kleihauer test, even rhesus-positive women.

C ✔ **Full blood count and liver function tests** – True. Maternal blood tests are important for assessing maternal health after fetal death. These tests are used to identify disseminated intravascular coagulation, maternal sepsis and haemorrhage. They can also identify conditions associated with stillbirth such as obstetric cholestasis and the complications of pre-eclampsia.

D Maternal thrombophilia screen – False. Although commonly tested routinely for all stillbirths in many centres in the UK, national guidelines only recommend testing in women who have delivered a stillborn with IUGR or evidence of multiple thrombi in the placenta. Even though there is an association with the condition and stillbirth, it remains uncertain whether thrombophilia is a direct cause of stillbirth.

E ✔ **Postmortem of the baby and placental examination** – True. Postmortem examination of the fetus and placenta is recommended to all patients diagnosing the cause of stillbirth. Written consent must be obtained for autopsy and karyotyping to be performed. If the parents do not give consent, this test is absolutely contraindicated. Parents who do consent to this investigation must be informed that, despite investigation, it is still likely that no cause may be identified.

> **💬 Key Point**
>
> There are multiple investigations that can be offered after a woman has experienced a stillbirth. However, often these do not indicate a specific cause or inform future pregnancies.

> **🔍 Important Learning Points**
>
> - Many stillbirths remain unexplained even after investigation. Causes may be related to the mother, fetus or placenta.
> - The optimal method for diagnosing stillbirth is real-time ultrasonography, often augmented with colour Doppler of the fetal heart and umbilical cord.
> - The management of a pregnancy affected by stillbirth and subsequent pregnancies following this require

obstetrician-led management and may vary depending on the woman's wishes. The key areas are birth, investigations and psychosocial management.

- It is important to investigate the underlying cause of the stillbirth to determine if any steps can be taken in subsequent pregnancies to reduce the risk of recurrence.

15 OBSTETRIC EMERGENCIES

CORD PROLAPSE

Q1: What is the average drop in fetal pH for every minute that the umbilical cord is compressed during a cord prolapse?
The correct answer is D. 0.04.

Normal cord pH at birth is considered to be around 7.25. There is significant risk of long-term neonatal morbidity and mortality below a pH of 7.0. Intrapartum stressors such as hyperstimulation, infection and, in this case, cord prolapse can cause increasing hypoxia and acidosis either due to reduced blood supply from the placenta or increased metabolic demand. During these stressors, the pH will drop by 0.04 every minute.

 Key Point

If bladder filling has been used as a strategy to elevate the presenting part in a cord prolapse, it is important to clamp the catheter once 500 mL has been instilled. It is essential that the bladder is then emptied just before any method of birth is attempted.

Q2: Answer true or false: Which of the following are risk factors for cord prolapse?

The main precipitating event for cord prolapse is rupture of membranes, whether this is spontaneous or iatrogenic. Therefore, it is essential that any clinician performing an ARM palpates the membranes vaginally prior to rupturing them to rule out the presence of the umbilical cord between the membranes and the presenting part of the fetus.

A ✔ **Raised liquor volume** – True. Polyhydramnios increases the amount of space in the uterus for the fetus to occupy. It is therefore more free to move and less likely to engage in the pelvis. Polyhydramnios also increases the risk of preterm rupture of membranes. If this occurs when the fetal head is not engaged in the pelvis, the umbilical cord could lie in the pelvis and prolapse through the cervix.

B ✔ **Multiple pregnancy** – True. In a multiple pregnancy, the uterus is greatly distended, and the positioning of the fetuses can mean poor pelvic engagement of the presenting part of the first fetus. However, during vaginal birth of twins, the highest risk of cord prolapse is for twin two, immediately after the birth of twin one, as there is more space in the uterus and it is easier for the cord to slip down before a presenting part of the fetus.

C ✔ **Low-lying placenta** – True. A low-lying placenta or placenta praevia not covering the cervical os are risk factors for cord prolapse. This is because the placenta can prevent the fetal presenting part from entering below the pelvic brim, so it is not engaged. This means there is increased risk of the cord presenting and prolapsing in the event of membrane rupture.

D Assisted vaginal birth – False. Assisted vaginal birth is not a risk factor for cord prolapse. An assisted vaginal birth is used to mimic spontaneous vaginal birth when there are some complications or delays in unassisted birth. To even attempt assisted vaginal birth, a prerequisite is that the fetal head is at a low station, so the cord cannot prolapse around it. Assisted vaginal birth may be used in the management of cord prolapse in some situations, but it is not a risk factor.

E Maternal chronic hypertension – False. This is not a recognised risk factor for cord prolapse. Chronic hypertension is defined as a maternal BP of more than or equal to 140/90 mmHg on two occasions before 20 weeks gestation.

 Key Point

The majority of risk factors predispose to cord prolapse by preventing the presenting fetal part having a close association with the pelvic brim. If there is a poor association, there is an increased space between the fetal presenting part and the pelvic brim, and therefore, there is an increased chance the cord can prolapse through.

Q3: Which maternal or fetal features may indicate a cord prolapse?
The correct answers are A. Fetal bradycardia **and E.** Fetal decelerations on CTG.

Cord prolapse should be suspected when there are abnormalities on a CTG, particularly if there is a sudden bradycardia shortly after rupture of membranes. A vaginal examination is needed to then assess and make the diagnosis.

A ✔ **Fetal bradycardia** – Correct. This is one of the classic signs of cord prolapse which can be identified by auscultation in low-risk women or on CTG in high-risk labours. When cord prolapse occurs, the cord can be compressed in the birth canal. When this happens, fetal hypoxia can occur, which, in turn, causes bradycardia. Once this is detected, it is vital to act quickly: a vaginal examination must be performed to exclude cord prolapse. A persistent fetal bradycardia for any reason will require urgent delivery to reduce the chance of fetal morbidity and mortality.

B Maternal tachycardia – Incorrect. Maternal tachycardia does not classically indicate cord prolapse. For cord prolapse, there are likely to be no maternal symptoms. Maternal tachycardia can indicate other problems such as sepsis, shock or anxiety. It is important to monitor and investigate the cause of maternal tachycardia.

C Maternal abdominal pain – Incorrect. This is not an indicator for cord prolapse. It is possible that the woman will have no symptoms or signs if she has a prolapsed cord.

D Fetal accelerations on CTG – Incorrect. This is not a risk factor for cord prolapse. Fetal accelerations are seen on a CTG as rapid increases in fetal heart rate above the baseline with onset to peak of the acceleration less than 30 seconds long. They are a reassuring sign, as they rarely occur with fetal distress and are usually associated with spontaneous fetal movements.

E ✔ **Decelerations on CTG** – Correct. An acute change in the CTG, particularly if this has occurred after membrane rupture, should raise the suspicion of cord prolapse. Prolonged fetal bradycardia is the most common and worrying CTG feature, as it demonstrates acute compromise. If the cord prolapses, it may initially only be compromised during contractions as the cord is compressed, with easing of the compression after the contraction. This can lead to slowing of the fetal heart rate (decelerations), which can then recover. However, if not identified and managed, the prolapsed cord will become increasingly compromised, leading to increasing fetal distress and CTG deteriorations. So where there are signs of fetal distress on a CTG, review must include a vaginal exam to assess for cord prolapse.

Key Point

It would be unlikely that a woman would say that she feels a cord prolapse. It is most commonly diagnosed following observation of an abnormal fetal heart trace, leading a health professional to perform a vaginal examination and subsequently feel a prolapsed cord.

Important Learning Points

- Cord prolapse is an obstetric emergency characterised by descent of the umbilical cord through the cervix to the level of, or past, the presenting fetal part.
- Like any obstetric emergency, the midwives, obstetricians, anaesthetists and neonatologists are all required to achieve an effective outcome for mother and child. The most senior team members should be called for obstetric emergencies.
- Several techniques can be adopted to assist in improving fetal oxygenation and reducing umbilical cord vasospasm.
- The mainstay of management is to deliver the fetus as quickly and safely as possible.

SHOULDER DYSTOCIA

Q1: If shoulder dystocia is suspected, what is the first position or manoeuvre to encourage the woman to adopt?
The correct answer is B. McRoberts manoeuvre.

Shoulder dystocia is an obstetric emergency needing immediate attention. Each manoeuvre should be attempted for a maximum of 30 seconds, as this is an emergency where seconds count. Evidence recommends the use of McRoberts position as the initial position to try, as it is the most effective. McRoberts manoeuvre alone has been quoted to have success rates of up to 90%.

A Left lateral decubitus position – Incorrect. Use of the left lateral decubitus position may be used during obstetric spinal anaesthesia. In this position, the mother is stable and on a hard surface, so the spinous processes can be easily visualised and palpated to allow for safe anaesthesia.

B ✔ **McRoberts manoeuvre** – Correct. In this manoeuvre, the mother has to lie flat on her back without pillows or support. Her legs are then hyperflexed, bringing her knees up toward her ears. Routine traction from assistants on each leg can help the mother keep this position. The aim of McRoberts is to increase the anteroposterior diameter of the pelvic inlet and to optimise vaginal access for assisted delivery.

C Lithotomy position – Incorrect. In the lithotomy position, the patient's feet are held up in the air, with their knees above the hips. The patient's legs are often held in stirrups to assist. This is the position used in medical examinations, assisted vaginal births and surgical procedures of the lower pelvis.

D Zavanelli manoeuvre – Incorrect. Although this is a manoeuvre that can, in rare situations, be used in shoulder dystocia, it is not the first line, as it poses a high mortality risk to both the mother and fetus. The principle of the manoeuvre is to push the fetal head back within the birth canal and to sustain this position until a caesarean is performed.

E Squatting position – Incorrect. Squatting in labour can expand the pelvic bony dimensions and facilitate birth. While women often adopt the squatting position during labour, it is not recommended for management of shoulder dystocia.

Key Point

The acronym HELPPER can be useful for remembering how to manage shoulder dystocia.
- Help – call for the obstetric emergency team immediately.
- Evaluation for episiotomy – is this required and appropriate to allow more room for internal manoeuvres?
- Legs – move both legs into the McRoberts position.
- Pressure – suprapubic pressure applied and in a rocking motion.
- Posterior arm – attempt to remove the posterior arm.
- Enter – to attempt internal manoeuvres.
- Roll over – move onto all fours, where manoeuvres can be attempted again in this position.

Q2: A 26-year-old woman with a BMI of 31 kg/m² had a planned caesarean in her first pregnancy for placenta praevia. She is currently in labour and requires assistance with forceps to aid in the birth of the baby. She has an epidural in place for analgesia. From the options above, which factor is the most important risk factor for shoulder dystocia?

The correct answer is A. Assisted vaginal birth.

Evidence suggests that assisted births are more likely to be complicated by shoulder dystocia across all fetal weight groups. The causal relationship is unclear, however, since it is unknown if it is the assisted birth itself that causes the increased incidence in shoulder dystocia or whether it is factors that have caused the need for an assisted birth in the first place.

Q3: You have been called to see a woman in active labour. This is her first pregnancy, and, despite being diagnosed with gestational diabetes, she has had an uneventful pregnancy. She is asking for an epidural to assist in pain control, as the pethidine she received several hours ago has not been sufficient. From the options above, which factor is the most likely increase her risk of shoulder dystocia?

The correct answer is D. GDM.

The prevalence of gestational diabetes is increasing in our population. This is due to the increased incidence of obesity, an older pregnant population and enhanced antenatal detection. Gestational diabetes is thought to increase the risk of shoulder dystocia, based on the positive correlation between diabetes and fetal macrosomia.

Q4: If a woman with known type 2 diabetes becomes pregnant, based on the options above, what complication can occur that increases the risk of shoulder dystocia?

The correct answer is E. Macrosomia.

Diabetic mothers are more likely to have larger babies, which inherently will face difficulty when delivering the baby through the birth canal, but the nature of fetal fat distribution is different in babies of diabetic women. These babies are more likely to have greater shoulder and abdominal growth, making it harder for them to navigate the maternal pelvis and more likely that they will have a complicated birth.

 Key Point

Although prediction of shoulder dystocia is difficult, there are factors which may indicate an increased risk of dystocia occurring.

Q5: Answer true or false: Which of the following are recognised complications of shoulder dystocia for the baby?

If a neonatal doctor is not in attendance at a birth complicated by shoulder dystocia and there is a suspicion of injury, *the baby should be reviewed by a neonatologist as soon as possible. This is in addition to the routine baby check that is undertaken between 6 and 72 hours after birth.*

A Bulbar palsy – False. This palsy refers to impairment of the cranial nerves IX, X, XI and XII. This injury is caused by a lower motor neuron lesion in the medulla oblongata or brainstem. It is therefore not a complication of shoulder dystocia.

B ✔ **Brachial plexus injury** – True. Brachial plexus injuries can be divided into two major types: Erb palsy and Klumpke palsy. Erb palsy is the more common of the two and involves nerve roots C5 to C7 causing 'winging' of the scapula and the classic 'waiter tip' posture. Klumpke palsy involves C7, C8 and T1 and classically forms a 'claw' deformity of the hand.

C Femur fracture – False. Babies affected by shoulder dystocia can suffer from a fractured clavicle or humerus but not from a fractured femur. This is because the presenting part of the fetus in shoulder dystocia is the head. Once this is stuck, significant pressure may be placed on the clavicle and humerus as the obstetrician assists the birth. The baby's legs are not the part of the anatomy that is stuck in the birth canal during shoulder dystocia.

D ✔ **Clavicle fracture** – True. An x-ray can be performed to confirm this injury; however, it can be detected clinically by crepitus over the clavicle or obvious misalignment of the baby's shoulder. Fracturing the clavicle intentionally is a recognised method used to deliver a baby with shoulder dystocia when other methods have failed.

E Bells palsy – False. This palsy occurs due to an idiopathic dysfunction in cranial nerve VII. As the head is safely delivered in shoulder dystocia, the cranial nerves should not be injured.

 Key Point

Every child should have a 'routine baby check' after birth. Babies that are born in traumatic circumstances, such as births complicated by shoulder dystocia, may need closer investigation and observation by the paediatric team.

Important Learning Points

- Despite the many risk factors for shoulder dystocia, it can occur in women with no risk factors.
- Shoulder dystocia is diagnosed at the time of birth and requires senior multidisciplinary management.
- It is an obstetric emergency where seconds count, as a previously uncompromised baby can become acidotic as a result of hypoxia in 7 minutes.
- There are several methods that can be used to assist in the delivery of the baby: they are positional, internal and external. The McRoberts position is the most common, with a 90% success rate.
- Communication with the mother is vital in such an emergency. If possible, both the obstetrician and midwife need to explain the severity of the situation and what they are doing to assist the birth.

RETAINED PLACENTA

Q1: Which maternal conditions contraindicate the use of ergometrine in the active management of the third stage of labour?
The correct answers are B. Severe hypertension and **D.** Severe cardiac disease.

Ergometrine is an adrenergic, dopaminergic and serotonin receptor agonist. Due to this mode of action, ergometrine has several contraindications. Syntometrine (ergometrine plus oxytocin) is a commonly used drug given in the third stage of labour if the mother opts for active management. These substances assist in uterine contraction and the expulsion of the placenta from the uterus. If the use of ergometrine is contraindicated, women should receive only oxytocin to assist in the active management of the third stage of labour.

A Severe diabetes – Incorrect. Maternal diabetes can be problematic for many women who become pregnant. Careful glycaemic control is required throughout pregnancy and labour to ensure that many fetal and maternal complications are minimised. Maternal diabetes is not a contraindication for the use of ergometrine. Ergometrine has no effect on blood glucose levels.

B ✔ **Severe hypertension** – Correct. This is a recognised contraindication to the use of ergometrine. Ergometrine has numerous known side effects, including hypertension. Its use is contraindicated in women with known severe hypertension, as it can cause extremely high acute BP, potentially resulting in a stroke. It should be used with caution in women with mild to moderate hypertension. If the use of ergometrine is contraindicated, women should receive only oxytocin to assist in the active management of the third stage of labour.

C Multiple sclerosis – Incorrect. This is not a contraindication to the use of ergometrine in the third stage of labour.

D ✔ **Severe cardiac disease** – Correct. Ergometrine should not be used in women with risk of heart failure. Ergometrine can cause hypertension, arrhythmias, dizziness and circulatory shock.

E Sepsis – Incorrect. There is no contraindication to ergometrine use in sepsis, though it should be used cautiously in cases of severe sepsis due to its widespread vasoconstrictive action.

> **Key Point**
>
> Syntometrine is a medication used to assist in uterine contraction and actively manage the third stage of labour. It is important to recognise its contraindications.

Q2: What can cause a retained placenta?
The correct answers are A. Uterine atony **B.** Multiple pregnancy and **C.** Placenta accreta.

The main causes of retained placenta are important to recognise.

A ✔ **Uterine atony** – Correct. Normally, during a contraction, the uterus compresses the muscular vasculature. Therefore, after birth, a contracted uterus can assist in haemostasis and will assist in the separation of the placenta from the uterine wall. If there is uterine atony, there is an increased risk of PPH and retained placenta.

B ✔ **Multiple pregnancy** – Correct. Due to the overdistension of the uterus in multiple pregnancies, there is increased risk of uterine atony, which is the leading cause of retained placenta. For this reason, active management of the third stage is always advised for multiple pregnancies.

C ✔ **Placenta accreta** – Correct. Placenta accreta describes the abnormal implantation of the placenta into the myometrium. Due to this unusually deep attachment, women are at risk of retained placenta, as there can be problems with the placenta detaching. If this occurs, there is also increased risk of PPH and emergency hysterectomy.

D Assisted vaginal birth – Incorrect. There is no association between this and retained placenta. Operative birth is associated with problems such as maternal lower genital tract trauma.

E Oxytocin use in labour – Incorrect. This is not associated with retained placenta. Synthetic oxytocin is indicated in several situations such as inefficient contractions. Oxytocin can be used to induce labour, assist delivery and prevent PPH in the third stage of labour.

Q3: Answer true or false: Which of the following are recognised complications of retained placenta for the woman?
The correct answers are A. Uterine atony and **C.** PPH.

The key complications of retained placenta are important to know and to counsel women about.

A ✔ **Uterine atony** – Correct. As well as being a possible cause of a retained placenta, there is a risk of uterine atony after the placement has been manually removed. The uterus may need mechanical (bimanual compression) or pharmacological (uterotonics) support to ensure good tone, and therefore, haemostasis is achieved.

B DVT – Incorrect. There is no association between this and retained placenta. Women are at increased risk of a DVT in the postnatal period, and having a surgical procedure at this time can also increase the risk further. A careful venous thromboembolism assessment is vital for all postnatal women.

C ✔ **PPH** – Correct. Due to the lack of uterine contractions and thus atony when a women has a retained placenta, the risk of PPH can be high. If the woman is actively bleeding, she will need swift management in theatre to avoid a major haemorrhage.

D Obstetric anal sphincter injury – Incorrect. There is no association between this and retained placenta.

E Pneumonia – Incorrect. This is not associated with retained placenta. Endometritis, however, is; it is routine practice to provide women with antibiotic cover if they are diagnosed with a retained placenta to reduce this risk.

 Key Point

There are three forms of placenta accreta (abnormally invasive placenta) with increasing severity:

- Placenta accreta – the placenta invades abnormally into the uterus but only superficially into the myometrium.
- Placenta increta – the placenta invades more deeply into the myometrium.
- Placenta percreta – the placenta invades through the myometrium and penetrates the outer serosal layer of the uterus. It may even invade further into adjacent structures such as the bladder or bowel.

Important Learning Points

- An important step in the management of a retained placenta is to determine whether it is associated with a PPH.
- Manual removal of a placenta should be performed in an operating theatre, with adequate analgesia provided for the woman.
- Antibiotics given at the time of manual removal reduce the incidence of postnatal sepsis.

POSTPARTUM HAEMORRHAGE

Q1: For primary PPH to be diagnosed, up to what time after birth would the haemorrhage have to occur?

The correct answer is B. Less than 24 hours.

PPH is a major cause of maternal mortality worldwide, occurring in around 10% of women. It is estimated in low and middle income countries that PPH is responsible for up to 60% of maternal deaths. Work is ongoing to find cost-effective and simple measures that can be undertaken in resource-poor countries to reduce the impact that PPH has.

Key Point

A primary PPH is diagnosed if the bleeding occurs any time between the time of birth and 24 hours afterward. From 24 hours postdelivery to 6 weeks afterward, any excessive bleeding is classified as a secondary PPH.

Q2: From the options above, which option carries the highest risk of causing a PPH?

The correct answer is F. Placenta praevia.

Placenta praevia increases the risk of PPH approximately 15 times. The risk factors for PPH can be divided into antenatal and intrapartum factors. The important role during the antenatal period is to identify any possible risks of PPH, minimise them where possible and counsel the mother about her risk factors for this obstetric emergency. This should be done in conjunction with any apparent risk factors that arise during labour and birth.

Q3: A woman with known type 2 diabetes and trigeminal neuralgia is pregnant with twins. From the options above, which answer carries the greatest risk for PPH for this patient?

The correct answer is B. Multiple pregnancy.

Multiple pregnancies are picked up early in antenatal scanning. In a multiple pregnancy, the uterus is greatly distended, increasing the chance for uterine atony. Uterine atony is the leading cause of PPH worldwide.

Q4: From the options above, which mode of birth carries the highest risk of PPH?

The correct answer is H. Emergency caesarean section.

An emergency caesarean carries approximately nine times the risk of PPH in comparison to a vaginal birth. An emergency caesarean is indicated in several situations including: fetal distress, cord prolapse, uterine rupture and failed induction of labour. Planned caesarean birth carries an approximately four times increased risk, whilst assisted vaginal birth carries an approximately two times increased risk.

Q5: A 45-year-old woman with a past medical history of hyperthyroidism and menorrhagia has been admitted to hospital by her midwife. She is at 34 weeks gestation with her first child. Her midwife has noticed that the patient's BP has been increasing over the past few weeks, and now there is protein in her urine. From the options above, which answer is a risk factor for PPH in this patient?

The correct answer is C. Pre-eclampsia.

Pre-eclampsia is a maternal medical condition characterised by hypertension and proteinuria. There are several risk factors for the development of pre-eclampsia, including nulliparity, chronic hypertension, obesity, diabetes and multiple gestation. A lot is known about the condition, but its pathogenesis remains unclear. Amongst other mechanisms, it is thought to affect the endothelium and signalling pathways that control clotting. Changes in thrombin are thought to result in problems with maternal clotting, thereby predisposing to bleeding and PPH. HELLP syndrome, which is associated with pre-eclampsia, can develop quickly.

Q6: A 23-year-old woman has just had her first child by assisted vaginal birth. Her obstetrician decided to use forceps to assist in the safe and quick birth of a baby girl. The midwife has noticed that despite the use of synthetic oxytocin, the woman has a retained placenta. From the options above, which answer is a risk factor for PPH in this patient?

The correct answer is L. Retained placenta.

A retained placenta carries approximately a five times increased risk of PPH, whilst, as stated previously, an assisted vaginal birth carries approximately two times increased risk. There are several causes of retained placenta, including uterine atony, trapped placenta and placenta accreta.

> ### Key Point
>
> Women with significant risk factors for a PPH should be advised to labour and give birth in an obstetrician-led unit.

Q7: Answer true or false: Which of the following are causes of PPH?

Ultimately, it is most important to consider the four Ts when assessing causes for PPH – tone, trauma, tissue and thrombin. In an emergency, having a mnemonic can help develop efficient, systematic care.

A ✔ **Uterine atony** – True. Uterine atony is the inability of uterine contraction after birth. Uterine contraction needs to occur directly after birth, and this contraction needs to be sustained. Uterine haemostasis depends predominantly on myometrial contraction and prostaglandin production and less on the coagulation cascade. Failure of contraction of the uterine myometrium can lead to excessive continuous bleeding.

B ✔ **Coagulopathy** – True. Coagulopathies can cause bleeding due to impairment in the clotting process. Coagulopathies can arise from genetic disorders, such as von Willebrand disease or haemophilia. They can also develop from an acute insult, such as DIC in major obstetric haemorrhage or severe sepsis.

C Sepsis – False. PPH and sepsis have common predisposing factors, such as a retained placental fragment, which increase the risk of both bleeding and endometritis. However, sepsis is not a causative factor for PPH. Secondary PPH is commonly associated with infection, often in the form of endometritis, which may be caused by retained products. Treatment of secondary PPH is similar to primary PPH, with the addition of antibiotics. If uterotonics and antibiotics are unsuccessful, surgical evacuation of the uterus is commonly performed.

D ✔ **Lower genital tract lacerations** – True. As with any laceration, there is the chance that, if severe enough, major blood loss can occur. Pregnancy is a hypervascular state: blood volume significantly increases, and new networks of blood vessels are created. This increases the probability of a significant bleed.

E ✔ **Retained placental fragments** – True. Retained placenta can prevent the uterus from contracting, causing blood loss. The placenta during pregnancy has been receiving a large amount of blood flow to provide nutrients to the fetus. If it does not detach, it may continue to receive blood. If the placental fragments remain *in situ* for a prolonged period, they can become a source of infection, which can develop into sepsis and DIC.

> ### Key Point
>
> The most common cause of PPH is uterine atony. Sufficient uterine muscle contraction is essential to effectively clamp down on the large vascular supply to the uterus at term and prevent major blood loss.

> ### Important Learning Points
>
> - PPH is defined as either primary or secondary depending on when the haemorrhage occurred after delivery.
> - PPH is a significant cause of maternal morbidity and mortality globally.
> - To tackle PPH, it is vital to assess women at booking, considering their risk factors and medical history.
> - Early recognition of the compromised patient is vital, with careful monitoring in high-risk patients.

AMNIOTIC EMBOLISM

Q1: In a life-threatening emergency, when no G&S has been performed, what blood can be given to the woman?

The correct answer is D. O-negative blood.

Patients who are having elective surgery will have a G&S taken, ensuring that their blood type will be fully analysed and stored. If the need for a blood transfusion arises, the hospital blood bank will have a record of their blood type (Table 17.3) and, therefore, the blood they would need to receive. A routine crossmatch, where nonurgent blood is required, takes around 40 minutes to perform, which will fully analyse the blood sample. An emergency crossmatch can take around 5 minutes. This ensures that blood is ABO compatible (Fig. 17.2) but no other antibody compatibility. In an extreme emergency, when no information is available regarding the patient's blood type, O-negative blood is given.

A B-negative blood – Incorrect. Around 2% of the population has this blood type. People with this blood type have the B antigen, but no rhesus antigen, with anti-A antibodies in the plasma.

B O-positive blood – Incorrect. This is one of the more common blood types but is not given in an emergency. It can be given to anyone who is rhesus positive, regardless of ABO blood group. However, in an urgent emergency, the person's rhesus status may not be known; hence, this blood type cannot be used.

C AB negative blood – Incorrect. This is the rarest blood group in the UK. This blood is used to manufacture plasma.

D ✔ **O-negative blood** – Correct. Less than 10% of the UK population has blood type O negative. It is the universal donor, meaning this blood can be given to anyone, as it has neither A or B antigens. It is the only safe option when a patient's blood group is unknown or would take too long to arrive.

E B-positive blood – Incorrect. Around 8% of the population has this blood type. People with this blood type have the B antigen and the rhesus antigen, with anti-A antibodies in the plasma.

Donor   **Recipient**

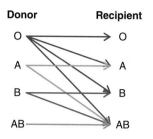

Fig. 17.2 Blood Types as Donors.

 Key Point

Table **17.3**	Blood Group Types	

BLOOD GROUP	ANTIGENS ON RED BLOOD CELL	ANTIBODIES IN PLASMA
A	A	Anti-B
B	B	Anti-A
AB	A and B	None
O	None	Anti-A and anti-B

Q2: Answer true or false: Which of the following blood products are typically used in the management of DIC?

The chain of events in DIC can be summarised as inappropriate and diffuse activation of the coagulation system. This leads to widespread thrombosis, ultimately causing haemorrhage, as the clotting factors are exhausted. It is a serious and life-threatening complication of multiple obstetric emergencies, but it may also occur in a nonobstetric setting. Ultimately, to treat DIC, the underlying cause must be treated. Prior to this, interim blood products can be used as part of intensive supportive treatment.

A ✔ **Fresh frozen plasma (FFP)** – True. In women with a prolonged prothrombin time and activated partial thromboplastin time, FFP has an important role where there is evidence of bleeding. FFP contains multiple clotting factors and is therefore indicated in DIC where these factors are likely to have been depleted.

B Packed red cells – False. Red cells are not consumed during the clotting cascade. Therefore, replacement is not needed to correct DIC. However packed red cells are often needed in the event of haemorrhage caused by DIC.

C ✔ **Cryoprecipitate** – True. Cryoprecipitate contains primarily fibrinogen, but also von Willebrand factor and factors VIII and XIII. Cryoprecipitate is indicated when the fibrinogen levels are low.

D ✔ **Platelets** – True. Platelets will be consumed during coagulation, so replacement may be necessary to correct an ongoing active haemorrhage.

E Albumin – False. Albumin has no place in the management of DIC.

 Key Point

If untreated, DIC can progress to multiorgan failure, hence the importance of timely diagnosis and management.

Q3: Which vessels are thought to be involved in carrying amniotic fluid to the maternal pulmonary system?

The correct answers are C. Inferior vena cava and **D.** Pulmonary arteries.

For an amniotic embolism to enter the lungs, it is thought that the embolism enters the maternal system through the venous system. It is therefore key to remember that pulmonary arteries carry deoxygenated blood, and like a PE, it is the venous system that is affected in an amniotic embolism.

Key Point

Amniotic embolism is a rare occurrence; however, it is an important differential to consider in patients presenting with shortness of breath or collapse. Remembering the key principles of ABC management, and to call for senior help quickly, remain most important.

Important Learning Points

- Amniotic fluid embolism is a rare occurrence.
- Rapid senior multidisciplinary management must occur to improve the mortality and morbidity of both the woman and fetus.
- Diagnosis is usually clinical and often a diagnosis of exclusion.

MATERNAL COLLAPSE

Q1: What is the first action to take?
The correct answer is D. Call for help.

If you are alone, it is important to raise the alarm of a maternal collapse. When you review a patient who has collapsed, it is important to check to see whether they are responsive. If a patient is responsive, then you can call for help and place them into the recovery position. If a patient is unresponsive, call for help and then assess for signs of life to confirm the seriousness of the situation, as you may then need additional help from specialist resuscitation teams.

A Check for a carotid pulse – Incorrect. This is part of the initial assessment of the collapsed patient but not the first step you should perform.

B Call for the senior clinician – Incorrect. Your senior clinician is not always the nearest person and may be far away. In the event of a maternal collapse, you need extra pairs of hands for assistance; this can be any healthcare professional.

C Check the BP – Incorrect. This is part of the assessment of the critically unwell patient but should not be part of your initial assessment.

D ✔ Call for help – Correct. If there is a maternal collapse, you will need assistance for management, raising the alarm and contacting the correct teams.

E Count the respiratory rate – Incorrect. Initial assessment of the collapsed woman should include checking for respiratory effort; this does not mean the respiratory rate. Waiting a minute to count this could waste crucial time needed for resuscitation.

Key Point

In any emergency in medicine, call for help early.

Q2: If the initial assessment shows she has no respiratory effort, which answer best describes who needs to be called for support?

The correct answer is E. The cardiac arrest, obstetric and neonatal teams.

It is important you know the names of the resuscitation teams in your hospital; each hospital will have slightly different teams and may have different names for them. You will always need the cardiac arrest team in the event of maternal collapse as well as the obstetric team. The hospital cardiac arrest team will ensure that an anaesthetist is present to maintain the airway as well as other general physicians. The obstetric team needs to be called, as not only is the woman under their care, but their expertise will be needed to perform an emergency caesarean if required. The neonatal team may be needed depending on the gestation of the fetus. The hospital intensive care team is important in the postarrest care of a patient if the resuscitation attempt is successful.

Key Point

To manage an obstetric arrest, a multidisciplinary group of professionals is needed. It is important to acknowledge this and ask for assistance early, as this will improve both maternal and neonatal outcome.

Q3: A 24-year-old woman has consented for a planned caesarean birth. This is her first pregnancy; she has never been in hospital before or had any operations. She has had a spinal anaesthetic and has been prepped for the operation, including having antibiotic cover. Just as the procedure is about to start, she becomes unstable, tachycardic, tachypnoeic and hypoxic. From the options above, which cause of maternal collapse is most likely?

The correct answer is K. Anaphylaxis.

This patient is demonstrating some of the signs of anaphylaxis. She is likely to have little medical history, having never been in hospital before, and has just been given antibiotics. Another cause of maternal compromise in this situation is a high spinal block, which can block the neurological supply to the diaphragm and heart. During a caesarean, an amniotic fluid embolus can occur shortly after membrane rupture, and haemorrhage is more common at caesarean than vaginal birth.

Q4: A 32-year-old woman in her first pregnancy has presented to delivery suite with abdominal pain and feeling generally unwell. She is 36⁺⁶ weeks pregnant and looks unwell. On initial examination, she is hypotensive and tachycardic and has a tender, firm abdomen. She rapidly becomes unresponsive. From the options above, which cause of maternal collapse is most likely?

The correct answer is F. Placental abruption.

Placental abruption is where the placenta partially separates from the uterus before birth. Classically, it presents with sudden-onset pain, a tender uterus and signs of maternal shock. Vaginal bleeding is not always evident, but there can be massive blood loss into the uterus, and this commonly leads to DIC.

[See 'Antepartum Haemorrhage' on page 297.]

Q5: A 27-year-old woman in her third pregnancy with known gestational diabetes has just had a normal vaginal birth. The birth was uncomplicated, with an active third stage and a one-off temperature of 37.9°C. She is feeling generally unwell. She is responding to voice, is pyrexial, tachycardic, hypotensive and tachypnoeic and has normal saturations. From the options above, which cause of maternal collapse is most likely?

The correct answer is B. Severe sepsis.

Sepsis can usually be identified before a patient becomes too unwell. Signs in this woman include the temperature in labour and the change in her vital signs. Sepsis is a severe, but reversible, cause of collapse. Patients usually respond well with fluid resuscitation and antibiotics. It is important to determine the cause and treat both mother and baby accordingly.

Key Point

The initial assessment of maternal collapse is the same, no matter what the cause. Good resuscitation skills will allow time for the diagnosis to be made. Once this has occurred, specific and tailored management can be given to the woman.

Important Learning Points

- Maternal collapse can be an obstetric emergency. Swift recognition and assessment of the patient are vital to ensure good outcomes.
- The ABCDE approach should be used to assess the patient.
- If maternal resuscitation is needed, the cardiac arrest, obstetric and neonatal teams need to be called.

16 POSTNATAL COMPLICATIONS

VENOUS THROMBOEMBOLISM

Q1: Which of the following factors is considered the most significant predictor of the risk of VTE in pregnancy?

The correct answer is D. Previous VTE during pregnancy.

It is important to be able to identify the women who are at increased risk of VTE during pregnancy, as appropriate prophylaxis can then be initiated.

All the options in this question are risk factors for VTE, but a previous VTE in pregnancy is most concerning since it is an unprovoked oestrogen-dependent VTE, and unprovoked VTEs are associated with the highest risk. Previous VTE following thrombophilia or surgery are both associated with significant yet smaller increases in risk. Immobility and smoking are both associated with an increased risk but individually would not require thromboprophylaxis.

> **Key Point**
>
> Perform and regularly update VTE risk assessments using validated measures in order to target management.

Q2: Antenatal warfarin use is associated with which of the following?

The correct answers are A. Stillbirth, **B.** Fetal haemorrhage, **C.** Cardiac abnormalities, **D.** IUGR and **E.** Spontaneous miscarriage.

Warfarin crosses the placenta, and exposure between the 6th and 12th weeks of gestation is associated with fetal warfarin syndrome. Bone formation in the fetus is affected, as it is a vitamin K-dependent process; the manifestations are variable, but the most characteristic feature is nasal hypoplasia. However, the effects can range widely.

A ✔ Stillbirth – Correct. Stillbirth is reported at a rate of approximately 15% to 20% with warfarin. This may be caused by a variety of mechanisms, including those listed as other options in this question.

B ✔ Fetal haemorrhage – Correct. Placental transfer of warfarin later in the pregnancy can result in fetal haemorrhage. The risk of haemorrhage in the fetus is higher than in the mother. This is due to the impaired hepatic metabolism and renal excretion of warfarin and its metabolites in the fetus, in addition to reduced fetal production of vitamin K-dependent clotting factors.

C ✔ Cardiac abnormalities – Correct. Cardiac abnormalities, including aortic coarctation and situs inversus, have also been reported following early warfarin exposure.

D ✔ IUGR – Correct. Warfarin is one of several drugs that are associated with IUGR. Others include steroids and phenytoin.

E ✔ Spontaneous miscarriage – Correct. Miscarriage, similar to stillbirth, is also reported at a rate of 15% to 20%. The definition of miscarriage is pregnancy loss before 24 weeks gestation. Pregnancy loss after 24 weeks is a stillbirth.

> **Key Point**
>
> LMWH should be used as an alternative to warfarin wherever possible in pregnant women.

Q3: Answer true or false: Which of the following are contraindications to using LMWH?

Although LMWH is recommended as prophylaxis in women at high risk of VTE, it is important to weigh the potential benefits against the risks. This is often not a straightforward decision and may require joint decision-making with multiple specialists.

A BP increase from 110/70 to 160/90 – False. The BP needs to be above 200/120 mmHg to contraindicate LMWH use because this increases the risk of bleeding. Although this is a significant rise in BP and should be investigated, it is not classified as uncontrolled hypertension.

B Previous PPH losing approximately 1 L of blood – False. PPHs can occur for a plethora of reasons. In the absence of other risk factors for further haemorrhage, LMWH is not contraindicated. If there is current active antenatal or postpartum bleeding, LMWH would be contraindicated.

C ✔ Women with von Willebrand disease – True. Von Willebrand disease is a common inherited bleeding disorder in which platelet aggregation is impaired and is a contraindication to LMWH therapy.

D ✔ Severe liver disease – True. Severe liver disease, particularly with an elevated prothrombin time or known varices, is a contraindication for LMWH due to the existing increased bleeding risk.

E ✔ Severe renal disease – True. Severe renal disease with an estimated glomerular filtration rate of less than 30 mL/min/1.73 m^2 is a contraindication for LMWH. This is because the elimination route of LMWH is via the renal system. Hence, the half-life of LMWH would increase substantially in patients with severe renal failure. In such cases, should LMWH have to be used, it may be necessary to prescribe a reduced dose.

> **Key Point**
>
> In women who are at risk of bleeding, careful consideration of the risks and benefits of anticoagulation prophylaxis is required, and LMWH may be contraindicated.

> **Important Learning Points**
>
> - Pregnant women are at increased risk of developing VTE, particularly in the postpartum period.
> - PEs are the most common direct cause of maternal death in the UK.
> - Many of these events can be prevented with thorough risk assessment and appropriate thromboprophylaxis.
> - In the majority of cases, LMWH is the prophylactic agent of choice in pregnancy due to the risks of teratogenicity associated with warfarin. Warfarin can be used safely in the postnatal period and while breastfeeding.

BACTERIAL SEPSIS FOLLOWING PREGNANCY

Q1: What investigation would be most useful when trying to determine the cause of the infection in Mairi's case?

The correct answer is A. Wound swab.

Identifying the causative organism in a case of sepsis would be most useful for guiding antibiotic therapy. However, it should never delay initiation of treatment.

A ✔ **Wound swab** – Correct. Wound swabs should be sent for microscopy, culture and sensitivity. This will identify the causative organism and allow antimicrobial therapy to be altered to more specific antibiotics after initial empiric therapy.

B White blood cell count – Incorrect. Although this should be performed, it will only indicate the presence of an inflammatory response. It will not provide information regarding the cause of the infection.

C Serum lactate – Incorrect. Although this should be performed, it will only indicate the presence of tissue hypoperfusion and guide management. It will not provide information regarding the cause of the infection.

D Abdominal CT – Incorrect. Although this may be useful if an abscess or deep tissue infection is being considered, it would not be the first-line investigation in a patient who appears to have cellulitis as her source of sepsis and would not identify the causative organism.

E Tissue biopsy – Incorrect. Although this may be useful if an abscess or deep tissue infection is being considered, it would not be the first-line investigation in a patient who appears to have cellulitis as her source of sepsis.

 Key Point

Specific investigations should be performed based on the suspected source of infection – but the results should not delay empirical antibiotic therapy. Although isolation of an organism from the wound is useful, the organism causing systemic infection should ideally be confirmed in blood cultures, as there is a chance that they may be different. Blood cultures should therefore be taken in all septic patients.

Q2: An aminoglycoside antibiotic.

The correct answer is F. Gentamicin.

Gentamicin is an aminoglycoside, meaning that it works by affecting bacterial ribosomes so that they are unable to produce proteins. It is a broad-spectrum antibiotic that is commonly recommended to be given as a one-off dose (in addition to other antibiotics) in conditions including endometritis, acute pyelonephritis and toxic shock syndrome.

Q3: A glycopeptide commonly used in MRSA-positive patients.

The correct answer is L. Vancomycin.

Vancomycin is a glycopeptide that is a very broad-spectrum antibiotic commonly considered first line in conjunction with clindamycin in cases of MRSA sepsis. Vancomycin levels are monitored due to dangerous side effects such as ototoxicity, nephrotoxicity and neutropenia.

Q4: An antibiotic which is a folate antagonist.

The correct answer is K. Trimethoprim.

Trimethoprim is an antibiotic commonly used to treat lower urinary tract infection. However, it is a folate antagonist which is known to be teratogenic in the first trimester of pregnancy. It should therefore be avoided in the first trimester of pregnancy.

Q5: Only covers anaerobic bacteria and protozoa.

The correct answer is H. Metronidazole.

Metronidazole is cytotoxic to anaerobes and protozoa. It is not usually first-line empirical treatment for sepsis in the postpartum period. Nonetheless, it can be used in combination with other antibiotics in cases of severe sepsis of unknown origin where the patient has a penicillin allergy.

Q6: An antibiotic which should be avoided in penicillin-allergic patients and also in PPROM.

The correct answer is C. Co-amoxiclav.

Co-amoxiclav contains amoxicillin (a penicillin) and clavulanic acid (a beta-lactamase inhibitor). Its use should therefore be avoided in patients with known penicillin allergy. Co-amoxiclav is also potentially associated with an increased risk of necrotising enterocolitis in neonates and should thus be avoided in PPROM.

 Key Point

It is important to remember that patterns of resistance vary regionally, and local guidelines should therefore be consulted regarding antibiotic prescribing.

🔍 Important Learning Points

- Women are at increased risk of sepsis in the postnatal period.
- Sepsis is associated with a high mortality.
- Rapid initiation of treatment with antibiotics and fluid resuscitation is vital.

PERINEAL TRAUMA

Q1: What degree of perineal trauma has this woman sustained?

The correct answer is B. Second degree.

Correctly classifying the degree of trauma sustained is important, as it affects the management.

Perineal damage which involves the perineal muscle but spares the anal sphincter is a second-degree tear. Involvement of the anal sphincter classifies the tear as either third or fourth degree, and a superficial tear affecting only the perineal skin is a first-degree tear.

A First degree – Incorrect. A first-degree tear would not involve the perineal muscles but would be limited to the perineal skin.

B ✔ **Second degree** – Correct. A second-degree tear involves the perineal muscles but not the anal sphincter.

C Third degree, classification A – Incorrect. A third-degree tear would involve the anal sphincter, and a classification A tear would be limited to less than 50% of the sphincter.

D Third degree, classification B – Incorrect. A third-degree tear would involve the anal sphincter, and a classification B tear would involve more than 50% of the sphincter.

E Third degree, classification C – Incorrect. A third-degree tear would involve the anal sphincter, and a classification C tear would include the internal anal sphincter.

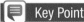 **Key Point**

First- and second-degree tears are common following vaginal birth, whereas third- and fourth-degree tears are much rarer.

Q2: Which of the following make up the bulk of the pelvic diaphragm?

The correct answer is D. Levator ani.

The perineum refers to both an external region and an internal compartment. The internal compartment is surrounded by the pelvic cavity and the pelvic diaphragm, and the external surface of the perineum overlies this, extending between the mons pubis and the intergluteal cleft. The pelvic diaphragm is important for maintaining the position of pelvic organs. The pelvic diaphragm, or pelvic floor, is made up of the levator ani, coccygeus muscle and fascial layers. It separates the pelvic cavity from the perineum. Levator ani is made up of three components: the iliococcygeus, pubococcygeus and puborectalis muscles. The perineal muscles play an important role in the maintenance of bowel and urinary continence and in sexual function. They converge to form the perineal body, a fibromuscular mass which is crucial for the integrity of the pelvic diaphragm.

A Bulbospongiosus muscle – Incorrect. The bulbospongiosus muscle is a superficial perineal muscle which, in women, covers the vestibular bulb of the vagina. It supports the perineal body and pelvic floor, contributes to erection of the clitoris and closes the vagina.

B Deep transverse perineal muscle – Incorrect. The deep transverse perineal muscles support and fix the perineal body or pelvic floor.

C External anal sphincter – Incorrect. The external anal sphincter is a perineal muscle which surrounds the margin of the anus and is important for maintaining faecal continence.

D ✔ **Levator ani** – Correct. The pelvic diaphragm, or pelvic floor, is made up of the levator ani, coccygeus muscle and fascial layers.

E Superficial transverse perineal muscle – Incorrect. The superficial transverse perineal muscle runs between the ischial tuberosity and the perineal body and sits posterior to the bulbospongiosus muscle.

 Key Point

The perineal muscles are important for maintaining faecal and urinary continence, sexual function and the integrity of the pelvic diaphragm.

Q3: Answer true or false to the following statements.

Women are likely to have concerns about the risk of perineal trauma and will often have come across a lot of information from friends and the media about risks and prevention. It is therefore important to discuss perineal trauma comprehensively if women are worried and to ensure they are aware of both the risks and possibilities.

A ✔ **Women with a previous history of severe perineal trauma should be informed that their risk of perineal trauma is not increased in comparison to nulliparous women** – True. The rate of repeat severe trauma in subsequent pregnancies is similar to the original incidence (6%). However, it should be noted that the risk of flatus or faecal incontinence with a repeat third-degree tear is higher than with the first-third degree tear (up to 15%).

B ✔ **Antenatal perineal massage has been found to reduce the incidence of perineal tears** – True. Perineal massage from 24 weeks of gestation onward reduces the risk of requiring perineal suturing.

C ✔ **Postoperatively, laxatives should be administered after a third-degree perineal repair** – True. Laxatives are recommended during the postoperative period for a third- or fourth-degree tear, as constipation can disrupt the repair and cause wound dehiscence. A short course of antibiotics and early physiotherapy are also advised for third- and fourth-degree tears. For first- and second-degree tears, none of these treatments are necessary after repair.

D Women who have had a fourth-degree perineal tear in a previous pregnancy should be offered a prophylactic episiotomy – False. Planned episiotomy is not recommended in the UK. The decision to offer episiotomy should be based on the clinical situation. Each pregnancy and birth is different, so the subsequent birth may occur easily without any perineal injury. However, as with any birth, if the delivering midwife or obstetrician is concerned about the risk of perineal tearing, an episiotomy can be offered.

E When episiotomy is indicated, a medial incision should be made – False. UK guidance states that an episiotomy incision should be made mediolaterally, as this is associated with a reduced risk of anal sphincter injury (third-degree tears) compared to medial incisions. Medial incisions are routinely performed in some countries, as it is felt these incisions are easier to repair.

Key Point

It is important that women are given accurate information about their risk of perineal trauma, as well as methods of reducing this risk and of reducing complications.

Important Learning Points

- Perineal trauma is common following vaginal birth.
- All women should be assessed for perineal trauma following vaginal birth.
- Third- and fourth-degree tears are rare and require surgical repair by an experienced obstetrician.

MASTITIS

Q1: Which isotype of antibodies is predominantly transferred to the newborn baby in breast milk?

The correct answer is A. IgA.

The drive behind campaigns promoting breastfeeding is partially based on the antibodies expressed in breast milk, which help the newborn's immature immune system. IgA is the isotype of antibody that is produced in the highest concentration in breast milk. It is particularly high in the colostrum, and IgA levels remain high for at least 7 months postpartum. IgG is also produced in breast milk, though not in as great a quantity as IgA. IgG is the only isotype of antibody that can cross the placenta, and it provides the fetus with immune protection in utero.

Key Point

Breastfeeding has multiple benefits, including that it is monetarily free, there is no need to sterilise bottles carefully, and it does not need preparation like formula. It is readily available and constantly at the correct temperature. In addition, it is nutritionally well balanced, it enables bonding between mother and baby, and it possesses the immunological benefits as outlined.

Q2: Which organism is most commonly isolated from breast milk in infective mastitis?

The correct answer is B. Staphylococcus aureus.

An awareness of the common underlying organisms in different infections is useful, as it will help you to understand and remember empirical antibiotic choices.

A *Streptococcus pyogenes* – Incorrect. *S. pyogenes* is a common cause of superficial and deep skin infections and would be an important differential to consider. *S. pyogenes* is the cause of group A streptococcal infections.

B ✔ *Staphylococcus aureus* – Correct. *S. aureus* is the most common bacteria isolated from breast milk in clinical cases of mastitis. Determining the cause of infective mastitis is important to enable the most appropriate antibiotics to be prescribed.

C *Staphylococcus epidermis* – Incorrect. *S. epidermidis* is a common skin commensal which makes up part of the normal skin flora. It can be problematic for people who have an indwelling urinary catheter but is unlikely to be the cause of a clinical infection in the breast.

D *Neisseria gonorrhoea* – Incorrect. More commonly, *N. gonorrhoea* causes genital and urinary tract infections. It rarely causes mastitis.

E *Escherichia coli* – Incorrect. More commonly, *E. coli* causes gastroenteritis and urinary tract infections. However, rarely, virulent strains can cause mastitis.

Key Point

Staphylococcus aureus is a Gram-positive cocci. It is a common cause of skin and respiratory infections.

Q3: Answer true or false to the following statements regarding mastitis.

Often women are given support during the first few days of breastfeeding following birth, as it can be a difficult time for the mother. This will help develop and reinforce good technique as well as attempt to prevent complications such as mastitis. It is important that women are given accurate information about mastitis, methods of reducing their risk and management options.

A ✔ **The risk of mastitis is increased by tight-fitting bras** – True. Tight-fitting bras are thought to increase the risk of mastitis because they may restrict milk flow.

B Women with mastitis should stop breastfeeding – False. Women should be advised to continue breastfeeding from the affected breast in order to prevent abscess formation associated with sudden cessation. Support should be given to help continuation of breastfeeding, and if women are unable to breastfeed, they should be encouraged to express milk. There is no evidence that breastfeeding with mastitis will harm the infant.

C ✔ **An episode of mastitis following a previous pregnancy increases the risk of mastitis in the current postpartum period** – True. Mastitis in a previous pregnancy or a previous episode of mastitis in the current pregnancy increases the risk of a recurrence.

D ✔ **Using only one position to breastfeed increases the risk of mastitis** – True. Changing position whilst breastfeeding can facilitate effective drainage of the breast milk and, hence, reduce the risk of mastitis.

E Mastitis can only develop with broken skin, for example, cracked nipples – False. Although broken skin on the breast, such as cracked nipples, may be important as a source of entry of bacteria causing mastitis, it is not the only aetiological factor.

> **Key Point**
>
> Women presenting with mastitis should be advised to continue breastfeeding.

> **Important Learning Points**
>
> - Mastitis is common in breastfeeding women but is usually self-limiting, requiring only conservative therapy.
> - Presenting symptoms include pain, swelling, heat and a lump in the breast.
> - Abscesses are the most worrying complication, and if suspected, these can be confirmed by ultrasound.

POSTNATAL MENTAL HEALTH

Q1: Which is the following is lithium known to increase the risk of most significantly?

The correct answer is B. Cardiac abnormalities.

Lithium is a mood stabiliser used in the management of bipolar affective disorder and some cases of severe depression. Women taking lithium should be carefully counselled regarding contraception and should ideally discuss their medication prior to conceiving, as lithium is most problematic in the first trimester. Women who are well and not at high risk of relapse will usually be advised to stop lithium and should be offered an antipsychotic as an alternative. Women who are unwell or at high risk of relapse may consider changing to an antipsychotic medication, stopping lithium and restarting in the second trimester or may choose to continue with lithium treatment.

A Oral cleft – Incorrect. Oral cleft abnormalities are associated with the use of lamotrigine (9 cases per 1000 pregnancies).

B ✔ **Cardiac abnormalities** – Correct. Lithium is associated with an increased rate of fetal heart defects (60 cases in 1000 pregnancies compared to 8 cases in 1000 pregnancies in the general population). A specific abnormality associated with lithium teratogenicity is the Ebstein anomaly, an abnormal formation of the tricuspid valve which results in a smaller right ventricle and is often associated with an atrial septal defect.

C Neural tube defects – Incorrect. Neural tube defects are increased with both sodium valproate (100 to 200 cases per 10,000 pregnancies) and carbamazepine (20 to 50 cases per 10,000 pregnancies) use compared to the general population (6 cases per 10,000 pregnancies).

D Gastrointestinal defects – Incorrect. This is not a specific complication reported with the use of mood stabilisers.

E Respiratory defects – Incorrect. This is also not a specific complication reported with the use of mood stabilisers. A rare side effect of taking lithium outside of pregnancy is chest tightness.

> **Key Point**
>
> Caution should be taken before prescribing mood stabilisers in women of reproductive age, and they should be appropriately counselled about contraception, the risks of pregnancy when taking these medications and the risks of abrupt withdrawal of medication.

Antidepressants are one of the treatment options for postnatal depression. Match the drug with the corresponding class.

Antidepressants may be considered for women with depression during pregnancy and the postpartum period. It is important to know which antidepressants may cross the placenta and which are present in breast milk. All antidepressants carry the risk of withdrawal or toxicity in neonates; in most cases, these effects are mild and self-limiting.

Q2: Fluoxetine.

The correct answer is C. Selective serotonin reuptake inhibitors (SSRIs).

Fluoxetine is the safest SSRI during pregnancy. SSRIs taken after 20 weeks gestation are associated with an increased risk of neonatal pulmonary hypertension, but the actual risk is very low, and if it does occur, it is usually mild and transient. Both fluoxetine and citalopram are present at relatively high levels in breast milk. Paroxetine, another SSRI, should not be taken during pregnancy, as it is associated with fetal heart defects.

Q3: Moclobemide.

The correct answer is B. Monoamine oxidase inhibitors.

There is little evidence of any fetal effects with moclobemide use during pregnancy, and low levels are present in breast milk. It is not a commonly used antidepressant in the general population due to potentially fatal interactions with common medications and certain foods.

Q4: Mirtazapine.

The correct answer is E. Noradrenaline and specific serotoninergic antidepressants.

Mirtazapine is an antidepressant and is commonly used as a second-line treatment when SSRIs have failed to control symptoms. Current data indicate that the risks of fetal malformation are not significantly increased above normal incidence. The limitations of the safety data should be communicated to women and a risk-benefit analysis performed when making decisions surrounding prescribing.

Q5: Amitriptyline.

The correct answer is A. Tricyclic antidepressants (TCAs).

TCAs have lower known risks during pregnancy than other antidepressants but are associated with a higher mortality in overdose and are therefore rarely used during pregnancy and the postpartum period. Amitriptyline is no longer recommended as an antidepressant agent but may be encountered with patients who take it for neuropathic pain, to aid sleep or because they have been stable on it since before recommendations changed.

Q6: Venlafaxine.

The correct answer is D. Serotonin and noradrenaline reuptake inhibitors.

Venlafaxine is usually a second- or third-line therapy in patients who have not responded adequately to SSRI therapy. Risks with venlafaxine include hypertension at high doses, higher toxicity in overdose than SSRIs and some TCAs and increased difficulty in withdrawal. As with all medication, these risks should be balanced with the risks of deterioration in mental health when off medication.

 Key Point

Antidepressants would be considered in a woman with a moderate episode and a history of depression, a severe episode or an episode unresponsive to psychological treatment.

Q7: Answer true or false: Which of the following are risk factors for puerperal psychosis?

Although some risk factors for puerperal psychosis are known, many women who are affected will not have any of these. This can be particularly difficult, as symptoms most commonly develop around 2 weeks after birth, by which point most women will be discharged and at home, where they may struggle to access appropriate support.

A ✔ **Having a sister who developed puerperal psychosis** – True. Although the aetiology of puerperal psychosis is still not well understood, there is generally believed to be a genetic component. Therefore, women who have had a first-degree relative affected are at a higher risk, and this should be noted and followed up at the booking appointment.

B ✔ **Previous history of bipolar disorder** – True. The patient in this scenario has a known diagnosis of bipolar disorder. Therefore, those involved in the care of her pregnancy should have increased the surveillance and support surrounding her regarding the higher risk of puerperal psychosis.

C ✔ **Previous history of schizoaffective disorder** – True. Any mental health problem that is associated with psychosis, such as schizoaffective disorder, schizophrenia or bipolar disorder, places women at a higher risk of puerperal psychosis.

D Low maternal age – False. The risk of puerperal psychosis is not greater in young mothers. Puerperal psychosis can occur in women of any age and from any socioeconomic background, so predicting those at high risk is difficult.

E ✔ **Having puerperal psychosis in a previous pregnancy** – True. The risk of recurrence is thought to be up to 50%. Therefore, women who have had puerperal psychosis in a previous pregnancy are at a very high risk. A higher level of support and surveillance should be given, often with the involvement of a psychiatrist as part of the multidisciplinary team early on in the pregnancy to ensure that if psychosis does reoccur, then treatment can be offered immediately.

 Key Point

Women at high risk include those with a previous episode of puerperal psychosis or a preexisting mental health condition that involves psychosis. The risk of being affected has been documented to be between 25% and 50%.

Important Learning Points

- Deaths associated with psychiatric conditions make a significant contribution to overall maternal mortality.
- Any psychiatric disorder can complicate pregnancy and the postnatal period and may present as a new episode or as a recurrence of a preexisting condition.
- Psychotropic medications should not be prescribed to women of childbearing age without appropriate counselling. This counselling should cover contraception (prior to pregnancy), risks in pregnancy and risks of stopping medication.
- The threshold for psychological drug intervention is reduced in pregnancy in order to reduce risks associated with psychotropic drug use.
- Postpartum psychosis is an emergency, usually requiring hospital admission.

18 Medical Ethics in Obstetrics and Gynaecology

Ethics is a broad term encompassing sets of principles that govern the conduct of groups and individuals within a society. Medical ethics analyses the moral principles that govern medical practice; this applies to teaching, political, governance, research and clinical aspects of medical practice.

THE PILLARS OF MEDICAL ETHICS

There are several different approaches to medical ethics, the most popular and widely used being based on the idea of the four pillars of medical ethics: autonomy, beneficence, nonmaleficence and justice. The four pillars are key principles that can be applied as a framework for medical ethics for any doctor, regardless of their personal, moral or religious beliefs. When used, they help doctors to provide care that is ethically acceptable to patients and society as a whole, although bare in mind that patients and doctors may have differing attitudes to models for care.

AUTONOMY

Autonomy is the principle that each person should be able to make their own decisions about all aspects of their medical care including ensuring that they are not being coerced by anybody (including their medical team). The individual also needs to have enough information to make a fully informed choice by understanding all implications of the offered treatment. Respect for patient autonomy also means that a person is free to decide against any treatment proposed by their medical team, even if that decision will cause their condition to worsen. The importance of autonomy in modern clinical practice was highlighted in the 2010 Department of Health paper that stated part of their ongoing strategy for the NHS would be to make shared decisions making the norm *'no decision about me without me'*.

BENEFICENCE

The principle of beneficence refers to the moral obligation to act for the benefit of others. Beneficence requires doctors to practice medicine at the highest standard they can to ensure the greatest level of care and benefit for their patient. The WHO defines health as 'a state of complete physical, mental and social well-being and not merely the absence of disease'. Therefore, a doctor seeking to apply the principle of beneficence is obligated to do more than simply treat the presenting symptom or disease, but to both view and treat the patient holistically. Outside of clinical care, the principle of beneficence also ought to have an impact on a doctor's conduct; doctors should act in a way that encourages trust and respect in the profession.

NONMALEFICENCE

Nonmaleficence is the principle that doctors have a duty to avoid unnecessary harm to their patients. The most extreme outworking of this is the duty of a doctor not to kill their patient (although globally different moral positions are taken on euthanasia), but it also includes a doctor's duty not to cause unnecessary pain or suffering. The vast majority of medical interventions come with either some accepted actual harm or risk of harm. This could be very minor (for example, pain at the needle site following a blood test) or very significant (for example, the risk of a bowel injury sustained during a caesarean). Nonmaleficence worked out practically then means the doctor must weigh up the good caused by the proposed action (or decision not to act) and balance it with the harm or risk of harm to ensure the balance falls in the favour of good rather than harm for the patient.

JUSTICE

In the context of medical ethics, justice is the principle of providing fair, equitable and appropriate treatment to all patients. This can refer to a doctor's moral obligation to interact with and care for all of their patients in the same nonjudgmental manner, contextualised to the patient's individual needs, which may vary depending on their previous experience of healthcare, and their underlying values. Discrimination should not occur based on protected characteristic such as ethnicity, sexual orientation, religion, health beliefs or actions.

More commonly relevant to clinical practice is the principle of distributive justice. In the NHS, healthcare resources are generally distributed on the basis of need. But because it is a healthcare system that seeks to provide care, free at the point of access to all who need it, yet is a system with finite resources, the decisions around how to justly use these resources can be complicated. Allocation of finite resources and decisions over which treatments to fund all come under the principle of distributive justice. In the UK, the National Institute of Clinical Excellence primarily uses a model of cost effectiveness to determine which treatments are commissioned and can be prescribed within the NHS. A threshold of £20-30,000 per Quality Adjusted Life Year (QALY) is used to assess this. There is also a moral duty of the individual doctor to ensure their own practice uses these resources in a fair manner (for example, recommending the most cost-effective treatment or not ordering unnecessary investigations).

ETHICS IN CLINICAL PRACTICE

Far from being an academic exercise, medical ethics is directly relevant to the practice of medicine in all specialties. The principles of autonomy, beneficence, nonmaleficence and justice are used daily in clinical practice for all doctors, whether they are conscious of it or not.

However, obstetrics and gynaecology is a speciality where the need to apply medical ethical principles is often more obvious. The following cases look at how the four principles can be applied in obstetrics and gynaecology.

A CASE IN OBSTETRICS

'A 27-year-old woman is admitted to the hospital delivery suite in active labour. She is progressing well until there is a fetal bradycardia. The fetal heart rate has remained less than 100 bpm for 6 minutes, so the decision is made for a category one caesarean section. The doctor explains to the woman that her baby is at high risk of a poor outcome and therefore needs immediate birth. The woman declines the caesarean because she wants to have a vaginal birth and is fearful of having an anaesthetic.'

AUTONOMY

This woman, like all people, has the right to make her own decisions about her treatment, free from coercion or control from others. This means that her consent is morally and legally necessary for the caesarean to go ahead. It does not matter if her decision seems illogical or even morally wrong to the medical team; it is still hers alone to make.

Under the principle of autonomy, the doctor is morally obligated to support her decision. However, to ensure she is truly acting autonomously, the doctor must make sure that she is able to give informed consent. This involves making sure that she is aware of the potential outcome of her decision – in this case, that her baby could be born in very poor clinical condition with the risk of hypoxic ischaemic encephalopathy or with no signs of life. The team also need to explore the woman's concerns regarding anaesthetic, provide accurate information and alternatives as this may be an important factor in her decision making. The doctor needs to explain this clearly in language she can understand while also refraining from bullying and coercing her into accepting the medical opinion. This can practically be very difficult, as in such cases, there is often very limited time to safely deliver (as every minute, the risk of irreversible fetal hypoxia increases), so the doctor must be mindful of their own emotions when having these important but time-pressured discussions. The doctor must also be aware of differing values around birthing practice, and recognise the value of having a vaginal birth for the women concerned may be different to what the doctor might perceive.

Should the woman and the doctor still have different views on whether a caesarean should take place, then the automony of the women is more important than the opinion of the doctor. Without consent, the caesarean should not take place.

BENEFICENCE

The aim of the doctor is to do good, and in a case like this, it seems like the obvious good would be to save the life of the unborn baby. However, the fetus has no legal rights until they are born, and so in obstetrics, the woman is always the medical team's first concern. This means that when following the principle of beneficence, the doctor needs act for her benefit first. Whilst increasing the possibility of a healthy baby being born may be the only thing that matters for some women, others may see any risk reduction from a caesarean as small, at the expense of other things of value, like for example a more 'natural' birth, having more family around, and potentially going home faster. A reluctance to have caesarean immediately is not a rejection of any intervention – other interventions could be considered, and an agreement could be made as to what the threshold for operative intervention might be, for example agreeing a particular time limit.

NONMALEFICENCE

There are potential physical and psychological risks to a pregnant woman associated with any birth, be it vaginal or caesarean. In this situation the timing of delivery is a key factor, with the health and life of the baby at risk. At this point the unborn baby does not have legal rights which would require this woman to act, so as we have discussed her autonomy is not altered by the risk to the baby. The doctor must however make sure they have adequately counselled on the potential risks of each action (and the risks of inaction) to avoid causing maleficence by omission of information for the woman to make an informed decision. By preparing appropriately for all eventualities, such as preparing theatre for a caesarean birth, the healthcare team reduce the risk of an error (active maleficence).

JUSTICE

It is important to recognise that women giving birth and doctors often have deep disagreements. However, it is still imperative that the women concerned is treated in a 'fair, equitable and appropriate' manner. This means that the doctor is still bound to treat the woman with respect and compassion, not blaming or punishing her for her decision. It may be the case that the baby is born healthy, but if not, it is important that just care also applies to the baby and family.

A CASE IN GYNAECOLOGY

'A couple in their late 30s have been trying to get pregnant for the last 2 years, with no success. They have been referred to the fertility clinic, as they wish to have IVF. The male partner has one child from a previous relationship, and the female partner has a BMI of 38, so they are informed that they do not meet the eligibility criteria for IVF treatment on the NHS. They do not have the funds to pay for private treatment.'

AUTONOMY

In this case, this couple has made the decision that they wish to have IVF treatment to have a baby. Making this decision is an example of them exercising their autonomy, of them 'self-ruling', but they require the assistance of the medical team to actually achieve this. The team is telling the couple that they cannot facilitate the decision they have made; doesn't this mean the medical team is denying them their autonomy?

While a patient's right to autonomy is vitally important, it is not absolute. A patient cannot demand a treatment and force the medical team into complying based on their right to autonomy. There is also the ethical question raised about whether people have a right to have a child; advances in fertility treatments mean that there are many people who are parents now who would not have been otherwise. But does this mean that everyone who wishes to have a child should be able to demand that they are helped to do so in the way they wish (therefore via IVF instead of surrogacy or adoption)? There is no easy answer to this, but the distress caused by infertility should not be forgotten, so whatever the doctor's personal feelings, their response should always remain compassionate.

BENEFICENCE

In this case, there is a seemingly obvious way that the doctor could bring about good for their patients by facilitating the couple to have IVF and therefore have a baby. You could argue that this is the role of the doctor under the principle of beneficence, but this ignores the nuances of the case. A doctor has a duty to act for the good of all their patients, not just the one who sat in front of them in a particular outpatient clinic. This means that they need to work within guidelines and systems that exist for a reason. A doctor's duty is not just to grant the wishes of their patient without considering the wider picture, no matter how sympathetic they may feel towards a particular patient.

There are still ways a doctor can fulfil their duty to the principle of beneficence in this case. IVF may not be this couple's only option, so a doctor can bring about good for them by fully investigating whether any other treatment option might be appropriate. Alternatives like surrogacy or adoption may also be explored.

NONMALEFICENCE

The distress felt by those who wish to become parents but are unable to for whatever reason can be immense and should not be underestimated. It is therefore easy to see how some might argue the best way to avoid harm in this case would be to help this couple proceed with IVF. This would avoid the harm of the ongoing and significant psychological distress caused by their childlessness while also honouring the principle of beneficence.

But as discussed earlier, the doctor must function and practice within the system of the NHS, meaning their focus must be broader than one couple. A doctor therefore also has a duty to avoid harm by respecting referral and eligibility criteria that exist to protect both patients and the NHS.

IVF itself raises ethical issues, in particular the issues surrounding creation, storage, use and disposal of embryos. There are many that would view embryos as human life, and within some doctrines, worthy of similar legal protection given to a child that has been born. This means that some doctors may feel like their duty to the principle of nonmaleficence extends to embryos created as part of IVF, and therefore, they cannot in all good conscience get involved in the field of IVF. While doctors are, of course, permitted to have their own ethical opinions, IVF is a legal and expected treatment option, so as with termination care, a doctor must not deny an eligible person from receiving the treatment, even if it is not them delivering it. There are also additional side effects that come with infertility treatments (for example egg harvesting, hormone injections), and risks to the mother associated with IVF, like for example multiple pregnancy.

JUSTICE

In this case, the principle of distributive justice is more applicable. IVF is an expensive treatment with variable chances of success; the NHS quotes success rates of 35% for women under 35 years, with steadily decreasing percentages as the woman's age increases. In a healthcare system with finite resources that cannot spend unlimited money on every treatment for every person, eligibility criteria are required to safeguard the resources. This is a way to try to make the healthcare system more just for everyone, with a doctor needing to play their role in that by not attempting to bypass checks that are there for a reason.

In fact, the issue of whether fertility treatments should be available on the NHS at all is a source of ethical debate. There is no universally agreed right to a child, so is infertility actually a disease that requires treatment? Should the money spent on fertility treatments be spent on something else such as oncology treatments or dialysis? On the other hand, if fertility treatments are only available to those able to pay for them, does this mean that the ability to have a child is limited to those who are more socioeconomically well off, thereby being discriminatory? All these questions relate to how best to apply the principle of justice to everyday clinical practice.

THE ROLE OF THE OBSTETRICIAN AND GYNAECOLOGIST IN SOCIETY

Being a doctor is a difficult job but also an incredibly privileged one. Doctors are respected and valued members of society and extremely well trusted by the general population. It is vital for doctors to live up to the trust placed in them by the general population and to strive to act ethically and with their patient's best interests at heart at all times.

This duty belongs to doctors in all specialties, but the obstetrician and gynaecologist perhaps have an additional role. As laid out in the Royal College of Obstetricians and Gynaecologists training curriculum, one of the professional identities of an obstetrician and gynaecologist is a champion for women's health. This includes both health promotion and practicing in a way that is nondiscriminatory and inclusive to women from all parts of society. An obstetrician and gynaecologist should see themselves as an advocate for women and women's health, as well as recognising that their influence could reach far beyond the labour ward or operating theatre.

SUMMARY

Medical ethics play an important part in all aspects of the practice of medicine. The four pillars approach to medical ethics, using the principles of autonomy, beneficence, nonmaleficence and justice, can be used to work through the ethical issues of a particular case and give guidance to a doctor about how they can best fulfil their ethical duties in their everyday clinical practice.

KEY REFERENCES

Beauchamp, T.L., Childress, J.F., 2009. Principles of biomedical ethics, 6th ed. Oxford University Press, New York.

Gillon, R., 1994. Medical ethics: four principles plus attention to scope. British Medical Journal, 309 (6948), 184–188.

Nisselle, P., 2013. *Doctor's orders vs patient choice* [online]. Available from: https://www.medicalprotection.org/uk/articles/doctors-orders-vs-patient-choice [accessed 7 June 2022].

Royal College of Obstetricians and Gynaecologists, 2020. *Core curriculum for obstetrics and gynaecology. Definitive document* [online]. Available from: https://www.rcog.org.uk/media/j3do0i1i/core-curriculum-2019-definitive-document-may-2021.pdf [accessed 9 June 2022].

Varkey, B., 2021. Principles of clinical ethics and their application to practice. Medical Principles and Practice, 30 (1), 17–28.

19 Careers in Obstetrics and Gynaecology

Obstetrics and gynaecology (O&G) is a specialty that slightly differs from those in other hospital departments. It may be housed in a separate building, and it often runs alongside the workings of a general hospital rather than being fully integrated into it. Uniquely, it comprises elements of surgery, medicine, paediatrics, radiology and genetics. For many in this speciality, this breadth of subject area is one of its most attractive features. It combines the adrenaline rush of labour ward emergencies with the relatively more relaxed and finesse of routine gynaecology surgery and everything in between. The service users demographics are highly varied, covering all age ranges. Many of the women you see will not be unwell, just pregnant! In obstetrics, you will usually be part of an extremely happy time when a baby is born and couples become parents for the first time, but this is matched occasionally with the other extreme: tragedy when something goes wrong.

To be an effective O&G doctor, you will require excellent communication, good teamwork ability and efficient time management skills. You need to be able to make rapid and effective decisions, as this is a time-critical specialty where minutes really do count. You must be able to communicate as effectively with a grumpy, disengaged mum as you will with an informed and confident woman with menstrual issues. Gynaecological problems can be particularly challenging, as many women feel embarrassed and sensitive about having to seek medical advice. It is important to be able to put people at ease and be able to show empathy and give appropriate reassurance.

THINGS YOU CAN DO AT MEDICAL SCHOOL TO LEARN MORE ABOUT OBSTETRICS AND GYNAECOLOGY

- Try to spend time in an O&G placement at both a teaching hospital and a district general hospital to see the differences in O&G services provided.
- Ask to help assist at a caesarean birth instead of passively watching from afar.
- Try to experience as wide a range of deliveries as possible – from pool births to assisted vaginal births to emergency caesarean sections.
- Make sure you are easily available within the department and people know that you are interested. The difficulty with obstetrics for a medical student is that things happen quickly, and if you are not on the ward, it is unlikely people will remember to call you. To see as much as possible, stay on the labour ward and take books or work to do during calm times. Good things come to those who wait. Consider working a night shift, as there are often fewer people around and more opportunities to get involved.
- Attend events organised nationally and locally to promote O&G as a career. For example, in the UK, the Royal College of Obstetricians and Gynaecologists (RCOG) runs a careers day.

THINGS YOU CAN DO AT MEDICAL SCHOOL TO ENHANCE YOUR CAREER PROSPECTS IN OBSTETRICS AND GYNAECOLOGY

- Get involved in an O&G audit during your placement.
- Review a local guideline during your O&G placement.
- Consider planning an elective with an O&G theme.
- Undertake special, student selected or extended study modules in O&G.
- Liaise with national and international societies that promote O&G. For example, in the UK, you can register with the RCOG website for email updates about a career in O&G. You can also join the British Undergraduate Society of Obstetrics and Gynaecology (BUSOG), or your medical school may have its own O&G society.
- Intercalated degrees also exist that either cover elements of women's health or are entirely focused on this subject.
- Try to get involved with some research or teaching related to O&G.
- Consider writing up an O&G case report if you see any particularly interesting or challenging cases.
- Try to present at a conference with any of the extra-curricular work that may have given you interesting results.
- Think about submitting work to other O&G publications. Organisations like RCOG often have essay competitions specifically for medical students.
- Contact us about being involved in the next edition of this book!

THINGS YOU CAN DO AS A JUNIOR DOCTOR TO LEARN MORE ABOUT OBSTETRICS AND GYNAECOLOGY

- Apply for a post in O&G as part of your junior doctor rotations, or, if this is not possible, apply for a 'taster' week.
- Attend career days for junior doctors aimed at those interested in O&G.
- Use the many resources available online to explore career options in O&G; this may include the careers prospectus on the RCOG website.
- Talk to current trainees in your local O&G department.

THINGS YOU CAN DO AS A JUNIOR DOCTOR TO ENHANCE YOUR CAREER PROSPECTS

- Take obstetrics membership examinations; you do not need to be in a training programme to sit the first exam.
- Consider undertaking a basic practical skills course in O&G.
- Take advantage of any opportunities to become involved in O&G projects or audits running in your local department.
- Show commitment to the specialty by attending extra clinical sessions over and above the expected working commitments.
- Apply for prizes and awards for junior doctors. There may be essay competitions and research awards for example.

Most of the these ideas are focussed on trainees based in the UK, but the principles can be taken into any setting. Get involved in projects in your local O&G department, and talk to the consultants about what opportunities there may be available for you. If you are keen and show dedication to the specialty, people will often be very receptive. Almost every country in the world that trains doctors has a national organisation for O&G; many of these are affiliated with, or have links to, the RCOG. Many have student or junior doctor branches, and if they don't, try to set one up!

CAREER PATHWAYS IN OBSTETRICS AND GYNAECOLOGY

Many of these pathways overlap and encompass elements of several specialty areas. For example, maternofetal medicine is combined as one specialty area in some hospitals; they are not mutually exclusive. In some of the more competitive areas, such as gynaecological oncology and reproductive medicine, undertaking a period of research may be necessary to secure a subspecialty training position. As demonstrated, O&G can be a very varied specialty with no set pathway; rather, the potential exists for subspecialisations, along with a variety of activities within the job.

ADJUNCTS TO A CAREER IN OBSTETRICS AND GYNAECOLOGY

There are many ways to supplement a career in O&G, including those that are nonclinical or more community based in nature. These may start as areas of interest alongside your clinical role but may, in some cases, become the central focus of your career.

AN OVERVIEW TO THE TRAINING PATHWAY IN THE UK

After completing 2 years of foundation training, an individual in the UK undergoes a minimum of 7 years of specialty training (ST1 to ST7) in O&G. There is a central core curriculum, and the programme is divided into basic, intermediate and advanced levels of training. Once these individuals reach advanced training, they will start to develop more specific skills in the areas that they want to practice in the future, in Advanced Training Skills Modules (ATSM) or by applying for subspecialty training (Table 19.1). The subspecialty training programmes are gynaecological oncology, maternal and fetal medicine, reproductive medicine and urogynaecology. There is also an academic curriculum with more focus on research; therefore, training can be very varied (Table 19.2).

There are three exams during the training pathway:
- Part 1 Membership of the Royal College of Obstetricians and Gynaecologists (MRCOG) – a pass is required to move from ST2 to ST3, and this covers basic sciences relevant to O&G.
- Part 2 (multiple choice) and part 3 (OSCE) MRCOG – these need to be attained to move from ST5 to ST6, which assesses clinical knowledge and practical application of that knowledge (Fig. 19.1).

Table 19.1   Career Pathways in Obstetrics and Gynaecology

CAREER PATHWAY	LOCATION	MAIN TOPIC AREAS	SPECIFIC SKILLS REQUIRED
Fetal medicine	Hospital based	Prenatal diagnosis, genetics, paediatrics, in utero surgery	Ultrasound scanning and counselling
Maternal medicine	Hospital based	General medicine in an obstetric setting	May require additional postgraduate examinations to be taken, good knowledge base as broad and varied subject area, the ability to liaise well with physicians
Labour ward management	Hospital based	Practical skills in emergency birth, managing emergency scenarios	Good organisation, leadership and time management skills and a liking for an adrenaline rush!
Benign gynaecology	Hospital based	Menstrual issues, endometriosis and pelvic pain	Laparoscopic skills, understanding of psychosocial patient issues
Gynaecological oncology	Hospital based	Pelvic cancer surgery, colposcopy and hysteroscopy	Good surgical skills, enjoyment of long, complex theatre cases
Urogynaecology	Hospital based	Pelvic organ prolapse surgery and management of urinary incontinence	Good surgical skills, but also requires excellent medical knowledge
Reproductive medicine	Hospital based	Subfertility treatments including IVF	Ultrasound scanning, surgical skills, understanding of psychosocial patient issues
Paediatric or adolescent gynaecology	Hospital based	Genetics, embryology, paediatrics	Sound anatomy and multidisciplinary working, sensitive communication skills, not offered in all hospitals
Community gynaecology	Community based	Sexual health, contraception and termination services	People and communication skills
Early pregnancy management	Hospital based	Management of early pregnancy complications including ectopic pregnancy	Ultrasound scanning and counselling

IVF, In vitro fertilisation.

Table 19.2   Adjuncts to Careers in Obstetrics and Gynaecology

CAREER PATHWAY	LOCATION	MAIN TOPIC AREAS	SPECIFIC SKILLS REQUIRED
Humanitarian and charity work	Overseas	Predominantly obstetrics but some gynaecology, particularly fistula repair and emergency gynaecology; may involve working in challenging situations with little access to resources typical in high income economies	An enjoyment of travel and team working and the ability to adapt to manage with whatever is available
Healthcare politics	Nonclinical	An interest in improving healthcare on a more national level	Useful to have had some form of background in healthcare before pursuing this route, as it may allow better insight into the challenges
Medical education	Nonclinical	Can be on a local or national level coordinating medical student teaching and assessment	Patience and an interest in the next generation of doctors
Hospital management	Nonclinical	Providing appropriate services for the local community accessing medical care; has an aspect of the job regarding budgeting and finances, due to limited resources	Useful to have had some form of background in healthcare before pursuing this route, as it may allow better insight into the challenges

Table 19.2 Adjuncts to Careers in Obstetrics and Gynaecology—Cont'd

CAREER PATHWAY	LOCATION	MAIN TOPIC AREAS	SPECIFIC SKILLS REQUIRED
Public health	Community based	Responsible for the health of the country by communicating important health information to the general population and managing some national and international health issues	Team working and knowledge of statistics
Pharmaceutical and medical devices industries	Usually nonclinical	Usually involvement in large multinational companies, helping to create and test new drugs and equipment	Experience of clinical trials and an interest in business
Academic O&G	University based	Obstetric and gynaecological research; multiple roles within the university setting including teaching, lecturing and pastoral roles	Ability to combine both research and clinical training
Primary care physician with special interest in gynaecology	Community based	Primary care physician with a special interest in gynaecological issues	Primary care physician training

O&G, Obstetrics and gynaecology.

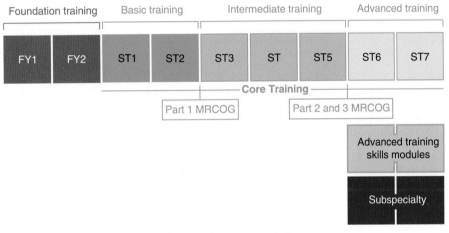

Fig. 19.1 The Training Pathway in the UK.

Index

Page numbers followed by "*f*" indicate figures, "*t*" indicate tables.